UICC International Union Against Cancer

MANUAL OF
CLINICAL ONCOLOGY

Seventh Edition

GW00762683

UICC International Union Against Cancer

MANUAL OF CLINICAL ONCOLOGY

Seventh Edition

Editor
Raphael E. Pollock

Associate Editors
James H. Doroshow
James G. Geraghty
David Khayat
Jin-Pok Kim
Brian O'Sullivan

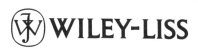

WILEY-LISS

A JOHN WILEY & SONS, INC., PUBLICATION

New York • Chichester • Weinheim • Brisbane • Singapore • Toronto

For ordering and customer service, call 1-800-CALL-WILEY.

Library of Congress Cataloging-in-Publication Data:
Library of Congress Cataloging-in-Publication Data is available.

ISBN 0-471-23828-7

Printed in the United States of America.

10 9 8 7 6 5 4 3 2 1

CONTENTS

Preface   ix

Contributors   xi

1. **The Natural History and Biology of Cancer**   1
   George T. Bryan, Mark R. Olsen, and H. Ian Robins

2. **Carcinogenesis**   19
   Suryanarayana V. Vulimiri and John DiGiovanni

3. **The Molecular Basis of Cancer**   45
   Karol Sikora

4. **Genetic Predisposition to Cancer**   63
   Gordon B. Mills, Paula Rieger, Mary Anne Watt, Christie Graham,
   and Rebecca Pentz

5. **Tumor Immunology**   99
   George E. Peoples, Alexander R. Miller, and Timothy J. Eberlein

6. **Cancer Epidemiology**   131
   Peter Boyle

7. **The Chemoprevention of Cancer**   163
   Fadlo R. Khuri, Anita L. Sabichi, Waun Ki Hong, and Scott M. Lippman

8. **Screening and Early Detection**   181
   David A. Sloan

9. **Cancer Diagnosis**   201
   James G. Geraghty and Albrecht Wobst

10. **The Role of Cancer Staging in Evidence-Based Medicine**   215
    William J. Mackillop, Peter Dixon, Mary K. Gospodarowicz, and Brian O'Sullivan

11. **Principles of Surgical Oncology** 235
Michael J. Edwards

12. **Principles of Radiation Oncology** 251
John N. Waldron and Brian O'Sullivan

13. **Principles of Medical Oncology** 275
James H. Doroshow

14. **Bone Marrow Transplantation** 293
George Somlo

15. **Biostatistics and Clinical Trials** 307
*Richard Sylvester, Patrick Therasse, Martine Van Glabbeke,
and Françoise Meunier*

16. **Skin and Melanoma Cancer** 325
B.H. Burmeister, B.M. Smithers, M.G. Poulsen, D. Kennedy, and D.B. Thomson

17. **Head and Neck Cancer** 341
Brian O'Sullivan, Jonathan Irish, Lillian Siu, and Anne Lee

18. **Endocrine Tumors** 359
Jeffrey A. Norton

19. **Lung Cancer** 385
David Payne and Tsuguo Naruke

20. **Liver Cancer** 407
Zhao-You Tang

21. **Esophageal Carcinoma** 425
Douglas E. Wood, Eric Valliéres, and Carlos A. Pellegrini

22. **Cancer of the Stomach** 439
Jin-Pok Kim

23. **Cancer of the Pancreas** 453
Douglas B. Evans, Robert A. Wolff, and James L. Abbruzzese

24. **Cancer of the Colon and Rectum** 477
Hermann Kessler and Jeffrey W. Milsom

25. **Breast Cancer** 491
Umberto Veronesi, Virgilio Sacchini, Marco Colleoni, and Aron Goldhirsch

26. **Cancer and Precursor Lesions of the Uterine Cervix**   515
    Michele Follen Mitchell, Guillermo Tortolero-Luna, Diane C. Bodurka,
    and Mitchell Morris

27. **Gynecologic Cancer**   537
    J. L. Benedet and D. M. Miller

28. **Cancer of the Prostate**   563
    Louis J. Denis and G.P. Murphy

29. **Non-Prostate Tumors Genitourinary Cancer**   575
    Mary K. Gospodarowicz

30. **Tumors of the Central Nervous System**   607
    Charles J. Vecht

31. **Soft Tissue Sarcomas**   621
    Peter W.T. Pisters, Brian O'Sullivan, and Raphael E. Pollock

32. **Lymphomas**   641
    M. A. Gil-Delgado, S.A.N. Johnson, and D. Khayat

33. **The Leukemias**   661
    Frederick R. Appelbaum

34. **Pediatric Malignancies**   689
    Ruby Kalra and Judith K. Sato

35. **AIDS-Related Malignancies**   709
    Anil Tupule and Alexandra M. Levine

36. **Cancer in the Elderly**   723
    Riccardo A. Audisio, Vittorina Zagonel, and Lazzaro Repetto

37. **Oncological Emergencies**   731
    Mark R. Olsen and H. Ian Robbins

38. **Pain Management**   745
    Betty R. Ferrell

39. **Nutrition**   757
    Brian I. Labow and Wiley W. Souba

40. **Rehabilitation of the Cancer Patient**   779
    Aileen M. Davis and Marlene Carno Jacobson

41. Quality of Life in Oncology   **791**
  Vittorio Ventafridda

Index   **805**

■ PREFACE

The 7th Edition of the *International Union Against Cancer (UICC) Manual of Clinical Oncology* builds on a long and successful tradition of providing a concise presentation of the oncology disciplines as they apply to contemporary multimodality management of the cancer patient. The target audience for this effort consists of medical students, physicians-in-training, and practicing physicians throughout the world. In the current era, we are witnessing rapid emergence of molecular insights into the genes and their cognate proteins that drive tumor inception, proliferation, and dissemination. Consequently, our understanding of the treatment for these diseases is likewise undergoing change.

Contained within this small manual is a core of knowledge that will introduce the critical sciences underlying our current multimodality oncology treatment programs. Each disease site chapter presents readily accessible information about diagnosis, staging as per the 5th Edition of the *UICC TNM Classification of Malignant Tumors*, the relevant multimodality therapies, as well as rehabilitation and follow-up strategies. Much of the material presented differs from earlier editions of this manual, and this is reflected in the work of many new experts who have contributed to this effort.

In that this manual is translated into many languages, our hope is that this book can provide a common and unifying core of oncology understanding to all who are interested throughout the world. Appropriately, our patients expect that we will consider all available relevant knowledge and apply it to their disease problem. For ourselves, we should settle for nothing less than this standard. On behalf of the editorial board and co-authors, we appreciate your interest and willingness to accept this challenge.

Raphael E. Pollock
Head, Division of Surgery
Professor and Chair, Department of Surgical Oncology
University of Texas
M. D. Anderson Cancer Center
Houston, TX
USA

James L. Abruzzese
University of Texas
M.D. Anderson Cancer Center
Houston, Texas, USA

Frederick R. Appelbaum
Fred Hutchinson Cancer Research Center
Seattle, Washington, USA

Riccardo A. Audisio
General Surgery–Multimedia
Milan, Italy

J.L. Benedet
BC Cancer Agency
& University of British Columbia
Vancouver, Canada

Diane C. Bodurka
University of Texas
M.D. Anderson Cancer Center
Houston, Texas, USA

Peter Boyle
European Institute of Oncology
Milan, Italy

George T. Bryan
University of Wisconsin
Madison, Wisconsin, USA

B.H. Burmeister
Queensland Radium Institute
and Princess Alexandra Hospital
South Brisbane, Australia

Marco Colleoni
European Institute of Oncology
Milan, Italy

Aileen M. Davis
Mount Sinai Hospital
Toronto, Canada

Louis J. Denis
Algemeen Ziekenhuis Middelheim
Antwerp, Belgium

John DiGiovanni
University of Texas
M.D. Anderson Cancer Center
Smithville, Texas, USA

Peter Dixon
University of Toronto
Princess Margaret Hospital
Toronto, Ontario, Canada

James H. Doroshow
City of Hope National Medical Center
Duarte, California, USA

Timothy J. Eberlein
Brigham and Women's Hospital
Boston, Massachusetts, USA

Michael J. Edwards
James Graham Brown Cancer Center
University of Louisville
Louisville, Kentucky, USA

Douglas B. Evans
University of Texas
M.D. Anderson Cancer Center
Houston, Texas, USA

Betty R. Ferrell
City of Hope National Medical Center
Duarte, California, USA

James G. Geraghty
City Hospital
Nottingham, United Kingdom

M.A. Gil-Delgado
Salpetriere Hospital
Paris, France

Aron Goldhirsch
European Institute of Oncology
Milan, Italy

Mary K. Gospodarowicz
University of Toronto
Princess Margaret Hospital
Toronto, Ontario, Canada

Christie Graham
University of Texas
M.D. Anderson Cancer Center
Houston, Texas, USA

Waun Ki Hong
University of Texas
M.D. Anderson Cancer Center
Houston, Texas, USA

Jonathan Irish
Princess Margaret Hospital
University of Toronto
Toronto, Ontario, Canada

Marlene Carno Jacobson
Sunnybrook Health Science Centre
North York, Ontario, Canada

S.A.N. Johnson
Taunton and Somerset Hospital
Taunton-Somerset, United Kingdom

Ruby Kalra
City of Hope National Medical Center
Duarte, California, USA

D. Kennedy
Queensland Radium Institute
and Princess Alexandra Hospital
South Brisbane, QLD, Australia

Hermann Kessler
The Cleveland Clinic Foundation
Cleveland, Ohio, USA

David Khayat
Salpetriere Hospital
Paris, France

Fadlo R. Khuri
University of Texas
M.D. Anderson Cancer Center
Houston, Texas, USA

Jin-Pok Kim
Inje University Seoul
Paik Medical Center
Korea Gastric Cancer Center
Seoul, Korea

Brian I. Labow
Massachusetts General Hospital
Boston, Massachusetts, USA

Anne Lee
Pamela Youde Nethersole Eastern Hospital
Hong Kong, China

Alexandra M. Levine
University of Southern California
Los Angeles, California, USA

Scott M. Lippman
University of Texas
M.D. Anderson Cancer Center
Houston, Texas, USA

William J. Mackillop
Kingston General Hospital
Kingston, Ontario

Françoise Meunier
EORTC Data Center/Central Office
Brussels, Belgium

Alexander R. Miller
University of Texas
M.D. Anderson Cancer Center
Houston, Texas, USA

D.M. Miller
University of Texas
M.D. Anderson Cancer Center
Houston, Texas, USA

Gordon B. Mills
University of Texas
M.D. Anderson Cancer Center
Houston, Texas, USA

Jeffrey W. Milsom
The Cleveland Clinic Foundation
Cleveland, Ohio, USA

Michelle Follen Mitchell
University of Texas
M.D. Anderson Cancer Center
Houston, Texas, USA

Mitchell Morris
University of Texas
M.D. Anderson Cancer Center
Houston, Texas, USA

G.P. Murphy
Pacific Northwest Cancer Foundation
Seattle, Washington, USA

Tsuguo Naruke
National Cancer Center
Tokyo, Japan

Jeffrey A. Norton
University of California, San Francisco
San Francisco, California, USA

Brian O'Sullivan
University of Toronto
Princess Margaret Hospital
Toronto, Ontario, Canada

Mark R. Olsen
University of Wisconsin
Madison, Wisconsin, USA

Carlos A. Pellegrini
University of Washington
Seattle, Washington, USA

Rebecca Pentz
University of Texas
M.D. Anderson Cancer Center
Houston, Texas, USA

George E. Peoples
University of Texas
M.D. Anderson Cancer Center
Houston, Texas, USA and
Uniformed Services
of the Health Sciences
Bethesda, Maryland, USA

Peter W.T. Pisters
University of Texas
M.D. Anderson Cancer Center
Houston, Texas, USA

Raphael E. Pollock
University of Texas
M.D. Anderson Cancer Center
Houston, Texas, USA

M.G. Poulsen
Queensland Radium Institute
and Princess Alexandra Hospital
South Brisbane, QLD, Australia

Lazzaro Repetto
IST-National Institute for Cancer Research
Genoa, Italy

Paula Rieger
University of Texas
M.D. Anderson Cancer Center
Houston, Texas, USA

H. Ian Robbins
University of Wisconsin
Madison, Wisconsin, USA

Anita L. Sabichi
University of Texas
M.D. Anderson Cancer Center
Houston, Texas, USA

Virgilio Sacchini
European Institute of Oncology
Milan, Italy

Judith K. Sato
City of Hope National Medical Center
Duarte, California, USA

Karol Sikora
WHO Cancer Control Programme
Lyon, France and
Imperial College School of Medicine
Hammersmith Hospital
London, United Kingdom

Lillian Siu
The University of Texas Science Center
at San Antonio
San Antonio, Texas, USA

David A. Sloan
University of Kentucky
Lexington, Kentucky, USA

B.M. Smithers
Royal Brisbane Hospital
South Brisbane, QLD, Australia

George Somlo
City of Hope National Medical Center
Duarte, California, USA

Wiley W. Souba
Massachusetts General Hospital
Boston, Masschusetts, USA

Richard Sylvester
EORTC Data Center/Central Office
Brussels, Belgium

Zhao-You Tang
Zhongshan Hospital
Shanghai Medical University
Shanghai, P.R. China

Patrick Therasse
EORTC Data Center/Central Office
Brussels, Belgium

D.B. Thomson
Queensland Radium Institute
and Princess Alexandra Hospital
South Brisbane, QLD, Australia

Guillermo Tortolero-Luna
University of Texas
M.D. Anderson Cancer Center
Houston, Texas, USA

Anil Tupule
University of Southern California
Los Angeles, California, USA

Eric Vallières
University of Washington
Seattle, Washington, USA

Martine Van Glabbeke
EORTC Data Center/Central Office
Brussels, Belgium

Charles J. Vecht
University Hospital Rotterdam
Rotterdam, The Netherlands

Umberto Veronesi
European Institute of Oncology
Milan, Italy

Vittorio Ventafridda
European Institute of Oncology
Milan, Italy

Suryanarayana V. Vulimiri
University of Texas
M.D. Anderson Cancer Center
Smithville, Texas, USA

John Waldron
University of Toronto
Princess Margaret Hospital
Toronto, Ontario, Canada

Mary Anne Watt
University of Texas
M.D. Anderson Cancer Center
Houston, Texas, USA

Albrecht Wobst
European Institute of Oncology
Milan, Italy

Robert A. Wolff
University of Texas
M.D. Anderson Cancer Center
Houston, Texas, USA

Douglas E. Wood
University of Washington
Seattle, Washington, USA

Vittorina Zagonel
Centro di Riferimento Oncologico, INRCCS
Aviano, Italy

CHAPTER 1

THE NATURAL HISTORY AND BIOLOGY OF CANCER

GEORGE T. BRYAN, MARK R. OLSEN, and H. IAN ROBINS

University of Wisconsin
General Clinical Research Center
Madison, WI USA

Detection, diagnosis, prognosis, and employment of appropriate and effective therapies for cancers are major elements in medical practice. Knowledge of the natural histories of cancers is critical to the medical practitioner, whatever his or her specialty, to maximize for patients opportunities for survival with high quality of life. Thus, the pathologist needs an intimate knowledge of the natural histories of cancers to aid in diagnosis. Surgical, radiation, and medical oncologists require detailed knowledge for planning and integrating appropriate therapies. Oncologic epidemiologists need an understanding of the natural histories of cancers to design and analyze meaningful population-based investigations. Oncologic psychiatrists, oncologic nurses, and psychosocial workers must comprehend the natural histories of cancers to enhance quality of life of involved patients and their families. Finally, the cancer laboratory scientists must understand the elements of the natural histories of cancers to design and conduct relevant laboratory studies, and to develop novel therapies. In this chapter, the major characteristics and principles regarding natural histories of cancers are presented.

INTRODUCTION

Available evidence indicates that cancers are not new diseases. Dinosaur fossils have exhibited lesions compatible with the diagnosis of cancer. The earliest drawings or writings from many ancient civilizations in all parts of the world have provided descriptions of cancers. Bone cancers and urinary bladder cancers have been identified

Manual of Clinical Oncology, 7th edition, Edited by Raphael E. Pollock
ISBN 0-471-23828-7, pages 1–17. Copyright © 1999 Wiley-Liss, Inc.

in Egyptian mummies. Writings of Hippocrates contained descriptions and recommended therapeutic procedures for cancers. It is clear from these writings that ancient physicians were aware that cancers exhibited spatial and temporal characteristics of progression, and ultimately led to death.

The natural histories of cancers describe (and in part explain) the progressive steps and stages of cancer evolution in individuals and populations. The natural history is often called biologic progression, and more recently has been linked to molecular progression. Each of the more than 150 to 200 diverse forms of cancer diseases has a unique natural history. This evolution, from beginning to termination, varies with the genetic characteristics of the host, the cell of origin, the tissue of residence, the carcinogenic factors affecting the cell and tissue of origin, host defense and enabling factors, and coexisting morbid entities. Thus, the origin and development of cancers are thought to have multietiologic factors and progress through multiple stages of evolution prior to and subsequent to their clinical detection and diagnosis.

CANCER AS A CELLULAR DISEASE

The fundamental unit of organization of all biologic entities is the cell. In multicellular organisms, cells are organized into tissues and organs. In these structures cells are bound together by a secreted intercellular substance (e.g., collagen, proteoglycans, etc.). Growth of cells may occur by an increase in the number of cells, an increase in the size of cells, or both. In higher animals, growth in cell number usually exceeds growth in size. Growth in cell number is the most significant component of human development. The average human adult is composed of about one quadrillion (10^{15}) cells derived from a single fertilized ovum. After humans reach maturity, the number of cells present remains essentially constant (Fig. 1.1). Maintenance of cellular constancy, however, is a very dynamic process. Cell division occurs at a brisk rate, and approximately one trillion (10^{12}) human cells die each day, and must be replaced. The most active sites of cellular replication occur in the gastrointestinal tract, bone marrow, and skin. Thus, in the adult animal or human, the number of new cells produced is equal to the number of cells that die (Fig. 1.1). This basic equation is fundamental to our understanding of normal and abnormal cellular growth.

Three subgroups of cells comprise every cell population (Fig. 1.2). Cycling cells occupy the first group, continuously proliferating and moving from one mitosis to the next. Terminally differentiated cells that irreversibly leave the growth cycle, and are destined to die without dividing again, comprise the second group. The third subpopulation of nonproliferating cells are not cycling and do not divide, but can reenter the cell cycle if an appropriate stimulus is applied (G_0 cells). During their normal cycling processes, proliferating cells progress through four different phases defined as G_1, S, G_2, and mitosis.

Nonproliferating (G_0 cells) are normally present in most tissues of living animals. For example, in the liver most cells are in the G_0 phase. If, however, approximately two thirds of the liver is removed surgically, the remaining nonproliferating (G_0) cells will reenter the cell cycle, proliferate, and restore the liver to its approximate original size. A similar phenomenon occurs in bone marrow. Knowledge of this is important to radiation and medical oncologists, who often introduce therapeutic procedures for the treatments of cancers that deplete maturing bone marrow cells, and stimulate protected (G_0) stem cells to reenter the cell cycle and eventually repopulate the bone marrow.

Growth in number of any population of cells can occur by any one of three mechanisms (Fig. 1.2). In the first, shortening of the length of the cell cycle results in more cells being produced per unit time. In the second, decreasing the rate of cell death will also result in more cells being produced. In the third, moving G_0 cells into the cell cycle will result in more cells produced per unit time. Each of these mechanisms appears important in normal and cancer cell growth.

The cell cycle of all cells, normal as well as cancerous, may be characterized by the time required to double the cell population (cell doubling time). In normal cells this doubling time is well regulated and controlled. In human cancers and their distant progeny, or metastases, however, the cell and volume (or mass) doubling times may be widely variable and relatively autonomous. In the fastest growing neoplastic diseases (e.g., Burkitt's lymphoma), a mean volume doubling time of less than 3 days is present. Intermediate is a volume doubling time of 17 days for Ewing's sarcoma, and at a slow extreme is a volume doubling time of more than 600 days for certain adenocarcinomas of the colon and rectum. The cell and volume doubling times of cancers are real measures of aggressiveness of a cancer, because they are dynamic measurements. Other measurements such as the mitotic index or the degree of anaplasia may be visualized by a pathologist at the level of light microscopy, but provide less sensitive measures of cancer aggressiveness.

CANCER AS A TEMPORAL DISEASE

Each cancer, and each patient bearing a cancer, exhibit a chronologic record of significant events. These events are set in motion by a process called initiation that results in significant, irreversible changes in a host cell, usually a stem cell, leading to development of cancer. If attempts to alter these processes are not made, or if they are made but fail, eventually clinical cancers will result that will lead to the death of the host. The summation of these temporal processes is designated as the natural history or biologic progression of a cancer (Fig. 1.3).

The temporal growth of a cancer proceeds through two phases. The first phase is called the preclinical phase (latent period or tumor induction time). During this period a number of now recognizable molecular and cellular events occur in a chronologic order that eventually results in the production of a cancer that can produce symptoms and can be clinically detectable. The duration of this preclinical phase may be as short as a few months after initiation (e.g., Burkitt's lymphoma), or as long as many years (e.g., colon, lung, urinary bladder cancers). It has been estimated that the mean preclinical phase for most human cancers may be 15 to 20 years, and may be as long as 40 to 50 years. During the preclinical phase it is not possible t recognize any molecular or cellular abnormalities suggestive of cancer. The pa

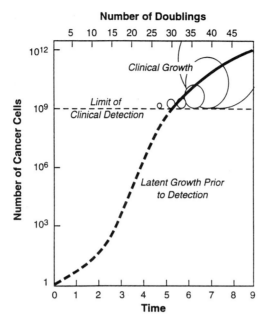

FIGURE 1.3. Growth curve of a hypothetical cancer. This diagram emphasizes that the preclinical phase (latent period) of growth occupies the majority of time (75%) of development of a cancer, and that by the time a cancer is diagnostically detectable it is very late in its natural history. Approximately 30 volume doublings have occurred prior to development of symptoms or signs leading to diagnosis. During the clinical phase of growth with only a few additional volume doublings the cancer burden to the host becomes overwhelming. The larger number of cell doublings prior to diagnosis permit time for development of micrometastases, as well as resistant clones of malignant cells. (Adapted from Tannock, 1992.)

will have no signs or symptoms of the latent progressive disease processes. Estimates exist that the preclinical phase may occupy as much as 75% of the time course of the natural history of a developing cancer. The insidious nature of this preclinical phase permits a developing cancer to grow to an approximate size of 1 cm^3, with a content of about 1 billion (10^9) cancer cells prior to development of symptoms or signs of illness permitting diagnosis. About 30 volume doubling progressions from the initial viable initiated cancer cell are necessary to produce a cancer mass containing 1 billion (10^9) cancer cells (Fig. 1.3). As a crude estimation it is recognized that the accumulation of 10^{13} cells in a given patient usually correlates with a lethal event. During the latter portion of the preclinical phase, small cancers may develop micrometastases in other sites or organs of the host.

In this regard, Fig. 1.4 relates tumor doubling to size. If a cancer has metastasized prior to the time it has reached a detectable size, that is, prior to 20 to 25 doublings, surgical cure is not possible, raising the specter of the need for effective adjuvant therapies to be discussed later. Tumor doubling time also has significant implications for cancer screening as is also highlighted by Fig. 1.4.

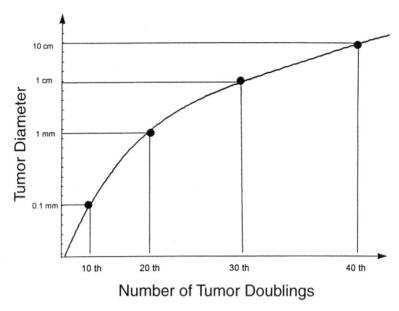

FIGURE 1.4. Number of tumor doublings versus tumor diameter (log scale): Note: The difference between exponential Gompertzian changes are minimal between the 30th and the 40th doubling.

The clinical phase of the natural history of a cancer begins at the point when the cancer is definitively diagnosed. It is at this point that symptoms may appear in a patient, and at which therapy is required in an attempt to cure or palliate the patient who has cancer. Knowledge concerning the clinical phases of cancers is much more comprehensive. This later phase generally occupies only the last portion ($\sim$ 25%) of the natural history of an individual cancer; if the cancer is not successfully eradicated during this phase, a patient will die.

CANCER ETIOLOGY

In experimental animals it is possible to produce a wide variety of detectable cancers by single or multiple applications of individual cancer-causing substances, or complete carcinogens (e.g., chemical carcinogens, ultraviolet or X-radiations, or viruses). In experimental animals it is also possible to use combinations of exposures to two or more chemical carcinogens, radiations and chemical carcinogens, or chemical carcinogens and viruses to produce cancers in high frequency. In humans, examples of exposures to a single carcinogen (e.g., cyclophosphamide producing urinary bladder cancer) resulting in a subsequent neoplasm do exist. In most instances, however, it appears that exposures to multiple types of cancer-causing agents in a concurrent or sequential manner is responsible for the cancers subsequently diagnosed. Examples of multiple causation factors include cigarette smoking and asbestos exposure, and tobacco abuse and alcohol consumption.

CANCER AS A MULTISTAGE DISEASE

The term *carcinogenesis* is used to describe the cascade of events that convert a normal cell, usually a stem cell, into a cancer. It is visualized currently as a multistage process propelled by genetic damage and epigenetic changes (Fig. 1.5). At least six stages have been described depicting the sequential chronologic events in carcinogenesis: *initiation, growth, promotion, conversion, propagation,* and *progression* composed of the processes of invasion and metastasis. These terms describe operational concepts, not well-understood molecular and cellular mechanistic events. At present, most of the available information concerns initiation, promotion, and progression. Much less information is available regarding the other three stages—growth, conversion, and propagation.

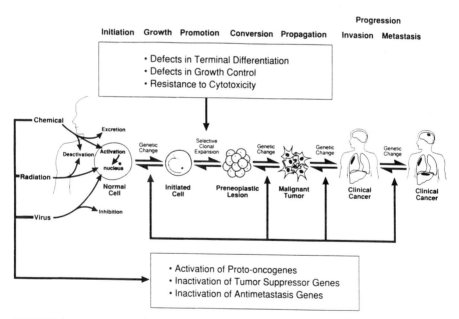

FIGURE 1.5. Multistage, temporal model of cancer development. This diagram presents six stages of cancer development and depicts their time of occurrence in relationship to progression from a normal cell to a malignant clinical cancer. Characteristics of evolving cancer cells and crucial molecular events involved in carcinogenesis are shown in the boxes. (Modified from Weisburger and Horn, 1991, and Shields PG, Harris CC [1993] Principles of carcinogenesis: Chemical. In: DeVita VT Jr, Hellman S, Rosenberg SA (eds) *Cancer—Principles & Practice of Oncology*, 4th edition, Vol. 1. JB Lippincott, Philadelphia, pp. 200–212.)

Initiation

The stage of cancer initiation begins in cells, usually stem cells, through mutations from exposures to incomplete carcinogens (e.g., chemical, ultraviolet, or X-radiations, or viruses). Initiating agents are capable only of beginning this first stage. Initiating agents are believed to change irreversibly the base composition or structure of component nuclear DNA and through this process begin the cancer development. Mutated cells may exhibit an altered responsiveness to their microenvironment and a selective growth advantage, in contrast to surrounding normal cells. It is also recognized that many potential initiation events are reversed by cellular DNA repair mechanisms and that mutations in nonexpressed DNA sequences may be "silent," or nonfunctional. A number of characteristics describe the initiation stage of cancer. This process appears to be rapid, completed within fractions of seconds. Only single steps are required to confer initiation, and the process appears to be irreversible. At present, no threshold has been identified for the stage of initiation. Initiated cells may also have a diminished responsiveness to intercellular and intracellular signals that maintain their structure and regulate homeostatic growth. In the present environment in which humans reside, much exposure to potential initiation agents is inevitable, and their effects may be additive. In the general circumstances of human exposure, initiated cells are not usually identifiable or visible. It has been suggested that during the course of an individual's lifetime many of the cells in his or her body may undergo the process of initiation, but those initiated cells either may not progress further, may die, or may be neutralized by immunologic mechanisms.

Growth

Following initiation, a stage of growth, or selective clonal expansion, of initiated cells may also occur. This may be facilitated by physical alteration of the normal microenvironment (e.g., wounding of mouse skin or urinary bladder, or partial hepatectomy in rodents), chemical agents (e.g., phorbol esters on mouse skin, or rat liver and phenobarbital exposures), microbial agents (e.g., influenza virus enhancement of rodent lung carcinogenesis, or hepatitis virus in human liver carcinogenesis), or other inflammatory processes. Detailed information concerning this phase is not yet available. Given that the subsequent stage of tumorigenesis, promotion, also involves clonal expansion of an initiated cell population, the two stages may be thought of as a continuum rather than as discrete temporal events.

Promotion

The stage of cancer promotion involves alteration of gene expression, selective clonal expansion, and proliferation of initiated cells. A schemata of experiments in mouse skin demonstrating characteristics of initiation and promotion is presented in Fig. 1.6. Application of a single dose of an initiator chemical alone (X) at a dose too low to produce neoplasms by itself is not followed by subsequent development of tumors enumerated in these experiments as papillomas or carcinomas (Fig. 1.6, line 1). In contrast (line 2), a similar exposure to an initiator followed by repeated

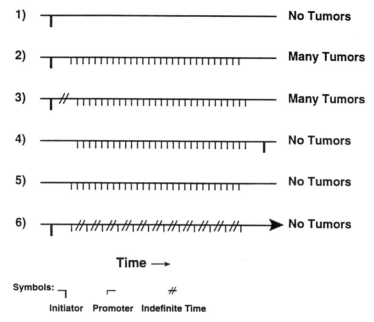

FIGURE 1.6. Illustration of experiments conducted in mouse skin demonstrating characteristics of initiation and promotion. Each numbered line (1, 2, 3, 4, 5, and 6) represents the single application (or no application) of an initating agent (heavy |). The multiple vertical lines (light |) represent multiple consecutive applications of a promoting agent. Passage of time without initiator or promoter treatment is indicated by //. The designation "tumors" refers to the production of murine skin papillomas or carcinomas. Consult text for detailed discussion of experiments. (Modified from Pitot, 1985.)

exposures to a promoting agent results in the presence of many tumors. The irreversibility or "memory" of the initiating event is illustrated in line 3. With the passage of time following application of the initiating chemical (which can be up to 1 year) before exposure to a promotional agent, tumors develop. It is clear that initiation must precede (line 4) and is an absolute requirement (line 5) for tumor production, respectively. Finally, promotion is not additive, but may be reversible, as passage of time between repeated applications of the promoting agent creates a situation in which no tumors develop (line 6). A similar series of events has been studied in other rodents and found to be applicable (e.g., rat colon, rat liver, rat urinary bladder). Thus, the promotion stage exhibits characteristics of reversibility, it is prolonged in duration, it may require multiple steps, a dosage threshold may be present, it appears to be nonadditive, and it results in grossly visible neoplasms. The extent of human exposures to promoting agents may be variable. It appears clear that the several features of initiation and promotion that have been identified emphasize that they are distinct and different stages. Many of the characteristics of initiation and promotion have been known for more than 50 years, and have been referred to as two-stage carcinogenesis in which tumor initiation (mutation) is followed by tumor promotion (epigenetic changes). Recent concepts have been modified as it is viewed that two-stage carcinogenesis, although conceptually important, is too simplistic. Other data suggest that there may be six or more independent mutational events preceding the formation of cancer.

Conversion

The next stage of cancer development, that is, conversion, relates to the entrance or the emergence of potentially reversible small nests of cancer cells that begin their irreversible course toward clinical malignancy. At present, this stage resides in the realm of hypothesis as little data are available to clearly define it. It has been speculated that, in contrast to stages of initiation and promotion, external factors have little to contribute to this stage of cancer evolution. It is believed more likely that internal factors residing in the microenvironment of the emerging irreversible cluster of cancer cells may influence this process. In any event, this stage appears to signal the presence of an irreversible cancer. It must be pointed out that at this stage the presence of cancer is not detectable in the host. It is highly likely that such a cancer consists of cell clusters of fewer than 10 to 1000 cells, a number too low to be detected by any available qualitative or quantitative methods of analysis.

Propagation

Following the stage of conversion, the microscopic cancer undergoes a stage of propagation characterized by growth of the expanding clusters of cancer cells resident in a particular tissue. External environmental factors appear to have little influence on this process, and it may be more related to the presence or absence of certain internalized host factors (e.g., estrogens and breast cancer). The time of propagation may be as short as a few months, or may require many years of evolution. During this stage the expanding cancer mass may increase from 1000 to 1,000,000 cells in composition, but is still too small to be seen by available analytic methods. For most cancers, no external symptoms or signs are produced during the stage of progression that would alert the patient or the physician to the presence of a preclinical cancer.

Progression

The last and sixth stage is called progression. It is characterized by additional enlargement of the primary cancer mass, the breaking off of cells from this mass and movement into adjacent tissues and organs, and the penetration of individual cancer cells or small clumps of cells into the circulatory system with transport of these and entrapment in distant tissues and organs. These entrapped cancer cell clumps often establish residence in the new tissue sites and continue to grow, a process known as metastasis. A most characteristic feature of progression is the development of measurable changes in nuclear karyotype. Accompanying the change in karyotype is increase in growth weight of the cancer mass, increasing cellular autonomy, invasiveness, and metastatic capacity. The stage of progression concludes the preclinical phase of cancer evolution, and provides a transition into the clinical phase of cancer formation. If cancers can be diagnosed prior to the time of formation of generally nondetectable micrometastases, then cures by means of surgery, or where appropriate, radiation therapy, may occur with a high degree of frequency. However, if micrometastases occur prior to the diagnosis of cancer, then cures of such cancers occur much less frequently. Attempts to control metastatic cancers must then rely upon systemic forms of therapy including enhancement of host immunologic defense mechanisms, external biologic and immunologic therapies, or the introduction of chemical or hormonal modes of therapies.

THE MALIGNANT NATURE OF CANCER: INVASION AND METASTASIS

If cancers grew only with the formation of solitary masses of increasing size with the passage of time, treatment of these lesions would be relatively easy. Cures in high frequency could be produced by surgery or radiation therapy. However, it is the properties of invasion and metastasis (Fig. 1.7) formation accompanied by the absence of regulation of cell replication and karyotypic instability that distinguishes cancers, and makes them lethal. Fig. 1.8 provides a schematic illustration of the various stages of the metastatic process. Knowledge concerning the process of invasion is scanty. It appears to be associated with a defined series of events including increased mobility of malignant cells, capacity for proteolysis of tissue and organ support structures (e.g., collagen), and "loss of contact inhibition." Normal cells grow in vitro as a cellular monolayer, and retain contact inhibition, that is, when dividing normal cells contact other normal dividing cells, the process of division ceases. Cancer cells grown in vitro, however, have lost this capacity to be inhibited in growth on contact with other cells, and thus cells continue to pile up during cell division. In addition, the ability of cancer cells to stimulate neovascularization, or the formation of new blood vessels to supply the tumor, appears to be critical to successful establishment of metastatic lesions.

A metastasis is defined as one or more cancer cells spreading from a site of origin, moving to a new site, and continuing its growth process at this new site some finite distance from the original primary growth of the cancer. It is this process of metastasis formation that gives cancers their potential for lethality. Cancer cells can metastasize by implantation, by local extension into adjacent tissues and organs, or by invasion and passage through the blood circulatory and lymphatic systems (Fig. 1.8). When cancer cells enter the bloodstream, they lodge in small distal capillaries where they then invade through the capillary wall and grow in the new tissue of residence. This is the major route of metastasis formation. A similar process may occur when cancer cells invade the lymphatic systems. Cancer cells have been demonstrated to be present in the bloodstream during the stage of progression, and it appears that the number of cancer cells present in the bloodstream is proportional to the size of the primary cancer. However, the number of circulatory cancer cells is believed to far exceed the number that give rise to actual metastatic lesions. It has been estimated

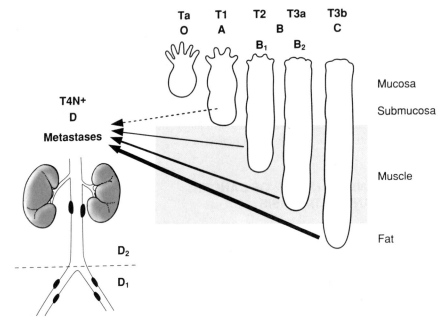

FIGURE 1.7. Illustration of the spatial progression of a hypothetical cancer arising in a hollow viscus. The specific model represented compares the Tumor Metastasis Nodes (TMN) and the older Marshall–Jewett systems for the classification of urinary bladder cancer. Progressive invasion of the developing cancer through normal mucosa, submusoca, muscle, and fat of the involved organ is portrayed. Metastasis formation at early and late stages of cancer development is depicted by arrows. (Modified from Fair WR, Fuks ZY, Scher HI [1993] Cancer of the bladder. In: DeVita VT Jr, Hellman S, Rosenberg SA (eds) *Cancer—Principles & Practice of Oncology*, 4th edition, Vol. 1. JB Lippincott, Philadelphia, pp. 1052–1072.)

that the ratio of new metastatic lesions formed may be 1 for every 10,000 cancer cells entering the bloodstream. Entrance of cancer cells into the lymphatics is the second major route of distant cancer cell metastasis formation. This mode of spread of cancer cells into local lymphatic channels may sometimes block these channels and lymph nodes. This blockage of regional lymph nodes forms the basis for "en bloc" cancer surgery. At one time it was believed that lymph nodes served as filters for cancer cells. However, experimental investigations have demonstrated that cancer cells can pass through lymph nodes. Development of metastases in lymph nodes first occurs in the subcapsular space of the node. In certain types of cancers, the number of lymph nodes involved by metastases is a critical measure of prognosis and likelihood of the development of other metastases found to be involved.

Local extension of tumor growth may be impeded by other body tissues or organs (e.g., bone, cartilage, or the presence of a serosa). Cancers spreading by local extension often follow paths of least resistance (e.g., blood vessels, nerves, tissue planes). Where cancer cells have free access to serosal cavities (e.g., the abdominal cavity with cancer of the ovary), cells may be disseminated in the free fluid, and may

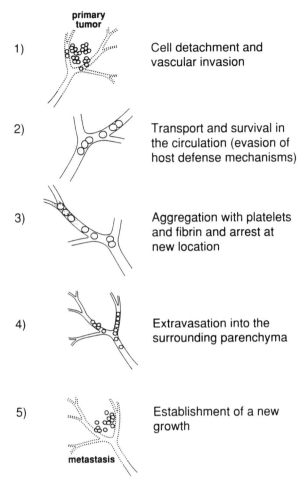

1) Cell detachment and vascular invasion

2) Transport and survival in the circulation (evasion of host defense mechanisms)

3) Aggregation with platelets and fibrin and arrest at new location

4) Extravasation into the surrounding parenchyma

5) Establishment of a new growth

FIGURE 1.8. Conceptual illustration of various stages of the metastatic processes occurring in vascular and lymphatic channels. (Modified from Hill, 1992.)

subsequently implant distant from the ovary of origin into the abdominal serosa or mesentery. It has been demonstrated that implantation of cancer cells may occur during the process of surgery if a scalpel, other instruments, or surgical gloves become covered with cancer cells. These cells may be transferred to another part of the body or the wound. This mode of spread has led to the development of meticulous cancer surgical techniques such as the "no touch" techniques used to minimize the problem of this method of transfer. Occasionally metastases may become evident later in a surgical scar formed following a cancer operation. Such metastases, in addition to direct introduction by the surgical process, may also occur because cancer cells circulating in the bloodstream or lymph channels became lodged in damaged capillary structures of the wound and continue to proliferate.

Knowledge of routes of spread of particular cancer types provides the basis for staging or measuring the extent of disease in individual patients during the clinical phase of cancer growth and development. This knowledge is also applied to design of appropriate therapies for patients classified as having identical stages of cancer.

Patterns of sites of metastases differ considerably for different primary cancers, and for different parts of a particular organ in which a cancer arises. Certain organs appear prone to metastasis formation depending upon the site of the primary cancer, whereas very few metastases occur in some organs (e.g., muscle, skin, thymus, and spleen). From many organs bearing a cancer, the lung capillaries are the first to receive venous blood, as well as lymphatic fluid through the thoracic duct, and thus the lungs are common sites for metastases. It has been demonstrated experimentally in mice that it is possible to select cancer cells that have specific predilections for growth as metastases in particular organs, so-called organotropism.

Detailed knowledge concerning the most significant mechanisms responsible for the occurrence of metastases is incomplete, but has been advancing rapidly. By the time the cancers develop to the stage of progression, cellular karyotypic instability has advanced, and individual cancer cells within a cancer mass have become heterogeneous with respect to each other. Significant changes in the properties of cancer cells (e.g., cell-to-cell adhesion) have occurred favoring successful metastatic development. Although metastases may be produced by single cancer cells, it appears more probable that they are produced by clumps of similar cells. Knowledge has been rapidly advanced indicating that host immunologic integrity is significantly compromised as cancers develop through stages of propagation and progression. These alterations in host immunologic mechanisms facilitate continued cancer growth and metastasis formation. In addition to alterations in immunologic mechanisms, clotting mechanisms may be significantly perturbed, leading to a predisposition for intravascular clot formation. This may be due to secretion of procoagulant mediators by tumors, increased platelet counts, and abnormalities in the production of clotting factors by the liver. Experimental studies have been directed toward development of interventions designed to enhance immunologic mechanisms, restore coagulation functions, and inhibit unrestricted growth of cancer cells.

In addition, many clinical investigations have been conducted exploring the use of effective cancer chemotherapies as "adjuvants" to surgery or radiation therapy. These so-called "adjuvant" therapies have been directed at patients with known cancers, but not known to harbor clinical evidence of metastasis formation. Use of these therapies has been partially successful in patients with breast and colon cancers, but not yet successful in many other malignant diseases. Such adjuvant therapies may be limited by a variety of factors including: (1) cancer cell heterogeneity, that is, populations of cells within a given cancer resistant to the antineoplastic therapy; and (2) an adequate biologic milieu to deliver therapy (e.g., lack of a microvasculature to deliver chemotherapy, or tissue hypoxia creating resistance relative to ionizing irradiation). In addition cancer regrowth after effective therapy in both the adjuvant and metastatic setting often heralds the emergence of a neoplasm resistant to therapy. This concept is illustrated in Fig. 1.9.

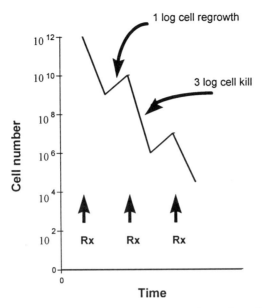

FIGURE 1.9. The relationship of therapy (RX) and regrowth to cell numbers. If one assumes that a population of cancer cells does not evolve resistance to a given RX then a constant proportion of cell is destroyed with each cycle of treatment. To produce a cure cell killing must exceed regrowth.

CANCER GROWTH

Characteristics of the preclinical phases of cancers as multistaged diseases have been described. As symptoms or signs of cancer formation and evolution are not at this time detectable, almost no information is available concerning the in vivo growth characteristics of developing cancers. Information concerning in vivo growth of cancers has thus been obtained from observations of patients in the clinical phase of cancer development. These observations suggest that cancers exhibit exponential and Gompertzian growth (Fig. 1.1 and 1.4). Mature cancers exhibit relatively uncontrolled growth behavior, and in contrast to normal cells, lose their responsiveness to normal intracellular and extracellular growth control mechanisms. Initial cancer cell growth behavior appears to be exponential, but as the cancer becomes larger in size, and perhaps outgrows its vascular supply and source of micronutrition, the growth rate decreases with time. Thus, a growth curve can be described by an equation relating size and time, a so-called Gompertzian curve. In addition, clinical cancers may exhibit circumstances in the natural process in which the cancer seemingly decreases temporarily in size before again becoming progressive in growth. The growth behavior of clinical cancers may "wax and wane," but eventually they resume their progressive and relentless natural history that may lead to death of the host.

CLINICAL SEQUELA OF MALIGNANCY

As cancer masses increase in size, they can destroy and invade surrounding normal tissues, compromising their function and causing severe and difficult to control local pain. Most advanced cancers cause death because of established metastases and progression in new metastatic locations. Metastases in vital organs (e.g., liver, lung, bone marrow, or brain) severely compromise organ function and lead to various symptoms depending upon the organ involved. In addition to direct effects of cancers in sites of primary origin, or in sites of metastasis formation, cancers may have indirect effects of clinical significance. These include impairment of nutritional balance, significant metabolic disturbances, continued immunologic compromise, progressive weakness of the host, and enhanced susceptibility to life-threatening infections. Exact mechanisms producing such effects are not clearly understood, but may be related to the production of toxins by the continually expanding and heterogeneous cancer burden, or may involve the trapping of certain essential nutritional elements (e.g., essential amino acids, vitamins) by the expanding cancer at the expense of the host. For example, certain cancers elaborate specific hormones that mimic the action of normal body hormones. Antidiuretic hormone (ADH) and adrenal corticotropic hormone (ACTH) may often be produced by lung cancers, and the elaboration of these hormones may result in significant metabolic derangements. A frequent accompaniment of advancing cancer is suppression of appetite and a distaste for food. These effects may be mediated by a hormonelike substance elaborated by the growing cancer. The secretions of such known and unknown hormones and the resultant clinical effects are called "paraneoplastic syndromes" and often may be the most dominant and visible effects of advanced cancers in humans.

SUMMARY CONSIDERATIONS

During the past two decades rapidly advancing knowledge of the natural histories of cancers and the specific characteristics of their stages have developed from biologic, cellular, and molecular levels of investigations, and the interdigitation of these three levels of comprehension. These new understandings have provided more specific methods designed to prevent cancer formation in the preclinical phase, and to enhance management of these diseases in patients in the clinical phase. The concept of irreversibility of action by initiating agents has led to major efforts to limit human exposures to these agents (e.g., limiting radiation exposure from diagnostic radiology procedures; limitation of ultraviolet light from sunlight; and limitation of exposures to known human chemical carcinogens in the workplace, in pharmaceutical products, and in dietary sources). Additional efforts at removing exposures to promotion agents have led to educational efforts to limit exposures to cigarette smoke, use of smokeless tobacco, and reduction of excess dietary fat. A search for agents designed to modify the stage of promotion has led to the new science of cancer chemoprevention exemplified by the use of vitamin A and its chemical analogs (e.g., 13-cis-retinoic acid and inhibition of continued development of upper airway cancers). An understanding of the karyotypic instability present in the stage of progression and its relationship in some circumstances to actions by oncogenic viruses has led to development of immunization methods (e.g., hepatitis B vaccination and attempts to prevent hepatic cancers). Attempts have been made to inhibit the formation and growth of metastases by interfering with altered blood coagulation processes as well as by development of antiangiogenic therapies. Finally, adjuvant chemotherapy treatments have been actively designed in attempts to inhibit formation of metastases in patients with early clinical cancers. New knowledge concerning the natural histories of how cancers evolve should enable design of novel approaches to cancer control.

ACKNOWLEGMENTS

George T. Bryan and H. Ian Robins were supported in part by grant RR03186 from the National Institutes of Health. Mark R. Olsen was supported by NIH Training Grant R25-CA47785.

FURTHER READING

Baserga R (1993) Principles of molecular cell biology of cancer: The cell cycle. In: DeVita VT Jr, Hellman, S, Rosenberg, SA (eds) *Cancer—Principles & Practice of Oncology*, 4th edition, Vol. 1. JB Lippincott, Philadelphia, pp. 60–66.

Buick RN, Tannock IF (1992) Properties of malignant cells. In: Tannock IF, Hill RP (eds) *The Basic Science of Oncology*, 2nd edition. McGraw-Hill, New York, pp. 139–153.

Fidler J (1997) Molecular biology of cancer: Invasion and metastasis. In: DeVita VT Jr, Hellman S, Rosenberg SA (eds) *Cancer—Principles & Practice of Oncology*, 5th edition. Lippincott–Raven, Philadelphia, pp. 135–152.

Hill RP (1992) Metastasis. In: Tannock IF, Hill RP (eds) *The Basic Science of Oncology*, 2nd edition. McGraw-Hill, New York, pp. 178–195.

Kastan MB (1997) Molecular biology of cancer: The cell cycle. In: DeVita VT Jr, Hellman S, Rosenberg SA (eds) *Cancer—Principles & Practice of Oncology*, 5th edition. Lippincott-Raven, Philadelphia, pp. 121–134.

Pitot HC (1985) Principles of cancer biology: Chemical carcinogenesis. In: DeVita VT Jr, Hellman S, Rosenberg SA (eds) *Cancer—Principles & Practice of Oncology*, 2nd edition, Vol. 1. JB Lippincott, Philadelphia, pp. 79–99.

Scher HI, Shipley WU, Herr HW (1997) Cancer of the bladder. In: DeVita VT Jr, Hellman S, Rosenberg SA (eds) *Cancer—Principles & Practice of Oncology*, 5th edition. JB Lippincott, Philadelphia, pp. 1300–1322.

Tannock IF (1992) Cell proliferation. In: Tannock IF, Hill RP (eds) *The Basic Science of Oncology*, 2nd edition. McGraw-Hill, New York, pp. 154–177.

Weisburger JH, Horn CL (1991) The causes of cancer. In: Holleb AI, Fink DJ, and Murphy GP (eds) *American Cancer Society Textbook of Clinical Oncology*. The American Cancer Society, Atlanta, GA, pp. 80–98.

Yuspa SH, Shields PG (1997) Etiology of cancer: Chemical factors. In: DeVita VT Jr, Hellman S, Rosenberg SA (eds) *Cancer—Principles & Practice of Oncology*, 5th edition. JB Lippincott, Philadelphia, pp. 185–202.

CHAPTER 2

CARCINOGENESIS

SURYANARAYANA V. VULIMIRI and JOHN DIGIOVANNI

Department of Carcinogenesis
Science Park—Research Division
University of Texas M. D. Anderson Cancer Center
Smithville, TX 78957, USA

BACKGROUND AND HISTORICAL PERSPECTIVE

The roots of carcinogenesis date back to the 18th century. Human exposure to certain chemicals or substances was first related to an increased incidence of cancer independently by two English physicians. John Hill, in 1761, observed an increased incidence of nasal cancer among snuff users. Shortly thereafter Percival Pott, in 1775, observed that chimney sweeps had an increased incidence of scrotal cancer and attributed this to the occupational exposure to soot and coal tar. It was not until a century and a half later, in 1918, that two Japanese scientists, Yamagiwa and Ichikawa, confirmed these earlier observations by demonstrating that multiple topical applications of coal tar to rabbit ears produced skin carcinomas. The importance of the latter experiment was twofold: (1) it was the first demonstration that a chemical or substance could produce cancer in animals, and (2) it confirmed Percival Pott's initial observation and established a relationship between human epidemiology studies and animal carcinogenicity. In the 1930s Kennaway and co-workers isolated a single active carcinogenic chemical from coal tar and identified it as benzo[a]pyrene, a polycyclic aromatic hydrocarbon (PAH) resulting from the incomplete combustion of organic molecules.

The concept that cancer involves an alteration in the genetic material of a somatic cell (somatic mutation theory) was first introduced by Theodor Boveri in 1914.

Manual of Clinical Oncology, 7th edition, Edited by Raphael E. Pollock
ISBN 0-471-23828-7, pages 19–43. Copyright © 1999 Wiley-Liss, Inc.

Boveri suggested that cancer was related to chromosome abnormalities. In 1934, Furth and Kahn isolated single cell clones from a tumor and found that injection of these cells into a healthy host could reproduce the original disease, thus demonstrating that cancer is a stable heritable cellular alteration. In the 1950s and 1960s, James and Elizabeth Miller observed that a wide variety of structurally diverse chemicals could produce cancer in animals and suggested that they required metabolic activation to reactive electrophilic intermediates. In addition, they suggested that the common factor among the diverse chemical carcinogens was the ability of their reactive intermediates to bind covalently to nucleophilic centers on proteins, RNA, or DNA. The Millers termed this the electrophile theory of chemical carcinogenesis. Since then, many carcinogens have been shown to require metabolic activation to reactive electrophilic intermediates that bind covalently to cellular macromolecules. In 1964, Brookes and Lawley demonstrated that covalent binding of carcinogenic PAH to DNA correlated best with carcinogenic potency. Subsequently, many chemical carcinogens were shown to bind covalently to DNA in various animal model systems and to produce mutations in both prokaryotic and eukaryotic cells. These types of chemical carcinogens are referred to as genotoxic carcinogens.

It is important to note that not all chemicals that induce cancer in experimental animal systems directly damage DNA or produce mutations, that is, they are not genotoxic. Such "nongenotoxic" carcinogens are detected usually after chronic administration of relatively high doses to experimental animals. Many of these types of chemicals induce proliferation in specific target tissues either directly via a specific mechanism or indirectly as a result of cellular toxicity. Based on the knowledge that cancer is a multistep process, which is discussed in more detail in a later section, many of these "nongenotoxic" carcinogens could be considered as *cocarcinogens* or *tumor promoting* agents. These types of agents, although not directly carcinogenic per se, either enhance the action of a carcinogenic agent (cocarcinogen) or create an environment (tumor promoter) that allows genetically altered cells to grow into a tumor.

For the purposes of the current chapter, the term *carcinogenesis* is defined as a process wherein the normal physiologic function of living cells is altered, resulting in abnormal and uncontrolled growth of a particular organ or tissue. The newly formed mass of tissue, which is morphologically and genetically different from normal tissue and has autonomous growth, is called a *neoplasm*. An agent that either induces or causes a series of genetic or epigenetic events in normal cells resulting in a significant increase in the incidence of a neoplasm of a given or multiple histologic type compared with normal untreated individuals, irrespective of whether the control individual has a high or low incidence of neoplasms of that kind, is termed a *carcinogen*.

HUMAN CANCER

As shown in Fig. 2.1, epidemiologic studies indicate that a majority of human cancers occur as a result of exposure to environmental agents or factors. Environmental

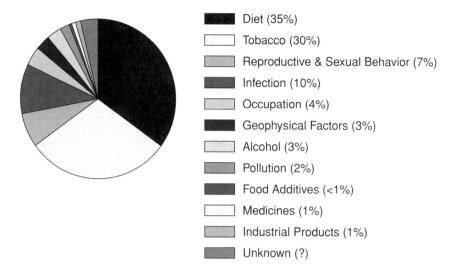

FIGURE 2.1. Factors contributing to the incidence of human cancer. Adapted from Doll R, Peto R (1981).

factors include smoking; diet; cultural and sexual behavior; occupation; exposure to radiation (natural or medical); and exposure to agents or substances in air, water, and soil. Elucidation of the relationship between exposure to a particular environmental factor and incidence of a specific cancer in a given community has been aided through studies of specific populations that have been stratified according to a number of variables including occupation, race, and lifestyle. Although cancer incidence is associated to a major extent with cigarette smoking and exposure to dietary substances, human carcinogenesis in many cases may involve an interaction among several etiologic factors.

TYPES OF HUMAN CARCINOGENS

Human carcinogens can be divided into three main categories: (1) physical carcinogens; (2) biologic carcinogens; and (3) chemical carcinogens. Examples of each type of carcinogenic agent are given in the following sections. In addition, specific types of cancers associated with exposure to these carcinogens are given. In some of the examples, the evidence for carcinogenicity in humans is considered sufficient (see further discussion in the section on Identification and Classification of Human Chemical Carcinogens), whereas in some examples the association is weaker (as noted).

Physical Carcinogens

Physical carcinogens include radiation, films and fibers, and chronic irritation. One of the most widely studied physical carcinogens is ultraviolet (UV) light. Skin cancers, such as squamous cell carcinoma (SCC), basal cell carcinoma (BSC), and malignant melanoma (MM), are all correlated with increased UV exposure. In particular, the incidence of skin cancer is higher in sunny regions of the world, among outdoor workers in general, in people with fair complexions, and on most sun exposed areas of the human body. Episodes of sunburn exposure in childhood or in early adolescence may contribute to an increase in skin cancer incidence. Ionizing radiation, induced by exposure to electromagnetic particles, such as γ-rays, X-rays, or photons, is also known to cause cancer in humans. Examples of occupations in which exposure to ionizing radiation resulted in bone marrow cancers include watch dial painters exposed to ^{224}Ra and underground mine workers exposed to radon. Medical radiation exposure is yet another source of occupational exposure to ionizing radiation. Exposure to asbestos fibers in humans leads to the induction of malignant mesothelioma and bronchogenic carcinoma. Induction of malignant mesothelioma appears to be dependent more on the size and structure of the fiber as opposed to its composition. Chronic irritation or trauma resulting from long-lasting wound or sore is considered a potential cause of cancer although a direct involvement in human cancer incidence is not shown unequivocally. Examples of chronic irritation are lip cancer in pipe smokers; moles in locations on the body subject to chronic irritation such as the belt region or the back of the neck; oral cancers in betel nut or tobacco chewers; and lung cancer in foundry or quarry workers or people exposed to other types of fibers such as silica fibers. However, in many of these latter cases, additional exposure to other potential carcinogenic agents may confound the establishment of direct associations.

Biological Carcinogens

Certain biologic agents have been shown to be associated with specific human cancers, including viruses, parasites, and bacteria. For example, Epstein–Barr virus (EBV) is associated with Burkitt's lymphoma and is also associated with Hodgkin's lymphoma. Chronic infection with hepatitis B virus has been linked to liver cancer in some parts of Asia and Africa. Papilloma virus infection has been implicated in cervical cancer. Other biologic agents such as parasites have been found to be associated with specific cancers. For example, associations between *Schistosoma haematobium* and bladder cancer have been noted in parts of Egypt and Africa, and liver flukes (*Clonorchis* and *Opisthorchis*) have been associated with bile duct cancer. Among bacteria, infection with *Helicobacter pylori* has been associated with gastric cancer in humans. The relationship between these latter infectious agents and cancer may not be direct, and they may be acting more like a cocarcinogenic and/or tumor promoting stimulus.

Chemical Carcinogens

As shown in Fig. 2.1, the majority of human cancers are associated with exposure to chemicals in the diet, tobacco smoke, pollution, medicinal agents, industrial products, etc. Based on studies in experimental animals as well as exposed human populations, chemical carcinogens may be divided into three major classes: (1) organic chemicals, (2) inorganic chemicals, and (3) hormones. Organic chemicals that are carcinogenic in man include PAHs such as benzo[a]pyrene which is found in tobacco smoke, combustion emissions, and coal tar. PAHs are associated with both lung cancer and skin cancer. Hemangiosarcoma of the liver is associated with exposure to vinyl chloride, another example of an organic chemical carcinogen. Aromatic amines were known to induce cancer in humans long before they were shown to be carcinogenic in animals. For example, 2-naphthylamine, used in the chemical and dye industry, induced bladder cancer in essentially 100% of workers involved in its purification. A final example of an organic chemical carcinogen is benzene, which induces acute myelogenous leukemia after prolonged exposure.

Inorganic carcinogens that are carcinogenic in humans include arsenic, nickel, and chromium. Arsenic, found in the copper mining and smelting industry, is associated with skin, lung, and liver cancer. Chromium and chromates, which are used in the tanning and pigmenting industry, and nickel are also associated with cancers of the nasal sinus and lung.

The last major category of chemical carcinogens are the hormones. Although the hormones discussed in this chapter are in fact organic chemicals, they are discussed separately because their mechanism(s) may be more like those of "nongenotoxic" carcinogens. In addition, other polypeptide growth factors (e.g., insulinlike growth factors, growth hormone, transforming growth factor-α, etc.) that are carcinogenic in experimental animals belong to this category. A dramatic example of hormonal carcinogenesis in humans involves the use of the synthetic estrogenic compound diethylstilbesterol in pregnant women to avert a threatened spontaneous abortion. A small percentage of the female offspring of mothers treated with diethylstilbesterol during pregnancy developed clear cell carcinomas of the vagina, usually within a few years after puberty. The use of oral contraceptives that contain synthetic steroidal estrogens as the predominant or sole component results in the development of liver cell adenomas. In addition, prolonged use of oral contraceptives has been associated with increases in the incidence of premenopausal breast cancer in some but not all epidemiologic studies. The administration of estrogens unopposed by progestin is associated with a significantly increased risk of the development of endometrial carcinoma. Androgenic steroids, usually in the form of synthetic congeners of testosterone, are associated with hepatocellular carcinomas in humans treated for extended periods of time. Finally, recent evidence has suggested that endometrial cancer may be induced by long-term treatment with the antiestrogen tamoxifen.

Because the majority of human carcinogens are chemical in nature, the remainder of this chapter is devoted to chemical carcinogenesis.

IDENTIFICATION AND CLASSIFICATION OF HUMAN CHEMICAL CARCINOGENS

The primary factors involved in the determination of carcinogenic potential are hazard identification and risk estimation, which form the basis of cancer risk assessment. Traditionally, carcinogen identification involved epidemiologic detection of human cancer risks and provided the original evidence that certain chemicals can be carcinogenic to humans. At present, animals are used as surrogates for human exposure to identify agents that pose a potential risk for human cancer induction. Because the purpose of these studies is to detect agents that might under some conditions of exposure result in human cancer development, the trend has been toward the use of the most sensitive species and endpoints. In addition, the maximum tolerated dose (MTD) of a compound is administered for a majority of the life span of the animal to ensure that if any carcinogenic hazard exists, it will be detected. At present, the primary factor used in risk assessment for human cancer is tumor incidence in 2-year bioassays in rodents. The 2-year rodent bioassay is performed by chronically administering a compound and assessing the incidence of tumors at all sites. The dose of the compound is the MTD and one half the MTD. In addition, both a solvent-treated control and an untreated control are included. The compound is administered by the route through which human exposure is most likely to occur. Animals with a low spontaneous tumor incidence result in the lowest background on which to detect an increased tumor incidence. In addition, the animal should be susceptible but not hypersensitive to the tested effect. The two strains typically used in these studies are the B6C3F1 mouse and the F344 rat. Both of these animals have high spontaneous rates of certain tumor types, limiting their predictive value and utility in risk estimation for these sites. The number of animals is minimally set at 50 per dose per sex per species to approach statistical relevance for the dose–response data needed for use in risk assessment.

Based on weight of evidence for carcinogenicity from epidemiologic studies in humans and from the results obtained in animal studies, human carcinogens are classified into five major groups by the Environmental Protection Agency (EPA) and the International Agency for Research on Cancer (IARC). These groups are as follows: Group 1: Human Carcinogen, where there is sufficient epidemiologic evidence in humans to indicate that a particular agent is carcinogenic (e.g., aflatoxin, benzene, estrogens); Group 2A: Probable Human Carcinogen, where there are limited human data and sufficient animal evidence to show that an agent is carcinogenic (e.g., benz[a]anthracene, diethylnitrosamine, polychlorinated biphenyls); Group 2B: Possible Human Carcinogen, where there are inadequate or no human data, but sufficient animal data showing that the agent in question is carcinogenic (e.g., styrene, 2,3,7,8-tetrachlorodibenzo-p-dioxin [TCCD], urethane); Group 3: Not Classifiable as to Human Carcinogenicity, where there is a lack of or an inadequate amount of human as well as animal data to show that an agent is carcinogenic (e.g., 5-azacytidine, diazepam); Group 4: Noncarcinogenic to Humans, where there is lack of evidence in humans and no evidence for carcinogenicity of the putative agent in at least two adequate animal tests in two different species (e.g., caprolactam).

Table 2.1 lists those chemicals for which there is currently sufficient evidence for carcinogenicity in humans.

TABLE 2.1. Chemical Carcinogens Implicated in Human Cancer

Occupation/Exposure	Carcinogen	Target Organ
Cigarette smoke	PAHs, aromatic amines, nitrosamines, free radicals	Lung, trachea, bronchii, larynx, pharynx, mouth, esophagus, bladder, prostate, cervix
Betel quid and tobacco chewers	N-nitrosamines	Mouth
Alcohol	Ethanol	Esophagus, liver, oropharynx, larynx
Hormones	Diethylstilbestrol	Vagina, uterus
Miners, insulation material producers, shipyard and dockyard workers	Asbestos	Lung, trachea, bronchii, pleura, and peritoneum
Mineral product workers	Chromium, nickel, arsenic	Lung, trachea, and bronchii
Organic chemical plants	Bis(chloromethyl)-ether, chloromethyl methyl ether	Lung, trachea, and bronchii
Foundry workers	Mustard gas, iron and steel	Lung, trachea, and bronchii
Coke plant workers, gas workers, and painters	Benzo[a]pyrene, β-naphthylamines, coal carbonization products	Lung, trachea, and bronchii
Aluminum plant workers	Benzo[a]pyrene and tar volatiles	Lung, trachea, and bronchii
Leather and wood industry	Leather dust, wood dust	Nasal cavity and sinuses
Copper mining and smelting workers, arsenic miners; vineyard, asphalt, coal tar, pitch workers	Arsenic and coal carbonization products, asphalt, coal tar and pitch	Skin on lips and scrotum
Gasoline, rubber industry	Benzene	Bone marrow
Dye manufacturing	4-Aminobiphenyl, auramine, 2-naphthyl-amine, benzidine, magenta	Bladder
Rubber manufacturing, gas workers	Coal carbonization products, 2-naphthyl-amine	Bladder
Aluminum plant workers	PAHs and tar volatiles	Bladder
Vinyl chloride producers	Vinyl chloride	Liver
Diet	Aflatoxin-B1	Liver
Charbroiled meat	Heterocyclic amines (PhIP)	Colon
Drugs	Cyclophosphamide, melphalan	Bone marrow and bladder
	Azathioprine	Bone marrow and skin
	Chlornaphazine	Bladder
	Methoxypsoralen with UV light	Skin
	Phenacetin	Renal pelvis
	Thorotrast	Liver

CHEMICAL CARCINOGENS AND METABOLIC ACTIVATION

Depending on their chemical nature, chemical carcinogens can be classified as either *direct* or *indirect* acting. In both cases, a chemically reactive intermediate is formed that covalently binds to cellular macromolecules of which DNA is the most important cellular target. *Direct carcinogens* are agents that are highly chemically reactive without the need for metabolic activation (e.g., β-propiolactone, aziridine, cyclophosphamide, bis(chloromethyl) ether, ethylene oxide, methyl methane sulfonate, nitrogen mustard derivatives). These carcinogens spontaneously decompose to produce a highly reactive electrophilic intermediate that can alkylate DNA and produce base modifications (e.g., O^6-alkylguanine, N^7-alkylguanine). *Indirect carcinogens* are agents that require metabolic activation to reactive electrophilic intermediates that can also bind covalently to DNA (e.g., PAHs such as benzo[*a*]pyrene). In the case of indirect chemical carcinogens, the unmetabolized compound is referred to as the *parent compound* or *carcinogen*. The parent carcinogen (e.g., benzo[*a*]pyrene) is inactive per se and requires metabolic activation to an intermediate metabolite called a *proximate carcinogen* (e.g., benzo[*a*]pyrene 7,8-diol) that is further metabolized to an *ultimate carcinogen* (e.g., benzo[*a*]pyrene-7,8-diol-9,10-epoxide) to exert its carcinogenic activity. Both direct and indirect carcinogens covalently modify DNA, producing adducts with the DNA bases (i.e., guanine, adenine, cytosine, and thymine).

The metabolic activation of chemical carcinogens is carried out primarily by the flavin-containing monooxygenases or cytochrome(s) P450 enzymes (a class of enzymes that display a characteristic absorbance maximum at 450 nm when reduced with carbon monoxide) present in the endoplasmic reticulum of most cells. The cytochrome(s) P450 superfamily consists of many enzymes that play a central role in both metabolic activation and detoxification of a variety of xenobiotics, including drugs, chemical toxicants, and carcinogens. To date, 12 P450 gene families comprising over 100 enzymes have been identified in mammalian species. Cytochrome P450 families are classified by percent similarity of the amino acid sequence of the proteins. For example, there is <35% similarity between any two families of cytochrome(s) P450 in the amino acid sequence. Each P450 gene family can be divided into several subfamilies. Those P450 genes considered to be in the same subfamily have more than 68% homology. The cytochrome(s) P450, or phase I enzymes as they are called, carry out oxidation, reduction, oxygenation, dealkylation, desulfuration, dehalogenation, and hydroxylation reactions, which convert nonpolar or hydrophobic carcinogens into more hydrophilic or polar compounds through the formation of more reactive intermediate metabolites. For example, cytochrome(s) P450 enzymes metabolize PAHs such as benzo[*a*]pyrene, into an array of metabolites, including phenols, quinones, epoxides, and dihydrodiols. In addition, through extensive studies performed during the 1970s and 1980s, it is now known that benzo[*a*]pyrene is metabolically activated by cytochrome P450 1A1 and the enzyme epoxide hydrolase, in a two-step reaction, to the dihydrodiol epoxide metabolite mentioned in the preceding paragraph. This dihydrodiol epoxide metabolite, of which several isomers are produced, is the ultimate mutagenic and carcinogenic metabolite of this carcinogenic compound.

From many other studies it is known that aromatic amines such as benzidine, which contain a primary or secondary amine group, are metabolically activated through N-hydroxylation by P450 1A2 followed by esterifcation resulting in a reactive ultimate carcinogenic metabolite that can covalently modify DNA. Nitrosamines, such as the tobacco-specific nitrosamine 4-(methylnitrosamine)-1-(3-pyridyl)-1-butanone or NNK, are activated by P450 2B1 in a one-step reaction to an unstable, hydroxylated intermediate that spontaneously decomposes to a carbonium ion capable of alkylating DNA. On the other hand, nitrosamides such as methylnitrosourea do not require metabolic activation and decompose nonenzymatically at physiologic pH to generate a reactive electrophile similar to the nitrosamines. All of these chemical carcinogens and their reactive intermediates (formed directly or indirectly via metabolic activation) are shown in Table 2.2.

As noted previously, the oxidation of indirect carcinogens, known generally as phase I metabolism, in most cases renders them more hydrophilic and prepares them as substrates for the conjugating enzymes, known as phase II metabolizing enzymes. These enzymes conjugate the metabolites produced during phase I metabolism with a variety of small ligands and include methyl transferases, sulfotransferases, glucuronyltransferases, and glutathione-S-transferases (GSTs). Of particular importance is conjugation with glutathione (GSH) catalyzed by GSTs. In general, conjugation reactions lead to less toxic/carcinogenic and more readily excretable metabolites; however, this is not always the case, as seen with aromatic amines such as benzidine in the example given earlier and in Table 2.2. Both acetylation and sulfation of the N-hydroxyl substituent introduced during the phase I metabolism by P450 1A2 lead to more chemically reactive and ultimate carcinogenic metabolites.

It should also be stressed that pathways other than those involving mixed-function oxidases such as the cytochrome(s) P450 may be involved in the metabolic activation of chemical carcinogens. In this regard, cyclooxygenase-dependent cooxidation of carcinogens may be important for the metabolic activation of certain aromatic carcinogens in some extrahepatic tissues, especially the urinary bladder.

CARCINOGEN–DNA ADDUCTS, MUTATIONS, AND CARCINOGENESIS

As noted in the previous section, chemical carcinogens are either inherently chemically reactive or are metabolically activated to form electrophilic intermediates that react covalently with nucleophilic sites in DNA and form carcinogen–DNA adducts, now generally considered the first step in the process of cancer induction. As noted previously, DNA adducts are usually formed between reactive carcinogen metabolites and the bases of DNA. Depending on the structure, DNA adducts may be categorized as: (1) bulky, such as those adducts produced by PAH and aromatic amines, or (2) nonbulky, such as those produced by alkylating agents. PAH carcinogens react primarily with guanine and adenine (e.g., benzo[a]pyrene diol-epoxide reacts principally at the exocyclic amino group of both guanine [N^2] and adenine [N^6] whereas

TABLE 2.2. DNA Reactive Intermediates of Chemical Carcinogens

Parent Carcinogen	Classification	DNA-Reactive Intermediate

Benzo[*a*]pyrene — Indirect — Benzo[*a*]pyrene-7,8-diol-9,10-epoxide

H_2N—⬡—⬡—NH_2 — Indirect — *N*-Acetyl benzidine Nitrenium ion

4-(Methylnitrosamino-)-1-(3-pyridyl)-1-butanone (NNK) — Indirect ⟶ — $CH_3N=NOH$ + Methanediazohydroxide

4-(3-Pyridyl)-4-oxo-butanediazohydroxide

N-methyl-*N*-nitrosourea — Direct — $CH_2N_2^+ [\longrightarrow CH_3^+(?)]$

alkylating agents are less specific and react at different sites and with all DNA bases. In addition, reactive oxygen species (ROS), produced as a result of carcinogen exposure, can lead to oxidative DNA damage (e.g., 8-hydroxyguanine, thymine glycol). Finally, several endogenous forms of DNA damage include simple base modifications resulting from processes such as depurination, deamination, depyrimidination, single-strand breaks, and alkylation. Oxidation of DNA bases can also be produced during normal cellular processes.

Using benzo[a]pyrene again as an example, the major DNA adduct formed in target tissues is a specific isomer of its reactive diol epoxide metabolite, (+)-*anti*-BPDE, bound through *trans* addition of the exocyclic amino (N^2) group of deoxyguanosine [(+)-*anti*-BPDE-N^2-dGuo]. With regard to other types of chemical carcinogens such as the direct acting alkylating agents, UV light, ionizing radiation, aromatic amines, nitrosamines, psoralens, and other chemicals, considerable information is also known about their interaction with DNA in target tissues in vivo and the DNA adducts that are associated with their carcinogenic activity. For example, O^6-alkylguanine and O^4-alkylthymine are the DNA adducts most closely associated with carcinogenicity by alkylating agents, whereas cyclobutane dimers have been associated with the carcinogenic properties of UV light.

Carcinogen–DNA adducts have been demonstrated in both target tissues for carcinogenesis (e.g., liver, lungs, bladder, skin, etc.) and nontarget tissues (e.g., white blood cells, lymphocytes, uroepithelial cells, buccal epithelial cells) in experimental animals and humans. In experimental animal systems, extensive research has shown that the presence of a given carcinogen–DNA adduct in a particular target tissue correlates with the biologic effect of that carcinogen. However, the ability of a carcinogenic agent to induce cancer depends on many factors including, but not limited to, the extent of DNA repair capacity of that cell, tissue, and/or experimental animal or individual. In addition, the rate of cell replication can influence the ultimate response of a tissue or cell to a carcinogen–DNA adduct. For example, patients with xeroderma pigmentosum (XP) exhibit a deficiency in repairing dimers induced by UV exposure, making them vulnerable to development of skin cancers. Cell replication in the presence of carcinogen DNA damage is generally considered to be the time when such damage produces critical effects (e.g., cytotoxicity, mutagenesis).

Extensive studies of different carcinogenic compounds have revealed a strong correlation between mutagenicity and carcinogenicity. Thus, carcinogens, by virtue of their ability to form specific DNA adducts, can induce a spectrum of mutations. The spectrum of mutations induced by chemical carcinogens include point mutations, frameshift mutations, (e.g., deletions/insertions), chromosomal aberrations, aneuploidy, and polyploidy with varying degrees of specificity that are usually dose dependent. The efficiency and spectrum of mutational activity of chemical carcinogens are assayed using both bacterial and mammalian cell systems or in cell free systems in vitro. As an example, DNA reactive metabolites of benzo[a]pyrene are mutagenic (inducing base pair and frameshift mutations) in both bacterial and mammalian systems. The overall spectrum of mutations arising from the (+)-*anti*-diol epoxide of benzo[a]pyrene [(+)*anti*-BPDE] is similar in bacterial and mammalian systems; the most frequent mutations are GC→TA transversions, although AT→TA and GC→CG mutations are also seen. Mutagenesis of the (+)-*anti*-BPDE metabolite was very recently examined in bacteria with site-directed vectors containing a single (+)*anti*-BPDE-*trans*-N^2-dGuo adduct. Depending on the sequence context around the DNA adduct, G→T, G→A, and G→C mutations were obtained.

Many chemical carcinogens can alter the primary sequence of DNA, as noted previously, causing mutations. Furthermore, specific genes found in normal cells, termed proto-oncogenes, have been identified as target sites for chemical carcinogens. Certain chemical carcinogens can produce mutations in these proto-oncogenes, thereby activating them to dominant transforming genes that have the ability to transform certain cells in vitro. The function and role of the protein products encoded by proto-oncogenes and oncogenes and the covalent interactions of chemical carcinogens with proto-oncogenes are being studied extensively. In addition, another family of genes, known as tumor suppressor genes, is involved in the carcinogenic process and certain tumor suppressor genes, such as the gene *p53*, have been shown to be targets for carcinogenic agents. Mutations in these genes induced by carcinogens lead to inactivation of the gene.

ONCOGENES AND TUMOR SUPPRESSOR GENES INVOLVED IN HUMAN CANCER

Oncogenes

Certain normal cellular genes, termed proto-oncogenes, appear to be target genes for chemical carcinogens and their alteration is strongly associated with tumor formation and carcinogenesis. Proto-oncogenes function in a tightly regulated manner to control normal cellular proliferation and differentiation. However, when these genes are altered by a mutation, sequence deletion, virus integration, chromosome translocation, gene amplification, or promoter insertion, they have the ability to transform cells in vitro. The altered forms of these genes are called oncogenes

Proto-oncogenes can be activated to oncogenes either qualitatively or quantitatively. Qualitative changes include alterations in the coding region of the gene such as point mutations. The best example of oncogenes that are activated by such a mechanism is the *ras* family of genes. For example, studies in many experimental animal model systems of chemical carcinogenesis have shown that the *ras* genes are activated by point mutation. Evidence has been obtained that the point mutations in the *ras* genes are related to the type of carcinogenic agent used. For example, in hallmark studies by Barbacid and co-workers, rat mammary carcinomas induced by methylnitrosourea contained an activated c-Ha-*ras* gene with a point mutation in codon 12 (G^{35} →A transition mutation), whereas with 7,12-dimethylbenz[*a*]anthracene-induced mammary carcinomas, A^{182} →T transversion mutations in codon 61 were observed. Quantitative changes include gene amplification (increase in the number of copies of a given gene) leading to overexpression, or chromosomal translocation of a proto-oncogene leading to aberrant expression of the proto-oncogene. The best example of these processes involves the *myc* family. Amplification of *myc* in human or murine carcinomas, leukemias, or sarcomas is a late, progression related event.

In Burkitt's lymphoma and mouse plasmacytoma the c-*myc* gene is translocated and inserted near an immunoglobulin locus. According to one model, such a juxtaposition allows for the deregulation of c-*myc* expression that is no longer under proper cellular regulation but rather under the control of the immunoglobulin promoter and is therefore constitutively expressed. However, the actual mode(s) of such deregulation is not fully understood. Translocation of c-*myc* from chromosome 8 to an immunoglobulin region in either chromosome 14, 22, or 2 is a consistent feature found in the great majority of Burkitt's lymphoma tumor biopsies or cell lines derived from these tumors.

A large number of cellular oncogenes (>50) have been identified. Most oncogene protein products appear to function in one way or another in cellular signal transduction pathways. Signal transduction pathways are used by the cells to receive and process information and ultimately to effect a biologic response. These pathways often consist of external signals, receptors, transducer proteins, second messengers, amplifier proteins, and internal effectors, all of which are involved in the regulation of cellular function and/or gene expression. Table 2.3A lists some of the known oncogenes and their functions. Note that oncogenes fall into six main categories, all of which are molecules involved in signal transduction, including: (1) growth factors; (2) growth factor receptors; (3) nonreceptor tyrosine kinases; (4) serine–threonine kinases; (5) G proteins/GTPases; and (6) nuclear proteins.

Tumor Suppressor Genes

Tumor suppressor genes and the proteins they encode function as negative regulators of cell growth. Their function is in direct contrast to the dominant transforming oncogenes which act as positive regulators of cell growth. Accordingly, tumor suppressor genes have been termed anti-oncogenes, recessive oncogenes, and growth suppressor genes. When tumor suppressor genes are lost by deletion or inactivated by point mutation they are no longer capable of negatively regulating cellular growth. Generally, if one copy of the tumor suppressor gene is inactivated, the cell is normal, but if both copies are inactivated, loss of growth control can occur and cancer can develop. The concept that loss of genetic material is involved in carcinogenesis comes from somatic cell fusion experiments. When a tumor cell is fused with a normal cell many of the resulting hybrids are nontumorigenic. These experiments suggest that the normal cell is contributing genes to the tumor cell that impose normal growth restraints on the latter and that cancer is a recessive trait. Subsequently, it was determined that these tumor cells contain specific chromosome deletions and such deletions are "corrected" in the normal–tumor cell hybrids because the previously deleted chromosome is now contributed by the normal cell. Further, by using microcell fusion experiments that allow for the selective introduction of specific chromosomes or a portion of a chromosome into these tumor cells it can be determined which chromosome or portion of a chromosome suppresses the tumorigenic phenotype and restores normal growth control. Additional evidence has come from the work of Knudson, who postulated that two mutational events are necessary for the development of retinoblastoma. This work led to the eventual identification of

TABLE 2.3. Oncogenes and Tumor Suppressor Genes Involved in Carcinogenesis

A. Oncogenes Identified from Human or Animal Studies

Functional role	Oncogenes
Growth factors	*wnt-2, wnt-1, wnt-3, hst, fgf-5, TGF-α, sis*
Growth factor receptors	*erbB, fms, kit, met, neu (erbB-2), ret, ros, trk*
Cytoplasmic tyrosine kinases	*bcr-abl, fes, jak,*
src family	*src, frg, fyn, hck, lck, lyn, yes, yrk*
Serine–threonine kinases	*mos, PKC-β1, PKC-γ, PKC-ε, PKC-ζ, raf*-1
G binding protein with GTPase activity	Ha-*ras*, Ki-*ras*, N-*ras*
Nuclear proteins	
Thyroid hormone receptor	*erb A*
Transcription factor	*ets, fos, jun,*L-*myc, myc,* N-*myc, rel, tal-1*

Adapted from Bowden, 1997.

B. Human Tumor Suppressor Genes

Tumor Suppressor Gene Involved	Condition	Human Cancer
p53	Li–Fraumeni syndrome (hereditary)	Sarcomas, leukemia, breast and brain cancers
	Nonhereditary	Lung, breast, colon, esophagus, liver, bladder, ovary, sarcoma, brain, all solid tumors, lymphomas, leukemias
WT-1, U'	Wilm's tumor	Nephroblastoma
MSH-2, PMS-2, PMS-1, hMLH-1	Hereditary nonpolyposis Colorectal cancer (Lynch syndrome)	Adenomas and adenocarcinomas in the right and transverse colon
3p25	Von Hippel–Lindau syndrome (VHL)	Hemangioblastomas of the central nervous system and retina, renal cell carcinoma, and pheochromocytoma
APC, MCC	Familial adenomatous polyposis (FAP)	Large bowel adenomas and adenocarcinomas
NF-1	Neurofibromatosis	Neurofibroma
RB-1	Retinoblastoma	Retinoblastoma
BRCA-1	Familial breast carcinoma	Breast cancer
MENI	Multiple endocrine neoplasia type 1	Pancreatic endocrine tumors, and pituitary adenomas
DCC	Deleted in colon carcinoma	Adenomatous polyps in colon

Adapted from DiGiovanni, 1997 and Pitot and Dragan, 1996.

the retinoblastoma gene and the discovery that both copies of the gene (two mutational events) are inactivated and/or deleted in retinoblastoma tumors. This deletion involves a specific locus termed Rb.

A number of other tumor suppressor genes have been identified through the analysis of families with inherited cancer syndromes, the most notable being *p53* in Li–Fraumeni syndrome. Table 2.3B lists a number of tumor suppressor genes, hereditary syndromes associated with the loss of function of the specific gene, and the type of tumor involved. The *p53* tumor suppressor gene is quite unique. In addition to being associated with Li–Fraumeni syndrome, this tumor suppressor gene is either mutated or deleted in many different types of human cancers. It has been shown to be a target of several types of carcinogens. In particular, a strong relationship between UV exposure and *p53* mutations exists with regard to human skin cancer. Epidemiologic and clinical studies have implicated UV radiation in sunlight as the agent responsible for the induction of most human skin cancers. Analysis of a large number of skin tumors (including both basal cell carcinoma and squamous cell carcinoma) has revealed the presence of UV signature mutations (i.e., $C \rightarrow T$ and $CC \rightarrow TT$) in various exons of this gene at a relatively high percentage (60 to 100% of tumors). In addition, *p53* mutations have been detected in sun damaged skin prior to the development of any tumors, suggesting that loss of *p53* may be an early event in human skin cancer. Other very recent studies have shown that mutational hotspots in the *p53* gene found in lung cancers are hotspots for the formation of DNA adducts by the reactive diol epoxide metabolite of benzo[*a*]pyrene. These data support the hypothesis that the *p53* gene may be an important target for human chemical carcinogens. The extent to which other tumor suppressor genes might be targets for chemical carcinogens remains to be determined.

MULTISTAGE CARCINOGENESIS

The concept of the multistage nature of the carcinogenic process dates back over 70 years to studies by Deelman, who found that wounding led to the appearance of skin tumors in mice that had been first treated with a carcinogenic tar. These, and other early studies, suggested a role for cell proliferation and hyperplasia in tumor development and skin carcinogenesis. In their hallmark article in 1944, Friedewald and Rous first defined the terms initiation and promotion after utilizing a two-stage protocol for the development of skin tumors in rabbits. They demonstrated that "latent" tumor cells initiated in rabbit skin by one treatment with 3-methylcholanthrene (MCA) could be "forced" or "promoted" to reveal themselves by subsequent treatment of the skin with agents that did not themselves initiate neoplastic change (e.g., turpentine, chloroform, wounding). The discovery of croton oil as a potent promoting agent led Mottram and others to ultimately develop the two-stage protocol of mouse skin tumorigenesis as it is generally used today. In his early experiments, Mottram (1944) elicited skin tumors by treating the backs of mice with a single, subcarcinogenic dose of benzo[*a*]pyrene and followed this with repeated topical applications of croton oil, obtained from the seed of *Croton tiglium*. The concept of multistage carcinogenesis is particularly important in terms of human cancer for several reasons. First, outside of occupational settings, human exposure to chemical carcinogens occurs at very low dose levels that, alone, are insufficient to produce cancer. Second, there is considerable evidence from both human epidemiologic as well as experimental animal studies that certain human carcinogens exhibit a strong tumor promoting activity. Tobacco smoke is an example of a human carcinogen with a strong tumor promoting activity component. Finally, many components of the human diet appear to influence cancer in humans through a tumor promotion effect.

The multistage nature of the carcinogenic process was first established using the mouse skin model of chemical carcinogenesis. The characteristics, based on our current understanding of the carcinogenic process in this model, are used to highlight the concepts and general mechanisms involved in multistage carcinogenesis. Epidermal neoplasia can be induced in mouse skin by two different protocols, that is, complete carcinogenesis and two-stage carcinogenesis protocols. In the first protocol, a single large dose or more commonly, multiple low-dose application of a genotoxic carcinogen (e.g., benzo[a]pyrene), is used to induce tumors on the backs of susceptible strains of mice. In two-stage carcinogenesis protocols, subcarcinogenic doses of a carcinogen (e.g., benzo[a]pyrene or 7,12-dimethylbenz[a]anthracene) are followed by multiple applications of a noncarcinogenic agent that possesses the ability to induce epidermal hyperplasia [e.g., 12-O-tetradecanoylphorbol-13-acetate (TPA) or benzoyl peroxide (BzPo)]. In the two-stage model of mouse skin carcinogenesis, three mechanistic stages can be define: *initiation*, *promotion*, and *progression*. The characteristics of each one of these stages is described in the following sections. Figure 2.2 shows the mouse skin model of multistage carcinogenesis and summarizes the major events that occur during the three mechanistically distinct stages described previously.

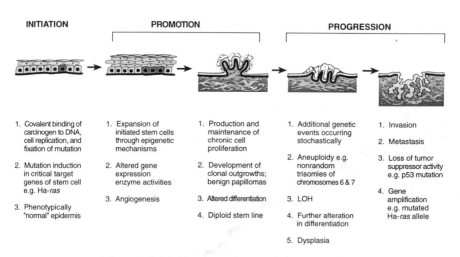

INITIATION	PROMOTION		PROGRESSION	

1. Covalent binding of carcinogen to DNA, cell replication, and fixation of mutation

2. Mutation induction in critical target genes of stem cell e.g. Ha-*ras*

3. Phenotypically "normal" epidermis

1. Expansion of initiated stem cells through epigenetic mechanisms

2. Altered gene expression enzyme activities

3. Angiogenesis

1. Production and maintenance of chronic cell proliferation

2. Development of clonal outgrowths; benign papillomas

3. Altered differentiation

4. Diploid stem line

1. Additional genetic events occurring stochastically

2. Aneuploidy e.g. nonrandom trisomies of chromosomes 6 & 7

3. LOH

4. Further alteration in differentiation

5. Dysplasia

1. Invasion

2. Metastasis

3. Loss of tumor suppressor activity e.g. p53 mutation

4. Gene amplification e.g. mutated Ha-*ras* allele

Figure 2.2. Multistage carcinogenesis in mouse skin.

Initiation

The initiation stage of multistage carcinogenesis in mouse skin is effected by a single, subcarcinogenic dose of either a direct acting [e.g., N-methyl-N'-nitro-N-nitrosoguanidine (MNNG)] or indirect acting (e.g., benzo[a]pyrene or 7,12-dimethylbenz[a]anthracene) carcinogen. During initiation, chemical carcinogens such as MNNG or benzo[a]pyrene either spontaneously decompose or are metabolically activated to a reactive intermediate as described previously. The reactive carcinogenic intermediates then react with the DNA of epidermal cells of the skin to form DNA adducts. It is generally believed that the target cells for tumor initiation in this model system are epidermal stem cells and that DNA adducts produce mutations in a critical gene(s) involved in controlling epidermal proliferation and/or differentiation. In the mouse skin model, the Ha-*ras* gene appears to be a critical target gene for some skin tumor initiators such as the PAHs. Mutations in certain codons of this gene (e.g., G^{38} of codon 13 for benzo[a]pyrene; A^{182} of codon 61 for 7,12-dimethylbenz[a]anthracene) lead to its activation. The presence of mutations in Ha-*ras* appears to confer a selective growth advantage on skin epidermal cells such that these cells undergo clonal expansion during the early phase of the tumor promotion stage. The hallmarks of skin tumor initiation in this model system are twofold: (1) the initiation stage is phenotypically silent, that is, the initiated skin behaves as normal skin unless it is challenged with chemical tumor promoters or other types of promoting stimuli such as wounding; and (2) the initiation stage is cumulative and irreversible, that is, one can fractionate the initiating dose without loss of tumor initiation and one can delay the start of tumor promotion without loss of tumor initiation. These latter points helped contribute to our initial understanding that the early stages of carcinogenesis in this model system were irreversible and involved a stable alteration in genetic material.

Promotion

The promotion stage of mouse skin carcinogenesis occurs as a result of exposure of the initiated skin to repetitive promoting stimuli. Because most tumor promoters are not genotoxic, this stage of carcinogenesis is believed to occur primarily through epigenetic mechanisms. The endpoint of the promotion stage in the mouse skin model is the formation of squamous papillomas, which are exophytic, noninvasive lesions consisting of hyperplastic epidermis folded over a core of stroma. Tumor promoting stimuli are very diverse in this model system and include various chemicals such as the phorbol esters (e.g., TPA), organic peroxides (e.g., BzPo), and okadaic acid. In addition, UV light, repeated abrasion, full thickness skin wounding, and certain silica fibers when rubbed on the skin all function as skin tumor promoters. The tumor promotion phase of multistage carcinogenesis involves the clonal expansion of initiated cells. By definition and observation, tumor promoting agents are not mutagenic like carcinogens but rather cause an alteration of the expression of genes whose products are associated with hyperproliferation, tissue remodeling, and inflammation. At some point, the developing papilloma constitutively expresses these genes and thus becomes tumor promoter independent. The identification of the mechanisms by which tumor promoters elicit altered gene expression has been intensively pursued over the last decade, particularly because the identification of these critical events offers a target for chemoprevention strategies (see the section on Inhibition of Chemical Carcinogenesis).

The mouse skin model of multistage carcinogenesis is an excellent paradigm in which to study molecular alterations associated with the various stages of tumor development. This is particularly true with regard to tumor promotion, a process that occurs in other organs and species including humans as noted previously. In mouse skin, among the most potent and by far the most studied chemical tumor promoters are the phorbol esters. In fact, TPA has been the prototypical promoter used for many years. A hallmark of the tumor promotion stage of mouse skin carcinogenesis is that it is reversible in the early stages. However, once the papillomas that develop acquire additional genetic changes that allow them to grow autonomously, tumor promotion is no longer reversible.

Changes in gene expression can occur directly as a result of tumor promoter action on skin epidermal cells as well as indirectly as a result of the paracrine action of a factor secreted from a nonepithelial skin cell. These paracrine factors may be produced as a function of direct tumor promoter action on the secreting cell or as a result of activation of the secreting cell by a keratinocyte factor elicited in response to tumor promoters.

Changes in the expression of genes as a consequence of external stimuli usually result from the activation, or sometimes inactivation, of specific signal transduction pathways. Major insights into the mechanism of action of tumor promoters has come from the recent elucidation of the signaling pathways extant in cells. The nature of the initial interaction of tumor promoters with the cell depends on the type of promoter. For some, such as TPA, specific receptors, which are one or more of the isoforms of protein kinase C, have been identified. Others, such as okadaic acid, are potent inhibitors of phosphatases, causing a net increase in the level of phosphorylated proteins, an effect similar to the activation of kinases. For yet other promoters, for example, BzPo, it is not known what pathways they alter. However, for compounds such as BzPo, it is known that free radicals, including ROS, play a role in their tumor promoting action. Regardless of the disparity in initial signaling events, the key biologic and molecular changes elicited by tumor promoters (including increased DNA synthesis, induction of ornithine decarboxylase [ODC], induction of growth factors and cytokines, and increased production of eicosanoids) are all similar. Further, the elicited production and secretion of growth factors, cytokines, and eicosanoids activate additional signaling pathways via receptors specific for these molecules. This overall alteration of signal transduction and gene expression creates the environment sufficient for the selection and growth of the initiated cell population. Some of the growth factors and cytokines whose expression is altered by tumor promoting stimuli include: (1) transforming growth factor-α (TGFα); (2) transforming growth factor-β; (3) interleukins 1 and 6; (4) tumor necrosis factor-α; (5) granulocyte macrophage colony stimulating factor; (6) vascular endothelial growth factor; and others.

Progression

Tumor progression or malignant conversion, as it is sometimes referred to in this model system, occurs when papillomas convert into SCCs. Most, if not all, SCCs that appear during a two-stage carcinogenesis protocol in mouse skin arise from preexisting papillomas.

The hallmark of tumor progression in the mouse skin model is the accumulation of additional genetic changes in cells that comprise premalignant papillomas. Because all SCCs arise from preexisting papillomas, these lesions can be considered true premalignant lesions. Several genetic alterations have been linked to tumor progression in the mouse skin model system. For example, nonrandom trisomies of chromosomes 6 and 7 have been associated with the progression of papillomas to SCCs. γ-Glutamyltranspeptidase expression is elevated in SCCs, as is expression of $\alpha6\beta4$ integrin and keratin 13. Elevated expression of certain proteases (e.g., stomelysin), TGFβ, and inactivation of the *p53* tumor suppressor gene occurs in some SCCs. Loss of the normal Ha-*ras* allele also occurs in later stages of progression. In addition, many of the changes in gene expression detected in papillomas persist in SCCs and may also contribute, in a permissive way, to the malignant phenotype of these tumors.

In concluding this section on multistage carcinogenesis it should be emphasized that studies from using the mouse skin model have shown that the carcinogenic process results from a series of stepwise changes that involve both genetic and epigenetic processes.

MULTISTAGE CARCINOGENESIS AND HUMAN CANCER

The multistage model of carcinogenesis in mouse skin has, for more than 50 years, provided a conceptual framework from which to study the carcinogenesis process. Many concepts now currently applied to other tissues and model systems, including cell culture models for multistage carcinogenesis and transformation, were originally derived from the mouse skin model. That these concepts also apply to human cancer has been confirmed by epidemiologic studies indicating that human carcinogenesis also occurs via a multistep process involving initiation and promotion mechanisms. A convincing example of multistage carcinogenesis in humans has also been presented by Vogelstein and colleagues. In this regard, human colorectal carcinoma can be shown to occur via a multistep process at the molecular level. First, all of the colorectal tumors examined, including the smallest adenomas, are clonal in origin. These adenomas also exhibited DNA hypomethylation, which is hypothesized to lead to chromosomal defects resulting in loss of tumor suppressor genes. Among the chromosomal deletions known to occur in human colorectal carcinoma, those at 5q, 17p, and 18q occur most commonly. These genetic alterations appear to occur sequentially during tumor progression; deletions at 5q and activation of the K-*ras* gene often precede allelic deletion at chromosomes 17p and 18q. These results suggest a model in which the acquisition of a *ras* gene mutation coupled with the loss of several tumor suppressor genes (including the *p53* gene on chromosome 17p) leads to human colorectal tumorigenesis. Thus, the multistep nature of human tumorigenesis may involve the activation of proto-oncogenes as well as the inactivation of one or more tumor suppressor genes. As indicated previously, the multistage model of mouse skin carcinogenesis also involves a number of sequential cellular, biochemical, and genetic events. Although the exact sequence of events may differ between tissues and species, the overall concept appears to be directly applicable to human cancer.

MODIFYING FACTORS IN CARCINOGENESIS

Table 2.4 lists some of the general factors that modify the carcinogenic process not only in experimental animals but in humans as well. A few of these factors are discussed in this section.

The ability of an individual to metabolize chemical carcinogens can be influenced by simultaneous exposure to other chemicals or by genetic constitution or both. Many dietary and environmental chemicals that humans are exposed to can increase or decrease the activities or amounts of the enzymes that activate [cytochrome(s) P450] or detoxify (conjugative or phase II enzymes) chemical carcinogens. For example, certain chemicals found in vegetables (e.g., isothiocyanates) can enhance the detoxification and excretion of certain chemical carcinogens. In addition, certain chemicals called polyphenols, which are found in green tea, can block carcinogen activation through inhibition of metabolizing enzymes and thereby block carcinogenesis. Some of these types of chemicals are being studied as potential chemopreventive agents as discussed in the next section.

Population studies have identified variants in genes encoding phase I and phase II metabolizing enzymes that can significantly influence individual cancer risk. Because these variants have a much higher frequency than the more rare allelic losses or

TABLE 2.4. General Factors or Modifiers of Chemical Carcinogenesis

Exposure to other chemical carcinogens
Capacity to metabolize carcinogens
DNA repair capacity
Age
Sex
Hormonal
Immunologic status
Trauma
Radiation
Viral
Diet, nutrition, and lifestyle
Genetic constitution

variants associated with cancer syndromes, they may account for a significant component of the attributable risk of cancer in human populations. For example, certain variants in cytochrome(s) P450, GSTs, and acetyltransferases have been shown in some epidemiologic studies to be associated with increased risk for specific cancers. As a specific example, a significant number of studies have shown an increased risk of lung cancer in smokers who lack the GSTM1 allele. Because GSTM1 is important for detoxifying certain types of reactive carcinogenic intermediates, the lack of this enzyme may be detrimental in an exposed population.

Another important determinant of whether a cell becomes initiated by a chemical carcinogen or not is DNA repair. Inhibition of the excision repair system allows a greater chance that the carcinogenic damage will not be repaired, thus a greater likelihood of mutation induction and cancer initiation. A number of genetic diseases including xeroderma pigmentosum (XP), Fanconi's anemia, Bloom's syndrome, ataxia–telangiectasia, and porokeratosis Mibelli are associated with DNA repair defects. Individuals afflicted with one of these heritable syndromes have a higher if not invariable incidence of cancer, and this increase in susceptibility to certain types of cancer is attributed to a compromise in their ability to repair DNA damage. For example, in XP patients, the oversensitivity of the skin to UV light leads to skin cancer, a consequence of a defect in the ability of cells in these individuals to excise UV-induced DNA damage. In addition, other studies have provided evidence that variation in DNA repair capacity within the general population can also influence the risk of skin and other types of cancer.

Diet, nutrition, and lifestyle are important modifying factors of carcinogenesis in humans. Dietary intake (fat, protein, calories) has been associated with cancers of the breast, colon, endometrium, and gallbladder. Considerable experimental evidence has demonstrated that carbohydrates and lipids are effective promoting agents in the development of neoplasms in several tissue types and in different species. Elevated risks of several neoplasms in humans result from excessive intake of alcoholic beverages. Because all types of alcoholic beverages are implicated in the various studies supporting these claims, ethanol and its metabolites appear to be the critical components of these beverages. Ethanol is metabolized directly to acetaldehyde, which has been shown to be mutagenic. However, no evidence exists that ethanol or alcoholic beverages are complete carcinogens in any system. In contrast, chronic ethanol administration after initiation may act to enhance hepatic carcinogenesis in rats. Ethanol, when given simultaneously with a carcinogenic agent, acts as a cocarcinogen in several other organs in experimental animals. In support of the promoting action of ethanol in humans, risk of cancer of the oral cavity and pharynx increases markedly when an individual smokes tobacco and abuses alcoholic beverages. Further, individuals who have been infected with the hepatitis B virus and drink alcoholic beverages excessively are prone to a more rapid appearance of hepatic neoplasms. In general, it appears that many diet and/or lifestyle associated cancers result not from direct carcinogenicity of the dietary or lifestyle factor, but rather that these factors act as cocarcinogens and/or tumor promoters and thus either modify the action of other carcinogens or promote the development of spontaneously initiated cells.

INHIBITION OF CHEMICAL CARCINOGENESIS

Chemoprevention (administration of one or several naturally occurring or synthetic anticarcinogenic compounds) or dietary intervention is a means of cancer control when the disease results from exposure to environmental carcinogenic agents. Micronutrients present in food are the most desirable class of cancer chemopreventive agents because epidemiologic studies suggest that consumption of fresh fruits and yellow–green vegetables reduces the human cancer incidence and mortality due to stomach, colon, breast, prostate, and even lung and bladder cancers. A wide range of such micronutrients present in food have been shown to possess potent cancer chemopreventive effects in experimental animal models of carcinogenesis. Fruits, vegetables, common beverages, and several herbs and plants have been shown to be rich sources of cancer chemopreventive agents. At present, about 30 classes of chemicals with cancer chemopreventive effects have been described that may have practical implications in reducing cancer incidence. Moreover, the existence of a wide chemical diversity of chemopreventive agents enhances the likelihood that a variety of approaches can be made to cancer chemoprevention using these compounds.

In addition to identifying potentially useful inhibitors of cancer development, cancer chemoprevention studies have also been important in increasing the understanding of the mechanisms of carcinogenesis. For example, agents such as antioxidants, protease inhibitors, mixed function oxidase inhibitors, prostaglandin synthesis inhibitors, and antiinflammatory agents, among others, have been shown to inhibit carcinogenesis, suggesting the involvement of these events or pathways in the carcinogenesis process.

Given the multistage nature of carcinogenesis and our advancing knowledge of the critical processes involved at each stage, strategies for the inhibition of chemical carcinogenesis have focused on stopping the carcinogenic process at the earliest possible point in the pathway through mechanism-based approaches. As shown in Fig. 2.3, potential targets for the inhibition of the initiation stage include: (1) modifying carcinogen activation by inhibiting the enzymes responsible for that process; (2) enhancing carcinogen detoxification by altering the activity of detoxifying enzymes; (3) directly scavenging DNA-reactive electrophiles; and (4) enhancing DNA repair processes. Targets for blocking the processes involved in the promotion stage of carcinogenesis include: (1) scavenging ROS; (2) altering the expression of genes involved in cell signaling, proliferation, apoptosis, and differentiation; and (3) decreasing inflammation. Examples of chemopreventive agents used in the antiinitiation and antipromotion/progression strategies shown in Fig. 2.3 are summarized in Table 2.5.

It should be noted in Table 2.5 that most of the chemopreventive agents that are currently undergoing clinical trials in human populations target primarily the tumor promotion stage of the overall carcinogenesis process. In this regard, two fundamental concepts of carcinogenesis in humans, "multistage carcinogenesis" and "field cancerization," have influenced clinical researchers in applying cancer chemoprevention to patients. In studying the process of multistage carcinogenesis in humans and two-stage carcinogenesis in rodents, it is accepted that exactly when initiation takes

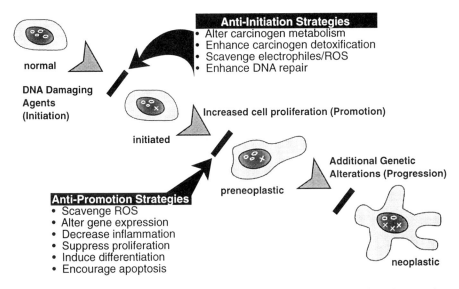

Figure 2.3. Antiinitiation and antipromotion strategies for the inhibition of carcinogenesis

TABLE 2.5. Examples of Chemopreventive Agents that Target Tumor Initiation and Promotion Stages of Carcinogenesis

Prevention Strategy	Example
Tumor initiation	
Alter carcinogen metabolism	Epigallocatechnin gallate (EGCG), selenium, phenethylisothiocyanate (PITC), indole-3-carbinol
Enhance carcinogen detoxification	Oltipraz[a], diallylsulfide (DAS), EGCG, glucarolactone
Scavenge electrophiles	EGCG, ellagic acid
Enhance DNA repair	?
Tumor Promotion	
Scavenge ROS	Antioxidants (e.g., vitamins C[a] and E[a])
Alter gene expression	Retinoids (e.g., 4-hydroxyphenyl-retinamide[4-HPR][a])
Decrease inflammation	Sulindac[a], vitamin C[a], vitamin E[a], piroxicam[a], glycyrrhetinic acid, ibuprofen
Suppress proliferation	Difluoromethylornithine (DFMO)[a], 8354 dehydroepiandrosterone (DHEA)[a], selenium[a], tamoxifen
Induce differentiation	Retinoids (e.g., 4-HPR, 13-cis-retinoic acid[a]), calcium[a]
Encourage apoptosis	DHEA[a]

[a] Agents currently in human clinical trials; ?, effective chemopreventative agents that work primarily through altering DNA repair processes are not known.

place in human cells is unknown. However, once a cell is initiated, it is an irreversible process. In contrast, tumor promotion requires repeated exposure and is a reversible process (at least in its early stages). In addition, growth of benign tumors can be arrested by preventive agents. Finally, tumor progression is characterized by an irreversible change of tumors from benign to malignant, and then further malignant changes such as metastasis that are often observed in the process of human carcinogenesis may occur. Thus, inhibition of tumor promotion, rather than of initiation or tumor progression, has been considered the more practical way to apply chemoprevention strategies.

The term "field cancerization" signifies multiple carcinogenesis in an area of epithelium preconditioned by an as yet unknown carcinogenic agent. The high recurrence rate in oral cancer supports this concept. For example, cancers of the aerodigestive tract and the lung are typical examples of field cancerization. The cases of "field cancerization" are 5% of the annual incidence of second primary cancers in patients with squamous carcinomas of the head and neck. Thus, many clinical trials involving potential chemopreventive agents are aimed at preventing the occurrence of second primary cancers.

Among the agents listed in Table 2.5 are some considered highly effective, including all-*trans*-*N*-(4-hydroxyphenyl)retinamide (4-HPR), a retinoid that alters gene expression and tissue differentiation processes; 2-difluoromethylornithine (DFMO), a suicide inhibitor of the proliferation associated enzyme ODC; piroxicam, a long-acting nonsteroidal antiinflammatory agent; oltipraz, and inducer of phase II metabolic enzymes; and dehydroepiandrosterone (DHEA), an adrenal steroid with antiproliferative activity. Other compounds showing more limited activity include ibuprofen, another nonsteroidal antiinflammatory agent; the DHEA analogue 8354 (a 16-fluoro analogue); tamoxifen, which is a well-known antiestrogen that has been clinically used in the adjuvant chemotherapy of breast cancer; and glycyrrhetinic acid isolated from licorice root which has antiinflammatory activity and weak antilipoxygenase activity.

Although targeting the tumor promotion stage of the carcinogenic process appears to be a highly effective strategy aimed at the chemoprevention of human cancer, agents that target the initiation stage should not be abandoned. Although it is likely that tumor promotion plays an important role in human carcinogenesis, there are clear examples of complete carcinogenesis through repetitive exposures to carcinogenic agents (e.g., tobacco smoke, UV light). In addition, humans are constantly exposed to low levels of carcinogens through air, water, and food. Except for very unusual situations, humans are likely not exposed to sufficient quantities of carcinogens in single doses to lead to carcinogenesis or even initiation. Any modifying factor that reduces the effective dose of a carcinogen (i.e., DNA adducts) in a specific target tissue may have a dramatic effect on overall cancer incidence, especially if the initiation process requires cumulative exposure to reach a threshold. Therefore, understanding specific dietary constituents that may reduce or block metabolic activation or DNA adduct formation of carcinogens is an important goal. Such information could lead to the development of specific chemopreventive agents, to specific dietary recommendations regarding food containing substantial quantities of certain types of of chemicals, or to approaches using mixtures of agents (e.g., a broad spectrum P450 inhibitor plus an antioxidant and/or an electrophile trapping agent) that block more than one stage of the carcinogenic process.

FURTHER READING

Bowden GT (1997) Proto-oncogenes as potential targets for the action of carcinogens. In: Sipes IG, McQueen CA, Gandolfi AJ (eds) *Comprehensive Toxicology*, Vol. 12, Elsevier Science, New York, pp. 55–81.

DiGiovanni J (1992) Multistage carcinogenesis in mouse skin. *Pharmacol Ther* 54:63–128.

DiGiovanni J (1997) Genetic determinants of cancer susceptibility. In: Sipes IG, McQueen CA, Gandolfi AJ (eds) *Comprehensive Toxicologyp53*, Vol. 12, Elsevier Science, New York, pp. 425–451.

Doll R, Peto R (1981) *The Causes of Cancer*. Oxford University Press, Oxford, England.

Escobar MR (1989) Oncogenic viruses. In: Sirica AE (ed) *The Pathobiology of Neoplasia*. Plenum Press, New York, pp. 81–109.

Fujiki H, Komori A, Suganuma M (1997) Chemoprevention of cancer. In: Sipes IG, McQueen CA, Gandolfi AJ (eds) *Comprehensive Toxicology*, Elsevier Science, New York, pp. 453–471.

Mulcahy T (1989) Radiation carcinogenesis. In: Sirica AE (ed) *The Pathobiology of Neoplasia*, Plenum Press, New York, pp. 111–129.

Pitot HC, Dragan YP (1996) Chemical carcinogenesis. In: Klaassen CD (ed) *Casarett and Doull's Toxicology: The Basic Science of Poisons*, 5th edition, McGraw-Hill, New York, pp. 201–267.

Smart RC (1994) In: Hodgson E, Levi PE (eds) *Carcinogenesis, Introduction to Biochemical Toxicology*, 2nd edition, Appleton & Lange, Norwalk, CT, pp. 381–414.

CHAPTER 3

THE MOLECULAR BASIS
OF CANCER

KAROL SIKORA

WHO Cancer Control Programme
Lyon, France
and
Imperial College School of Medicine,
Hammersmith Hospital
London, England

DEFINITION OF CANCER

Worldwide, one person in three will develop cancer. The disease can be defined as a disorder of growth and is caused by the accumulation of somatic genetic changes that can interfere with the intricate growth control processes of the cell. Unicellular organisms must respond to changes in their environment that favor growth, competing effectively with surrounding cells for resources, and continuing to divide until the nutrient supply is exhausted. Multicellular organisms have had to evolve mechanisms to control individual cellular activities. Complex signaling mechanisms have arisen so that cell growth and differentiation is coordinated and the internal environment maintained. A failure in cellular coordination can result in a single cell competing with its neighbors for space and nutrients, which can disrupt and eventually destroy the whole organism. Cancer is the term used to describe this event, and various types have been documented in many different species.

The clinical presentation of any cancer depends on the tissue type affected and the location but usually involves an expanding tumor mass. This causes symptoms through local invasion, local expansion, or the production of biologically active molecular products such as hormones or cytokines. Each tumor type has its own nat-

Manual of Clinical Oncology, 7th edition, Edited by Raphael E. Pollock
ISBN 0-471-23828-7, pages 45–61. Copyright © 1999 Wiley-Liss, Inc.

TABLE 3.1. Properties of Transformed Cells

Loss of contact inhibition
Reduced requirement for growth factors
Capacity to divide indefinitely
Anchorage independent growth
Ability to grow from a single cell
Ability to grow in immunocompromised animals

ural history depending on the anatomic site of the primary lesion, anatomic routes of spread, and the speed with which the cancer cells can metastasize.

Cancer cells can be cultured and grown in large numbers in the laboratory. Such transformed cells are the in vitro counterpart of normal cells. For many years comparisons were made between the biologic properties of normal and transformed cells. Morphologic and behavioral observations were essentially descriptive. As our understanding of the molecular mechanisms has increased so has the ability to analyze the genetic changes that lead to the physiologic abnormalities. The properties of transformed cells are shown in Table 3.1.

THE CLONAL NATURE OF CANCER

Genetic marker studies show that the vast majority of tumors arise from a single parental cell and are thus clonal (Table 3.2). In addition, numerous epigenetic events may create an environment conducive to change from the normal pattern of cell division, such as chronic inflammation or persistent stimulation of the immune system. Virtually all solid tumors and the majority of hematologic malignancies display abnormalities in the chromosomal karyotype that is inherited by the entire population of tumor cells. These abnormalities may involve the translocation, deletion, or addition of parts of chromosomes or indeed whole new chromosomes.

The first clear evidence that many tumors are indeed clonal came from studying the glucose-6-phosphate dehydrogenase (G6PD) gene in populations that have G6PD deficiency caused by a structural mutation within this gene that is on the X

TABLE 3.2. Evidence for the Clonal Nature of Cancer

Analysis of X-linked heterozygotes
Karyotype analysis
Specific translocations and deletions
Immunoglobulin gene rearrangements
T cell receptor gene rearrangements
Specific oncogene mutations
Specific tumor suppressor gene mutations

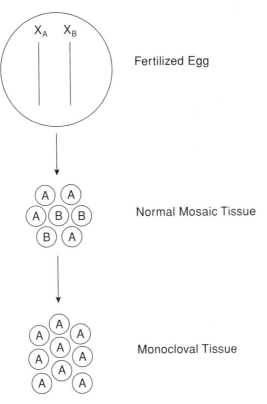

Fertilized Egg

Normal Mosaic Tissue

Monocloval Tissue

FIGURE 3.1. The clonal origin of tumors. The X-linked marker G6PD can be inherited in two forms, A and B. A heterozygote female has a mosaic of cells, some expression A and some B depending on which X chromosome is active in each somatic cell. A tumor expresses only one variant if it is of clonal origin.

chromosome. This condition is common in Africa and is inherited in two forms, A and B, readily identifiable by simple electrophoretic analysis. The cells of a woman who is heterozygous or G6PDA/B are a mosaic containing either the A or the B gene. Cancers arising in such heterozygotes express only one G6PD allele and are therefore monoclonal (Fig. 3.1).

Other evidence for monoclonality can be found in lymphomas where clonal rearrangements of immunoglobulin or T cell receptor genes take place early in lymphoid differentiation, providing another unique marker to demonstrate tumor monoclonality. More recently the clonal nature of human tumors has been confirmed by the direct analysis of mutation oncogenes in tumor suppressor genes using fluorescent in situ hybridization (FISH) in which fluorescent probes specific to certain DNA sequences can be hybridized to a specific chromosome.

ONCOGENES

The original evidence that specific genes have a role in carcinogenesis came from studies on RNA tumor viruses. These small entities possess only three genes, two coding for structural proteins and the third for reverse transcriptase—the enzyme that produces a DNA copy of the viral RNA allowing its genetic material to be incorporated into the host's genome. The addition of a fourth gene gives these viruses the ability to induce tumors rapidly in vivo and also to transform in vitro. These transforming sequences were termed viral oncogenes (v-*onc*). Surprisingly, it was subsequently shown that viral oncogenes share common sequences with the cellular genes, which were thus termed cellular oncogenes (c-*onc*).

This raised the problem of whether viruses cause cancer or whether they "hijacked" cellular genes involving growth control. Several pieces of evidence have clearly shown that the latter explanation is correct. Viruses carrying v-*onc* genes reproduce less efficiently than normal viruses. The extensive involvement of c-*onc* genes in normal cellular growth and differentiation indicates the likely origin of oncogenes. Cellular oncogenes do not usually possess transforming potential in the native state and the term *proto-oncogene* is used to distinguish them from genes with the ability to transform. This complicated nomenclature has arisen because the viral genes were named after the tumors in which they were first described. For example, v-*src*, one of the first genes studied, causes sarcoma in chickens whereas v-*sis* causes a sarcoma in monkeys.

Control of cell growth and development is a complex process. Oncogenes and their encoded proteins have been shown to be involved at each level of this process and alterations to this finely balanced system result in unregulated growth. Growth factors are extracellular proteins that act as growth modulators and possess several properties that indicate an involvement in carcinogenesis. Some growth factors will transform normal cells in vitro. Conversely in some systems the induction of cell transformation can result in an increased production of growth factor. The observation that growth factors can both initiate and be a product of transformation suggests the possibility of self-perpetuating positive feedback loops with unregulated cell division as the consequence. This phenomenon, termed autocrine secretion, has been implicated in various situations involving rapid growth such as wound repair and embryogenesis as well as malignant transformation. Both transformation and growth factor stimulation result in similar biochemical changes such as increased tyrosine phosphorylation and altered cellular lipid metabolism. One oncogene, c-*sis*, has been shown to code for a known growth factor—platelet-derived growth factor (PDGF).

Several oncogene-encoded proteins form part of a cell surface receptor. The presence of the appropriate growth factor switches the receptor on, with a resultant increase in tyrosine kinase activity within the cell. The kinase can also be upregulated by an internal regulatory region allowing responses to intracellular events. The consequence of increased kinase activity is a hallmark of transformed cells.

Small alterations in the receptor can produce defects in the regulation of tyrosine kinase activity. An example of this is c-*erbB-1*, which encodes for the cellular receptor of epidermal growth factor. The equivalent viral gene v-*erbB*, which has transforming activity, encodes a receptor with a truncated external domain. In addition there are internal alterations in the regulatory region. Transformation can occur by the viral gene assuming a locked on configuration, tricking the cell into rapid growth. The second mechanism is an alteration in tyrosine kinase activity. An example of this is the c-*fms* oncogene which encodes the receptor for colony-stimulating factor CSF-1 in differentiating macrophages. The transforming viral gene v-*fms* possesses enhanced kinase activity compared with its cellular counterpart.

Several oncogenes act as intracellular messengers—part of the signal transduction cascade taking signals from the cell's surface to the nucleus. The *ras* family of oncogenes are perhaps the best studied. These gene products have structural similarities to proteins termed G and N proteins that control adenylate cyclase activity. Products of *ras* genes have also been shown to have GTPase activity. These proteins are all thought to be important in the second messenger system. An example of the complexity of oncogene-controlled signaling mechanisms is shown in Fig. 3.2.

Several oncogenes such as *myc*, *myb*, *fos*, and *jun* code for nucleus-associated proteins. Their precise location and function are an area of intense research. These gene products may act as transcription factors controlling the binding of RNA polymerase to DNA, thus regulating gene expression. These oncogenes can be divided into two

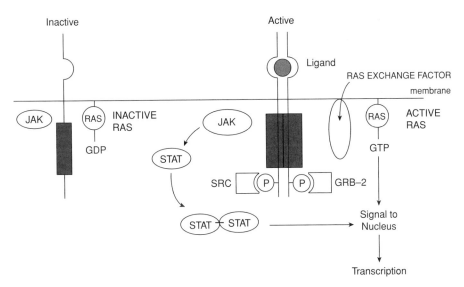

FIGURE 3.2. Examples of oncogene-controlled signal transduction. Binding of a growth factor ligand to its cognate receptor leads to receptor dimerization and activation of the tyrosine kinase internal domain. The phosphotyrosine residues that result in turn stimulate a variety of signaling molecules including docking proteins such as GRB-2 which activates *ras*, the *src* gene product, and JAK (Janus kinases). The latter phosphorylate latent transcription factors (signal transducers and activators of transcription, STAT) leading to dimerization and nuclear translocation.

TABLE 3.3. Functional Classes of Oncogenes

Function	Oncogene	Oncoprotein
Growth factors	*sis*	PDGF B
	hst	FGF related factor
Receptor tyrosine kinases	*erB*-1, 2, -3, -4	EGFR and variants
Kinases	*fms*	Mutant CSF-1 receptor
Nonreceptor	*src*, *yes*	Signal transducers
Tyrosine kinases	*fgr*, *fps*	
Membrane	H-*ras*, K-*ras*	Signal transducers
G proteins	N-*ras*	
Transcription factors	*fos*, *jun*	Gene expression
	myc	Control
Apoptosis blocking factors	*bcl*-2	Blocks *myc*-induced apoptosis

operational classes—those involved in the activation of cellular proliferation in response to growth factors and those regulating differentiation.

Transcription factor proto-oncogenes involved in cellular proliferation are members of the immediate early gene family whose expression is rapidly activated when growth-arrested cells are exposed to mitogens. Immediate early genes encode proteins that are committed to initiating a cascade of events that lead a cell through G_1 into the S phase of the cell cycle. Cellular activation by growth factors does not always involve the stimulation of transcription factor synthesis. Some onco-proteins such as the rel family—members of the NfkB family of proteins—are expressed in resting cells but are prevented from activating transcription by cytoplasmic inhibitors. Stimulation with growth factors leads to the release of rel proteins from cytoplasmic inhibitors with subsequent nuclear translocation and transcriptional activation.

TUMOR SUPPRESSOR GENES

The first evidence of the existence of tumor suppressor genes came from cell fusion experiments. Fusing normal cells with tumor cells leads to a loss of some or all malignant features. Over time some cells regain their malignant potential and this correlates with the loss of particular chromosomes or parts of chromosomes. Further evidence that tumor suppressor genes exist comes from cytogenetic studies that have shown consistent karyotypic abnormalities, particularly deletions, in a variety of human cancers. Analysis of restriction fragment length polymorphisms has enabled the examination of regions of chromosomal loss that are not visible microscopically. Using this method it is possible to map precisely the loci that have lost heterozygosity (termed loss of heterozygosity [LOH] analysis) and hence are the likely sites for tumor suppressor genes. It is interesting to note that some loci appear to be associated with tumors of a restricted histologic type (eg13q and retinoblastoma), whereas others have been associated with a wide variety of malignancies (Table 3.4). Some

TABLE 3.4. Inherited Syndromes Predisposing to Cancer

Disease	Chromosome	Cancer
Familial adenomatous polyposis	5q	Colorectal
Retinoblastoma	13q	Eye
Li–Fraumeni	17q	Various
Tuberous sclerosis	9q	Neurofibroma
Multiple endocrine neoplasia I	11q	Parathyroid, pancreas
Multiple endocrine neoplasia II	10q	Thyroid, pancreas
Von Hippel–Lindau disease	3	Germ cell, angiomas
Neurofibromatosis 1	17q	Gliomas

aberrations are associated with tumor progression or a more advanced stage of malignancy and some tumors have been shown to have multiple allelic loss.

Retinoblastoma

The conceptual basis for the genetic study of tumor suppressor genes came from a series of epidemiologic studies of retinoblastoma, Wilms' tumor, and neuroblastoma. These rare childhood tumors were of interest in that 10 to 30% of patients presented with bilateral disease. Bilateral tumors arose at an earlier age than the more common unilateral cancers and in some cases were associated with a positive family history. It was predicted that two rate-limiting genetic events or hits were required for tumor development.

Children with a genetic predisposition for cancer had inherited the first hit and only one additional genetic event was needed for cancer to arise. In contrast the sporadic cases required two hits, so that bilateral tumors were extremely unlikely to occur and the unilateral tumors that did occur presented much later. Subsequent studies have suggested the two-hit model could be explained by the inactivation of both alleles of a tumor suppressor gene typically with a point mutation in the first allele followed by gross chromosomal deletion or rearrangement affecting the second allele.

Inherited Cancer Syndromes

There is compelling epidemiologic evidence of an increased risk of cancer among first-degree relatives of individuals with a similar cancer. In the minority of cancer patients, genetic factors may be the primary determinant. In others, cancer may develop because an inherited factor increases susceptibility to environmental carcinogens. An increasing number of genes causing familial cancer syndromes have been mapped and several have been identified. These are usually recognized by a clinical phenotype such as multiple colonic polyps in familiar polyposis coli or by laboratory tests such as detection of structural chromosomal abnormalities. The syndromes may be autosomal dominant, recessive, or X-linked. Clustering of common cancers in families can be attributed to chance occurrences or shared environmental factors such as diet. A genetic cause for cancer is suggested by early age at onset, multiple tumors or bilateral disease, and a pattern of familial clustering compatible with a Mendelian segregation of the cancer.

At the molecular level two forms of cancer susceptibility gene can be distinguished in high-risk patients. In the first type the inherited susceptibility is caused by a mutation in genes involved directly in tumorigenesis such as an oncogene or tumor suppressor gene. In the second type, the predisposition to cancer is a secondary effect, for example, in DNA repair disorders where defective DNA repair results in the increased accumulation of mutations in widespread regions of the genome, including those involved in growth control.

None of the dominant oncogenes have yet been implicated in inherited human cancer but both recessive tumor suppressor genes and DNA repair defects may have an inherited predisposition. Li–Fraumeni syndrome is a disease affecting young patients and is inherited in an autosomal dominant manner. There is a predisposition to develop multiple tumors such as soft tissue sarcomas, leukemia, and breast and brain cancers. It is now known that this syndrome results from the germ line transmission of the mutant allele of the tumor suppressor gene *p53*. This defect has subsequently been seen in a variety of nonhereditary adult solid tumors and is thought to be the most common genetic abnormality seen in human cancer.

For genetic disorders in which there is an increased predisposition to cancer it is increasingly important to identify the genetic factors that interact with environmental carcinogens. The identification of those factors causing genetic syndromes is likely to lead to novel treatments such as gene therapy as well as the early identification, monitoring, and prevention of common cancers even if there is no background genetic defect.

DIFFERENTIATION

An important aspect of the malignant phenotype is the loss of the capacity to differentiate. This is well illustrated in the leukemias. Each type of leukemia arrests blood cell differentiation at a different stage, which provides a clinicopathologic basis for the classification of these diseases. A small group of oncogenic transcription factors have been demonstrated to be inhibitors of blood cell differentiation rather than activators of stem cell proliferation. Two leukemias, one experimental and one clinical, are good examples of this.

The oncogene v-*erbA* was discovered in an acutely transforming retrovirus that causes a leukemia in chickens. V-*erbA* is a fusion protein of the thyroid hormone receptor and the viral *gag* gene and transforms cells in conjunction with the v-*erbB* oncogene coexpressed by the same virus. Normal thyroid hormone receptors are transcription factors located in the nucleus. In the absence of thyroid hormone (T3) they act to suppress expression from genes that have T3 response elements in their promoters. In the presence of T3, expression from these genes is strongly activated.

V-*erbA* has lost the ability to respond to T3 and acts as a constitutive repressor. The effect of an infection of chicken bone marrow stem cells with a retrovirus is to arrest differentiation in the erythrocyte lineage, presumably by blocking the expression of erythrocyte specific genes that normally respond to T3. In clinical studies retinoic acid is an effective treatment for the human malignancy acute promyelocytic leukemia (PML) by forcing terminal myeloid differentiation. Like the T3 receptor the receptor for retinoic acid is a transcription factor located in the nucleus that regulates differentiation. Intriguingly, all cases of PML have a chromosomal translocation involving the α-retinoic acid receptor (RAR-α). As a result PML cells express a fusion gene comprised of truncated RAR-α sequences and a gene on the reciprocal chromosomes. The effect of this abnormal protein is to arrest myeloid differentiation in cells exposed to physiologic levels of retinoic acid. Higher, therapeutic levels of retinoic acid overcome this block, which may reflect the fact that leukemia cells are heterozygous for the translocation. Normal receptors encoded by the nontranslocated RAR-α allele are probably functionally repressed by the fusion gene so that higher levels of retinoic acid are required for activation.

GENOMIC INSTABILITY

A search for sites of LOH using markers containing simple tandem repeats (STRs) or minisatellites revealed a rather surprising finding. In several patients with colorectal cancer an expansion of the number of repeats was observed rather than the expected loss of chromosomal material. The explanation for this observation relates to the action of the DNA polymerases.

During replication of the billions of nucleotides that constitute the human genome occasional errors occur. STRs are particularly prone to error because of the tendency of the polymerase to slip, missing the occasional nucleotide in repeated sequences. Normally this does not matter as there is a system of repair enzymes that recognize the mismatch created in the newly synthesized strand and replace the whole segment by matching it to the template strand. In cancer cells that have a tendency for STR instability there is loss of function mutation in genes that either recognize the mismatch or are involved in repairing it (called MSH-1 and MSH-2 for Mat S homologue after homologous genes in yeast). When these genes were mapped their positions were very close to those of polymorphic markers that pinpointed the chromosomal sites of several cancer predisposition genes, Lynch syndrome 1 (nonpolyposis inherited colon cancer) and Lynch syndrome 2 (inherited colon, breast, and uterine cancer). It has recently been confirmed that mutations in the MSH-1 and MSH-2 genes are present both in affected individuals in Lynch syndrome cancer families as well as in cancers arising in individuals without a family history.

THE CELL CYCLE

The ability of oncogenes to stimulate self-proliferation in tumor suppressor genes to inhibit cell proliferation demonstrates that these genes have key roles in the regulation of the cell. The cell cycle is divided into a series of phases. The cell replicates its DNA during the S or synthetic phase and divides during the M or mitotic phase. Between these phases of the cell cycle are two G or growth phases; G_1 precedes S and G_2 precedes M (Fig. 3.3). The boundaries between G_1 and S and G_2 and M are "checkpoints." They cannot be traversed until the conditions are appropriate. During G_1 the cell is preparing for DNA replication, a process that requires a large repertoire of gene products from enzymes involved in nucleotide biosynthesis to the DNA polymerases themselves. The M phase is set in motion during G_2. Proteins such as tubulin, required for the formation of the mitotic spindle, are synthesized so that physical division of the cell can take place. Progression of cells through the cell cycle is governed by a set of protein kinase complexes involving regulatory subunits called cyclins and catalytic subunits called cyclin-dependent kinases (CDKs). The level of each member of the cyclin family peaks at a different phase of the cell cycle—cyclin D in early G_1, cyclin E at the G_1–S boundaries, cyclin A during S phase, and cyclin B at the G_2–M boundary. Each cyclin interacts with several characteristic CDKs so that each phase is distinguished by a particular pattern of cyclin expression in a restricted set of CDKs.

To traverse the G_1–S checkpoint and enter S phase the cell must integrate multiple signals from the external environment and growth factor receptors play a large part in this. However, the internal environment of the cell, particularly the integrity of the genome, is also a key determining factor for S phase entry. Exposure to radiation or

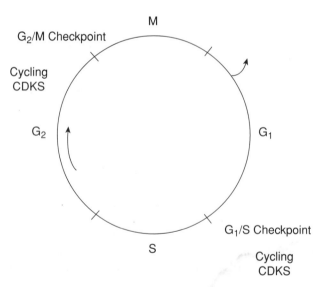

FIGURE 3.3. The cell cycle. The cell enters mitosis (M) and then either G_1, when protein RNA synthesis occurs, or moves out of the cycle to the resting phase G_0. The S phase, during which DNA synthesis occurs, follows G_1 and the cell ceases DNA synthesis in G_2 before moving into mitosis. Control is exerted by the interacting cyclins and cyclin-dependent kinases (CDKs) at the checkpoints at the G_1–S and G_2–M boundaries.

cytotoxic drugs leads to cell cycle arrest, as DNA repair rather than replication is a priority for the cell exposed to these agents. This has a clear survival advantage for the organism, as an attempt to replicate the genome in the presence of DNA damage would have disastrous consequences for the cell. Initial studies of *p53* and *pRb* emphasized a potential role in growth factor mediated cell cycle arrest by peptide growth factors such as TGF-β.

The discovery that cells that can express mutated *p53* did not show cell cycle arrest after irradiation indicates an important function of *p53* in the cellular response to DNA damage. Radiation stabilizes the *p53* protein and stimulates *p53*-dependent transcription. One of the genes transcriptionally activated by *p53* encodes the protein *p21*, which interacts with the cyclin–CDK complexes that are formed during G_1 to inhibit CDK activity and prevents cell cycle progression so that DNA repair can take place. Several other inhibitors that function similarly to *p21*, such as *p16*, have recently been identified. Mutation in the *p16* gene has been found in a number of cancers, suggesting that loss of expression in CDK inhibitors can also lead to unregulated cell proliferation.

APOPTOSIS

If DNA is irreversibly damaged by radiation or chemical insult the cell undergoes a process called programmed cell death or apoptosis. Apoptosis is an energy-requiring process characterized by morphologic changes, nuclear condensation, plasma membrane blebbing, and the action of an endonuclease that digests DNA into small fragments. The presence of the cell death pathway has been appreciated only relatively recently. Clearly the integrity of a multicellular organism benefits from the selective suicide of cells with damaged genomes. Apoptosis must therefore represent a major protective mechanism against cancer. Given this, it is not surprising that several oncogenes and anti-oncogenes impact on the rate of apoptosis. DNA tumor virus T antigens that target R6, such as adenovirus E1A, sensitize normal diploid cells to apoptoptic stimulae such as radiation. This may be due to the effect on c-*myc*, as overexpression of this gene also increases the rate of apoptosis. In contrast, T antigens that target *p53* such as E1B inhibit apoptosis. Similarly it is becoming clear that a number of cellular factors such as BCL-2 also act to inhibit apoptotic cell death. Cells also contain apoptotic inducers such as the Bax protein which physically and functionally interacts with BCL-2. Thus *p53* has a dual role in response to DNA damage, both inhibiting cell cycle progression and being critical for the onset of apoptosis of DNA damage. From this it can be readily seen that cells that contain mutations in *p53* will replicate despite the presence of DNA damage. Although many cells will not survive this a subpopulation of cells with greatly deranged genomes results, with a consequential exacerbation of the malignant phenotype.

DNA damage with an inappropriate oncogene expression is not the only stimulus that activates apoptosis. Programmed cell death is critically important to normal embryogenesis, occurring for example in the web spaces between digits during the formation of the hands and feet and when T cell clones are being deleted from the immune repertoire due to recognition of self antigens. The recent observation that some growth factors such as the insulinlike growth factors act as cell survival factors as distinct from growth factors is beginning to suggest that apoptosis may be a process that could be accelerated or inhibited by hormones in a therapeutically meaningful way.

CLINICAL APPLICATIONS

Although there have been dramatic advances in the management of patients with several types of cancer we are still limited by the lack of selectivity of many of our drugs when used against common solid tumors. Although surgery and radiotherapy can be effective in treating localized disease, the frequent occurrence of metastasis means that some form of systemic therapy is vital if the chances of cure are to be increased. Most anticancer drugs have been identified by screening large numbers of chemicals for heir antiproliferative effects on cells followed by trials on animal tumors. Our rapidly increasing knowledge of the molecular genetics of cancer has led to a new phase in the design of drugs that are able to selectively counter the abnormal growth processes involved. Further, by understanding the details of the molecular pathogenesis of malignancy it is likely that diagnosis or screening can be made more effective. This will increase the rate of cancer detection.

Prognosis

At present there are indications that new technologies are having an impact on the diagnosis and separation of patients in different prognostic categories.

In chronic myeloid leukemia, for example, reagents that can identify the fusion product of the c-*abl* gene with the *bcr* gene are proving valuable in monitoring the effectiveness of intensive chemotherapy in bone marrow transplantation aimed at eradication of the last remaining clone of malignant cells. In breast cancer, antibodies that detect the overexpression of the c-*erbB-2* gene product are proving useful as indicators of prognosis. The chances of a woman surviving 5 years after surgery

TABLE 3.5. Oncogenes and Prognosis

Tumor	Gene	Prognostic Lesion
Lung adenocarcinoma	K-*ras*	Point mutation
Breast cancer	*erbB*-1	Overexpression
	erbB-2	Overexpression
	myc	Amplification
Myelodysplasia	N-*ras*	Point mutation
	K-*ras*	Point mutation
Neuroblastoma	N-*myc*	Amplification

are considerably reduced if the presence of high levels of this surface receptor is detected immunohistologically on tumor biopsies. This group of patients may benefit from the use of intensive chemotherapy given shortly after the diagnosis has been made. As important, it may help to identify groups of patients who have a very good prognosis in whom chemotherapy is not beneficial. Recent evidence has shown that certain types of *ras* mutations are associated with outcome in lung cancer and gastrointestinal malignancies. These examples suggest that reagents that detect oncogene mutations and expression may soon become routine tools to gauge prognosis and guide cancer treatment. As yet the prognostic significance of abnormalities in tumor suppressor gene expression is unclear but as with oncogenes many studies are now underway.

Screening

Population screening to detect mutations that predispose to cancer may be possible in the future, with particular emphasis on individuals with several relatives affected by cancer. Carriers of defined cancer predisposing mutations could be specifically targeted for early detection, for example, colonoscopy and mammography, prevention, and the administration of cancer preventing agents. Examples of cancer preventing drugs include retinoids and tamoxifen in the case of women at risk for breast cancer and prostaglandin synthesis inhibitors in patients with familial adenomatous polyposis. Definitive identification of carriers would be a significant advance over the current need for regular screening of all members of an affected family when only a proportion are in fact at risk. a

Treatment

The major problem in cancer treatments is undetected metastatic disease at the time of primary therapy. For many of the common tumors current systemic treatments are inadequate and there have been essentially few advances over the last 50 years.

The key problem in the effective treatment of patients with solid tumors is the similarity between tumor and normal cells. Local therapies such as surgery and radiotherapy can succeed, but only if the malignant cells are confined to the area treated. This is true in approximately one third of cancer patients. For the majority, some form of systemic selective therapy is required. Although many cytotoxic drugs are available, only a small proportion of patients are actually cured by their use. The successful treatment of Hodgkin's disease, non-Hodgkin's lymphoma, childhood leukemia, choriocarcinoma, and germ cell tumors have just not materialized for the common cancers such as those of the lung, breast, or colon. Despite enormous efforts in new drug development, clinical trials of novel drug combinations, the addition of cytokines, high-dose regimens, and even bone marrow rescue procedures, the gains in survival have been marginal.

The next decade should see a new golden age of drug discovery. This will not be based on empirical screening programs as in the past, but on logical drug design using molecular graphics to produce novel structures that will interfere with specific biologic processes vital for growth. These will include blocking and stimulating therapies for signal transduction pathways; inactivators of oncogene products; the use of high-throughput screens to discover small molecules to mimic tumor suppressor genes; transcription control inhibitors for specific genes; selective activators of apoptosis; and cell cycle inhibitors and effective antimetastatic drugs. It is also likely that direct genetic intervention will be possible for the treatment and perhaps even prevention of cancer.

GENE THERAPY

The main problem facing the gene therapist is how to get new genes into every tumor cell. If this cannot be achieved then any malignant cells that remain unaffected will emerge as a resistant clone. At present ideal vectors are not available. Despite this drawback, there are already more than 250 protocols accepted for clinical trial in cancer patients worldwide, the majority in the United States. The ethical issues are fairly straightforward, with oncology providing some of the highest possible benefit–risk ratios. Several strategies are currently under investigation.

Genetic Tagging

The use of a genetic marker to tag tumor cells may help in making decisions on the optimal treatment for an individual patient. The insertion of a foreign marker gene into cells from a tumor biopsy and replacing the marked cells into the patient prior to treatment can provide a sensitive new indicator of minimal residual disease after chemotherapy.

Enhancing Tumor Immunogenicity

The presence of an immune response to cancer has been recognized for many years. The problem is that human tumors seem to be predominantly weakly immunogenic. If ways could be found to elicit a more powerful immune stimulus, then effective immunotherapy could become a reality. Several observations from murine tumors indicate that one reason for weak immunogenicity of certain tumors is the failure to elicit a T helper cell response. This in turn releases the necessary cytokines to stimulate the production of cytolytic T cells which can destroy tumors. The expression of cytokine genes such as interleukin-2 (IL-2), tumor necrosis factor (TNF), and interferon in tumor cells has been shown to bypass the need for T helper cells in mice. Similarly clinical experiments are now in progress. Melanoma cells have been prepared from biopsies and infected with retrovirus containing the *IL-2* gene. These cells are being used as a vaccine to elicit a more powerful immune response.

Vectoring Cytokines to Tumors

Cytokines such as the interferons and interleukins have been actively explored for their tumorcidal properties. Although there is evidence of cytotoxicity, their side effects are profound, which limits the dose that can be safely administered. It is possible to insert cytokine genes into cells that can potentially home in on tumors and so release a high concentration of their protein locally. *TNF* genes have been inserted into tumor-infiltrating lymphocytes from patients with melanoma and given systemically.

Inserting Drug Activating Genes

The main problem with existing chemotherapy is its lack of selectivity. If drug activating genes could be inserted that would be expressed only in cancer cells then the administration of an appropriate prodrug could be highly selective. There are now many examples of genes preferentially expressed in tumors. In some cases, their promoters have been isolated and coupled to drug activating enzymes. Examples include α-fetoprotein in hepatoma, prostate-specific antigen in prostate cancer, and c-*erbB*-2 in breast cancer.

Such promoters can be coupled to enzymes such as cytosine deaminase or thymidine kinase, thereby producing unique retroviral vectors that are able to infect all cells but can be expressed only in tumor cells. These suicide (or Trojan horse) vectors may not have absolute tumor specificity but this may not be essential—it may be possible to perform a genetic prostatectomy or breast ductectomy—so effectively destroying all tumor cells as well as certain portions of normal tissue.

Suppressing Oncogene Expression

The downregulation of abnormal oncogene expression has been shown to revert the malignant phenotype in a variety of in vitro tumor lines. It is possible to develop in vivo systems such as the insertion of genes encoding for complementary (antisense) mRNA to that produced by the oncogene. Such antigenes specifically switch off the production of the abnormal protein product. Mutant forms of the c-*ras* oncogene are an obvious target for this approach. Up to 75% of human pancreatic cancers contain

TABLE 3.6. Suppression of Malignant Phenotype by Gene Transfer In Vitro

Gene	Tumor Cell Line
WT-p53	Colon, glioma, lung, breast, prostate, osteosarcoma, sarcoma, leukemia
RB-1	Retinoblastoma, prostate, osteosarcoma
nm-23	Melanoma
E-Cadherin	Breast, renal, prostate
rap-1A	*ras*-Transformed cells

a mutation in the 12th amino acid of this protein and reversal of this change in cell lines leads to the restoration of normal growth control. Clearly the major problem is to ensure that every single tumor cell becomes infected. Any cell that escapes will have a survival advantage and produce a clone of resistant tumor cells. For this reason future treatment schedules may require the repetitive administration of vectors in a similar way to fractionated radiotherapy or chemotherapy.

Replacing Defective Tumor Suppressor Genes

In cell culture malignant properties can often be reversed by the insertion of normal tumor suppressor genes such as *RB-1*, *TP-53*, and *DCC*.

Although tumor suppressor genes were often identified in rare tumor types, abnormalities in their expression and function are abundant in common human cancers. As with antigene therapy, the difficulty in this approach lies in the delivery of actively expressed vectors to every single tumor cell in vivo. Nevertheless clinical experiments are in progress in lung cancer where retroviruses that encode *TP53* genes are being administered bronchoscopically. Tumor regressions have been reported.

The challenges to making gene therapy an effective and broadly useful treatment modality are formidable, not only in terms of the limitations in efficiency and targeting of gene transfer vectors but also with regard to our incomplete understanding of control of gene transcription and the long-term consequences of constitutive expression of a transferred gene.

Over the short term further improvements will come from refining currently used vectors and the design of new generation vectors incorporating the most useful aspects of viral and synthetic systems, which can then be applied to a specific cancer target. In the longer term we envisage the construction of artificial chromosomes that could carry whole clusters of genes with their natural control elements into cells.

TABLE 3.7. Strategies for Cancer Gene Therapy

- Gene marking in BMT and to detect minimal residual disease
- Genetic immunomodulation

  - Cancer vaccines
  - Polynucleotide immunization

- Vectoring of biotherapeutic genes to tomors
- Increasing normal tissue tolerance
- Selective drug activation
- Somatic corection of genetic defect

  - Antisense to mutant oncogene
  - Expression of tumor suppressor gene

With this new technology also come new ethical responsibilities to ensure that these strategies are safe for patients and staff. There is no shortage of ideas and applications in this advancing field. There is every indication we should be optimistic for patients with otherwise unresponsive cancers that this treatment modality will make an impact in the near future.

FURTHER READING

Cox TM, Sinclair J (1997) *Molecular Biology in Medicine*. Blackwell Scientific, Oxford.

Macdonald F, Ford CHJ (1997) *Molecular Biology of Cancer*. Bios Scientific Publishers, Oxford.

Lemoine N, Cooper D (1997) *Gene Therapy*. Bios Scientific Publishers, Oxford.

Roth J, Christiano RJ (1997) Gene therapy for cancer: What have we done and where are we going? *J Natl Cancer Inst* 89:21.

Weinstein JN, Myers TG, O'Connor PM, et al. (1997) An Information-intensive approach to the molecular pharmacology of cancer. *Science* 275:343.

Zhang L, Zhou W, Velculescu VE, et al. (1997) Gene expression profiles in normal and cancer cells. *Science* 276:1268.

Genes VI, Lewin B (1997) Oxford University Press, Oxford.

Yarnold J, Stratton M, McMillan TJ (eds) (1997) *Molecular Biology for Oncologists*. Chapman & Hall, London.

CHAPTER 4

GENETIC PREDISPOSITION TO CANCER

GORDON B. MILLS, PAULA RIEGER, MARY ANNE WATT,
CHRISTIE GRAHAM and REBECCA PENTZ

University of Texas M. D. Anderson Cancer Center
Houston, TX 77030, USA

GENETIC CHANGES IN CANCER CELLS

Over the last 10 years, it has become clear that all cancer is caused by genetic changes in critical genes.[1,2] In general, the accumulation of five to nine genetic changes must occur within a given cell to allow the cell to acquire the characteristics needed to escape normal growth control mechanisms and to develop into a malignant tumor. These genetic changes preferentially occur in a subset of human genes related to cellular development, cell differentiation, cell proliferation, cell survival, cellular senescence, and genetic repair. The genes involved in the positive regulation of cell growth are generally designated oncogenes, whereas the genes involved in the negative regulation of cell growth are generally designated tumor suppressor genes. The genes involved in regulating genomic stability and DNA repair are also common targets for mutational inactivation and are frequently included with the more classically defined tumor suppressor genes. In tumors, oncogenes are generally activated by "gain of function" mutations or increased expression, whereas tumor suppressor genes are generally inactivated by "loss of function" mutations or decreased expression. For the full manifestation of tumorigenic potential, an additional set of genes must be activated to allow the development of a neovasculature and metastasis. Indeed, without the ability to induce neovascularization, a tumor cannot increase in size beyond a few millimeters, a size that is not usually clinically apparent or relevant. Further, the vast majority of cancers, if identified when restricted to the primary site prior to becoming competent to metastasize, would be cured by surgery or local therapy. Thus acquisition of the ability to induce neovascularization and to metastasize are critical components of the poor prognosis associated with cancer. Despite the poor prognosis

Manual of Clinical Oncology, 7th edition, Edited by Raphael E. Pollock
ISBN 0-471-23828-7, pages 63–97. Copyright © 1999 Wiley-Liss, Inc.

and outcome attributed to cancer, it is important to note that in developed countries more than 50% of all cancer patients are cured by current therapy, primarily surgery, and that the absolute number of individuals dying from cancer has recently begun to decrease.

GENETIC CHANGES IN TUMORS CAN BE INHERITED IN THE GERMLINE OR ACQUIRED BY SOMATIC CELLS

The majority of genetic changes leading to tumorigenesis are acquired by mutation of genes in somatic cells giving rise to what are commonly known as sporadic tumors. These changes can be the consequence of a number of insults including environmental toxins such as those in cigarette smoke, DNA damage due to ultraviolet radiation, or the low but significant spontaneous mutation rate associated with DNA replication and repair. Inherited germline genetic changes predispose a number of individuals to the development of cancer. Mutations in the currently identified inherited cancer predisposition genes (Table 4.1) are all relatively rare. However, as these genetic changes exhibit relatively high penetrance (high likelihood of an individual developing a tumor), they contribute to a significant number of cases of cancer. These inherited germline genetic changes probably play a major role in the development of about 5% to 10% of all solid tumors and a smaller proportion of cases of leukemia and lymphoma. Indeed, rare, highly penetrant cancer genes likely contribute to more than 35,000 cases of cancer of the bowel, breast, and ovarian cancer in the United States each year. Even for those unfortunate individuals who inherit an abnormality in a cancer predisposition gene, development of cancer is not inevitable. In most cases, additional mutations must occur to allow cancer development. Besides the rare, high penetrance cancer predisposition genes currently identified (Table 4.1), it is also likely that an additional set of relatively common, low penetrance cancer predisposition genes remain to be identified. The low penetrance class of cancer predisposition genes may have a modest effect on their own, may modify the action of the high penetrance cancer predisposition genes, or alternatively may play a role in the method by which the body metabolizes environmental or endogenous toxins. Indeed, the genes involved in the metabolism of cigarette smoke or toxins in the diet may greatly alter the propensity to develop lung, bowel, or other cancers. Thus, low penetrance cancer predisposition genes may contribute to a much higher proportion of cancers than do the high penetrance cancer predisposition genes currently identified.

STUDIES OF INDIVIDUALS WITH INHERITED PREDISPOSITION TO CANCER MAY IMPACT ON MANAGEMENT OF SPORADIC CANCER

Studies of cancer predisposition genes (Table 4.1) offer the opportunity to understand the molecular mechanisms that lead to the development of the more common sporadic tumors. Indeed, many of the genes mutated in the germline of high-risk patients undergo somatic mutations in sporadic tumors. Thus elucidation of the function of a cancer predisposition gene or development of a method to target specific growth regulatory pathways or DNA repair pathways influenced by cancer predisposition genes may result in novel therapeutic approaches applicable to both inherited and sporadic cancer patients.

Evaluation of chemoprevention or screening strategies in the general population is frequently hindered by the low number of cancer cases seen in these patients[3,4]. The low prevalence of most cancers makes it difficult to determine whether any chemoprevention or screening strategy has been successful. Studies of individuals with a high risk of developing cancer due to inheritance of a mutation in a cancer predisposition gene may provide "proof of concept" for evaluation of chemoprevention or screening strategies. This will greatly facilitate the identification of approaches that may impact the management of sporadic tumors in the general population. Indeed, family history is one of the criteria used to identify high-risk individuals for the ongoing tamoxifen-based breast cancer prevention trial (BCPT). Although studies of chemoprevention or screening of cancers in high-risk individuals may not be directly transferable to prevention of sporadic cancers, the precepts defined with high-risk individuals should at a minimum be able to aid in the design of smaller, targeted clinical trials of low-risk individuals. In many cases, population-based studies may not be feasible, thus forcing the application of information obtained from high-risk individuals to the general population without confirmatory studies.

IDENTIFICATION OF CANCER PREDISPOSITION GENES

In the past, the identification of cancer predisposition genes has been time consuming, requiring the acquisition and study of large families with a large number of cancers.[2] Once high-risk families are identified, region(s) of the genome that segregate with the phenotype are determined using restriction fragment length polymorphism (allele specific presence or absence of restriction sites) and polymorphic microsatellite sequences (allele specific regions in the genome containing short repeats such as CA, CAG, etc. of different lengths). The approach is based on the theory that areas of the genome will be linked with the cancer predisposition gene if they are located close together on the same chromosome. Incomplete penetrance and sporadic cancers could result in an incorrect interpretation of linkage analysis and, as happened in the search for the breast cancer-1 (*BRCA-1*) gene, can delay identification of the cancer gene. Heterogeneity or multiple similar syndromes, such as those caused by the *BRCA-1* and *BRCA-2* genes which both lead to a breast/ovarian syndrome, further complicate the search. Sometimes the region could be narrowed through identification of microdeletions or analysis of genetic crossovers in family members. Once the area of the genome most likely to harbor a cancer predisposition gene is delimited, a detailed physical map of the region is created usually using Pls, or artificial bacterial or yeast chromosomes. Genes within candidate regions are identified using the candidate gene approach of studying genes known to be located in the region, "exon trapping," direct DNA selection, and cross-species sequence con-

TABLE 4.1. Examples of Familial Cancer Syndromes with Identified Genetic Mediators

Syndrome	Responsible Gene	Chromosome Location	Potential Function	Common Tumors	Rare Tumors	Nonmalignant Manifestations
Li–Fraumeni	p53	17p13	Cell cycle apoptosis	Leukemia	Sarcomas	
Breast/ovary	BRCA-1	17q21	DNA repair (?)	Breast (early onset)	Prostate Bowel (?) Ovary	
Breast/ovary	BRCA-2	13q12	DNA repair (?)	Breast (early onset)	Male breast cancer Pancreas Ocular melanoma	
FAP/Gardner's	APC	5q22	Cell adhesion	Ovary Colon	Desmoid Small intestine Thyroid Liver	Colon Polyps Osteomas
HNPCC	MLH-1 MSH-2 PMS-1 PMS-2 GTBP	3p21 2p16 2q 7p 2p16	Mismatch repair Mismatch repair Mismatch repair Mismatch repair Mismatch repair	Colon Endometrium	Ovary Breast Renal Small bowel	
Gorlin's	patched/PTC	9q22	Receptor	Basal cell	Medulloblastoma Primitive neuroectoderm	Ovarian fibromas Developmental defects Hamartoma
MEN-I	MENIN	11q13	Unknown	Parathyroid Pituitary Enteropancreatic Adrenal	Pancreatic	
MEN-II	RET	10q11	Kinase	Medullary thyroid	Parathyroid Pheochromocytoma	Parathyroid Mucosal Neuromas Skeletal abnormalities Hirschsprung's

Syndrome	Gene	Location	Function	Tumor		Features
Cowden's	MMAC-1/PTEN	10q23	Phosphatase	Breast, Basal cell, Thyroid	Endometrium (?), Ovarian (?), Renal cell (?), Brain	Facial papules, Keratoses, Benign breast lumps, Trichilemmomas, Thyroid hypertrophy
RB	RB	13q14	Cell cycle progression	Retinoblastoma, Sarcoma	Melanoma	
Denys Drash/WAGR	WT-1	11p13	Transcription factor	Wilms' tumor		Gonadal abnormalities, Aniridia, Retardation
VHL	VHL	3p25	Unknown, RNA elongation (?)	Kidney, Adrenal, Neural		Retinal angiomas, Cysts
Hereditary papillary renal carcinoma	MET	7q32	Tyrosine kinase receptor	Kidney		
AT	ATM	11q23	DNA repair, PI3 kinase family	Leukemia	Breast	Ataxia, Telangiectasia
Peutz–Jaeger's	STK-11/LKB-1	19q13.3	Serine kinase	Colon	Sex cord stroma	Hamartomas, Hyperpigmentation
Dysplastic nevi syndrome	p16/15, CDK-4	9p21, 12q14	Kinase inhibitor, Cyclin dependent kinase	Melanoma	Melanoma	Dysplastic Nevi
NF-1	NF-1	17q11	Guanine exchange factor	Schwann cell, Glia	Adrenal	Café au lait, Neurofibroma
NF-2	NF-2	22q12	Cytoskeleton	Schwann cell		Café au lait, Neurofibroma

servation. Finally, once a candidate gene is identified, it is sequenced in a number of individuals and whether mutations to "track" with cancer in a family is determined. Those individuals, laboratories, and consortia that complete this process are to be commended on their dedication and tenacity.

This tedious positional cloning approach is being streamlined and in some cases supplanted by technology arising from the Human Genome Project. A high-density map of microsatellites and ESTs (expressed sequence tags) has already been assembled that will facilitate rapid localization of cancer predisposition genes. Ongoing studies within the Human Genome Project will soon lead to the chromosomal assignment of the approximately 100,000 genes in the human genome. By the year 2005, the complete human genome of 3 billion nucleotides will be sequenced. Indeed, the complete sequence of several simple genomes such as those for specific bacteria and yeast have already been ascertained. Further, once a cancer gene is localized to a chromosome area by linkage analysis, new technologies allow sequencing of a megabase of DNA to identify candidate genes. These changes are greatly simplifying the process of identifying cancer predisposition genes. Indeed, a new cancer predisposition gene is reported about once every few months.

CANCER PREDISPOSITION GENES REGULATE NORMAL CELL GROWTH, CELL SURVIVAL, OR GENOMIC STABILITY

The currently identified inherited cancer predisposition genes play roles in regulating cellular development, cell differentiation, cell proliferation, cell survival, cellular senescence, and genetic repair.[1,2] The known cancer predisposition genes can be subcategorized into four classes dependent on functional role and type of mutation (Table 4.2).

A small group of cancer predisposition genes would normally be classified as oncogenes. These cancer predisposition genes exhibit mutations resulting in a "gain of function" that increases the activity of the gene product or releases the gene product from normal regulatory control. In contrast to most cancer predisposition genes where the normal copy must be inactivated, gain of function mutations are sufficient for the development of cancer in the presence of a normal gene copy. Mutations in *RET* and *MET*, the only identified members of this family, result in early onset and a high penetrance of thyroid and other endocrine tumors as part of the multiple endocrine neoplasia II (*MEN II*) syndrome and of kidney tumors in the papillary renal carcinoma syndrome, respectively. The identified mutations in *RET* and *MET* appear to increase the tyrosine kinase activity of these transmembrane receptors. Whether additional "gain of function" mutations will be discovered awaits further investigation.

The majority of cancer predisposition genes undergo loss of function mutations (Table 4.2). For the effects of these genes to be expressed, the normal copy of the gene must be lost or inactivated. This class of cancer predisposition gene can be further subdivided into those genes that regulate cell cycle progression, apoptosis, and cellular senescence and those genes that detect or repair DNA damage.

TABLE 4.2. Classes of Identified Cancer Predisposition Genes

Gene	Syndrome	Gene Function
Gain of Function Mutations in Growth Regulators		
RET	MEN2	Tyrosine kinase receptor
MET	Hereditary papillary renal carcinoma	Tyrosine kinase receptor
Loss of Function in Growth Regulators		
p53	Li–Fraumeni syndrome	Cell cycle progression
RB	Retinoblastoma syndrome	Cell cycle progression
APC	Familial adenomatous polypi Gardner's	Cell adhesion
WT-1	WAGR/Denys Drash	Transcription factor
VHL	Von Hippel–Lindau	RNA extension ?
p15/16	Dysplastic nevi syndrome	Kinase inhibitor
CDK4	Dysplastic nevi syndrome	Cyclin-dependent kinase
patched	Basal cell/Gorlin's syndrome	Receptor
MMAC-1/PTEN	Cowden's syndrome	Phosphatase
Menin (unknown)	MEN1	Unknown
STK-11/LKB-1	Peutz–Jaeger	Serine kinase
NF-1	Neurofibromatosis	Guanine exchange factor
NF-2	Neurofibromatosis	Cytoskeleton
Regulators or Mediations of Genomic Stability		
MLH-1	HNPCC	Mismatch repair
MSH-2	HNPCC	Mismatch repair
PMS-1	HNPCC	Mismatch repair
PMS-2	HNPCC	Mismatch repair
GTBP	HNPCC	Mismatch repair
ATM	Ataxia–telangiectasia	DNA repair Phosphatidyl inositol Kinase family
p53	Li–Fraumeni	Apoptosis
BRCA-1 (probable)	Breast ovarian syndrome	DNA repair
BRCA-2 (probable)	Breast ovarian syndrome	DNA repair
NF-1	Neurofibromatosis	High mutational rate
Dominant Negative Mutations in Growth Regulators		
p53	Li–Fraumeni	Cell cycle progression

Many of the inherited mutations that result in predisposition to cancer result in the formation of an abnormal protein. The normal copy of the gene is usually lost, but not always. This raises the potential that mutations in at least some cancer predisposition genes result in the formation of a protein product that functions as a "dominant negative" by inhibiting the function of the normal gene copy. Transgenic and knockout animal models of *p53* suggest that at least some *p53* mutations inactivate the function of the normal p53 protein, resulting in an increased probability of developing tumors despite retention and expression of the normal allele. Additional studies will be required to determine if other cancer predisposition genes also demonstrate a dominant negative activity and allow expression of the phenotype despite the presence and expression of a normal allele.

It is theoretically possible to reverse the effects of loss of function of genes that directly regulate cell growth either by introduction of a normal copy of the gene by gene therapy or by using small molecules that mimic the function of the gene product. Indeed, given that tumors must undergo multiple genetic changes, it has been surprising and hopeful that a single intervention with gene therapy or with small molecules blocks tumor growth both in vitro and in animal models. However, tumors that occur as a result of abnormalities in genomic stability may not be amenable to this approach. As these tumors are likely to have acquired the multiple abnormalities required for complete expression of the tumorigenic phenotype, reversing the genetic abnormality that led to genetic instability may not be efficacious. Nevertheless, reintroduction of *p53* and *BRCA-1* into human tumor cell lines has resulted in reversal of the tumorigenic phenotype.[5] Whether this represents normalization of genetic instability or alternative functions of these genes remains to be elucidated.

WHY SPECIFIC TYPES OF TUMORS?

As indicated in Table 4.1, abnormalities in cancer predisposition genes result in a very discrete pattern of susceptibility to cancer. The reasons underlying the sensitivity in specific cell lineages and resistance in other cell lineages remain unknown. Our lack of understanding of why certain lineages develop cancer when a specific cancer predisposition gene is inactivated is best exemplified by two of the oldest known cancer predisposition genes, *p53* and *RB*. These genes are expressed in all cell lineages and are critical to the normal cell cycle progression in these cells. However, despite being expressed in every cell lineage, the Li–Fraumeni and RB syndromes affect only a few cell lineages (Table 4.1). The most likely explanation is one of redundancy. In this model, an additional mediator is expressed in many cell lineages that can partially replace the function of the deficient cancer predisposition gene. In susceptible lineages, either the redundant gene is not expressed or is unable to fulfill the redundant function. Perhaps the most cogent message from studies of "knockout" mice, which have been engineered to lack specific genes, is that many genes are not essential for embryogenesis and even normal adult function. As an example, the *src* proto-oncogene constitutes a significant proportion of the total protein in the platelet and is highly expressed in the brain. However, *src* knockout mice have apparently normal platelet function, brain function, and indeed normal function of most cells with the exception of the osteoclasts and osteoblasts that regulate bone structure. The only detectable phenotype in *src* knockout mice is osteopetrosis and failure of the tooth bud to form functional teeth. Thus in many cell types, a redundant pathway can replace the function that is normally fulfilled by the cancer predisposition gene, resulting in a highly selective pattern of tumor susceptibility.

ANIMAL MODELS

Animal models are being created for a number of the cancer predisposition genes using homologous recombination or "knockout" technology to delete the function of the murine homologues of the cancer predisposition genes. These models provide critical new information related to the functions of the cancer predisposition genes. However, in many cases, the murine knockout models do not faithfully recapitulate the human diseases associated with cancer predisposition genes. For example, although animals with aberrant *p53* function develop tumors at a higher rate than their normal counterparts, the patterns of tumors that develop are different from those observed in individuals with the Li–Fraumeni syndrome. In addition, deletion of both copies of *BRCA-1* or *BRCA-2* results in embryonal lethality in the mouse whereas humans who have inherited mutant copies of *BRCA-1* from both parents are developmentally normal. Nevertheless, the power of the knockout approach is, and will continue to be, to provide important new information related to the mechanisms of action of the cancer predisposition genes. Further, knockout mice will provide important models to assess the efficacy of methods for chemoprevention and for gene therapy or small molecule treatment of tumors.

MECHANISM OF LOSS OF FUNCTION OF THE NORMAL ALLELE

As noted previously, most of the cancer predisposition genes behave in a cellular recessive manner, requiring the loss of the normal allele for the aberrant phenotype to be expressed. Loss of normal alleles appears to be a fairly frequent process, making the inheritance pattern appear to be autosomal dominant with incomplete penetrance. Loss of function of the normal allele at the cellular level occurs as the consequence of a number of different processes. In some cases, a point mutation or small deletion or insertion occurs in the normal allele in a somatic cell, most commonly during cell division. More frequently, the normal allele is replaced with the abnormal allele through gene conversion or sister chromatid exchange. In other cases, the whole normal chromosome is replaced through chromosomal loss, chromosomal loss and reduplication, or nondisjunction.[1,2]

Replacement of the normal copy of the gene by an abnormal copy of the gene can be detected by an analysis of heterozygosity. The locus of interest is generally studied through polymerase chain reaction (PCR) analysis of highly polymorphic microsatellites. Frequently the different alleles inherited from each parent can be identified based on size as determined by the number of repeats in the microsatellite. Normal tissue will retain both copies (heterozygous) and demonstrate both sizes when assessed by gel electrophoresis. In contrast, the tumor will demonstrate only a single size on gel electrophoresis indicating the presence of a single allele or loss of heterozygosity (LOH).

In addition to genetic changes, epigenetic processes may also be important in inactivating the normal allele. The promoter regions of a number of genes are highly methylated and silenced. This occurs frequently from one or another parent, resulting in genomic imprinting with only one parental allele (the nonmethylated allele) being expressed. Through as yet unknown mechanisms, the normal allele for tumor suppressor genes can be inactivated by acquired methylation. This epigenetic phenotype is clearly a future target for therapies aimed at inhibiting or reversing the methylation process, thus normalizing gene function in tumors.

IDENTIFICATION OF INDIVIDUALS AT RISK FOR CARRYING INHERITED CANCER PREDISPOSITION GENES—THE IMPORTANCE OF PEDIGREE

Family history or a family "pedigree" remains the best screening approach for identifying individuals at high risk for developing cancer owing to the inheritance of a mutated cancer predisposition gene (Fig. 4.1). Indeed, prior to the identification and cloning of a number of the cancer predisposition genes, it was frequently possible to define an individual's risk based on family history and epidemiologic studies.[2] Thus the careful collection of a family history is the cornerstone of clinical cancer genetics (Table 4.3).

Validation of a patient's family history remains paramount and problematic. A patient may not be aware of all of the cases of cancer in a family. Age at onset, which is critically important, may not be readily available. Further, in many instances, family members have wrongly attributed death to a metastatic cancer site rather than to the original primary cancer. It is advisable to ask the patient to validate the family history or pedigree through discussions with a number of relatives. Historical reporting of some types of cancer such as breast cancer appears to be relatively reliable, whereas distinguishing between the many causes of abdominal cancer including bowel, ovary, uterus, cervix, or kidney is comparatively unreliable. Thus, an attempt should be made to obtain pathology reports on all reported cases of cancer. In some families, the number of evaluable individuals may be insufficient to allow a valid estimation of risk. Nevertheless, a properly collected family history provides an excellent initial screen for identifying high-risk individuals (Fig. 4.1). Collecting a family history should be a component of any initial patient visit with the pedigree updated at all subsequent visits. In the current litigious environment of the United States, a number of cases are either in the courts or have been settled in the patient's favor for "failure to diagnose" due to failure of a clinician to collect and evaluate a family history. The initial family history screen should be sufficiently detailed so as to determine whether an individual requires further investigation or should be referred to a high-risk clinic more familiar with dealing with such patients.

Although it is critical to obtain an accurate history of cancer in family members, it is also important to ascertain whether individuals in the family demonstrate other constitutional changes. As indicated in Table 4.1, individuals carrying germline mutations in the known cancer predisposition genes may demonstrate non-cancer-related phenotypic changes that are likely to indicate the presence of a cancer predisposition syndrome. For example, multiple bowel polyps would be suggestive of the multiple hamartoma syndromes associated with familial adenomatosis polypi

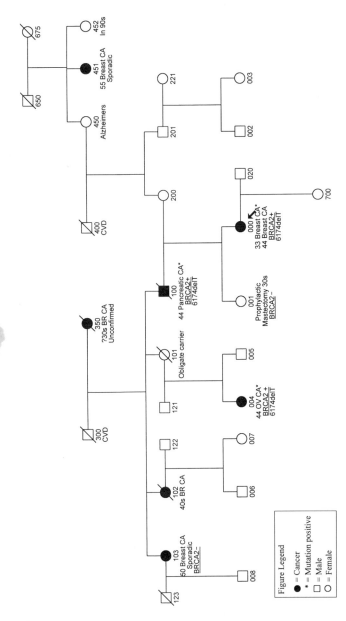

FIGURE 4.1. This is a typical *BRCA-2* family pedigree. There are a number of salient points demonstrated in this pedigree. The proband, 000, originally sought counseling because she was concerned about the potential risk her daughter, 700, might have for developing breast cancer. Individual 001 had a prophylactic mastectomy prior to testing negative based on her concern about her risk for developing cancer. Studies have shown that more than 95% of women who have had a prophylactic mastectomy have been very pleased with the outcome and "would do it again" or would "recommend the procedure to family members" under similar circumstances. Individual 101 died without developing a cancer. As both her daughter, 004, and her brother, 100, have tested positive for a mutation in *BRCA-2*, she would be an obligate carrier (must have the mutation in *BRCA-2*). This demonstrates that penetrance is <100% and that the phenotype can skip a generation. Individual 100 has tested positive for a mutation in the *BRCA-2* gene and passed it on to his daughter, 000. It is always important to assess the paternal side of the family as mutations in *BRCA-1* or *BRCA-2* have an equal likelihood of being passed by either the mother or the father. Individual 103 has a sporadic breast cancer in a family with a known mutation. The age at onset is later than for other individuals in the family. If this person had been tested first, it could have resulted in a false-negative result for the family.

73

TABLE 4.3. Characteristics Suggestive of the Presence of a Cancer Predisposition Gene in a Family Pedigree

Increased number of cancers
Unexpectedly early age of onset of tumors
Multiple tumors in a single individual
Rare tumors
Identifiable patterns of cancers predictive of a cancer syndromes
Nonmalignant manifestations of a cancer gene syndrome
Ethnic background or "founder" effects

(FAP)/Gardner's syndrome or Cowden's disease with associated mutations in *APC* or *MMAC-1/PTEN*, respectively. Hyperpigmentation might be a clue to the presence of a Peutz–Jaeger's syndrome with associated mutations in *STK-11/LKB-1* (Table 4.1).

When evaluating a family history, a number of characteristics suggest that a family is more likely to harbor a mutated cancer predisposition gene (Table 4.3). The first and foremost characteristic of a pedigree predictive of the presence of an inherited cancer predisposition syndrome is a higher than expected incidence of specific types of cancer in the family. Initially, the analysis should consist of looking for multiple cases of the same type of tumor such as breast cancer. However, as demonstrated in Table 4.1, the majority of cancer predisposition genes predispose individuals to the development of cancers in several different cell lineages. For example, an excess of breast and ovarian cancer would suggest that the family may carry an abnormality in *BRCA-1* or *BRCA-2* (Table 4.1). A high frequency of bowel and endometrial cancer would suggest that a family may have a mutation in the genes that make up the hereditary nonpolyposis colon cancer (*HNPCC*) syndrome (Table 4.1). It is important, however, to remember that familial clustering of cancers in common cancers such as bowel, lung, prostate, and breast can occur by chance or due to environmental influences so that a strong family history does not necessarily indicate the presence of a mutated cancer predisposition gene.

As noted previously, development of a sporadic tumor usually requires mutations in a number of different genes. This need for accumulation of mutations in a single cell results in most sporadic cancers occurring at a relatively late age. Tumors due to the inheritance of a cancer predisposition gene tend, however, to occur at an earlier age (Table 4.3). The most extreme examples are mutations in the *RB*, *p53*, *NF-1* and *NF-2*, *APC*, and *RET* cancer predisposition genes which predispose to childhood cancers (Table 4.1). Less extreme are those that induce a 10- to 20-year decrease in the peak age at onset such as breast cancer in families with mutations in *BRCA-1* or *BRCA-2*. It is important to remember that this is not always the case. For example, ovarian cancer does not appear to occur at a markedly younger age than usual in the breast/ovarian cancer syndromes.

The early onset of tumors due to genetic predisposition could be caused by inheritance of an abnormal gene which decreases the number of genetic changes that must accumulate in a single cell to result in tumor development. However, although important in many cases, this explanation is simplistic and does not explain the early onset induced by a number of cancer predisposition genes. For example, inactivation of *RB* may be sufficient to result in the development of retinoblastoma in the absence of any other mutation. Further, a number of the cancer predisposition genes such as *p53*; the mismatch repair genes involved in *HNPCC*, ataxia–telangiectasia mutated (ATM), and potentially neurofibromatosis-1 (NF-1); *BRCA-1* or *BRCA-2* are involved in the detection or repair of DNA damage. Inactivation of these genes can allow a more rapid accumulation of mutations in other important growth regulatory genes. Regardless of the mechanism, early onset of cancer remains a hallmark suggestive of the presence of a mutated cancer predisposition gene in a family.

Given that the chance of a single individual developing multiple primary tumors is relatively low, a history of multiple primaries in a single individual is sufficiently predictive of a mutated cancer predisposition gene to require a more thorough evaluation of the patient's pedigree (Table 4.3). Patients may have tumors in paired organs such as the breast, which would be suggestive of one of the breast/ovary syndromes or in the kidney, which could be suggestive of Wilms' tumor, papillary renal carcinoma, or Von Hippel–Lindau (VHL) syndromes. Further, primaries in multiple organs, especially if they cannot be explained by another mechanism, such as radiation- or chemotherapy-induced tumors, may be suggestive of the presence of a mutated cancer predisposition gene. A single patient with endometrial and colon cancer raises concern about the *HNPCC* group of familial predisposition genes. Similarly, both breast and ovarian cancer in a patient is strongly supportive of the presence of an inheritance of an abnormality in one of genes that predispose to the breast/ovarian syndromes (Table 4.1).

For the relatively common cancers such as bowel, lung, prostate, or breast, the presence of several cancers in the pedigree may be needed to raise a concern about whether a mutated cancer predisposition gene exists in a family. Indeed, in at least one study, the number of breast cancers in a family was found to be indicative of family size and number of evaluable individuals rather than of the likelihood of the presence of a mutated *BRCA-1* or *BRCA-2* gene. In contrast, the presence of one or two cases of relatively uncommon tumors such as sarcomas, retinoblastoma, male breast cancer, or schwannomas may be indicative of inheritance of mutations in the *p53*, RRBR, *BRCA-2*, or *NF-1* and *NF-2* cancer predisposition genes, respectively (Tables 4.1 and 4.3).

A number of cancer predisposition syndromes exhibit "founder" effects and are more common in certain ethnic groups (Table 4.3). Abnormalities in *BRCA-1* and *BRCA-2* are present in about 1/1000 individuals when assessed in a mixed population. Individuals of Dutch, Icelandic, French Canadian, or Ashkenazic Jewish origin may have, because of founder effects, as much as a 20-fold increase in the incidence of mutations in *BRCA-1* or *BRCA-2*. A similar increased incidence of a potential deleterious change in the *HNPCC* family of genes has been identified in individuals of Ashkenazic Jewish origin. Mutations within a specific ethnic background likely occurred by chance in a germ cell many generations ago, and owing to the limited effect of adult cancers on reproductive fitness were "fixed" and spread in that ethnic population. A knowledge of the patient's ethnic origin may provide an additional clue suggesting the presence of a mutated cancer predisposition gene, thus modifying the interpretation of the family pedigree. Further, as the genetic changes found in a given ethnic background are often limited to specific sites in the cancer predisposition gene, the patient's ethnic background could guide the genetic testing approach to be used.

GENETIC COUNSELING IN A HIGH-RISK CLINIC

The field of human clinical cancer genetics is changing rapidly with the discovery of new cancer predisposition genes and new options for care and management of high-risk patients (Tables 4.1 and 4.4).[6,7] Further, highly specialized skills are necessary to obtain and validate pedigrees, and to educate and counsel patients.[8,9,10] It is thus preferable to evaluate patients in a high-risk clinic that uses a multidisciplinary approach combining ancillary and medical staff with expertise in cancer genetics and in cancer care (Table 4.5). Because of the potential negative psychological sequelae of learning that one is either positive or negative for a mutation, inclusion of both psychologists and psychiatrists in the team is an important step. Support from individuals skilled in cancer screening, particularly diagnostic imaging and molecular diagnostics, is critical to the long-term success of the program. Finally, given the lack of consensus about appropriate approaches to the management of patients, concerns about genetic confidentiality, and the lack of precedents for many of the issues that arise, an ethicist should be available to provide support to the rest of the team.

An initial telephone triage can be conducted by clerical staff (Fig. 4.2). Questions can be readily designed that will determine whether there are an unusual number of cancer cases in the patient's background or whether unusual constitutional phenotypes, such as the high frequency of bowel polyps seen in FAP patients, are found in the family. A typical questionnaire designed to determine whether a family has at least a 10% chance of carrying an abnormality in the *BRCA-1* or *BRCA-2* breast cancer genes is provided in Table 4.6. If there is no evidence of an abnormal cancer predisposition gene in the family, the patient can be informed that there is no need to proceed with counseling. However, in many cases, these individuals request further reassurance. This can occasionally be accomplished by a telephone conversation with a genetic counselor or with a nurse practitioner (Fig. 4.2). If there is evidence of a potentially elevated risk, the information is not clear in the telephone triage, or the patient needs reassurance, the patient should be requested to fill out a detailed family history questionnaire and attend the clinic for genetic counseling. We find that this is best done by mailing the questionnaire to the patient prior to the scheduled visit. This approach allows patients to fill out the information at their leisure and to consult other relatives to produce as complete a pedigree as possible. The pedigree can then be assessed by the high-risk team in a "disposition conference" during which the need for clarification of the family history or for verification of pathology or clinical findings can be determined. A genetic counselor or nurse practitioner can assist the patient with this follow-up process, frequently by telephone (Fig. 4.2). If the disposition conference suggests that the patient is not at high risk, the patient can be informed and offered age-adjusted cancer surveillance. However, in most cases,

TABLE 4.4. Management of Selected Cancer Predisposition Syndromes

Syndrome Gene	Penetrance	Testing	Prevention	Screening	Prophylactic Surgery
Breast/ovarian *BRCA-1*	Breast, 40%–60% Ovary, 20%–40%	Management options may not be altered by test results.	No known chemoprevention methods	*Breast Cancer* Breast self-exam Begin age 20 Clinical breast exam Annual age 25 Mammography Annual age 30	Prophylactic mastectomy may decrease risk by 20-fold
BRCA-2	Breast, 30%–50% Ovary, 10%–30%	Test results have high false-negative rate. Full-length sequencing method of choice	Birth control pill decreases risk of ovarian cancer by approximately 50%. Tamoxifen may prevent development of breast cancer. Further research needed	*Ovarian Cancer* Transvaginal ultrasound Annual age 30 CA125 Annual age 30 *Prostate Cancer* Digital rectal exam Annual age 50	Prophylactic oophorectomy may decrease risk by 2- to 20-fold Further research needed
Cowden's *PTEN/MMAC-1*	Breast, 15% DCIS and ductal carcinoma Basal cell Thyroid Ovary Rare Renal cell Rare Brain Rare	Genetic testing now available	None known	*Breast Cancer* Breast self exam Begin age 20 Clinical breast exam Annual age 25 Mammography Annual age 30 *Basal Cell Carcinoma* Dermatological exams *Thyroid* Physical exam	Prophylactic mastectomy has been standard. May not be needed owing to low frequency and good outcome. However, may improve quality of life as patients have multiple lumps and biopsies.

(continued)

TABLE 4.4. (continued)

Syndrome Gene	Penetrance	Testing	Prevention	Screening	Prophylactic Surgery
Familial adenomatous polyposis (FAP) *APC*	Nearly 100%	Genetic testing part of the standard management of affected families	Ongoing clinical trials to evaluate the use of chemoprevention agents (e.g., NSAIDs) in this disease	Flexible sigmoidoscopy Begin annually 10–11 years Surveillance for extracolonic neoplasms, (e.g., upper gastrointestinal tract adenomatous polyps)	Prophylactic colectomy performed after appearance of adenomatous polyps
Hereditary non-polyposis colorectal cancer (HNPCC) *MLH-1, MSH-2, PMS-1, PMS-2, GTBP*	Colorectal cancer 60%–75% Metachronous colorectal cancer 30%–50% Endometrial cancer, 30%–40% Ovarian cancer, 3.5-fold increase (less than 10%)	Management options may not be altered by test results. Test results have high false-negative rate. Optimal testing method not yet defined	Ongoing clinical trials to evaluate the use of chemoprevention agents (e.g., NSAIDs) in this disease	*Colon Cancer* Colonoscopy every 1 to 3 years, Beginning at 20–25 years *Endometrial Cancer* Transvaginal ultrasound annually, at 20–25 years OR Endometrial biopsy Annually, at 20–25 year	Subtotal colectomy with ileorectal anastomosis should be considered in HNPCC-associated mutation carriers who have colon cancer and as prophylaxis in selected *HNPCC*-associated mutation carriers with adenomas at the time of surveillance.
MEN II *RET*	Lifetime risk of 90% for medullary thyroid cancer Parathyroid, 10%–20% Pheochromocytoma, 40%–60%	Genetic testing part of the standard management of affected families	None currently available	Pentagastrin Testing—historical	Thyroidectomy—generally done during childhood

TABLE 4.5. High Risk Clinic Multidisciplinary Team

Genetic counselor with additional training in cancer management
Nurse practitioner with additional training in genetics
Clinical geneticist
Medical oncologist
Surgical oncologist
Psychologist
Psychiatrist
Diagnostic imaging
Molecular diagnostics
Ethicist

the patient will still opt for a formal genetic counseling visit. At this visit, which usually takes several hours, the pedigree is evaluated and validated. More importantly, however, the patient is educated as to the significance of the pedigree, the specific aspects of clinical cancer genetics that are applicable to the patient, and the potential options for management (Table 4.4). Some clinics do an initial group educational session. At the first counseling visit, many individuals can be reassured that their risk is not significantly different from that of the normal population. Patients with a risk of carrying a mutation in a cancer predisposition gene can be offered management options that can range from no active management or "watchful waiting" to prophylactic surgery depending on the particular syndrome (Table 4.4). For patients with a significantly elevated risk (our standard is a 10% probability of carrying a mutation in a gene), the patient can be offered genetic testing for syndromes if available. However, genetic testing may be appropriate for lower risk individuals who are contemplating prophylactic surgery, individuals from specific ethnic groups, and for patients who "just need to know."

Many individuals are "information seekers" and want as much information as possible to guide future decisions (Table 4.7). Information about a person's chance of developing cancer may provide important directions for patient care. Further, high-risk patients have questions related to the best options for management (Table 4.4). Even when the best medical management option is not known, identifying one's risk and the potential options may provide empowerment, allowing the individual to make decisions based on the best information available. For many patients, awaiting the results of ongoing trials to define the best mode of care is not an option, as they feel that they must take action in the immediate future. Wanting to do all that is possible to remain cancer free for themselves or for their children can drive utilization of approaches that have not been medically proven to be beneficial. For example, preliminary studies suggest that prophylactic mastectomy may decrease the chance of developing breast cancer by up to 20-fold and in models may significantly increase lifespan.[11] The protective effect of prophylactic oophorectomy, although not carrying the same psychological overtones as prophylactic mastectomy, remains unclear, with estimates ranging from 2- to 20-fold. Although definitive studies have not been completed, many patients consider that there is sufficient evidence to justify pro-

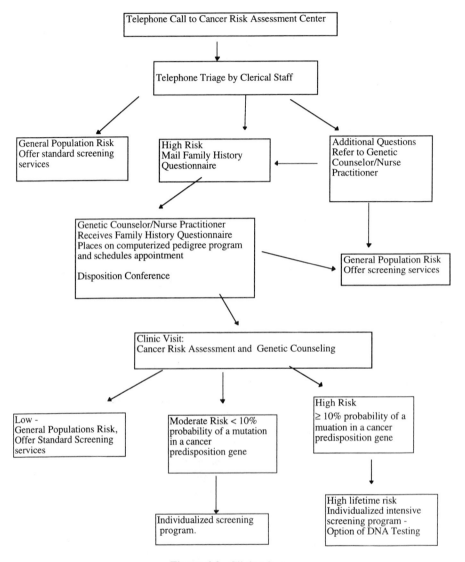

Figure 4.2. Clinic triage.

phylactic surgery in the breast/ovary syndrome. Concerns about risks for children and relatives is paramount for many individuals who have already developed cancer (Table 4.7).

It is important to realize that many individuals do not wish to attend a high-risk clinic or to undergo genetic testing (Table 4.7). Many patients are concerned about the potential for insurance and employment discrimination. There is major concern about potential genetic discrimination based on the founder effects and ethnic relationships observed with some of the cancer predisposition genes described previ-

TABLE 4.6. Predictors of at Least a 10% Probability of *BRCA1/BRCA2* Mutation in the Family

Non-Ashkenazi Jewish Heritage	Ashkenazi Jewish Heritage
At least one single breast cancer before age 40	At least one single breast cancer before age 59
At least two breast cancers before age 50	
Bilateral breast cancer before age 50	Bilateral breast cancer before age 50
Two or more ovarian cancers at any age	Two or more ovarian cancers at any age
Ovarian cancer and a breast cancer at any age	Ovarian cancer and a breast cancer at any age
A single person with breast and ovarian cancer	A single person with breast and ovarian cancer

The questions are designed to identify a 10% probability of the family testing positive for abnormalities in *BRCA-1* or *BRCA-2*. Many families have a much higher risk based on family history. The optimal use of these questions requires a detailed knowledge of all cases of breast and ovarian cancer. Factors that most strongly influence risk are ethnic background, cases of ovarian cancer, average age at onset of breast cancer, and early onset of breast cancer. In several studies, the number of breast cancers is not a strong predictor of the likelihood of testing positive. Cases of male breast cancer, pancreatic cancer, or prostate cancer may indicate a risk for testing positive for abnormalities in *BRCA-1* or *BRCA-2*.

The predicted 10% risk is for the family. A woman who has a breast or ovarian cancer has a risk equal to that for the whole family. For an unaffected family member, the predicted probability is determined by the relationship to an affected family member. In the case of an unaffected child or sibling of an affected member, the probability would be half (50%) of the predicted probability for the whole family. An unaffected grandchild of an affected family member would carry a 25% probability if his or her parent was also unaffected.

TABLE 4.7. High-Risk Clinic

Why to Seek Counseling
    Accurate up to date information applicable to patient's family history
    Empowerment
        Informed decisions
    May need less frequent screening
    Risks for self
    Risks for children
    Management options

Why Not to Seek Counseling
    Genetic discrimination
        Insurance
        Employment
    Lack of proven methods for screening and prevention
    Bad news and no news
    Costs
    Possibility of a false or inconclusive result
    Impact on family dynamics
    Psychological implications

ously. Many of the US State legislatures have passed "Genetic Discrimination" bills, which, combined with the Federal Health Insurance Portability and Accountability Act of 1996 (HIPAA) and the Americans with Disability Act, provide a degree of protection from genetic discrimination in the United States. Major concerns remain, however, particularly about discrimination for medical insurance based on family history, which, as noted previously, is a good indicator of risk and is not covered under many of the genetic discrimination laws. In contrast to the United States, the laws of several countries allow genetic testing by insurance companies as a prerequisite for obtaining certain types of insurance, usually life insurance. Although concerns about genetic discrimination are real, it has been difficult to document discrimination based on family history or genetic testing in high-risk cancer families.

A number of additional reasons dissuade individuals from obtaining genetic counseling (Table 4.7). A lack of awareness of the availability of genetic counseling, of a linkage between family history and risk of developing cancer, and of the individual's own family history may prevent utilization of genetic counseling facilities. In many of the cancer syndromes, the appropriate management is not yet known, decreasing enthusiasm about obtaining genetic counseling. Further, in many cases, individuals who prefer to remain ignorant of their risk are concerned that they will be told that they are at high risk. In some cases, the individual's understanding of the limitations of genetic testing dissuades them from obtaining genetic counseling. Finally, the cost of genetic counseling and of genetic testing is often prohibitive, particularly for those individuals who do not have insurance, whose insurance does not cover genetic counseling and testing, or who choose to avoid the risk of requesting payment from an insurance company owing to concerns about future genetic discrimination.

GENETIC TESTING

Genetic testing for many of the cancer predisposition syndromes remains controversial (Table 4.4). At a minimum, the patient must be counseled as to the ramifications of testing and the potential interpretation of test results. The patient must be informed of the potential of obtaining false-negative, false-positive, or uninformative results. The person counseling the patient should understand the limitations of the particular technology utilized (Table 4.8). The American Society of Clinical Oncologists does not recommend testing unless the results have the potential to alter the patient's medical management.[8] However, knowing one's mutation status, whether or not there are specific proven medical management options, may provide the patient with information that will improve his or her quality of life.

In most cases, genetic testing should be considered experimental and be performed under an informed consent approved by an institutional review board (see Appendix 1 for an example).[8,9,10,12] However, as genetic testing approaches are validated, appropriate management techniques developed, and safeguards against genetic discrimination put in place, genetic testing will likely become a component of general medical practice. An individual's risk of developing cancer will be one piece of the process in designing individualized screening and prevention programs.

TABLE 4.8. Selected Techniques for Identifying Mutations in Cancer Predisposition Genes

Technique	Description	Strengths	Weaknesses
Allelotyping	Restriction fragment polymorphisms or microsatellite analysis of DNA from multiple family members used to track mutation in family	If family of sufficient size, will faithfully predict carrier tatus. Independent of types of mutation	Applicable only to large families Difficult to obtain blood from multiple family members Sensitive to "sporadic" cancers
Single-strand conformational polymorphism (SSCP)	DNA is expanded using PCR. The DNA obtained is then heated to separate the complementary strands which are separated by gel electrophoresis. Altered DNA will produce a band that is higher or lower.	SSCP can detect 50%–75% of mutations, depending on the type. Technique is fast, multiple samples can be screened quickly for a relatively low cost. Readily detects deletions and insertions.	Technique lacks sensitivity. Difficult to detect point mutations. Can miss small inserts or deletions. Abnormalities must be confirmed by sequencing
Heteroduplex analysis	DNA is expanded using PCR. The DNA obtained is then heated and cooled to form homoduplexes (two normal strands or two mutant strands) or heteroduplexes (one mutant and one normal strand). The duplexes are then separated by gel electrophoresis. Homo- and heteroduplexes will migrate differently according to shape and size.	Same benefits as SSCP, Adds additional sensitivity by increasing the likelihood of seeing a mobility shift on the gel.	Technique lacks sensitivity. Abnormalities must be confirmed by sequencing.
Protein truncation test	Protein is produced by PCR linked to transcription and translation from DNA or reverse transcriptase (RT)-PCR linked to transcription and translation from RNA. Proteins are separated by gel electrophoresis based on size.	Detects mutations that introduce a stop signal (nonsense or frameshift mutations) that result in the production of a shortened protein. Once primers developed and validated, relatively easy to perform.	Will not detect other types of mutations. Low sensitivity RNA may be unstable due to introduction of stop codons leading to mRNA instability.

(continued)

83

TABLE 4.8. (*continued*)

Technique	Description	Strengths	Weaknesses
Direct sequencing	Sequences both copies of each gene being analyzed. This is considered the "gold standard" of testing.	Will detect all changes in the regions analyzed. Amenable to automation for processing large numbers of specimens.	Applicable only to relatively large sized exons. Abnormalities must be confirmed by sequencing. Expensive. Labor intensive. Slow. Misses regulatory mutations that are outside the region analyzed. Will miss large deletions. Polymorphisms difficult to distinguish from missense mutations
Allele-specific oligonucleotide testing	Uses hybridization to sequence specific oligonucleotides to detect mutations.	Rapid. In theory as efficient as direct sequencing. Once "CHIP" established relatively inexpensive	Emerging. Need to have oligonucleotide present for all possible mutations. Difficult to assess insertions and deletions
Functional assay	Assesses function of protein in model system such as yeast.	Sensitive. May distinguish polymorphism from mutation	Emerging. Assays will require validation
Protein levels	Detects differences in protein levels in normal cells due to a copy number effect.	Easily performed (Theoretical). Will detect all forms of mutations	Emerging. Requires extreme care to ensure ability to measure changes in protein expression in normal cells. Useful only for genes demonstrating copy number effects

A number of different techniques are utilized for genetic testing (Table 4.8). Mutations in cancer predisposition genes fall into two major categories that determine the difficulty and testing approaches that can be utilized. In many of the cancer predisposition genes, mutations cluster around specific "hot spots." In these cases, an analysis of specific regions of the cancer predisposition gene is sufficient to identify the majority if not all of the potential mutations. This appears to be the case for *RET* and *MET*, for example, but may also be true for a number of the other cancer predisposition genes. In these circumstances a number of approaches (Table 4.8) can be used to derive accurate results. In contrast, mutations are scattered throughout many of the cancer predisposition genes, requiring assessment of the complete regulatory and coding regions of the gene. Genetic testing is further complicated by the large size of many of the cancer predisposition gene. In these cases, the "gold standard" for genetic testing remains end-to-end sequencing, which is time consuming and expensive (Table 4.8). Unfortunately, even full length sequencing may not detect all mutations, with false-negative rates as high as 15 to 30% occurring in testing of the *BRCA-1* and *BRCA-2* genes. Whether the failure of sequencing to detect mutations is due to deletions of large areas of the gene that would not be detected by current sequencing approaches, mutations in regulatory regions outside of the regions currently assessed, silencing of the gene by promoter methylation, or additional as yet unknown mechanisms is unknown (Table 4.8). Many laboratories utilize a screening technique such as single-stranded conformational polymorphism (SSCP), heteroduplex analysis, or protein truncation testing (see Table 4.8) followed by sequencing of any regions demonstrating abnormalities in the screening test to identify mutations. These approaches may be considerably less sensitive than direct full length sequencing. To appropriately interpret the results to the patient, it is critical to know the mutation detection approach utilized by any testing laboratory and to understand the limitations of the technique.

Interpretation of testing results can be complex. Mutations that have been identified to track with disease in several families are the easiest to interpret. Clearly they predispose an individual to the development of cancer. Nevertheless, the degree of penetrance and age at onset of cancer induced by a particular mutation may vary between families and between individuals in a family. Mutations that result in a truncated protein generally can be expected to result in a predisposition to cancer. However, for example, a significant portion of the carboxyterminus of *BRCA-2* can be deleted with no apparent ill effect. Mutations that result in a change in the identity of a single amino acid (missense mutations) in the resultant protein product are most difficult to interpret. Such changes may represent polymorphisms of no or limited consequences. When the same missense mutation is found in a number of different cancer-prone families and is found to track with the disease, it likely predisposes to tumor development. When a missense mutation has not been seen before or has not been demonstrated to track with disease, the mutation must be categorized as being of "unknown significance." Further analysis of these missense mutations is required to determine if the mutation segregates with cancer or if it is found in a significant number of nonaffected individuals in the general population, making it a likely polymorphism. Mutations that result in a change in the nucleotide sequence without a change in protein sequence due to "third codon wobble" can generally be assumed to be without consequence. Mutations found in introns, particularly those in splice acceptor and donator sites, must be assessed further to determine whether they track with disease in several families. Similar examination is necessary for mutations in promoter regions.

Emerging technologies such as gene sequencing CHIPs (arrays of short nucleotide sequences on a solid matrix that can detect all potential sequences in a gene), tandem mass spectrometry (linking HPLC and mass spectrometry to give extremely accurate size measurement), and functional assays (assessing function of a patients gene in model systems such as yeast) may prove to be more accurate and less expensive than current approaches. More important, functional assays, such as studying function of the gene product in yeast, have the potential to distinguish significant mutations from polymorphisms.[13] These new technologies will need to mature prior to being instituted as "first line" approaches, replacing current sequencing technology. It is important to note, however, that *p53* sequencing CHIPs are commercially available and that CHIPs have been developed that can detect the majority of point mutations and small inserts even in large genes such as *BRCA-1*.

BAD NEWS AND NO NEWS

The interpretation and presentation of positive test results to the patient is relatively straightforward. The patient should be told that he or she is at an increased risk for the development of cancer and offered a menu of management options. The risk level should be presented so as to reflect the range of penetrance for abnormalities in the cancer predisposition gene and, where possible, the penetrance for the specific mutation. Where clinical studies have identified appropriate management options (Table 4.4),[6,7] they can be offered to the patient. However, where the appropriate medical approach has not been defined, the alternative options should be described to the patient in a nondirective manner, allowing the patient to make his or her own informed decision. It is important to note that the patient's decision will likely be tempered by her own exposure to family members who developed cancer and, despite extensive education during the counseling process, to her previous convictions and education.

The interpretation and presentation of test results that do not indicate the presence of a mutation is more complex, particularly if the individual tested does not have cancer. Indeed, it is preferable, but not always possible, to test a family member who is afflicted with cancer. However, even in families at high risk for cancer, sporadic cases of cancer, particularly common cancers such as breast cancer, can occur and confuse the issue (see individual 103 in Fig. 4.1). A failure to detect a mutation could be indicative that mutations in the tested genes are not present in the family. Alternatively, it may suggest that a genetic change is present in the family and was not inherited by the tested individual. A failure to detect a mutation in the cancer predisposition gene may indicate that the mutation is outside of the region tested, not detected by the technique used, or that a mutation is present in an as yet unidentified cancer predisposition gene that induces a similar syndrome. *BRCA-1* and *BRCA-2* (and potential BRCA-3, -4, -5, or -6) provide excellent examples. Full length sequencing for *BRCA-1* likely misses 15% of the mutations in *BRCA-1* and may miss as many as 30% of the mutations. Further, sequencing of *BRCA-1* alone will clearly miss all mutations in *BRCA-2* and any other related phenocopy syndromes. Thus, there is a high potential for false-negative results in testing. There is controversy as to whether a negative test result decreases the chance that a mutation is present in the family. Negative test results for a gene with a known false-negative test rate have been suggested to reflect a decrease in the probability that a mutation is present in the family inversely proportional to the false-negative rate. Conditional probability (a form of statistical analysis) suggests, however, that the predicted likelihood of a mutation in a cancer predisposition gene in a family based on family history is not altered by a negative test result. Rather, a negative test result suggests that the mutation in the family is not detectable by the technology utilized. Thus, in most cases, patients can only be given "bad news" (they have a genetic abnormality) or "no news" (we don't know if there is a genetic abnormality in the family). In either case, medical management and advice may not change markedly as a consequence of genetic testing. The patient, regardless of test results, may continue to be considered at high risk and would continue to be offered intensive screening or prophylactic surgery. Indeed, this lack of new options decreases the attractiveness of genetic testing for many patients (Table 4.7).

There are exceptions to the "no news" category. When the identity of the mutation present in a family is known, it is possible, with a high degree of accuracy, to determine whether any person in the family has or has not inherited the specific mutation. Thus, the patient could potentially receive "good news." Further, in cases where the likely location of a specific mutation can be predicted owing to the phenotype, hot spots accounting for the majority of inherited cases, or mutations prevalent in specific ethnic backgrounds, it may be possible to indicate that negative results essentially rule out the likelihood of a mutation being present in the tested gene in that patient. This may have important consequences for the patient, allowing decreased surveillance or potentially abrogating the need for prophylactic surgery (Table 4.7). It may have a major effect on the patient's concerns about reproduction and passing on a high risk to one's children.

PSYCHOSOCIAL CONSEQUENCES

There are many psychosocial implications associated with cancer predisposition testing.[14,15] Several factors such as beliefs about cancer and its prognosis, life history, and the level of fear and anxiety present, are known to influence how patients perceive personal risk and their comprehension of risk information. In the United States, uncertainties regarding the potential for genetic discrimination in insurance or by employers remains, despite the passage of legislation. Diligent measures within the clinical setting to safeguard patient information specific to genetic testing must be maintained and patients' wishes respected. The full spectrum of psychological reactions to the results of genetic testing has not yet been fully elucidated, and thus remains an area of active research. Assessment of family dynamics is important and should be discussed prior to initiation of testing, as results obtained by one family member may have potential impact upon others within the family. Some family members may wish to know their status, whereas others most definitely will not want to know. This can obviously lead to conflict within the family. Potential negative sequelae that may result from testing include heightened fear and anxiety, depression, changes in family relationships, guilt over transmission of a mutated gene, guilt over not receiving a mutated gene (survivor guilt), changes in functional status, and changes in body image and self-perception. Within the context of the patient's beliefs about health care and his or her cultural orientation, the multidisciplinary team must strive to support patients following provision of test results by reinforcing existing coping mechanisms, teaching new ones, providing the necessary information to empower patient decision making, and referring to mental health professionals when warranted. There are also potential benefits that may be obtained from testing. These include relief from the uncertainty of not knowing one's risk status, targeting of aggressive screening measures and prevention strategies to those at the highest risk, and providing information on the potential for children to have inherited a predisposition to develop cancer. It is important to reinforce that the presence of a mutated cancer predisposition gene within the family does not mean that all family members will inherit this mutation, or that they will develop cancer.

VARIATION IN PENETRANCE

The degree of penetrance and the severity of the syndromes associated with cancer predisposition genes can vary widely between families and between individuals in the same family. This makes it necessary in many cases to communicate the likelihood of developing cancer to a high-risk individual with a very wide confidence interval.

Within a family, the degree of penetrance may be altered by the presence of additional modifying genes found in the family. For example, individuals who have inherited specific *HRAS* alleles appear to be much more susceptible to the effect of inherited mutations in *BRCA-1*. Other low-penetrance, high-frequency genetic changes are likely important in the expression of the phenotype associated with cancer predisposition genes. The lifestyle of individuals may also play a major role. The frequency of development of ovarian cancer in carriers of mutations of *BRCA-1* and *BRCA-2* appears to be governed by the same reproductive characteristics as in individuals without abnormalities in *BRCA-1* or *BRCA-2*. Strikingly, and of potential theoretical and practical importance, use of the birth control pill for at least 5 years appears to decrease the chance of developing ovarian cancer by at least 50% in individuals with normal or mutant *BRCA-1* or *BRCA-2* genes. This suggests that changes in lifestyle or the use of chemoprevention approaches, such as the birth control pill, may have a major impact on the development of cancer in individuals who have inherited abnormalities in cancer predisposition genes. As mentioned previously, studies are underway to assess whether tamoxifen will decrease the chance that high-risk individuals will develop breast cancer. Once this trial is completed and the results correlated with *BRCA-1* and *BRCA-2* status, tamoxifen may be recommended for carriers of mutations in *BRCA-1* or *BRCA-2*. An additional criterion determining penetrance of specific cancer predisposition genes may be the extent of exposure to environmental toxins or stresses. Individuals with the *ATM* gene, and potentially mutations in the *HNPCC* genes, *NF-1*, *BRCA-1*, or *BRCA-2*, may be particular sensitive, for example, to the effects of various forms of radiation. The degree of exposure to sunlight or medical radiation may be critical to cancer development in these individuals.

The modifying effects on penetrance seen within a family can affect the penetrance of cancer predisposition genes between families. In addition, the type and location of the mutation also affects penetrance. Indeed, specific mutations in a number of the cancer predisposition genes result in markedly attenuated forms of the cancer syndrome. This is more likely to occur with missense (protein sequence change) than with truncating mutations. Thus, for many of the cancer genes, the risk of developing cancer must be communicated to the patient with wide confidence intervals.

The concept of incomplete penetrance is particularly important to communicate to the patient.[16] In our breast/ovarian cancer clinic, patients routinely overestimate their risk and are relieved to discover that developing and dying of cancer is not inevitable (Fig. 4.3). The bad news that they carry an abnormality in a cancer predisposition gene such *BRCA-1* or *BRCA-2* can be tempered by this knowledge.

Although it is possible to indicate to a patient what the expected frequency of cancer is for individuals with a given cancer predisposition syndrome, it is usually not possible to determine which individuals and, importantly, when a specific individual will develop cancer (Tables 4.1 and 4.4). Patients find it particularly difficult to relate statistical risks of developing cancer to their own likelihood of developing cancer in the near future or even in their lifetime. The patient's response to counseling is frequently driven by the patient's past experience as well as by his or her prior knowledge. These preconceptions have proven particularly recalcitrant to patient education.[14,15] Approaches ranging from intensive counseling to the development of interactive computer driven education programs are under investigation to provide more efficient and convincing patient education.

OUTCOME

Whether the prognosis for cancers that develop in high-risk individuals is different from that for sporadic tumors is not yet clear and likely depends on the specific cancer predisposition gene, as well as on the specific mutation in the family. Individuals with abnormalities in the genes comprising the *HNPCC* syndrome have an improved outcome for their bowel cancers independent of location, stage, and grade. This outcome is not likely due to increased surveillance but rather seems to reflect an intrinsic characteristic of the tumor. The effect of mutations in other cancer predisposition genes on outcome remains controversial. Although abnormalities in *BRCA-1* had been suggested to result in an improved outcome for ovarian cancer,[17]

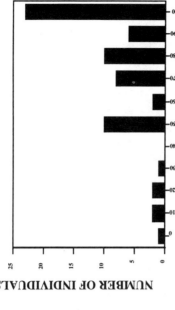

LIKELIHOOD OF DEVELOPING BREAST CANCER

LIKELIHOOD OF AN ABNORMAL GENE IN FAMILY

FIGURE 4.3. Patients attending a high-risk clinic were asked about their perception of likelihood for developing breast cancer (only patients without cancer) or the likelihood of there being a mutated cancer gene in the family (all patients). A subset of the patients were tested by full length sequencing for abnormalities in both *BRCA-1* and *BRCA-2*. The positive test rate was approximately 30%. It is important to note that a 30% test positive rate translates into at most a 15% chance of developing breast cancer. When the 10% risk of developing breast cancer in the general population is accounted for, it is clear that women attending the clinic greatly overestimate their chance of developing breast cancer. Importantly, even when a woman is told that she is positive for mutations in *BRCA-1* or *BRCA-2*, her risk is frequently lower than she perceived prior to coming to the clinic. Further, in general, these women greatly overestimate the chance that they carry a mutated cancer predisposition gene.

this has not been confirmed in subsequent studies. Breast tumors from patients with mutations in *BRCA-1* demonstrate pathologic and biochemical changes that predict that the outcome is likely to be worse than in the general population. It is important to note, however, that patients who develop tumors due to abnormalities in cancer predisposition genes have been treated with the same approaches as have patients who develop the more common sporadic tumors. It remains probable and even likely that specific therapeutic approaches will exhibit different efficacies in patients with inherited abnormalities in some cancer predisposition genes. Additional research is necessary to validate or refute this hypothesis.

THE FUTURE

Because cancer is a genetic disease, the identification of the genetic changes that occur in a patient's tumor has the potential to greatly improve management and outcome. Our emerging ability to readily assess the genetic changes required for tumorigenesis in each patient's tumor may soon allow the development of approaches for early diagnosis, mechanisms to determine prognosis for individual patients, identification of new targets for chemoprevention or therapy, characterization of intermediary markers for clinical trials, and individualization of patient therapy. This may greatly increase the response and cure rates for human tumors and ameliorate the suffering associated with cancer. Made possible by the technological revolution spawned by molecular genetics and the Human Genome Project, the realization of these lofty goals is much closer than most of us perceive. Indeed, the challenge may not be in our technical ability to identify and characterize the genetic changes associated with cancer, but rather in the development of the approaches necessary to apply the masses of genetic information that will be available from each patient to clinical management. We will need to develop the computer and information systems or "bioinformatics" that will allow us to integrate the information that will arise from this new field of "functional genomics" into patient care. The biggest threat to the next generation of oncologists may be to keep from being overwhelmed by the wealth of data that will be available on each patient's tumor.

Many of the genetic changes that occur in tumors have already been identified. Current technology allows us to assess a subset of these changes in any patient's tumor. However, with very few exceptions, this information is not yet sufficiently mature to alter how we treat cancer patients. Nevertheless, preliminary studies are very exciting. It is currently possible to detect mutations in the *ras* oncogene or *p53* tumor suppressor gene, by amplifying DNA from stool, blood, or urine of patients with bowel or bladder tumors. These results suggest that there is potential for the assessment of accessible bodily materials to identify genetic changes that occur early in the course of tumorigenesis. This may provide a whole new approach to early diagnosis, which remains the "holy grail" for improved cancer care and economics.

In the more immediate future, genetic mutations present in a specific patient's tumor will be assessed by detecting mutations in specific oncogenes or tumor suppressor genes using direct sequencing or "sequencing CHIPs" (multiple oligonucleotides with all possible sequences from a single gene on a matrix). Alternatively the messenger RNAs expressed by the tumor that reflects mutations in the tumor will be assessed by "profiling" using "arrays" (segments of cDNAs on a matrix) or "array CHIPs" (multiple oligonucleotides from different genes on a matrix). "CHIPs" have already been developed that will detect all of the common mutations in oncogenes such as *ras* or in tumor suppressor genes such as *p53* or *BRCA-1*, thus providing the ability to identify a mutation in a patient's tumor or germline. An assessment of mRNA expression patterns in tumor cells using arrays will provide an indirect indication of the specific oncogenes that are mutated by assessing the effect of the signaling or growth regulatory pathways activated in a specific tumor and the resultant increase in transcription of specific genes. Commercially available genetic arrays can assess the expression of at least 18,000 different genes. As only 20% of the 100,000 genes in the human genome are expressed in any cell lineage (i.e., approximately 20,000 genes), it is currently theoretically possible to create a tissue-specific DNA array that could assess expression of all genes relevant to a given cell lineage. Relatively small arrays assessing the expression of the even smaller fraction of genes of significance to tumor development in a given cell lineage or even potentially in all cell lineages will be developed. An example of a DNA array assessing the level of expression of 588 genes by an ovarian cancer cell line is demonstrated in Fig. 4.4. This demonstrates that a number of genes are expressed at relatively high levels in ovarian cancer, whereas others are expressed at relatively low levels. This pattern reflects genes induced by the genetic mutations in this particular ovarian cancer which includes mutation of *p53* and amplification of phosphatidyinositol $3'$-kinase.

Assessment of the genes expressed by a patient's tumor should allow evaluation of the patient's prognosis as well as individualization of therapy for each patient. We currently treat most tumors based on a relatively small set of criteria including stage, grade, histologic origin, volume and site of tumor, and the site and amount of metastases. This results in a "lumping" of patients into a fairly limited number of treatment modalities. "Molecular profiling" may offer the opportunity to better identify those individuals who do not need additional therapy, who will respond to a particular therapy, or who are best treated with investigational therapy. The evaluation of the large number of genes expressed by a specific cell and the need for the correlation of patterns of gene expression with eventual outcome has given rise to a new field of bioinformatics.

Even more exciting is the possibility that molecular therapeutics can be designed that will specifically target the genetic abnormality that occurs in an individual's tumors. Indeed, a number of therapeutic approaches that target abnormalities in genes involved in tumor development are in preclinical or early clinical evaluation. As we begin to understand the genetic changes that must occur during tumorigenesis in a particular cell lineage, it may be possible to derive cancer prevention approaches that will prevent or reverse these genetic changes and block the development of clinically evident cancers. Alternatively, it may be possible to normalize the function of aberrant genes by "gene therapy" that will reintroduce either the normal gene product or small molecules that mimic the normal function of the gene or bind to the aberrant

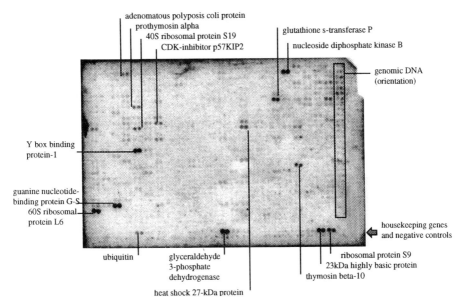

FIGURE 4.4. Gene expression in a human ovarian cancer cell line. Hybridization of OVCAR-3 cDNA probes to the Human Atlas Expression Array. Poly(A)+ RNA was isolated from serum-starved OVCAR-3 cells and used to generate ^{32}P-labeled cDNA probes. The probe sample was hybridized to the Atlas array according to the user manual. The membrane was exposed to a phoshpor-imaging screen overnight and the signal acquired using the Storm 860 system. The array consists of 588 different 200- 500-bp PCR-amplified cDNA fragments that have been spotted in duplicate on the membrane. Selected positive signals are indicated.

gene product. Indeed, small molecules that normalize the functions of some forms of the mutant *p53* tumor suppressor gene have been identified. This genetic revolution has the potential to alter the way in which we treat cancer, thereby greatly improving the outcome for those with this devastating disease.

SUMMARY

Five to ten percent of all cancers occur in individuals who have inherited mutations in cancer predisposition genes. Cancer predisposition genes have been identified that account for the majority of hereditary breast, ovary, and bowel cancers, as well as for a spectrum of less common tumors. Family history provides the cornerstone for identifying high-risk individuals. Genetic testing can then determine whether a high-risk individual carries a gene mutation. Identification of appropriate management approaches including chemoprevention, early detection, and prophylactic surgery are needed to decrease the physical and psychological suffering of individuals with a genetic predisposition to cancer.

FURTHER READING

1. Holland JF, Bast RC, Morton DL, et al. (1997) *Cancer Medicine*, 4th edition, Vol. 1, Williams & Wilkins, Baltimore, pp. 97–117.

2. Holland JF, Bast RC, Morton DL, et al. (1997) *Cancer Medicine*, 4th edition, Vol. 1, Williams & Wilkins, Baltimore, pp. 245–260.

3. Holland JF, Bast RC, Morton DL, et al. (1997) *Cancer Medicine*, 4th edition, Vol. 1, Williams & Wilkins, Baltimore, pp. 401–420.

4. Holland JF, Bast RC, Morton DL, et al. (1997) *Cancer Medicine*, 4th edition, Vol. 1, Williams & Wilkins, Baltimore, pp. 511–530.

5. Hot JT, Thompson ME, Szabo C, et al. (1996) Growth retardation and tumour inhibition by bRCA1. *Nat Genet* 12:298–302.

6. Burke W, Petersen G, Lynch P, et al. (1997) Recommendations for follow-up care of individuals with an inherited predisposition to cancer. *JAMA* 277:915–919.

7. Burke W, Daly M, Garber J, et al. (1997) Recommendations for follow-up care of individuals with an inherited predisposition to cancer. *JAMA* 277:997–1003.

8. Anonymous (1996) Statement of the American Society of Clinical Oncology: Genetic testing for cancer susceptibility. *J Clin Oncol* 14:1730–1736.

9. Anonymous (1997) Predisposition genetic testing for late-onset disorders in adults. *JAMA*, 278:1217–1220.

10. Geller G, Botkin JR, Green MJ, et al. (1997) Genetic testing for susceptibility to adult-onset cancer: The process and content of informed consent. *JAMA* 277:1467–1474.

11. Schrag D, Kuntz KM, Garber JE, et al. (1997) Decision analysis—Effects of prophylactic mastectomy and oophorectomy on life expectancy among women with *BRCA1* or *BRCA2* mutations. *N Eng J Med* 336:1465–1471.

12. Clayton EW, Steinberg KK, Khoury MJ, et al. (1995) Informed consent for genetic research on stored tissue samples. *JAMA* 274:1786–1792.

13. Humphrey JS, Salim A, Erdos MR, et al. (1997) Human *BRCA1* inhibits growth in yeast: Potential use in diagnostic testing. *Proc Natl Acad Sci USA* 94:5820–5825.

14. Lynch HT, Lemon SJ, Durham C, et al. (1997) A descriptive study of *BRCA1* testing and reactions to disclosure of test results. *Cancer* 79:2219–2228.

15. Lerman C, Narod S, Schulman K, et al. (1996) *BRCA1* testing in families with hereditary breast-ovarian cancer: A prospective study of patient decision making and outcomes. *JAMA*, 275(24):1885–92.

16. Struewing JP, Hartge P, Wacholder S, et al. (1997) The risk of cancer associated with specific mutations of *BRCA1* and *BRCA2* among Ashkenazi Jews. *N Engl J Med* 336:1401–1408.

17. Rubin SC, Benjamin I, Behbakht K, et al. (1996) Clinical and pathological features of ovarian cancer in women with germ-line mutations of *BRCA1*. *N Engl J Med* 335:1413–1416.

APPENDIX 1   MODEL INFORMED CONSENT FORM (THE "MAXI" MODEL)

Based on ASCO's Guidelines, the Consensus Statement (*JAMA*, 1997, 277:1467–1473), and Other Centers' Consents

Description of Research

Includes:

- How genetic counseling will be done. Suggested is a multistep process with two stages before the test is performed: (1) one explaining risks, benefits, alternatives; and (2) one obtaining consent or refusal for the test to be performed. After the test is performed, another genetic counseling session to deliver the results should occur.
- Type of analysis to be performed, cost of analysis, length of time for results to become available.
- Participants will be asked to contact other family members who may be at risk for this mutation. Participants are NOT giving consent for other members of their family to participate in this study. No family member will be contacted until he or she returns the "Consent by Relative to be Contacted" form.

Describe disposition of samples:

- Permission must be asked for banking samples for further research in cancer. Include the duration of the storage and plans, if any, for discarding the sample. Ask if participant agrees to be contacted about future research.
- If the sample is to be anonymized for banking, so inform the participant.
- If the banked samples will have individual identifiers, ask:
  1. Does the participant want to be recontacted if future genetic tests become available?
  2. Does the participant wish to be notified if unanticipated results of medical significance are found?

Risks, Side Effects, and Discomforts to Participants

- The risks associated with drawing blood are minimal. There may be discomfort and temporary bruising at the site. Infections can occur rarely.

Other Risks Associated with DNA Testing

- Some individuals may have emotional or psychological problems knowing that they have a gene that increases the risk for developing cancer. They may feel angry or shocked or deny that they have it. They may worry about their health, family, or employability. They may feel differently about themselves. They may worry about passing the alteration to their children. They may worry about medical costs or insurance. Finding that one does not carry the gene can also be upsetting, producing guilt as well as joy. Anyone experiencing these feelings will be offered supportive counseling.

- If an alteration in the gene is found, the participant will be encouraged to inform other family members who may also carry the mutation. However, the participant should be aware that not everyone will want or welcome the information when contacted. During the discussion, the participant may find out unwanted information about relatives. For example, someone may disclose that a family member is adopted. Therefore, sometimes relationships in families may be changed.

- Information regarding the participant's parents may be discovered in the course of this research project. For instance, adoption and/or issues of paternity (*fatherhood*) may be discovered. This information will not be revealed unless it has direct medical or reproductive implications for the participant.

- All test results will be kept in a confidential file separate from the medical record. The participant should realize, however, once he or she has been personally informed of a test result, regardless of whether or not it is entered into the medical record, he or she may be required to reveal the result as part of an application for health, life, disability or other insurance coverage. Some insurance companies may consider an inherited change in a gene to be a preexisting condition, and on that basis, may decide not to offer coverage, to limit coverage, or to charge a higher premium for coverage. The participant may want to review and adjust insurance coverage prior to testing.

- There may be risks to employment if employers learn of the potential for future health risks.

Limitation of DNA Testing

- If an alteration of a gene is found, it means that there is a higher chance of having a disease develop. It is not known when the disease will develop, if it does. (*Omit, if known.*)

- Not all the alterations of the gene that may increase the risk for cancer are known. There is a chance that an inherited alteration may be missed. It is not known what that chance is. Or, there may be another gene for breast and ovarian cancer that was not tested. (*Put in specifics of gene to be tested.*)

- Results of DNA testing can sometimes be unclear. (*Include reliability of test, if known.*) Therefore, the participant may go through the testing process and not have any more information about the personal risk to develop cancer.

- There is a possibility of errors at the laboratory. This risk may be minimized by testing two samples and comparing them for accuracy.

Potential Benefits

- There may be no direct benefit from being tested.
- If the test is positive, the participant will know that he or she is at high risk for the development of cancer. The participant will be able to discuss management options with the physician to best protect health. (*Specify what these are.*)
- Some people feel relief from the uncertainty of not knowing the risk for cancer. Knowing can help provide some control over what is to be done about the risk of cancer.
- Close relatives may also carry the gene mutation. If they know this, they can decide whether or not to pursue testing or special surveillance.

What It Means if an Alteration in the Gene Is Found

- The presence of an alteration means the participant is at increased risk of developing hereditary cancer. (*Specify medical options given this increased risk.*)
- (*Explain limited proof of efficacy for surveillance and prevention.*)
- (*Explain chance of passing alteration on to children.*)

What It Means if an Alteration in the Gene Is Not Found

- A hereditary form of the disease may still exist, as there may be other genes that can cause cancer.
- There is still the chance of developing the disease. (*Specify general population risk for specific disease. Specify accepted screening for general population.*)

Alternate Procedures or Treatments

The alternative is not to undergo testing, in which case the participant will not learn if he or she has an altered form of the gene. A genetic counselor may be able to provide an approximation of risk using family history.

CHAPTER 5

TUMOR IMMUNOLOGY

GEORGE E. PEOPLES

Department of Surgical Oncology
University of Texas M.D. Anderson Cancer Center
Houston, TX 77030, USA

Department of Surgery
Uniformed Services University of the Health Sciences
Bethesda, MD 20814, USA

ALEXANDER R. MILLER

Department of Surgical Oncology
University of Texas M.D. Anderson Cancer Center
Houston, TX 77030, USA

TIMOTHY J. EBERLEIN

Department of Surgery
Division of Surgical Oncology
Brigham and Women's Hospital
Boston, MA 02115, USA

Surgery, radiation, and chemotherapy have long been the mainstays to traditional cancer therapy; however, in recent years, biologic cancer therapy has emerged as a fourth arm to cancer treatment. This form of therapy induces, utilizes, and/or modifies the host immune system to more efficiently recognize and destroy cancer cells. The basic components, the mechanisms of action, and the communications of the immune system must be understood to fully appreciate biologic cancer therapies; therefore, these facets are reviewed briefly in this chapter. Basic science research into many apects of the immune system has produced immunotherapeutics such as cytokines, monoclonal antibodies, cellular therapies, vaccines, and gene therapies that are currently under investigation in clinical trials. A review of these new alternative forms of therapy is the fundamental purpose of this chapter.

Manual of Clinical Oncology, 7th edition, Edited by Raphael E. Pollock
ISBN 0-471-23828-7, pages 99–130. Copyright © 1999 Wiley-Liss, Inc.

THE IMMUNE SYSTEM

The immune system is composed of a wide array of cell types but lymphocytes provide the specificity of the immune response. The immune system can largely be divided into the humoral branch and the cellular branch, which differ in both effector cell type and mechanism of antigen recognition. The T lymphocyte is responsible for many of the functions of the cellular branch such as delayed type hypersensitivity (DTH) and rejection of grafts and tumors. The humoral branch is largely associated with B lymphocytes and the production of antibodies (Abs).

Cellular Immunity

Thymus-derived lymphocytes, or T cells, are all CD3$^+$ cells that recognize antigens via the T cell receptor (TCR). This receptor has a specificity that is analogous to that of the immunoglobulins. T cells can be divided into two major types: CD8$^+$ cytotoxic T lymphocytes (CTLs), which are capable of direct cellular killing, and CD4$^+$ T helper (Th) lymphocytes, which produce cytokines (Fig. 5.1). CD8$^+$ T cells interact with target cells expressing human leukocyte antigen (HLA) class I molecules on their cell surface. The HLA class I molecule is ubiquitously expressed on all cells and

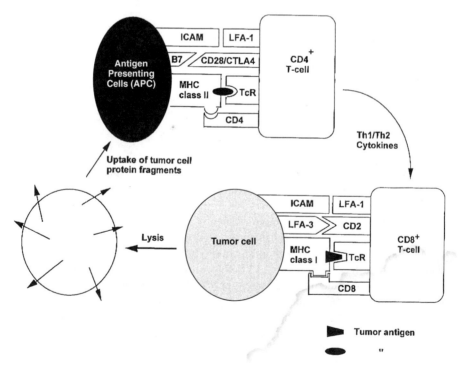

FIGURE 5.1. T helper cell binding to antigen presenting cells and cytotoxic T cell binding to tumor cells require specific MHC, adhesion, and accessory binding molecules.

presents short 8 to 10 amino acid peptides that have been processed from degraded endogenous self proteins or viral proteins. The CD8$^+$ T cell's TCR/CD3 complex specifically recognizes a single peptide/HLA complex and, along with secondary signals related to the interaction of an elaborate array of accessory molecules, is then triggered to destroy that cell by granule exocytosis. This process involves the release of cytolysin (perforin) and granzymes (serine protease containing granules), which leads to target apoptosis.

The CD4$^+$ T cell interacts with specialized antigen-presenting cells (APCs) such as macrophages, dedritic cells, and B lymphocytes that express HLA class II molecules (Fig. 5.1). HLA class II molecules present longer 12 to 20 amino acid peptides processed from exogenous proteins that have been taken up and processed by the APC. When a CD4$^+$ T cell's specific TCR has been activated, the cell begins to produce cytokines that enhance B cell antibody production, support T cell responses, and activate other immune cells. T helper cells can be further divided into subtypes based on their pattern of cytokine production, as well as the antigens that stimulate them and the immune responses that they support. Th1 cells promote cytotoxic cellular responses, DTH, and macrophage activation by secreting interleukin (IL)-2, interferon (IFN)-γ, and tumor necrosis factor (TNF)-β. Th2 cells support B cell responses and the production of IgG, IgA, and IgE Abs by secreting IL-4, IL-5, IL-6, and IL-10. Both subsets of CD4$^+$ cells produce TNF-α, IL-3, and granulocyte, macrophage colony stimulating factor (GM-CSF). Th1 cells are usually stimulated by infectious agents such as viruses and bacteria, whereas Th2 cells respond to allergens and parasites.

Natural killer (NK) cells are large granular cytotoxic lymphocytes that are distinct from T and B cells. NK cells participate in the host's first line of defense and are nonspecific. These cells are CD3$^-$ and do not express TCR. NK cells express the CD56 molecule that promotes cellular adhesion and the receptor for immunoglobulins (FcR). These cells participate in antibody-dependent cellular cytotoxicity (ADCC). NK cells are not target cell specific but demonstrate target cell selectivity by unknown mechanisms. Clearly, these cells are more cytotoxic for tumor cells and virally infected cells than for normal cells.

Humoral Immunity

"Bursa-equivalent" lymphocytes, B cells, are the major cell type of the humoral branch of the immune system. Whereas T cells are restricted to recognizing processed antigens from only protein sources and presented in the context of "self" HLA molecules, B cells can recognize unprocessed antigens and outside the context other molecules. Also, these antigens may be polysaccharides, nucleic acids, or proteins. Abs form tight, noncovalent complexes with specific antigens and act first as cell surface receptors. Once a B cell becomes activated by the binding of a cell surface Ab to its specific target antigen, the cell undergoes maturation to a plasma cell producing the specific immunoglobulin bound. The Abs are then soluble, secreted molecules that bind the target fixing complement, marking it for phagocytosis, or initiating ADCC.

All Abs are composed of two identical heavy and light chains that are covalently bound by disulfide bonds forming a Y-shaped molecule. There are five major classes of Abs, which differ in structure and function. IgG Abs are monomers with a γ-heavy chain and four subclasses. IgG Abs fix complement, cross the placenta, bind monocytes and neutrophils, and are the predominant Abs in secondary immune responses. IgM Abs are pentamers with a μ-heavy chain and two subclasses. IgM Abs fix complement, are involved in primary immune responses, and function as lymphocyte surface receptors and as accessory secretory Abs. IgA Abs are monomers with an α-heavy chain and two subclasses. Iga Abs predominate in secretions. IgD Abs are monomers with a δ-heavy chain. IgD Abs are thought to act as lymphocyte receptors. IgE Abs are monomers with ε-heavy chains. IgE Abs bind basophils and mast cells and are effectors of allergic and anaphylactic reactions.

The specificity of an Ab is determined by gene rearrangement in the variable domains of the heavy and light chains. Within these variable regions are three distinct widely separated areas that are hypervariable. These segments are called collectively the complementary determining regions (CDRs). When the polypeptide is folded, these CDRs are brought together to form the antigen binding site. The diversity of Abs is generated by gene rearrangements within the variable region genes, as well as in the D and J joining genes, of both the heavy and light chains in addition to the CDRs. The diversity and specificity of the TCR are similarly determined.

Cytokines

Cytokines may be defined as immunobiologically active molecules produced by defined cell populations that either enhance or suppress specific immunologic functions (Table 5.1). Certain cytokines enhance the expression of target antigens, HLA molecules (IFN-γ), or antigen-presenting cells (GM-CSF). Other biologicals may facilitate antigen presentation by providing accessory signals that enhance the ability of lymphocytes to respond to mitogenic stimuli (IL-1, TNF, IL-6, IL-7, IL-12). The absence of such accessory signals can lead to immunologic anergy. The cytokines IL-2 and IL-4 may augment T-cell proliferation and overcome the requirement for cellular cooperation in the generation of cytotoxic T-cell responses. Finally, lymphocytes and some tumors may produce molecules such as transforming growth factor (TGF)-β and IL-10 that suppress immune responses.

BIOLOGIC CANCER THERAPY

Several factors suggest the presence of host immune influences on cancer such as spontaneous regression, the latency period prior to metastasis or recurrence, and metastatic spread without known primary lesion. These observations have prompted much interest in immunotherapies, and these interests have led to the foundation of an ever expending field of research. Currently, biologic therapies attempt by many different strategies to induce specific immune responses against a cancer and provide long-term protective immunity. Prior to the recent accumulation of an enor-

TABLE 5.1. Cytokines and Their Actions

Cytokine	Source	Action	Upregulates	Downregulates	Clinical uses
IL-2	Activated lymphocytes	T cell proliferation; T and B cell activation; NK cell, macrophage activation; TIL, LAK, and CTL growth	TNF, IFN-γ, GM-CSF, IL-7		Melanoma, renal cell carcinoma
IL-4	Lymphocytes	B-cell stimulatory factor; T and B cell activation; macrophage, mast cell activation	HLA class II antigens Immunoglobulin expression	IL-1, IFN-γ, TNF, IL-6	Melanoma, renal cell carcinoma
TNF-α	T and B cells, macrophages, neutrophils, endothelial cells, tumor cells	B- and T-cell stimulator; inflammatory mediator; tumoricidal	HLA class I, IL-6 GM-CSF, ICAM-1		Melanoma, sarcoma (isolated hyperthermic limb perfusion) Mesothelioma
IFN-γ	Lymphocytes, T cells	Development of CTL, NK cells, macrophages	HLA class I and II antigens; Adhesion molecules		
IFN-α	Leukocytes	Increases activity of NK cells, macrophages; tumoricidal	HLA class I antigens, Tumor antigens		Adjuvant therapy for metastatic melanoma, renal cell carcinoma hematologic malignancies

(continued)

103

TABLE 5.1. (continued)

Cytokine	Source	Action	Upregulates	Downregulates	Clinical Uses
IL-1	Monocytes/macrophages, NK cells, fibroblasts, T cells, tumor cells	Inflammatory responses; endogenous pyrogen; prostaglandin release; T- and B-cell activation; fibroblast growth factor	T-helper responses, TNF, GM-CSF, IL-2, IL-2 receptor, IL-3, IL-4, IL-6, IL-7 ICAM-1		Platelet recovery after chemotherapy
IL-6	T and B cells, platelets, fibroblasts, macrophages, tumor cells	B cell growth factor; hepatocyte growth; stimulates acute phase reactants	HLA class I antigens		Melanoma
IL-7	Keratinocytes dendritic cells, T-cell subsets	Stimulator of lymphocyte growth and differentiation	IL-6	TCF-β	Melanoma
IL-12	B cells, monocytes/ macrophages	Lymphocyte stimulatory factor; tumoricidal	NK cells, IFN-γ, TNF, GM-CSF, IL-3	IL-4	Renal cell carcinoma
Colony-stimulating Factors					
IL-3	Activated lymphocytes	Hematopoietic growth factor			Bone marrow rescue
G-CSF	Monocytes/macrophages	Growth and differentiation of hematopoietic precursors			Bone marrow rescue
GM-CSF	T-cells, macrophages	Growth and differentiation of hematopoietic precursors	Antigen presenting cells, TNF, PGE-2		Bone marrow rescue

mous amount of information regarding the specifics of antitumor immune responses, investigators attempted nonspecific induction of the immune system and were encouraged by occasional tumor regression and even complete, durable responses in animal studies. These findings and the recent advances in our understanding of the immune system have led to many clinical trials of biologic therapies both specific and nonspecific in nature.

Cytokines

The use of cytokines that are known to have accessory function in the generation of T-cell-mediated immunity is a logical approach to cancer immunotherapy that has been studied in some detail. The hypothesis is that such signals could be lacking or deficient in the tumor-bearing host. Because T-cell recognition of antigen in the absence of accessory signals can lead to immunologic anergy, this pathway is of extreme importance. Systemic administration, or more elegantly, vaccination with cells expressing such cytokines, would be expected to be of benefit. In addition to modifying the in vivo inflammatory environment, cytokine transduction may cause other phenotypic changes in tumors. An autocrine action of cytokines may be linked to cell growth, secondary cytokine production, and the secreted extracellular matrix.

Inflammatory/T Cell Reactive Cytokines

IL-2   IL-2 is the most extensively studied cytokine to date. It is a lymphocyte secreted, 15-kDa glycoprotein produced in response to several stimuli (Table 5.1). Systemic administration of IL-2 alone and in combination with other cytokines has been studied in several trials, principally for patients with melanoma and renal cell carcinoma. As it has been studied for the longest period of time of any of the cytokines, data regarding the consistency of IL-2 responses are substantial. Most protocols involve high-dose bolus regimens of 720,000 international units (IU)/kg/8 h on days 1 to 5 and 15 to 19, repeated every 4 to 6 weeks. Other trials have involved lower doses (72,000 IU/kg), or continuous infusion therapy, and have demonstrated results similar to those of high-dose treatment schemes. The lower dosing schedules substantially reduce the toxicity associated with higher dose therapy which includes capillary leak syndrome, hypotension, azotemia, and metabolic acidosis. Toxicity seems related to induction of TNF-α, and the magnitude of this response appears to be genetically determined, resulting in individual variation in the clinical significance of the toxic response.

   Overall response rates of approximately 20% (approximately 20% of these are complete) have been achieved, evaluating a variety of dosing levels and schedules. Meta-analyses reveal that a survival advantage may be conferred to patients with excellent performance status compared to standard nonbiologic therapy. Combinations of IL-2 and IFN-α have been used in the treatment of renal cell carcinoma and melanoma, and have demonstrated responses similar to IL-2 alone. Adding cisplatinum to the IL-2 + IFN-α regimen may well enhance the antitumor response in patients with metastatic melanoma, and produced a 54% response rate in a recent trial. IL-2 has been tested in the treatment of a variety of hematologic malignancies, with occasional responses documented. The combination of IL-2 and melatonin has been evaluated in several clinical trials involving patients with hepatocellular carcinoma, non-small-cell lung cancer, and renal cell cancer. Objective responses have occurred in all disease types, some of which were improved compared to the use of IL-2 alone and associated with less toxicity.

IL-4 IL-4 is a lymphocyte-derived 20-kDa glycoprotein originally termed B-call stimulatory factor (Table 5.1). IL-4 is currently being investigated in clinical protocols involving patients with renal cell carcinoma and melanoma, and appears less effective in inducing antitumor responses than IL-2 in solid tumors, but may have more activity against hematologic malignancies, specifically B cell lymphomas and myelomas. Combinations of IL-2 and IL-4 have also been evaluated without significant responses to date.

TNF-α TNF-α is a 17-kDa protein first described as a serum component responsible for inducing hemorrhagic necrosis of certain tumors in vivo (Table 5.1). Systemically administered TNF-α alters the growth of some tumor cell lines in vitro and in vivo, perhaps by acting on tumor microvasculature. However, high systemic levels of TNF-α induce a septic-shock-like syndrome associated with tissue injury, organ failure, and cachexia. Clinical cancer trials have been largely disappointing; however, TNF alone or with IFN-α in hyperthermic isolated limb perfusion protocols for patients with melanoma and sarcoma have been associated with significant tumor responses and have obviated the need for amputation in some patients. Regional toxicity has also been reported, and has resulted in ischemic compartment syndromes in affected limbs.

IFN-γ IFN-γ is a 20-kDa glycoprotein demonstrating divergent properties in different tumor models (Table 5.1). This cytokine has been reported to promote tumorigenicity and metastatic potential in certain murine systems, whereas it has demonstrated antineoplastic activity in other models. Clinically, the most encouraging data have come from studies involving patients with malignant mesothelioma who demonstrated approximately 15% response rates to intrapleural therapy.

IFN-α IFN-α is another member of the IFN family, and is a leukocyte-secreted cytokine possessing tumoricidal effects (Table 5.1). The treatment of several human malignancies by IFN-α has been evaluated, particularly renal cell carcinoma, melanoma, and hematologic malignancies. IFN-α is currently recommended as an initial treatment for patients with hairy cell and chronic myelogenous leukemias, and is capable of inducing hematologic and karyotypic remissions in treated patients.

Recently, Kirkwood et al. from the Eastern Cooperative Oncology Group (ECOG) published the most compelling evidence to date regarding the efficacy of systemically administered IFN-α2b in patients with malignant melanoma. In a multicenter randomized trial comparing adjuvant high-dose interferon for 52 weeks to observation for the same period, a significant prolongation of relapse-free and overall survival was observed. The patients most likely to benefit from this therapy were individuals with regional lymph node metastases. The associated toxicity was significant, however, and a substantial proportion of patients could not tolerate full treatment dosing schedules, and/or experienced significant or life-threatening toxicity including myelosuppression, hepatotoxicity, and neurologic symptoms.

Combinations of IFN-α and standard chemotherapy agents have been evaluated in the treatment of several solid tumor types. Although occasional responses have been observed, the addition of IFN-α to established chemotherapy regimens has not produced dramatic changes in response rates, but does appear to alter the pharmacokinetics and toxicity profiles of many therapies, some adversely.

IL-1 IL-1 is a 17-kDa cytokine initially recognized for its effect as an endogenous pyrogen (Table 5.1). IL-1 expression is stimulated by endotoxin, exotoxins, TNF-α, and GM-CSF. This cytokine has been observed to induce cytotoxic effects in certain tumors, but its significant toxic side effects have limited its clinical utility. Antitumor effects of IL-1 administration have been disappointing, but combinations of IL-2 and IL-1 have suggested activity in phase II trials of patients with a variety of metastatic solid tumor malignancies. Further, IL-1 may play a role in enhancing platelet recovery following chemotherapy and has been studied in this capacity.

IL-6 IL-6 is a 25-kDa glycoprotein that has demonstrated significant antineoplastic activity in tumor-bearing mice, the effect of which was abrogated by sublethal irradiation of the animals (Table 5.1). In a melanoma model, IL-6 differentially regulated the growth of metastatic and nonmetastatic cells. IL-6 has been clinically evaluated both as a platelet growth factor and as an antineoplastic agent. It appears to function more effectively in the former role than in the latter. Results of current studies have been mixed in a variety of tumor types, although anecdotal reports of response by melanoma patients are encouraging. Toxicity of therapy includes anemia, neurologic symptoms, cardiac arrhythmias, and constitutional symptoms.

IL-7 IL-7 is a 25-kDa glycoprotein found to be a more potent generator of antitumor cytotoxic T cells in a murine model than IL-2 (Table 5.1). In addition, intratumoral injection of high doses of IL-7 resulted in decreased tumor growth and rejection in a proportion of animals treated. Mice that rejected tumors after IL-7 administration were found to be specifically immune to subsequent tumor challenge. Currently, there are no specific clinical protocols involving direct administration of IL-7. There is one phase I protocol evaluating IL-7 in a gene therapy tumor vaccine model for melanoma, however, that is discussed later in the section on gene therapy.

IL-12 IL-12 is a disulfide-linked heterodimer composed of 40- and 35-kDa subunits, both of which are required for biologic activity (Table 5.1). Because of this unique structure, IL-12 has a longer half-life (measured in hours) compared to other cytokines, and its longer duration of action may allow less frequent dosing schedules and possibly less associated toxicity. Recently, IL-12 was shown to stimulate T-helper subpopulation Th1 cells, which characteristically secrete IL-2, IFN-γ, and

TNF-β. Cells of the Th2 lineage are less affected by IL-12. Systemic and intratumoral administration of recombinant IL-12 to tumor-bearing animals caused growth inhibition of established primary and metastatic lesions that was at least partially dependent on CD8$^+$ cells. Mice were specifically immune to tumor rechallenge in certain systems. Clinical trials have recently been initiated, and responses in patients with metastatic renal cell cancer have been suggested.

Colony-Stimulating Factors

IL-3   In a comparison with several other cytokines, exogenous IL-3 administration was found to enhance the immunogenicity of irradiated tumor cells most significantly, including a nonimmunogenic tumor (Table 5.1). Clinical use has primarily involved bone marrow rescue with principal responses involving leukocytes and platelets. Combinations of IL-3 and other colony-stimulating factors are also ongoing.

Granulocyte Colony-Stimulating Factor (G-CSF)   G-CSF is an approximately 20-kDa glycoprotein that is not species specific, and, therefore, demonstrates biologic activity in human and murine models (Table 5.1). Clinical trials using this cytokine have demonstrated its efficacy in reducing the period of myelosuppression after chemotherapy for solid and hematologic malignancies, as well as in the setting of bone marrow transplantation.

Granulocyte, Macrophage Colony-Stimulating Factor (GM-CSF)   Clinical trials using this 22-kDa cytoline have reported increased peripheral granulocyte counts after myelosuppressive treatment in cytopenic patients (Table 5.1). GM-CSF may also act to enhance cytokine levels in treated patients, thereby promoting antineoplastic inflammatory responses.

Monoclonal Antibodies (MAbs)

Whereas a substantial number of investigations have focused on immunotherapy protocols designed to alter or enhance cell-mediated antitumor activity, manipulation of the humoral immune system represents a relatively underutilized area of inquiry. For decades, it has been known that tumors possess antigens that, although relatively weak immunogenically, may be recognized as foreign by the immunocompetent host. For certain tumors, Abs to these antigens have been identified that have been useful in clinical determinations of disease presence or recurrence as in the case of carcinoembryonic antigen (CEA) for assessing colorectal cancer, α-fetoprotein for testicular tumors and hepatocellular carcinoma, and prostate-specific antigen for prostate carcinoma.

MAb Production   MAbs are generated by fusing B lymphocytes to a murine myeloma cell line, resulting in a hybridoma that may produce large quantities of a single Ab type, each with unique specificity. MAbs have been evaluted as therapeutic as well as diagnostic tools in cancer therapy with varying degrees of success. MAb therapy is limited by physical characteristics of tumors, including variations in tumor vascularity and cellular density which often inhibits the ability of MAbs to sufficiently penetrate bulky tumors. Construction of Abs that recognize only tumor tissue and ignore nonneoplastic cells is difficult, also. Further, tumor antigen heterogeneity also impedes the ability of MAbs to generate clinically significant tumoricidal effects. Probably the most significant obstacle to MAb efficacy is the reaction to the murine component of the antibody which is recognized as foreign by human hosts, resulting in the generation of human antimouse Ab (HAMA) reactions that destroy circulating MAbs, and enhance their serum clearance. Attempts to reduce the immunogenicity of MAbs have included the use of antibody fragments that lack the Fc domain (the portion binding the effector cell). However, reduced binding affinity typically accompanies the loss of this portion of the antibody. Generation of human MAbs has been attempted, also.

MAb/Immunotoxins One strategy used to enhance the clinical efficacy of MAbs has been to combine antibodies with known cellular toxins to create immunotoxins. Several clinical trials have evaluated the use of various forms of ricin immunotoxins. Whereas antitumor responses have occurred in a minority of patients and have been transient, these immunotoxins have been associated with consistent toxic effects in patients that include fatigue/myalgias, capillary leak syndromes, elevation of hepatic transaminases, as well as bone marrow suppression. In two studies involving breast carcinoma patients, substantial neurotoxicity was observed, the etiology of which was attributed to cross-reactivity to antigens contained within neural tissue.

Bispecific MAbs Another strategy involves the construction of bispecific MAbs that target additional effectors of the immune system as well as tumor antigens. For example, some MAbs have dual specificity for tumor antigens and the CD3/TCR or the CD16/FcRIII receptor on NK cells. This technology has been used in clinical trials directed toward B cell neoplasms in certain patients, but disappointing results have been obtained thus far.

MAb/Conjugates Other MAb models have employed drug immunoconjugates in which the antibody is fused to a chemotherapeutic drug such as doxorubicin. Radioimmunoconjugates have also been created in which radioactive sources such as ^{125}I and ^{131}I have been combined with MAbs to elicit antineoplastic responses. Limitations common to all of these manipulations continue to be HAMA responses and host toxicity induced by cross-reactivity with rapidly dividing normal cells (bone marrow, etc.)

Clinical Results Results of clinical trials of MAbs have been disappointing overall, but a few responses have been noted. A murine IgM MAb JD118 specific for neoplastic B cells has been constructed and found to destroy human leukemia and lymphoma cells in the presence of human complement. An anti-CD19 MAb HD37 induced cell cycle arrest in several Burkitt's lymphoma cell lines in vitro and in a xenograft model. Also, treatment with an antiganglioside MAb caused objective antitumor responses in patients with metastatic melanoma as well as neuroblastoma. Finally, a large randomized trial demonstrated that adjuvant therapy with a murine MAb 17-1A recognizing a 37-kDa cell surface glycoprotein induced improved remission durations and extended overall survival in patients with resected, locally metastatic colorectal carcinomas. Although MAb therapy remains a theoretically intriguing focus of attention, it has yet to overcome the problem of significant toxicity and host inactivation.

Cellular Therapy

With the discovery of IL-2 and the ability to efficiently expand T cells in culture, the idea of cellular therapies became a true possibility. As has been previously discussed, systemic IL-2 induces an anticancer response but with high levels of toxicity. These findings stimulated interest in adoptive immunotherapy that involves the transfer of specific immune cells with antitumor activity to the tumor-bearing host with less anticipated toxicity. The vast majority of clinical experience has been gained from IL-2-generated lymphokine-activated killer (LAK) cells and more recently from tumor-infiltrating lymphocytes (TILs).

LAK Cell Therapy   LAK cells are a heterogeneous population of cells made up of T cells and NK cells harvested from the peripheral blood that develop antitumor activity after incubation in high doses of IL-2. The mechanism of selective cellular killing is unknown; however, these cells maintain their antitumor activity in vivo with exogenous IL-2 administration. LAK cells were first described in 1980, and clinical studies to determine the safety of infusional therapies were initiated shortly thereafter at the NCI. The first series was published in 1985 of 25 patients demonstrating the effectiveness of the therapy with regression of metastatic cancer of several histologies in some patients. The follow-up series of 178 consecutive patients treated with LAK cells at the NCI revealed a 14% complete response (CR) and 30% partial response (PR), with the best results seen in renal cell carcinoma (35% CR + PR), melanoma (21% CR + PR), and non-Hodgkin's lymphoma (57% CR + PR). Other institutions have reported variable results with response rates for melanoma (0 to 56%, composite = 18%), renal cell (0 to 50%, composite = 27%), lymphoma (0 to 100%, composite = 50%), and colorectal (0 to 100%, composite = 9%). The composite results are from pooled data from nine studies. The variability of results between institutions was likely due to differences in the numbers of infused LAK cells, the length of time cells were incubated in IL-2, and the dose and method of systemic IL-2 administration. The duration of response was usually less than 6 months; however, long-term CRs have been reported. Significant toxicity was reported in most studies related to the systemic IL-2. In a prospective randomized study between IL-2 alone and IL-2 + LAK, the latter resulted in an improved response rate, but only represented a statistically nonsignificant trend toward improved overall survival.

With the sentinel report in 1986 describing the enhanced antitumor activity of tumor-infiltrating lymphocytes (TILs), most of the clinical attention has shifted away from LAK cells. However, some recent reports have looked at new ways to develop LAK cells in IL-12 instead of IL-2, and new ways to use LAK cells such as in the treatment of myelodysplastic syndrome. The regional use of LAK cells has also been reported such as intraperitoneal or intrapleural administration and even intralesional therapy in neurologic malignancies.

TIL Therapy   TILs are reported to be 50 to 100 times more potent on a cell-to-cell basis than LAK cells in antitumor activity as demonstrated in animal models. TILs are derived from an individual's surgically resected tumor by cell separation. These T cells have been shown to be cytotoxic for the tumor cells, and this killing shown to be limited to the individual's tumor suggesting HLA restriction. In fact, it is now widely accepted that TILs recognize and lyse tumor cells by CD3–TCR interaction with HLA class I/peptide complexes on the tumor cell surface. Many of the involved TCRs, HLA class I molecules, and even peptides in this specific recognition are now known and the latter are being investigated in vaccine trials.

In 1988, the NCI reported the first clinical trial with TIL demonstrating complete and partial regression of melanoma in some patients. The follow-up series of 86 melanoma patients revealed a 34% CR + PR. This response rate is almost twice the composite response rate for LAK cells in melanoma and has been confirmed at other institutions with some variation in results. Similar to the LAK cell trials, variable results appear to be related to IL-2 dose and administration, TIL number, and most importantly TIL culture characteristics. Better results are seen with cultures grown over shorter periods of time, that are predominantly CD8$^+$, and that demonstrate in vitro antitumor activity.

In renal cell carcinoma, there does not appear to be a significantly improved response rate between TIL and LAK cells. Some response has been seen with TIL therapy in both the treatment of primary lung cancer as well as the often associated malignant effusions. Several groups have utilized TIL in ovarian cancer with and without chemotherapy with some success. Intraperitoneal TIL infusions + IL-2 resulted in some marginal clinical activity; however, the results with combination therapy are very promising with TIL + cyclophosphamide (14% CR and 57% PR) and TIL + cisplatinum (70% CR and 20% PR). TIL studies on other malignancies are currently underway.

Some limitations to TIL therapies include the need for surgically resected tumor and 4 to 6 weeks to grow TIL cultures. Some groups have overcome the necessity of surgery by isolating tumor-associated lymphocytes from malignant ascites and/or effusions. The culture expansion time can be decreased with nonspecific stimulation and cytokines but often at the expense of the tumor-specific cytotoxicity of the TIL. Because the latter is the best predictor of clinical response, the goal is efficient culture conditions with improved tumor reactivity. Current advances have included repeat in vitro stimulation with tumor cells and most recently with newly identified, HLA-presented, immunodominant peptides. In vitro peptide stimulation has resulted in TILs 50 to 100 times more potent than TILs grown conventionally. This enhanced efficiency may allow for clinically effective peripheral blood lymphocyte (PBL) cultures, obviating the need for surgically resected tumor. Other attempts to improve adoptive immunotherapy include in vivo stimulation with tumor immunization and subsequent harvest of the draining lumph nodes as the source of TILs. This method has been studied in preliminary clinical trials without apparent improvement in response. Some other groups have modified the TILs with transduced cytokine genes to enhance their potency whereas others are experimenting with combination therapies with other immunomodulators or chemotherapies. Clinical studies investigating these methods are being performed.

Vaccines

The concept of vaccinations against cancer analogous to antiviral vaccines has been intriguing researchers since the beginning of the field of biologic cancer therapy. Recent advances in the understanding of the immune response to tumors has brought this notion to clinical trial in many forms. All types of cancer vaccines have as a common denominator the need to induce a host immunologic response against specific antigens to rid or protect the host from the malignancy. The first step in vaccine development is to determine the specific antigens of concern (Fig. 5.1). Optimally, these antigens will efficiently stimulate a tumor-specific, tumor-protective immune response. The discovery of tumor-specific antigens (TSAs), expressed exclusively on tumors, and tumor-associated antigens (TAAs), expressed preferentially on tumors, has accelerated in the 1990s, leading to new candidate antigens for vaccines. Some groups argue that the exact antigens need not be known and favor whole tumor cell vaccines or viral oncolysates in order to induce an immune response against many tumor antigens, thus addressing the issue of heterogeneous antigen expression in the tumor. Despite these differences, all vaccine regimens require stimulation of the host with nonspecific immunoadjuvants to enhance the vaccine efficiency.

Immune Adjuvants and Immunomodulators   Immune adjuvants are substances that nonspecifically enhance the immune response to antigens. These substances can generally be classified as bacterial products, polysaccharides (glucans), immunogenic proteins (keyhole limpet hemocyanin, KLH), haptens, or synthetic products. The bacterial products are either cell wall components or intact organisms such as viable bacillus Calmette-Guerin (BCG), viable/Pen-G-inactivated Group A streptococcus (OK-432), or nonviable *C. parvum*. Haptens such as dinitrophenyl (DNP) or TNP either supply helper determinants or act as neoantigens. Purified or synthetic products such as muramyl dipeptides, trehalose, or endotoxins (lipid A) have also been studied. These substances can also be utilized in combination.

Immunomodulators are substances such as the interleukins, the colony-stimulating factors, and the interferons previously described. This group also includes levamisole and the thymic hormones. Levamisole is a synthetic antihelminthic with immunostimulatory abilities. This drug stimulates monocytes, macrophages, and neutrophiles in both chemotaxis and phagocytosis. It also augments IL-2-induced T cell proliferation and demonstrates Fc receptor activity. Levamisole has been studied as a single anticancer agent with variable results, but has been most extensively used in combination with 5-fluorouracil (5-FU) for the treatment of Dukes' C colon cancer. The thymic hormones include thymosins (α and β), thymosin fraction 5 (TF-5), and thymopoetin pentapeptide (TP-5). These substances have been shown to promote the proliferation/maturation of T cell precursors. Most of the research utilizing the thymic hormones has been in the area of restoration of the immune system after immunosuppression with chemotherapy or radiotherapy, and some survival advantage has been seen in non-small-cell lung, breast, and ovarian cancers.

The therapeutic benefit of most immune adjuvants and immunomodulators is dependent on their use in combination with other biologic therapies or chemotherapies with the notable exceptions of BCG in bladder cancer and IFN-α in hairy cell leukemia.

Whole Tumor Cell Vaccines (WTCVs)   The majority of clinical data on anticancer vaccines have been generated in WTCV studies, and all other vaccines are compared against these data. The theoretical advantages of a WTCV is that individual antigens do not need to be known. The latter requires an enormous amount of work and, theoretically, must be individualized in each cancer. Because the whole tumor cell is utilized, it should express all the possibly important antigens, and the tumor cell itself can act as an APC. The tumor cell can also be genetically altered to enhance its ability to express and present antigens. The theoretical disadvantages would include safety issues of introducing tumor cells into a patient. This concern is obviously less for patients who already have cancer but would be more of an issue in production of preventative vaccines, as would the source of tumor cells for the latter vaccine. Any alterations in the tumor cell to decrease its virulence for safety purposes may diminish its effectiveness as a vaccine. The whole tumor cell also expresses many irrelevant antigens, and the expression of the relevant antigens may be low. The tumor cell may also be an inefficient APC. For these and other concerns, it is not surprising that early clinical trials in melanoma with unaltered, irradiated, autologous WTCVs were disappointing (1 CR/64 patients in four studies). The addition of immunoadjuvants such as BCG and microbial antigens enhanced the performance of the WTCVs (10 to 20% overall response rates), and in one study of advanced melanoma by Seigler et al. utilizing a complicated regimen of BCG sensitization followed by vaccination with BCG and then finally autologous and allogenic WTCs, the disease-free survival (DFS) was 32% at 2 years. The results of this study are difficult to assess fully because of a high dropout rate and lack of controls.

Several studies have looked at combination therapy with WTCVs and chemotherapy in metastatic melanoma. Only one randomized study has shown an improvement in response rates in the biochemotherapy group, but this study had many protocol problems and many of the partial responders had mixed responses with progression of disease at other sites. Survival was not improved. The failure of these WTCVs is possibly related to overall tumor burden; therefore, several studies were designed to vaccinate patients rendered surgically free of disease but at a high risk of recurrence. The results of these studies have been mixed, with two of the studies being halted because tumors in the biochemotherapy group appeared to be recurring more frequently than in the control chemotherapy group. This observation did not prove to be true on subsequent follow-up, however. Morton et al. reported a 45% recurrence rate in a randomized surgery + WTCV group as compared to 59% in a surgery alone group. Survival was not affected, however, in these 95 patients. Other studies have likewise found no survival benefit to WTCV as compared to chemotherapy alone in advanced melanoma.

Some other tumor histologies have also been studied such as colorectal, renal cell, and non-small-cell lung cancer. Although it has been difficult to demonstrate an endogenous immune response in colorectal cancer save its responsiveness to the immunostimulator levamisole, several groups have attempted WTCVs after surgical resection for advanced disease. Hoover et al. reported a significant increase in 10-year DFS in patients vaccinated with BCG + autologous WTC in colon cancer but not rectal cancer. This finding had not been confirmed in the multiinstitutional, randomized ECOG trial at the time of the interim analysis; however, this study had many design and accrual difficulties. The studies in renal cell carcinoma to date show a few significant objective responders although tumor regression was rare. Perlin et al. showed a strong trend toward better DFS in non-small-cell lung cancer vaccinated with BCG + allogeneic WTC after surgery, but this was not yet significant.

Other attempts to improve WTCV have included the addition of the immunopotentiating cyclophosphamide to overcome immunologic tolerance and the modification of WTCV to make them more antigenic. Cyclophosphamide in low doses augments both humoral and cellular immunity as has been shown in many clinical studies demonstrating enhanced Ab and DTH responses to WTCV. However, this improvement in immune parameters has not translated into improved disease response rates. The xenogenization of tumor cells with animal proteins or viruses is thought to enhance the immune response to a tumor cell by adding T helper determinants or new immunogens. This form of WTCV modification has been studied with goat and rabbit globulins, as well as the Newcastle virus, without significant improvement in disease response rates over unmodified WTCVs, although some impressive durable responses have been seen. Berd et al. have reported that haptenization with DNP has shown a significantly improved DFS at 33 months as compared with their earlier results with an unmodified WTCV, although this is a nonrandomized study. Other clinical studies are underway with genetically modified WTCV and are discussed later in the section on gene therapy.

Viral Oncolysates Vaccines (VOVs)   The oncolytic property of viruses has been known for many years and has been shown to induce protective immunity in animals that survived the viral oncolysis. The same protective immunity for a specific tumor could be induced if animals were injected with the oncolysates, the products of viral oncolysis, prepared from the same tumor. The mechanism by which oncolysates induce an immune response is felt to be due to haptenization of tumor antigens with viral antigens. The theoretical advantages of VOVs include not needing to identify specific antigens, less safety concern than using whole tumor cells, preserved antigen diversity, and enhancement of antigenicity with viral haptenization. The theoretical disadvantages would include safety concerns over viral infection because these vaccines are inactivated when the virus is killed. Further, the VOVs include mostly irrelevant antigens and are derived mostly from cultured

MHC-unmatched cell lines, not from the patient's own tumor. Some of the earlier clinical studies were accomplished by in vivo preparation of the VOVs to overcome the latter concern by intralesional injection of the virus. This technique resulted in unpredictable results secondary to the lack of standardization between studies. More recent studies have utilized in vitro VOV preparations and have been performed in melanoma, colorectal, and ovarian cancer. Early in vitro VOVs produced minimal clinical response and resulted in toxicity associated with the influenza virus used in most of the VOVs. The change to vaccinina virus decreased the toxicity and revealed the best response in melanoma. The most extensively studied VOV for melanoma is the vaccinia melanoma oncolysate (VMO) prepared from four allogeneic melanoma cell lines. It has been shown to be well tolerated and resulted in a significantly improved DFS in phase II trials. Similar results have been reported by other groups. However, in a prospective, randomized phase III trial, there was no significant improvement in DFS or overall survival, although there were some encouraging trends toward improved survival on subset analysis.

Less information is available on VOV treatment of other tumor types. However, 9/40 ovarian patients had some clinical response to intraperitoneal influenza-modified allogeneic VOV, and 4/19 CR and 9/19 PR were seen in sarcoma patients treated with a combination of VOV + chemotherapy.

Tumor Antigen Vaccines (TAVs)   TAVs may be partially purified or highly purified/synthetic in nature. The pure antigen vaccines (PAVs) offer the best theoretical advantage over WTCVs by delivering the specific immunogenic antigen(s) that would induce an efficient, specific tumor-protective immunity without the irrelevant antigens or need of autologous or allogeneic tumor material. The PAVs could be easily and reproducibly manufactured, and delivered in high volumes safely. The obvious disadvantage is that effective TAA and/or TSA must be defined. A few of these antigens are known and clinical trials to test them just beginning. An intermediate form of vaccine between WTCVs and PAVs are partially purified vaccines (PPVs). These vaccines offer a theoretical advantage in that it is not necessary to know specific TAA and/or TSA, but are more selective than WTCVs, delivering fewer irrelevant antigens and are safer than the latter. PPVs have taken many forms such as soluble membrane extracts, autologous tumor protein polymer particles, and shed antigens. Clinical studies with extracts and protein polymers in melanoma demonstrated some clinical activity, but these studies were without controls. Melanoma-associated antigen (MAA) vaccines prepared by the collection and partial purification of shed antigens from multiple cultured melanoma cell lines have been reported by Bystryn et al. to increase the median DFS by 50% compared to pooled historical controls. Responders were accurately predicted by Ab and DTH responses, with the best results among those with both parameters. To date, this vaccine has not been evaluated in a prospective, randomized study.

Potential PAVs are becoming more common as more TAAs and TSAs are being described. Currently, in melanoma several protein products have been described as targets for cellular immunity. They include the MAGE-1 and MAGE-3 antigens presented by HLA-A1, and the HLA-A2-presented antigens derived from tyrosinase,

MART-1, and gp100/pmel 17. Ab responses have been reported to the protein gp75 and the gangliosides GM2 and GD2. These antigens are all being studied as PAVs in clinical trials. Preliminary studies with a MAGE-1-derived peptide vaccine have demonstrated induction of cellular and humoral responses in vivo; however, no clinical response data are available to date. In a prospective, randomized trial comparing vaccination of surgically free stage III melanoma patients with BCG or BCG + GM2, there was no significant increase in DFS or overall survival. However, there was a significantly improved DFI and overall survival in patients with anti-GM2 antibodies compared with those without. In an attempt to enhance the immunogenicity of GM2, a new conjugate with KLH is currently being tested by ECOG.

Much less work has been accomplished in epithelial tumors, but Ab responses have been shown to the Thomsen–Friedenreich antigen, and sialylated Tn overexpressed in epithelial tumors. Ab responses have also been described to p53 in several tumor histologies. Both Ab and CTL responses have been seen to viral transformation antigens in Hodgkin's disease and nasopharyngeal cancer (EBV) and cervical cancer (HPV). MUC-1, an antigen derived from the protein core of mucin molecules on the cell surface of epithelial tumors, has been described as a CTL target recognized in an HLA-unrestricted fashion. The latter fact has made this antigen the focus of several clinical trials because it may be universally applicable in epithelial tumors, although the mechanism of recognition is poorly understood.

The oncogene product HER2/neu has been demonstrated to be the target of both humoral and cellular immunity in many epithelial tumors such as ovarian, breast, pancreas, and non-small-cell lung cancer. Unlike MUC-1, the specific immunodominant peptides are presented in the context of HLA-A2, and induce a very specific, effective immune response. The PAV derived from HER2/neu may be very promising as 50% of the population is HLA-A2$^+$, and the HER2/neu antigen appears to be widely, and differentially, expressed in epithelial tumors. Clinical studies are just beginning, but animal immunizations against neu-derived peptides have induced both humoral and cellular immunity.

Gene Therapy

The concept of gene therapy focuses on the theory that the host response to tumorigenesis is deficient and might be improved given the introduction of either novel or excess levels of existing genes. A variety of strategies have been conceived to exploit this basic concept. Most gene therapy models have focused on melanoma and renal cell carcinoma because these two tumor types are considered more immunogenic than most other solid organ malignancies, and have demonstrated spontaneous regressions. Further, tumor antigens and cell-mediated immune responses to these neoplasms have been demonstrated in vitro and in vivo.

As previously discussed, biologic therapies for solid tumors originally concentrated on cytokines to augment host immune responses; likewise, early gene therapies have also concentrated on these substances. The large systemic doses of cytokines required to sustain biologically significant tissue levels have been associated with substantial toxicity and only modest antitumor responses. Therefore, searches for alternative delivery systems have resulted in multiple strategies to deliver relatively low, continuous concentrations of cytokines directly into tumor or effector cells by inserting the gene responsible for these protein products within a biologic (typically viral) vector capable of infecting designated target cells.

The introduction of novel genetic information (DNA) into eukaryotic cells has been accomplished by chemical, physical, and biologic means. Calcium phosphate transfection and electroporation are gene transfer techniques that have been useful in the laboratory but limited in their clinical application. The most widely used biologic gene transfer vehicles are modified RNA and DNA viruses. Murine retroviral vectors (RVVs) have been the most extensively studied. RVVs can transduce dividing cells, and allow stable integration of proviral sequences via a receptor-mediated process of endocytosis. This process is accompanied by certain limitations, however. Despite the introduction of safety features in viral and packaging systems, recombination events and the generation of wild-type virus are possible. There is also the absolute requirement for target cell replication at the time of retroviral infection to permit integration. Viral titers of moderate magnitude have been achieved.

Adeno-associated viruses (AAVs) and adenoviruses (AVs) represent two additional viral vectors that have been evaluated in gene transfer models. AAVs are single-stranded DNA (4.5kb) parvoviruses that are not pathogenic in humans and may integrate into the host genome at specific regions in chromosome 19. Recombinant AAV vectors allow the insertion of relatively small DNA constructs of up to 4 kb in size. AAV vectors may not require target cell replication for integration, and multiple concatemeric copies may be integrated per cell. High AAV titers also may be achieved.

Adenovirus-based vectors are currently being used for many gene transfer efforts because they combine the characteristics of high achieved titers and infection of nondividing cells with a broad host range and a tropism for epithelial tissue. Consequently, transduction efficiencies approach 80 to 90% of cells, in contrast to RVVs, which transduce between 5 and 20% of targets following multiple transduction attempts at high multiplicities of infection ratios. These viruses are composed of double-stranded DNA of approximately 35 kb. Recombinant adenovirus vectors may accommodate up to 7.5 kb of inserted DNA. Limitations of adenoviral vectors include the fact that proviral DNA is not integrated but rather episomally inserted into target cells, resulting in transient gene expression. Further, host immune reactions have been observed directed toward recognition of adenoviral proteins. These reactions have resulted in decreased gene expression and have necessitated repeated delivery of adenoviral vectors to the host.

Clearly, each vector system has advantages and disadvantages for use in different tumor models. A problem common to all vectors (although less so for adenoviral vectors) is that of low-level gene expression. Investigators have tried to optimize proviral gene expression using a variety of gene promoters and induction sequences. The cytomegalovirus (CMV) promoter has been used in a variety of systems with success in several tissue types. Regrettably, the CMV promoter also induces gene expression in nontargeted cells, and relatively low level expression in certain in vivo systems. To more precisely direct gene expression, tissue-specific promoters have been developed including the insulin promoter (for pancreatic islet cell transduction), the tyrosinase promoter (melanoma), the albumin promoter (liver), CEA promoter (GI tumors, breast, and lung adenocarcinomas), and the T cell receptor promoter (T lymphocytes). Although theoretically intriguing and logical, the use of these promoters in various viral constructs has not yet been demonstrated to be superior to nonspecific high-level promoters such as CMV in any models to date.

Target Cells for Gene Therapy

Lymphocytes   A variety of cells have been evaluated as targets of gene therapy. Early interest in activated lymphocytes was motivated by trials of LAK cells and TILs demonstrating antitumor activity in adoptive immunotherapy protocols. Initial studies of genetic modification of lymphocyte populations including Peripheral Blood Lymphocytes (PBL) seemed promising, and demonstrated successful transduction and selection of cells secreting proviral genetic elements. Rosenberg et al. at the NCI pioneered early efforts to transduce TILs, and initial reports suggested high-level gene expression, particularly of TNF. However, experience has demonstrated that lymphocytes are difficult to transduce with retroviral vectors because only a small percentage of cells are dividing during transduction and repeated transduction results in significant cell death. Similar difficulties exist with AAV vectors, and lymphocytes are impossible to transduce with AV constructs. Further, evidence of transcriptional silencing of gene products has tempered enthusiasm for transduction of lymphocytes. Finally, the debate continues on whether TILs selectively locate within tumors in greater numbers than PBL. Although the gene marking studies utilized to generate these data advanced the field in terms of quantitation of gene copy number within large groups of untransduced cells, the clinical ramifications of this effort have been minimal, except to move investigators away from transduction of mature lymphocytes. Stem cell and progenitor transduction has been attempted with greater efficiency than mature lymphocyte transduction and has been clinically successful in the treatment of patients with adenosine deaminase (ADA) deficiency. Certain models involving hematologic malignancies are currently being tested in clinical protocols involving the transduction of drug-resistance genes in hematologic and solid tumors utilizing retroviral vectors.

Fibroblasts   Given the recent findings that the particular properties of transduced cells do not necessarily affect antitumor effects, investigators have sought to transduce heartier cells that are easier to grow and maintain in vitro and in vivo. Several studies (principally involving IL-2 and IL-12) have evaluated the transduction of fibroblast cell lines such as NIH 3T3 cells and reintroduced transduced cells into a tumor-bearing host, either alone or in mixing experiments with tumor cells as vaccines. Transduction efficiencies have been high and antineoplastic responses have been observed. It may well be more cost effective and less labor intensive to maintain fibroblasts in culture than to attempt to grow tumor explants for ex vivo protocols.

Tumor Cells A variety of tumor cell lines are easily maintained in vitro and can maintain excellent growth kinetics despite multiple transduction attempts with cytokines and other types of genes. In addition, readministration of nondividing, irradiated tumor cells to patients has the theoretical advantage of stimulating a specific immune response in the host as in a vaccine model. Safety concerns of tumor growth following readministration have necessitated irradiation which still allows for continued proviral gene expression, albeit for shorter periods of time and at somewhat lower levels compared to nonirradiated cells. This model has been employed with varying degrees of success by many investigators, and is currently being evaluated in the majority of tumor-directed gene therapy clinical protocols.

Cytokines in Gene Therapy   The introduction and expression of cytokine genes in tumor cells may modify their phenotype and alter the tumor–host relationship. The introduction of virtually all inflammatory cytokines into tumors has been found to decrease tumorigenicity in vivo. Reduced primary tumor growth is largely due to the infiltration and activation of host effector cells. The composition and activity of the cellular infiltrate depends on the cytokine used, the amount produced, the ability of the host to generate responses, and inherent properties of the tumor. It has been difficult to demonstrate regression of established lesions in certain systems, likely owing to the fact that murine tumors appear to outgrow cytokine-transduced cells, thus exceeding the latter's ability to generate immunity in a short time period.

The initial response to tumor inoculation involves nonspecific inflammatory immune mechanisms both in the immunocompetent and the immunodeficient host. A major question yet to be resolved is how this initial response relates to the development of specific immunity that often follows primary tumor rejection. The mechanism of this "cross-talk" is unknown but presumably relates to the processing and presentation of antigens capable of generating target-specific tumor immunity. Gene therapy using cytokines as immunologic effectors has been attempted for virtually all known cytokines, with favorable in vivo and in vitro results in most systems. Rather than providing an exhaustive list that may be reviewed in other texts, a brief analysis of selected cytokine gene therapy models is provided.

IL-2 Gene-modified, IL-2-secreting tumors consistently have had dose-dependent decreased tumorigenicity irrespective of histology, immunogenicity, or metastatic potential without altering in vitro tumor growth or morphology. Nanogram levels (50 to 5,000 U/10^6 cells/24 h) of human IL-2 were produced in several engineered tumor cell lines. IL-2-transduced cells did not demonstrate changes in MHC antigens or adhesion molecules. An important observation is that IL-2-producing cells mixed in vitro with autologous or allogeneic lymphocytes generate enhanced in vitro lymphocyte cytotoxicity at levels that could not be reproduced by the addition of recombinant IL-2 to cultures. The growth of implanted tumors is inhibited when mixed with IL-2-producing cells injected at the tumor site, an effect not observed when the modified and unmodified cells are injected at sites remote from the tumor. This local "bystander" effect has been observed by several investigators.

T cells are not required for decreased in vivo tumorigenicity. IL-2-modified human and murine melanomas and sarcomas have retarded or absent growth in congenitally athymic (nude) mice, with such tumors generating a mononuclear cell infiltrate. In immunologically competent animals, IL-2-induced CD8$^+$ T-cell-mediated tumor rejection in a murine colon cancer model. Decreased tumorigenicity was shown to depend on NK cells in a nonimmunogenic murine fibrosarcoma and was associated with granulocyte activity in a murine breast carcinoma system.

The development of specific systemic immunity was reported in syngeneic animals rejecting weakly immunogenic tumors of varying histologies. At least one group has reported that an IL-2-dose-dependent window exists in the optimal generation of protective immunity to parental tumor challenge. The observation that tumor killing in the immunologically competent host occurred in the absence of CD4$^+$ cells led to a hypothesis that the T helper cell response may be insufficient (owing to unfavorable antigen–MHC complex presentation) to drive cytotoxic T cell generation against the tumor and that IL-2 could overcome this deficiency. Virtually all investigators have concluded that primary tumor rejection may be induced by nonspecific inflammatory responses (NK cells, neutrophils, or macrophages), but that T-cell-dependent systemic immunity develops in the same host.

IL-2 has been compared with several other inflammatory agents (IFN-γ, IFN-α, IL-7, GM-CSF) in tumor-directed gene therapy investigations. IL-2 was equal or superior to most other cytokines in the mediation of antitumor effects, particularly in T-cell-deprived animals. This finding, and the considerable clinical experience with this cytokine, has led to the development and approval of several clinical protocols studying the effects of IL-2-producing vectors and tumors.

IL-4   Despite the reported antiproliferative effects of IL-4, in vitro growth of IL-4-transduced tumors of several histologies producing 2,000 to 10,000 U/10^6 cells/48 h was not altered compared with implanted cells. IL-4-secreting cells were rejected after injection in immunocompetent and immunodeficient mice. This effect was reversed by administration of anti-IL-4 MAb. Reduced tumorigenicity was also demonstrated for untransduced murine melanoma and plasmacytomas when mixed with IL-4 producers before injection. Significant tumor regression was also observed in established plasmacytomas after intralesional injection of exogenous IL-4 or autologous tumor cells producing this cytokine.

IL-4-producing tumors in syngeneic mice induced the infiltration of eosinophils initially and the later accumulation of macrophages in several tumor models. Tepper et al. demonstrated that tumor rejection was abolished in syngeneic immunocompetent animals by depleting the hosts of mature granulocytes. Tumors were rejected in lymphocyte-depleted mice, but protective (T-cell-dependent) immunity against implanted tumor rechallenge was not observed, suggesting that nonspecific effectors were involved in primary tumor rejection, and confirming the requirement of T cells for the generation of immunologic memory. In two reports, the induction of systemic immunity was observed in immunocompetent animals rejecting IL-4-producing tumors. Tumor-specific immunity was completely abolished by MAb-depletion of CD8$^+$ cells and incompletely inhibited by CD4$^+$ cell depletion. The systemic immunity demonstrated in this model might have been due to enhanced tumor antigen presentation by the macrophage infiltrate induced by IL-4. Several clinical trials are currently in progress.

TNF-α   Several investigators have studied the properties of tumor cells lines engineered to produce TNF. TNF-transduced cells do not demonstrate altered cell growth or cell morphology in vitro. However, the efficiency of gene transduction of TNF-sensitive cells is low owing to cell death, suggesting that TNF-resistant cells are selected in such cultures. Deleterious host effects were not observed after injection of tumor cells producing TNF at levels <100 ng/10^6 cells/24 h; however, tumors producing much higher levels of this cytokine did demonstrate significant host toxicity and death. Inoculation of TNF-secreting tumors into syngeneic mice resulted in dose-dependent decreased tumorigenicity that was reversed by MAbs to TNF. Parental murine sarcomas were rejected by gene-modified cells injected at the same anatomic site, but not when the two cell types were implanted at different sites. Antineoplastic effects have been inconsistently observed in nude mice in certain models, but were reported in others.

The cellular infiltrate surrounding a TNF-producing murine plasmacytoma was predominantly composed of macrophages. Blankenstein et al. noted that the antitumor effect in this model was abolished by anti-type 3 complement receptor MAb that inhibited the migration of inflammatory cells such as neutrophils, NK cells, and macrophages. These findings emphasize the role of non-T-cell effectors in TNF-mediated antineoplastic responses. However, Asher et al. noted that immunologically intact animals experiencing complete regression of murine sarcomas were found to be specifically immune to subsequent tumor challenge and have a predominantly lymphocytic infiltrate. Selective depletion of CD4$^+$ or CD8$^+$ T cells completely abrogated the development of protective immunity in syngeneic mice. This finding documented the importance of T-cell-mediated immunity in this particular TNF-tumor model.

Asher et al. attempted to resolve the disparity between their findings and observations regarding the role of macrophages in inducing TNF-mediated antitumor responses by suggesting that secretion of a membrane-bound form of TNF might be incapable of recruiting other effectors. A therapeutic distinction between the membrane-bound and secretory forms of TNF was later described. Although both forms of TNF demonstrated biologic activity in vitro, only the secretory form reduced tumorigenicity in vivo. The mechanisms responsible for these divergent effects of the two TNF molecules remain unclear, but clinical protocols using secretory TNF gene-modified autologous tumors are in progress.

IL-7   Tumor models using cells engineered to secrete IL-7 in the range of 1 to 80 ng/10^6 cells/24 h demonstrated significant antineoplastic effects. No alterations of in vitro growth or cell morphology were observed in IL-7-secreting cells. An IL-7-producing melanoma cell line expressed lower levels of TGF-β messenger RNA and protein compared with untransduced or IL-2-transduced cells. Expression of melanoma antigens MAGE-1 and MAGE-3 was not altered by cytokine gene transfer. IL-7-transduced cell lines had decreased tumorigenicity in immunocompetent syngeneic mice. Animals rejecting these tumors were immunologically protected against tumor rechallenge. In nude mice, however, growth of gene-modified tumors was either unchanged or slightly decreased compared with parental cells. Histologic analyses of the cellular infiltrates surrounding these tumors in immunocompetent animals showed a predominance of lymphocytes, although eosinophils and basophils were also present. Specifically, increased numbers (fivefold greater) of $CD4^+$ and $CD8^+$ cells were recruited to IL-7-secreting tumor sites compared with parental tumors. Lymphocyte depletion analyses performed using MAbs to $CD4^+$, $CD8^+$, macrophages (anti-$CR3^+$) and NK cells were performed. Tumor rejection was inhibited by anti-$CD4^+$ MAbs in a plasmacytoma line, and dependence of the antitumor response on $CD8^+$ cells was demonstrated in a murine glioma model. Selective depletion of macrophages, but not NK cells, also inhibited tumor rejection, but to a lesser degree than treatment with MAbs for T cells.

Lymphocytes isolated from transduced tumors demonstrated significantly enhanced cytotoxicity toward parental tumor targets. Interestingly, allogeneic lymphocytes cocultured with IL-7-producing melanoma cell lines demonstrated increased cytotoxicity toward implanted tumors compared with untransduced cells; this could not be duplicated by the addition to culture of recombinant IL-7. This stimulation of in vitro cytotoxicity was comparable to that produced by IL-2-transduced cells of the same tumor cell lines. It appears that IL-7 acts primarily through T-cell-mediated mechanisms in generating antineoplastic effects, although its ability to downregulate TGF-β production may be a distinct component of its biologic activity. The relative importance of $CD4^+$ or $CD8^+$ cells in mediating tumor rejection may vary between particular tumors. Currently, Economou et al. are conducting a phase I clinical protocol involving vaccination of patients with melanomas with autologous-irradiated melanoma cells producing IL-7 contained within a retroviral construct. A few patients have been treated, but the results of therapy are as yet unreported.

IL-12 Recent reports have described the transfection of IL-12 into NIH/3T3 cells. These IL-12-producing fibroblasts were mixed with murine melanoma cells in syngeneic mice and reduced tumorigenicity in the majority of animals treated. IL-12-transduced murine colon carcinoma cells grew in a delayed fashion compared to unmanipulated tumors, and resulted in delay in the formation of pulmonary and hepatic metastases. Antitumor activity was also recently demonstrated in a murine fibrosarcoma model using a vaccinia virus vector. The question of which T cell subsets are most responsible for IL-12's antitumor effect is as yet unclear, as $CD4^+$ and $CD8^+$ cells appear to act differentially depending on the specific model tested.

GM-CSF Gene therapy efforts involving GM-CSF were evaluated in a murine model and compared to cytokine gene therapy involving at least nine other cytokines by Dranoff et al. The investigators used both live and irradiated genetically modified tumors producing high levels of GM-CSF (300 ng/10^6 cells/24 h) in syngeneic mice. This report was noteworthy in several respects. First, it demonstrated that vaccination of irradiated implanted tumors alone resulted in some degree of antitumor immunity.

Second, systemic murine toxicity was described, apparently induced by injection of tumor cells secreting high concentrations of this cytokine. Third, in contrast to many other investigations, systemic immunity was not conferred upon animals treated with live IL-2-producing tumors although these cells were the only type to be rejected in this comparative analysis. However, irradiated tumors producing GM-CSF alone and live cells secreting a combination of IL-2 and GM-CSF did induce resistance to subsequent tumor challenge. Finally, MAb depletion of several effector cell subsets demonstrated dependence on both CD4$^+$ and CD8$^+$ T cells for the establishment of systemic immunity induced by GM-CSF-secreting murine melanoma cells.

A recent report from Johns Hopkins on renal cell carcinoma patients randomized and treated prospectively with either a GM-CSF gene-transduced autologous tumor cell vaccine or a nontransduced autologous tumor cell vaccine demonstrated only one objective partial responder in 16 evaluable patients.

Tumor Suppressor Genes   The *p53* gene has been identified as a putative tumor suppressor gene. Tumor suppressors are recessively functioning genes both copies of which must be mutated to elicit phenotypic alterations supporting malignancy in the host. Therefore, it has been hypothesized that delivering one copy of the wild type (*wt*) gene could reverse a neoplastic process. The *p53* gene is mutated in a wide variety of tumors including head and neck squamous cell cancer, non-small-cell lung cancer, colorectal carcinoma, and premalignant conditions such as Barrett's esophagitis. The *p53* gene encodes a 393-amino-acid phosphoprotein that forms complexes with a series of viral proteins. Other areas within the gene interact with other proteins allowing *p53* oligomers to form, resulting in transactivation of gene expression. Wild-type *p53* appears to regulate the cell cycle and to control cell growth and proliferation, at least in part through the mechanism of apoptosis or programmed cell death. The *p53* gene also has a role in controlling transcriptional regulation and DNA replication. Mutated *p53* allows unregulated cell growth to occur, while restoring *wt-p53* restores cell cycle regulation and renders cells apoptotic or in G1 arrest.

A variety of viral constructs have been evaluated that contain *wt-p53* in several tumor systems. Roth et al. have demonstrated that retroviral vectors containing *wt-p53* can suppress in vivo and in vitro growth of human lung carcinoma cell lines that contain deleted or mutated *p53*. Conversely, tumor cell lines containing *wt-p53* are not significantly altered by the retroviral construct. The phenomenon of the bystander effect has also been observed in these studies as the growth of nontransduced cells was reduced following coculture with a transduced population.

Several models involving adenoviral vectors containing *wt-p53* have also been evaluated. Apoptosis has been observed in tumor cells whose genome contained mutated or deleted *p53* following transduction with adenoviral *wt-p53*. Constructs of *p53* have also been shown to act synergistically with cisplatinum in inducing apoptosis in human lung tumors grown in nude mice. These results have led to several clinical gene therapy protocols involving *wt-p53* introduced through a variety of delivery systems. Clinical responses have been modest to date, although the toxicity of therapy appears minimal. In addition, viral vectors containing related cell cycle control genes (*p21* and *p16*) are currently being evaluated, and may soon be used in clinical protocols.

Suicide Gene Therapy One gene therapy strategy that has been used with some degree of success in CNS tumor models involves so-called "suicide gene therapy." This technique involves the transduction of cells with a gene that can be killed by systemic administration of a compound toxic to all cells containing the gene or in proximity to it. Most commonly, the gene for the herpes simplex virus (HSV) driven by the thymidine kinase promoter has been introduced via both adenoviral and retro-viral vectors. Following transduction, the host is administered gancyclovir, which is toxic to all HSV-containing cells. Additional cell killing has been observed in non-transduced cells in proximity to the transduced population, suggesting a "bystander effect" in this model. This strategy is currently employed in more than 20 approved clinical protocols worldwide, most of which are directed toward treatment of brain tumors.

Costimulatory Molecules-B7 B7 is the ligand for the CD28 receptor of lym-phocytes. Antigen presentation to T cells and subsequent T cell activation depends on binding to CD28, yet most tumors lack B7 molecules on their surface. Murine models of B7 tumor transfection have demonstrated antineoplastic responses and the generation of systemic immunity. Gene therapy studies involving the delivery of B7 in patients with melanoma are currently underway. B7 is commonly confused with, but is structurally and functionally different from, the HLA-B7 molecule which is a major histocompatibility class I haplotype also being studied in gene therapy models involving patients with melanoma and colorectal cancer. This system utilizes nonviral, liposomally delivered gene constructs involving intratumoral injection. It has demonstrated some antineoplastic responses in melanoma patients, but no doc-umented responses in studies evaluating direct injection of liver metastases from colorectal carcinoma.

Antisense Gene Therapy Antisense gene therapy strategies involve the cre-ation of genetic sequences that are complementary to specific regions of RNA known to be critical for gene expression and transcription. Typically, regions of interest for antisense binding involve oncogene coding regions. Oncogenes act predominantly to promote neoplastic cell growth. Antisense constructs may be directed toward onco-genes, and may also be composed of oligonucleotides that bind to double-stranded DNA, thereby interfering with transcription. Other alternatives include antisense RNA, which may bind to single-stranded DNA or to mRNA and interfere with tran-scription, splicing, and translation.

Antisense oligonucleotides have been tested in phase II clinical studies, but effi-cacy has been limited by rapid host-induced degradation by nuclease in vivo. Anti-oncogenic oligonucleotides have been constructed to disrupt expression of *abl*, *fos*, *kit*, *myc*, *src*, and *ras* gene families, again with limited clinical consequence.

Roth et al. described a model in which an antisense RNA construct was used to induce tumoricidal activity in a human lung cancer cell line expressing K-*ras*. The anti-K-*ras* retroviral constructs reduced tumorigenicity of a cell line with a homozygous K-*ras* mutation in nude mice. These observations have led to clinical trials involving direct intratumor injection of anti-K-*ras* retroviral particles in patients with unresectable pulmonary malignancies. Also, an adenoviral anti-K-*ras* construct has been reported recently to have potent antitumor activity in murine models involving human cancer cell lines.

CONCLUSION

Biologic cancer therapies hold enormous promise, as many different forms of therapeutics from cytokines to vaccines have been shown to induce tumor regression in many human clinical trials. Although the response rates are not high, they are encouraging because the best results in trials in animals have been in small-volume disease and prevention, and not in the treatment of established large cancers. Because most of these therapies rely on the induction of the host immune responses, patients with end-stage, bulky disease and poor nutritional status may not respond optimally. Therefore, most biologic modalities may not have been adequately tested clinically to date. Further, more specific and possibly more potent therapies are just not entering clinical trial. Advances in biotechnology offer the promise of even more sophisticated therapeutics. The next generation of biologic therapies will most likely consist of multimodality biologic treatments targeting both humoral and cellular immunity against multiple tumor antigens.

SELECTED REFERENCES

Cytokines

Anderson CM, Buzaid AC, Grimm EA (1996) Interaction of chemotherapy and biological response modifiers in the treatment of melanoma. *Cancer Treat Res* 87:357.

Brunda MJ, Luistro L, Rumennik L, et al. (1996) Antitumor activity of interleukin-12 in preclinical models. *Cancer Chemother Pharmacol* 38(Suppl):S16.

Dutcher JP (1995) Therapeutic strategies for cytokines. *Curr Opin Oncol* 7:566.

Eggermont AMM (1996) Treatment of melanoma in-transit metastases confined to the limb. *Cancer Surv* 26:335.

Kirkwood JM, Strawderman MH, Ernstoff MS, et al. (1996) Interferon alpha-2b adjuvant therapy of high-risk resected cutaneous melanoma: The Eastern Cooperative Oncology Group Trial EST 1684. *J Clin Oncol* 14:7.

Kopp WC, Holmlund JT (1996) Cytokines and immunological monitoring. *Cancer Chemother Biol Resp Modif* 16:189.

Mosmann TR, Coffman RL (1989) Heterogeneity of cytokine secretion patterns and functions of helper T calls. *Adv Immunol* 46:111.

Parkinson DR (1995) Present status of biological response modifiers in cancer. *Am J Med* 99:6a–54s.

Platanias LC (1995) Interferons: Laboratory to clinc investigations. *Curr Opin Oncol* 7:560.

Tepper RI, Pattengale PK, Leder P, et al. (1989) Murine interkeukin-4 displays potent anti-tumor activity in vivo. *Cell* 57:503.

Veltri S, Smith JW II (1996) Interleukin-1 trials in cancer patients: A review of the toxicity, antitumor and hematopoietic effects. *Stem Cells* 14:164.

Monoclonal Antibodies

Greiner JW, Guadagni F, Roselli M, et al. (1996) Novel approaches to tumor detection and therapy using a combination of monoclonal antibody and cytokine. *Anticancer Res* 16:2129.

Jurcic JG, Scheinberg DA, Houghton AN (1996) Monoclonal antibody therapy of cancer. *Cancer Chemother Biol Resp Modif* 16:168.

Cellular Therapy

Aoki Y, Takakuwa K, Kodama S, et al. (1991) Use of adoptive transfer of tumor-infiltrating lymphocytes alone or in combination with cisplatin-containing chemotherapy in patients with epithelial ovarian cancer. *Cancer Res* 51:1934.

Chang AE, Yoshizawa H, Sakai K, et al. (1993) clinical observations on adoptive immunotherapy with vaccine-primed T-lymphocytes secondarily sensitized to tumor in vitro. *Cancer Res* 53:1043.

Goedegebuure PS, Douville LM, Li H, et al. (1995) Adoptive immunotherapy with tumor-infiltrating lymphocytes and interleukin-2 in patients with metastatic malignant melanoma and renal cell carcinoma: A pilot study. *J Clin Oncol* 13:1939.

Itoh K, Tilden AB, Balch CM (1986) Interleukin-2 activation of cytotoxic T-lymphocytes infiltrating into human metastatic melanomas. *Cancer Res* 46:3011.

Mule JJ, Shu S, Schwarz SL, et al. (1984) Adoptive immunotherapy of established pulmonary metastases with LAK cells and recombinant interleukin-2. *Science* 225:1487.

Rivoltini L, Kawakami Y, Robbins P, et al. (1996) Efficient induction of tumor reactive CTL from peripheral blood and tumor-infiltrating lymphocytes of melanoma patients by in vitro stimulation with the human melanoma antigen MART-1 peptide. *J Exp Med* 184:647.

Rosenberg SA, Terry WD (1977) Passive immunotherapy of cancer in animals and man. *Adv Cancer Res* 25:323.

Rosenberg SA, Spiess P, Lafreniere R (1986) A new approach to the adoptive immunotherapy of cancer with tumor-infiltrating lymphocytes. *Science* 223:1318.

Rosenberg SA, Packard BS, Aebersold PM, et al. (1988) Use of tumor-infiltrating lymphocytes and interleukin-2 in the immunotherapy of patients with metastatic melanoma, special report. *N Engl J Med* 319:1676.

Rosenberg SA (1992) The immunotherapy and gene therapy of cancer. *J Clin Oncol* 10:180.

Rosenberg SA, Lotze MT, Aebersold PM, et al. (1993) Prospective randomized trial of high dose interleukin-2 alone or with lymphokine activated killer cells for the treatment of patients with advanced cancer. *J Natl Cancer Inst* 85:622.

Rosenberg SA, Yannelli JR, Yang JC, et al. (1994) Treatment of patients with metastatic melanoma with autologous tumor-infiltrating lymphocytes and interleukin-2. *J Natl Cancer Inst* 86:1159.

Schoof DD, Gramolini BA, Davidson DL, et al. (1988) Adoptive immunotherapy of human using low-dose recombinant interleukin-2 and lymphokine-activated killer cells. *Cancer Res* 48:5007.

Vaccines

Linehan DC, Goedegebuure PS, Eberlein TJ (1996) Vaccine therapy for cancer. *Ann Surg Oncol* 3:219.

Immunoadjuvants and Immunomodulators

Akporiaye ET, Hersh EM (1995) Immune adjuvants. In: VT DeVita Jr, S Hellman, SA Rosenberg (eds). *Biologic Therapy of Cancer*, 2nd edition. Lippincott, Philadelphia.
Schultz N, Oratz R, Chen D, et al. (1995) Effect of DETOX as an adjuvant for melanoma vaccine. *Vaccine* 13:503.

WTCV

Berd D, Maguire HC Jr, McCue P, et al. (1990) Treatment of metastatic melanoma with an autologous tumor-cell vaccine: Clinical and immunologic results in 64 patients. *J Clin Oncol* 8:1858.
Berd D, Maguire HC Jr, Mastrangelo MJ (1993) Treatment of human melanoma with a hapten-modified autologous vaccine. *Ann NY Acad Sci* 690:147.
Hoover HC Jr, Bandhorst JS, Peters LC, et al. (1993) Adjuvant active specific immunotherapy for human colorectal cancer: 6.5 year median follow up of a phase III prospectively randomized trial. *J Clin Oncol* 11:390.
Mastrangelo MJ, Maguire HC Jr, Sato T, et al. (1996) Active specific immunization in the treatment of patients with melanoma. *Semin Oncol* 23:773.
Morton DL (1986) Adjuvant immunotherapy of malignant melanoma: Status of clinical trials at UCLA. *Int J Immunother* 2:31.
Perlin E, Oldham RK, Weese JL, et al. (1980) Carcinoma of the lung: Immunotherapy with intradermal BCG and allogeneic tumor cells. *Int J Radiat Oncol Biol Physiol* 6:1033.
Schlag P, Manasterski M, Gerneth T, et al. (1992) Active specific immunotherapy with Newcastle-disease-virus-modified autologous tumor cells following resection of liver metastases in colorectal cancer. *Cancer Immunol Immunother* 35:325.
Seigler HF, Buckley CE, Sheppard LB, et al. (1977) Adoptive transfer and specific active immunization of patients with malignant melanoma. *Ann NY Acad Sci* 277:522.

VOV

Freedman RS, Edwards CL, Bowen JM, et al. (1988) Viral oncolysates in patients with advanced ovarian cancer. *Gynecol Oncol* 29:337.
Hersey P (1992) Active immunotherapy with viral lysates of micrometastases following surgical removal of high risk melanoma. *World J Surg* 16:251.
Morton DL, Foshag LJ, Hoon DSB, et al. (1992) Prolongation of survival in metastatic malignant melanoma after active specific immunotherapy with a new polyvalent melanoma vaccine. *Ann Surg* 216:463.

Sivanandham M, Scoggin S, Tanaka N, et al. (1994) Therapeutic effect of a vaccinia colon oncolysate prepared with interleukin-2 gene encoded vaccinia virus studied in syngeneic CC-36 murine colon hepatic metastasis model. *Cancer Immunol Immunother* 38:259.

Wallack MK, Sivanandham M, Balch CM, et al. (1995) A phase III randomized, double-blind multiinstitutioinal trial of vaccinia melanoma oncolysate-active specific immunotherapy for patients with stage II melanoma. *Cancer* 75:34.

Wallack MK, Sivanandham M, Whooley B, et al. (1996) Favorable clinical responses in subsets of patients from a randomized, multi-institutional melanoma vaccine trial. *Ann Surg Oncol* 3:110.

TAV

Brichard V, Van Pel A, Wolfel T, et al. (1993) The tyrosinase gene codes for an antigen recognized by autologous cytolytic T lymphocytes on HLA-A2 melanomas. *J Exp Med* 178:48.

Bystryn J-C, Oratz R, Henn M, et al. (1992) Relationship between immune response to melanoma vaccine and clinical outcome in stage II malignant melanoma. *Cancer* 69:1157.

Bystryn JC (1995) Clinical activity of a polyvalent melanoma antigen vaccine. *Rec Results Cancer Res* 139:337.

Cox AL, Skipper J, Chen Y, et al. (1994) Identification of a peptide recognized by five melanoma-specific human cytotoxic T-cell lines. *Science* 264:716.

Disis ML, Gralow JR, Bernhard H, et al. (1996) Peptide-based, but not whole protein, vaccines elicit immunity to HER2/new, oncogenic self-protein. *J Immunol* 156:3151.

Fisk B, Blevins TL, Wharton JT, et al. (1995) Identification of an immunodominant peptide of HER-2/neu proto-oncogene recognized by ovarian tumor-specific CTL lines. *J Exp Med* 181:2709.

Gaugler B, Van den Eynde B, van der Bruggen P, et al. (1994) Human gene MAGE-3 codesfor an antigen recognized on a melanoma by autologous cytolytic T lymphocytes. *J Exp Med* 179:921.

Hollinshead A, Arlen M, Yonemoto R, et al. (1982) Pilot studies using melanoma tumor-associated antigens (TAA) in specific-active immunotherapy of malignant melanoma. *Cancer* 49:1387.

Hu X, Chakraborty NG, Sportn JR, et al. (1996) Enhancement of cytolytic T lymphocyte precursor frequency in melanoma patients following immunization with the MAGE-1 peptide loaded antigen presenting cell-based vaccine. *Cancer Res* 56:2479.

Jerome KR, Barnd DL, Bendt KM, et al. (1991) Cytotoxic T-lymphocytes derived from patients with breast adenocarcinoma recognize an epitope present on the protein core of a mucin molecule preferentially expressed by malignant cells. *Cancer Res* 51:2908.

Kawakami Y, Eliyahu S, Sakaguchi K, et al. (1994) Identification of the immunodominant peptides of the MART-1 human melanoma antigen recognized by the majority of HLA-A2-restricted tumor infiltrating lymphocytes. *J Exp Med* 180:347.

Livingston PO, Wong GY, Adluri S, et al. (1994) Improved survival in stage III melanoma patients with GM2 antibodies: A randomized trial of adjuvant vaccination with GM2 ganglioside. *J Clin Oncol* 12:1036.

Livingston PO (1995) Approaches to augmenting the immunogenicity of melanoma gangliosides: From whole melanoma cells to ganglioside-KLH conjugate vaccines. *Immunol Rev* 145:147.

Maeurer MJ, Storkus WJ, Kirkwood JM, et al. (1996) New treatment options for patients with melanoma: Review of melanoma-derived T-cell epitope-based peptide vaccines. *Melanoma Res* 6:11.

Peoples GE, Goedegebuure PS, Smith R, et al. (1995) Breast and ovarian cancer-specific cytotoxic T-lymphocytes recognize the same HER2/neu-derived peptide. *Proc Natl Acad Sci USA* 92:432.

Van der Bruggen P, Traversari C, Chomez P, et al. (1991) A gene encoding an antigen recognized by cytolytic T lymphocytes on a human melanoma. *Science* 254:1643.

Gene Therapy

Asher AL, Mule JJ, Kasid A, et al. (1991) Murine tumor cells transduced with the gene for tumor necrosis factor-alpha. *J Immunol* 146:3227.

Blankenstein TH, Qin Z, Uberla K, et al. (1991) Tumor suppression after cell-targeted tumor necrosis factor alpha gene transfer. *J Exp Med* 173:1047.

Descamps V, Duffour M-T, Mathieu M-C, et al. (1996) Strategies for cancer gene therapy using adenoviral vectors. *J Mol Med* 74:183.

Dranoff G, Jaffee E, Lazenby A, et al. (1993) Vaccination with irradiated tumor cells engineered to secrete murine granulocyte-macrophage colony-stimulating factor stimulates potent, specific, and long-lasting anti-tumor immunity. *Proc Natl Acad Sci USA* 90:3539.

Gunzburg WH, Salmons B (1996) Development of retroviral vectors as safe, targeted gene delivery systems. *J Mol Med* 74:171.

Mastrangelo MJ, Berd D, Nathan FE, et al. (1996) Gene therapy for human cancer: An assay for clinicians. *Semin Oncol* 23:4.

Miller AR, McBride WH, Hunt K, et al. (1993) Cytokine-mediated gene therapy for cancer. *Ann Surg Oncol* 1:436.

Rosenberg SA, Anderson WF, Blaese M, et al. (1993) The development of gene therapy for the treatment of cancer. *Ann Surg* 218:455.

Roth JA, Cristiano RJ (1997) Gene therapy for cancer: What have we done and where are we going? *J Natl Cancer Inst* 89:21.

Roth JA, Nguyen D, Lawrence DD, et al. (1996) Retroviral-mediated wild type *p53* gene transfer to tumors of patients with lung cancer. *Nat Med* 2:985.

Simons JW, Jaffee EM, Weber CE, et al. (1997) Bioactivity of autologous irradiated renal cell carcinoma vaccines generated by ex vivo granulocyte-macrophage colony-stimulating factor gene transfer. *Cancer Res* 57:1537.

Toloza EM, Hunt K, Miller AR, et al. (1997) Transduction of murine and human tumors using recombinant adenovirus vectors. *Ann Surg Oncol* 4:70.

Zhang WW (1996) Antisense oncogene and tumor suppressor gene therapy of cancer. *J Mol Med* 74:191.

Zhang Y, Mukhopadhyay T, Donehower LA, et al. (1993) Retroviral vector-mediated transduction of K-*ras* antisense RNA into human lung cancer cells inhibits expression of the malignant phenotype. *Hum Gene Ther* 4:451.

General

Clark JI, Weiner LM (1995) Biologic treatment of human cancer. *Curr Prob Cancer* 19:185.

Clark JW (1996) Biological response modifiers. *Cancer Chemother biol Resp Modif* 16:239.

Del Prete G, Maggi E, Romagnani S (1994) Human Th1 and Th2 cells: Functional properties, mechanisms of regulation and role in disease. *Lab Invest* 70:299.

DeVita VT, Hellman S, Rosenberg SA (eds) (1995) *Biologic Therapy of Cancer*, 2nd edition. Lippincott, Philadelphia.

CHAPTER 6

CANCER EPIDEMIOLOGY

PETER BOYLE

Division of Epidemiology and Biostatistics
European Institute of Oncology
Milan, Italy

Cancer is not a modern disease but has clearly existed for many centuries, although it is a more common phenomenon in humans today than in the past. To a large extent this is attributable to the relatively advanced age to which people now live as it is a disease that is more common in older than in younger people. Cancer has been reported in dinosaurs[1] and in Egyptian mummies[2]; it was described by writers in ancient Greece, Rome, and Persia; and it has been noted and discussed in medieval texts. The medical papyri of Edwin Smith, dating from about 2500 B.C., are devoted to surgical case histories, and number 45 in this series states:

> ...if thou examinest a [woman] having bulging tumours on [her] breast, it thou puttest thy hand upon [her] breast upon these tumours thou findest them very cool, there being no fever at all therein when thy hand touches [her], they have no granulation, they form no fluid, and they are bulging to thy hand. Thou shouldest say concerning [her], "One having bulging tumours. There is no treatment."
> —Translated by Professor James Breasted in 1930.

Another papyrus describes a tumor of the uterus treated by local vaginal application of fresh dates and limestone with and without pig's brain. Writings from ancient India (Auyruedic books) suggest that it was possible to diagnose cancer correctly over 2500 years ago but it was considered incurable. Tumors of the oral cavity, pharynx, esophagus, pelvis, and rectum are described but no mention is made of cervical, breast, lung, or bone cancers. The aphorisms of Hippocrates contain a variety of references to malignant disease: *"Every cancer not only corrupts the part it has seized*

Manual of Clinical Oncology, 7th edition, Edited by Raphael E. Pollock
ISBN 0-471-23828-7, pages 131–161. Copyright © 1999 Wiley-Liss, Inc.

but spreads further." Galen (131–200 A.D.) noted that *"cancerous tumors develop with greatest frequency in the breasts of women."* He described a tumor raised above the skin, extending along the lymphatic vessels radially on all sides and often with red streaks; such tumors may ulcerate and discharge a dark, reddish, foul-smelling secretion. Galen likened the lesion to a crab (*karkinos* in Greek and *cancer* in Latin). He recognized that surgery was the only chance of cure, and must be done at an early stage when excision of the whole lesion was possible.

The captured Greek physician Democedes was called upon King Darius of Persia to treat Atossa, the Queen, who had a lump in her breast that increased in size and eventually ulcerated. Modesty had prevented her showing it to anyone until it had reached a large size.

Little progress or mention was made of cancer until the 18th century, when Bernard Peyrihle proposed a viral theory of cancer. John Hunter gave a long account of surgery for cancers of the female breast, uterus, lips, and stomach and advised that tumors may be hereditary, and that palpitation of the mass should be gentle in case rough handling spread the disease. He noted that *"no cure has been found."* In 1775, Percival Pott[3] described the occupational cancer of the scrotum that occurred in chimney sweeps. In 1761, John Hill suggested that snuff was responsible for nasal cancer and polyps.[4] Prior to this, Ramazzini[5] had reported an excess of breast cancer in nuns in Padua.

Treatment advances came in the 19th century. In 1881, Billroth performed a successful gastrectomy for stomach cancer and in 1884, Godlee removed a brain tumor. William Marsden founded his Cancer Hospital in 1851 with two aims: care of the cancer patient and cancer research. The century closed with the discoveries of Roentgen and the Curies, which led to radiologic diagnosis and radiotherapy, and the work of Beatson on hormonal manipulation in breast cancer.

Different forms of cancer have been recognized and treated for centuries, but it is advances in civilization and the associated improvement in life expectancy that have contributed to making cancer such a common disease worldwide. In the United Kingdom in 1880 approximately half of the population died before 40 years of age; in 1980 this figure had decreased to around 3%. In 1880 in the United Kingdom, 25% of the population reached the age of 70 and in 1990 the corresponding figure was 70%.[6] More recently, the effective prevention of cardiovascular diseases led to an acceleration of the decline of premature mortality and an increase in life expectancy and, inadvertently, of cancer. More and more men and women today live to ages at which cancer is most common than ever before, a phenomenon that is not restricted to a handful of developed countries.

THE GLOBAL CANCER BURDEN

Estimates of the global cancer burden have been made for 1975,[7] 1980,[8] and 1985.[9] These estimates are for all forms of cancer but specifically exclude nonmelanoma skin cancer, which is poorly registered on incidence statistics and only infrequently fatal. In men there were an estimated 3.8 million cases in 1985. The most common form of cancer is lung cancer, with an estimated 667,000 cases in 1985 (Table 6.1). The estimated number of cases of lung cancer has increased by 44% over the 10-year period covered by these estimates. Other forms of cancer that have increased notably are colorectal cancer, prostate cancer, bladder cancer, melanoma, and lymphoma, particularly Non-Hodgkin's lymphoma (Table 6.1). Although some of these increases could be due to better precision in the estimation methodology, there is also likely to be a real etiologic component to these increases.

In women, it was estimated that there were 3.8 million cases of cancer in 1985. Breast cancer is the most common form of cancer, with an estimated 719,000 new cases in 1985 (Table 6.1). This is a large increase over the estimated 541,200 cases in 1975: an increase of 33% in 10 years. A similar increase has taken place in oral

TABLE 6.1. Estimated Annual Cancer Incidence Burden Worldwide (Numbers of New Cases and Rank Order) in Women and Men in 1975, 1980, and 1985

	Women					
	1975		1980		1985	
Mouth and pharynx	105,600	(6)	121,200	(8)	143,000	(7)
Esophagus	102,300	(7)	108,200	(9)	108,000	(10)
Stomach	260,600	(3)	260,600	(4)	282,000	(4)
Colorectal	255,600	(4)	285,900	(3)	346,000	(3)
Liver	76,700	(9)	79,500	(-)	101,000	(11)
Lung	126,700	(5)	146,900	(6)	219,000	(5)
Breast	541,200	(1)	572,100	(1)	719,000	(1)
Cervix	459,400	(2)	465,600	(2)	437,000	(2)
Lymphoma	91,300	(8)	98,000	(10)	135,000	(9)
Leukemia	75,400	(10)	81,300	(-)	96,000	(12)
All sites	2,901,800		3,100,000		3,774,200	

	Men					
	1975		1980		1985	
Mouth and pharynx	232,900	(4)	257,300	(4)	270,000	(5)
Esophagus	194,000	(6)	202,100	(6)	196,000	(7)
Stomach	421,700	(2)	408,800	(2)	473,000	(2)
Colorectal	251,200	(3)	286,200	(3)	331,000	(3)
Liver	182,500	(7)	171,700	(7)	214,000	(6)
Lung	464,300	(1)	513,600	(1)	667,000	(1)
Bladder	130,700	(8)	167,700	(8)	182,000	(8)
Prostate	197,700	(5)	235,800	(5)	291,000	(4)
Lymphoma	129,500	(9)	139,900	(9)	181,000	(9)
Leukemia	100,300	(10)	106,900	(10)	121,000	(10)
All sites	2,968,500		3,250,000		3,849,400	

Estimates of the global cancer burden have been made for 1975,[7] 1980,[8] and 1985.[9] These estimates are for all forms of cancer excluding nonmelanoma skin cancers.

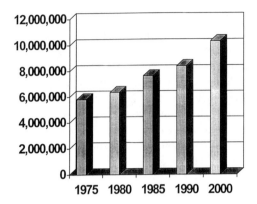

Figure 6.1. Estimated global cancer burden (numbers of new cases of cancer per annum).

cavity and colorectal cancer, and lymphoma. The largest relative increase of cancer in women has been in lung cancer, which increased from 126,700 in 1975 to 219,000 in 1985, an increase of 73%. This can almost entirely be explained by changes in smoking patterns in women in many parts of the world.[10]

The estimated number of new cases of cancer worldwide increased from 5.9 million in 1975, through 6.4 million in 1980, to 7.6 million in 1985 (Fig. 6.1). Assuming that the age-specific rates remain constant at the 1985 levels, it was estimated that there were 8.4 million new cases in 1990 and would be 10.3 million new cases in the year 2000.[9] It could be deduced that the number of new cases of cancer worldwide would have doubled between 1970 and 2000. Beyond 2000, the absolute numbers of cases of cancer will likely increase as the post-World War II "baby boom" generation reaches ages at which the age-specific rates of cancer start to increase.[11] In many countries this generation is the first whose numbers were not reduced by a great war and the first to have benefited from the advances in medical care and treatment witnessed in the second half of this century. Most members of this generation are still alive at age 50 compared to the same situation in many countries for the preceding generations.

This has important implications for public health as well as other health services around the world. There will be a need for more medical, nursing, and related staff to treat these patients; there will need to be more hospitals and treatment facilities available, and this will be a major expense for the near future as well as a major logistical problem. The implications for planning are that cancer control activities will need to increase to help reduce the mortality burden that is otherwise likely to materialize.

Geographic and Temporal Variation in Cancer Risk

The importance of acknowledging the large international variation in cancer occurrence throughout the world led to the designation of initial observations on cancer epidemiology as *geographical pathology*. There are still many interesting aspects to the geographic epidemiology of different forms of cancer worldwide.[12]

Lip cancer has for a long time been most common in the Prairie Provinces of Canada, although the high rates are declining. Cancer of the tongue is most common in India and cancer of the mouth is most common in France. Oral cavity cancer was the most frequent form of cancer in the mid-1800s[13] and the risks worldwide have dropped dramatically during this century; however, there has been a major increase in risk among successive generations of men born this century in central and eastern Europe[14] that is largely unexplained.[15] Nasopharyngeal cancer is rare in most Caucasian populations although exceptionally common in Chinese populations in Asia and elsewhere.

Perhaps more than any other form of cancer, *esophageal cancer* is characterized by an enormous range in occurrence throughout the world, with incidence rates as high as 200 per 100,000 in women and 165 in men in northern Gonbad in the Caspian region of Iran[16] and mortality rates of 211.2 in men and 136.5 in women of Linxian county in China.[17] These elevated levels are in marked contrast to those from Cluj County in Romania, where incidence rates around 1980 were 1.2 in men and 0.2 in women.[18] The highest risk areas of the world include the so-called Asian esophageal cancer belt stretching from the Caspian littoral in northern Iran, through the southern Republics of the (former) USSR, to eastern China[19]; this high-risk belt clearly extends into southern Republics of the former USSR. The cancer pattern of esophageal cancer in men in the European Community is dominated by the aggregation of *departments* in northwest France with similar and high rates of esophageal cancer mortality.[20]

The highest recorded incidence rates of *gastric cancer* in men are those from the Far East, with very high rates in males in Japan in Yagamata (95.5 in men and 40.1 in women) and in Hiroshima (83.1 in men and 35.9 in women) and in the Soviet Union.[21] Fairly high rates have also been reported from parts of China, Latin America, and central and eastern Europe.[22] In western Europe, age-standardized incidence rates are generally lower. Rates in northern Italy are substantially higher than in Ragusa in Sicily, a differential confirmed in studies of southern Italian migrants to the north of the country. In Africa, areas of high frequency have been reported in certain mountainous regions in Rwanda, southwest Uganda, and Tanzania, around Mt. Kilimanjaro. It is surprising to consider the difference in the incidence rate in men in Japan and to contrast this with the incidence rate reported in men in various white, or predominantly white, populations of the United States such as Iowa (6.6 per 100,000), Utah (5.6), and Atlanta (5.2). The most remarkable feature in the epidemiology of stomach cancer is the universal declining trend for both sexes characterized by a greater decline in western as compared to central and eastern Europe.

Primary liver cancer is very common in populations in Southeast Asia and Africa; it has been estimated that 44% of primary liver cancer is found in China.[9] The highest incidence rate in each sex is reported from Khon Kaen in Thailand, the rates being 97.4 per 100,000 in men and much lower in women (39.0). In men, extremely high rates are reported also from Qidong in China (72.1 per 100,000). The third highest rate is about half these two highest values and is reported from Bamako in Mali

(51.1). In women, the highest rates are found in similar population groups and the lowest rates in each sex generally are reported from developed countries. In China, primary liver cancer has a predominantly coastal distribution with incidence rates recorded in Shanghai of the same order as those reported from Hong Kong and Singapore. Immigrant Chinese in California exhibit much lower rates although these are substantially greater than among white populations residing in the same city. In adults, a large majority of liver cancers are hepatocellular carcinomas, cholangiocarcinomas being rare by contrast except in parts of Southeast Asia and around the shore of Lake Baikal in Siberia, in association with liver flukes (e.g., *Clonorchis sinensis, Opisthorchis viverrin*).[23] Most liver cancers in childhood are hepatoblastomas, rare tumors showing little worldwide variation.[24]

There is an unusual pattern of *larynx cancer* in men found in Spain with high rates also recorded in Italy, Poland, and France. The highest incidence rate of *lung cancer* observed in men are in several black populations of the United States including New Orleans (110.8), Central Louisiana (105.6), the San Francisco Bay Area (101.5), and Detroit (103.2). In SEER, rates in black men (99.1) are about 50% higher than in white men (61.3). The lowest incidence rates in men are from Indian, African, and South American populations, most of whom are among the less developed regions of the world. In women, the highest incidence rates are found among black and white populations of the United States and western Scotland. The lowest rates occur in the same populations as in men. This situation is quite deceptive and we should not be lulled into a false sense of security; the large inroads of the tobacco industry into the developing countries will, after the 20- to 40-year latent period between initiation of the habit and evidence of the full effects, have a major adverse impact on health in these countries from the early part of the next century.

Melanoma (of the skin) is an unusual form of cancer in that its incidence is increasing very quickly and it has a tendency to affect women more than men. In the past 4 decades, melanoma incidence has increased in all white populations of industrialized nations, with a 3% to 7% increase per year. For example, in the United States, in 1973, the melanoma incidence was 5.9 per 100,000 women, and reached 11.6 per 100,000 women in 1994.[25] In Europe, the increase is mainly noticeable among younger adults, and about 50% of melanomas now occur in subjects less than 55 years old, whereas the majority of most other solid tumors occur in those more than 60 years old. Although mortality from melanoma is also increasing in North America and Europe,[25,26] it is not increasing at the same pace as incidence; it seems that as melanoma incidence reaches high levels, mortality from melanoma tends to level off. So, in Australia, recent trends show a stabilization of mortality from melanoma.[27] This phenomenon could be partly due to better awareness of populations about melanoma, and many skin malignancies are being diagnosed at an earlier stage than 2 decades ago. Such an increase in incidence has not been reported for any other malignancy. It has not been noticed in other nonwhite populations, but among Japanese, an increase in melanoma incidence has been described, although the disease remains 10 times less frequent than in US white populations. In white populations, melanoma incidence in women is generally higher than in men, with, however, notable exceptions, such as in the United States.[25] The major difference resides in the lower mortality from melanoma in women as compared to men: in the United States, in 1994, mortality from melanoma was 3.5 per 100,000 in men as compared to 1.7 per 100,000 in women. The reason for the gender difference for melanoma mortality is unknown. If women tend to recognize that they may have a melanoma at an earlier stage than men, it does not explain the large difference in mortality from melanoma.

The highest incidence rates of breast cancer around the world around 1990 were generally found in Caucasian population groups in the United States (Table 6.2). Notable exceptions were that the highest incidence rate, by a considerable margin, was found in the European population of Harare in Zimbabwe; in Montevideo, Uruguay; and in the Jewish population of Israel born in America or Europe and Israel itself.

TABLE 6.2. Cancer of the Breast (ICD9 174/175)

Female Registry	Cases	Rate
Zimbabwe, Harare: European (1990–1992)	135	127.73
US, Los Angeles: nonhispanic white (1988–1992)	15,823	103.69
US, San Francisco: nonhispanic white (1988–1992)	9080	103.30
US, Hawaii: white (1988–1992)	856	96.54
US, Connecticut: white (1988–1992)	11,135	93.25
Uruguay, Montevideo (1990–1992)	3118	92.59
US, Seattle (1988–1992)	10,380	92.54
US, Detroit: white (1988–1992)	10,265	91.86
Israel: Jews born in Israel (1988–1992)	1802	90.47
US, Atlanta: white (1988–1992)	4253	89.92
Israel: Jews born in America or Europe (1988–1992)	4838	87.89
US, New Orleans: white (1988–1992)	2160	87.04
US, New Mexico: nonhispanic white (1988–1992)	2625	86.27
US, Central California: nonhispanic white (1988–1992)	4665	86.21
France, Isere (1988–1992)	2896	85.95
India, Bangalore (1988–1992)	1381	21.32
Israel: Non-Jews (1988–1992)	262	21.30
Uganda, Kyadondo (1991–1993)	126	20.75
Zimbabwe, Harare: African (1990–1992)	117	20.36
Japan, Saga (1988–1992)	657	19.14
India, Trivandrum (1991–1992)	156	18.82
Viet Nam, Hanoi (1991–1993)	504	18.22
India, Karunagappally (1991–1992)	56	15.13
Thailand, Chiang Mai (1988–1992)	477	14.62
China, Qidong (1988–1992)	371	11.19
Mali, Bamako (1988–1992)	100	10.24
Algeria, Setif (1990–1993)	118	9.47
India, Barshi, Paranda, and Bhum (1988–1992)	78	8.71
Thailand, Khon Kaen (1990–1993)	236	8.35
Korea, Kangwha (1986–1992)	23	7.11

Fifteen highest and fifteen lowest incidence rates per 100,000 person-years are shown (Parkin et al., 1997).

The highest 10% rates are between 80 and 100 per 100,000 and the lowest 10% are between 10 and 20 per 100,000 (Table 6.2). These lowest rates are reported form variety of non-Caucasian population groups in Africa and Asia.

Cancer of the cervix is the second most common form of cancer in women worldwide and the leading female cancer in sub-Saharan Africa, Central and South America, and Southeast Asia. The highest incidence rate is recorded in the African population of Harare, Zimbabwe (67.2 per 100,000), Belem in Brazil (64.8 per 100,000), and in Trujillo in Peru (53.5 per 100,000) (Table 6.3). In general, high incidence rates are recorded in regions of South America, Africa, and India (Table 6.4). Low incidence rates of cervix cancer are found in a variety of population settings. The highest incidence rates recorded previously around 1980 were in Re-

TABLE 6.3. Cancer of the Cervix Uteri (ICD9 180)

Registry	Cases	Rate
Zimbabwe, Harare: African (1990–1992)	295	67.21
Brazil, Belem (1989–1991)	931	64.78
Peru, Trujillo (1988–1990)	288	53.48
Uganda, Kyadondo (1991–1993)	248	40.76
India, Madras (1988–1992)	2540	38.91
Brazil, Goiania (1990–1993)	506	37.13
Colombia, Cali (1987–1991)	1061	34.41
New Zealand: Maori (1988–1992)	193	32.21
Argentina, Concordia (1990–1994)	108	32.05
Ecuador, Quito (1988–1992)	697	31.66
French Polynesia (1988–1992)	91	27.69
India, Barshi, Paranda, and Bhum (1988–1992)	252	27.45
Peru, Lima (1990–1991)	1294	27.27
India, Bangalore (1988–1992)	1732	27.21
Thailand, Chiang Mai (1988–1992)	864	25.63
Japan, Yamagata (1988–1992)	292	5.52
Switzerland, Basel (1988–1992)	98	5.44
Kuwait: Non-Kuwaitis (1988–1989, 1992–1993)	56	5.35
Israel: All Jews (1988–1992)	553	5.27
Spain, Zaragoza (1986–1990)	146	4.77
Spain, Navarra (1987–1991)	82	4.68
US, Hawaii: Chinese (1988–1992)	10	4.55
China, Tianjin (1988–1992)	454	4.39
Israel: Jews born in America or Europe (1988–1992)	187	4.07
US, Los Angeles: Japanese (1988–1992)	20	4.05
Finland (1987–1992)	893	3.62
China, Shanghai (1988–1992)	860	3.26
Israel: Non-Jews (1988–1992)	40	2.99
Italy, Macerata (1991–1992)	12	2.77
China, Qidong (1988–1992)	97	2.64

Fifteen highest and fifteen lowest incidence rates per 100,000 person-years are shown (Parkin et al., 1997).

TABLE 6.4. Estimate of the Proportion of Cancer Deaths that Will Be Found to Be Attributable to Various Factors

	Best Estimate	Range
Tobacco	30	25–40
Alcohol	3	2–4
Diet	35	10–70
Food additives	< 1	5–2
Sexual behavior	1	1
Yet to be discovered hormonal analogies of reproductive factors	Up to 6	0–12
Occupation	4	2–8
Pollution	2	1–5
Industrial products	< 1	< 1–2
Medicines and procedures	1	0.5–3
Geographic factors	3	2–4
Infective processes	10	1–?

[a]Refers to United Kingdom or United States cancer pattern, Source: Peto (1985).

cife in Brazil (83.2) and in the Pacific Polynesian Islanders (64.4); these rates are somewhat higher than the current highest. High incidence rates are seen in several large Indian cities. The rates are intermediate in eastern Europe, but much lower in North America, Australia, and northern and western Europe. In Europe, low rates are noted in Finland, Spain, and southern Italy. In the United States large differences are seen between ethnic groups, with a twofold difference between the black and white populations. Incidence is also lower in Japanese populations, but is higher in Hispanics and American Indians. Ethnic differences are also seen in New Zealand between the Maoris, the non-Maoris, and the Pacific Polynesian Islanders. Urban populations frequently show higher rates than rural populations. A decline in the incidence and mortality rates for cervical cancer has been observed virtually everywhere with the possible exception of countries of Central and South America. However, interpretation of temporal trends here is confused by the problems alluded to in previous publications of mortality trends.[28] Where effective national screening programs have been introduced, as in Finland, mortality has fallen substantially.[29] However, increases in mortality rates for women born around 1930 have been observed recently in New Zealand, Australia, and the United Kingdom,[30] suggesting greater exposure to risk factors, whether new or preexisting, in the more recent birth cohorts in these countries. Further, there is a tendency to see increasing mortality trends in some countries in Central and South America although a clear interpretation is hampered by uncertainties surrounding the quality of the data for individual rubrics.

The leading incidence rates of prostate cancer are reported from North America, but straightforward interpretation and comparison of incidence rates are currently distorted by wide international variation in the use of prostate specific antigen (PSA) testing. The highest incidence rates in the mid-1980s, before rates in many regions were altered by the impact of the introduction of aggressive case-finding policies, were reported from black population groups in Atlanta (102.0 per 100,000), the San Francisco Bay Area (95.6), Detroit (94.2), Alameda County (93.5), and Los Angeles (82.7).[9] The overall incidence rate among blacks in the SEER system in the United States was 82.0 per 100,000, which was considerably higher than the corresponding incidence rate in whites (61.8). The lowest incidence rates are recorded from populations in Asia and northern Africa. The highest rates of prostatic cancer have been recorded in the black population of the United States and are now higher than 100 per 100,000; the lowest incidence rates are around 1, indicating a 100-fold difference in the incidence of prostate cancer worldwide. In contrast to the distribution pattern of overt prostatic cancers, the frequency of the smaller noninvasive lesions denoted "latent" carcinoma does not appear to show much international variation.[31] The incidence of prostate cancer in blacks is much higher and often double that among whites in the same locality. Rates are intermediate, in the 30 to 50 range, in Canada, South America, Scandinavia, Switzerland, and Oceania, whereas more moderate rates, around 20, are seen in most European countries. Very low rates, below 10, are seen in China, Japan, India, and other Asian countries, as well as in the Middle East, but not in Israel, where rates are around 20, with the exception, however, of the non-Jewish population, among whom the rates are lower.

Five of the highest recorded incidence rates for *testis cancer* are recorded from Switzerland: Zurich (8.9 per 100,000), Vaud (9.3), Basel (8.8), St. Gall (10.1), and Neuchatel (9.0). Incidence rates continue to be high in Denmark (9.2), where elevated levels have existed for decades.[13] Low incidence rates are recorded in a variety of populations in Southeast Asia and northern Africa. Bladder cancer incidence is highest in Italy, Spain, France, and Switzerland. Five of the highest incidence rates (out of over 200) of *bladder cancer* are found in men in regions of Italy: Trieste (38.7 per 100,000), Genoa (38.3), Florence (35.2), Torino (36.2), and Varese (35.0). Other high rates are recorded from white population groups of the United States, Spain, and Denmark. Low incidence rates are recorded from populations of the developing world. In women, the incidence rates are much lower than in men: the highest in women (7.4) would rank 138th out of 166 in men. Rates for United States blacks are uniformly about half those in white Americans, apparently due in part to an under-reporting of early-stage tumors.[32] The lowest rates occur in Asia, notably in India. Rates in Japan are slightly higher.

In non-Hodgkin's lymphoma, the two- to three-fold excess incidence rate in adolescent boys compared to adolescent girls is difficult to explain but offers some potentially important etiological clues.[33]

CANCER CONTROL

Epidemiology provides compelling evidence that a large proportion of human cancer may be avoidable. Different populations throughout the world experience different levels of different forms of cancer and these levels change with time. Groups of immigrants acquire the cancer pattern of their new home, sometimes within decades (as demonstrated by immigrants to Australia)[34] or sometimes requiring generations, as in the case of breast cancer in Japanese immigrants to the United States. Further, groups of individuals in a community with some characteristic that differentiates them from other members of the same community (such as Seventh Day Adventists, Mormons, blacks in parts of the United States, etc.) have markedly different cancer patterns. From evidence such as this the environmental theory of carcinogenesis has developed[35,36] and it is widely held that upwards of 80%, and perhaps 90%, of human cancer may be attributable to environmental factors, defining "environment" in its broadest sense to include a wide range of lifestyle (sometimes) pooly defined aspects, including dietary, social, and cultural practices.

In theory, therefore, the large majority of human cancer diagnosed each year may be avoidable, but avoidable causes of many common cancers have not yet been clearly identified. A prerequisite of cancer prevention lies in identifying the determinants of cancer risk. Cancer control embraces a number of important elements with the aim of reducing the incidence of cancer and, failing primary prevention, reducing mortality either by finding disease at an earlier and more "curable" stage or by improving the survival stage-for-stage through improvements in therapy. A number of disciplines are involved in this pursuit including epidemiology, clinical science, behavioral science, and health education. It is a complex and at times uncoordinated package.

Primary Prevention

There are a number of risk factors that appear to be related strongly to common forms of cancer. Doll and Peto[36] estimated that upwards of 80% and perhaps even 90% of cancer deaths in a country such as the United States may be avoidable. Recent estimates indicate that the single largest avoidable cause is tobacco smoking (Table 6.4). It is important to consider cancer prevention strategies on a global basis. From such considerations, several possibilities exist to reduce the incidence of cancer.[37]

Tobacco   Tobacco smoking remains the largest single avoidable cause of premature death internationally and the most important known carcinogen to humans.[38] It is estimated that between 25% and 30% of all cancers in developed countries are tobacco related. For more than 30 years it has been clear that prevention of smoking would lead to substantial reductions in death associated with lung and other cancers, heart disease, bronchitis, emphysema, and a number of other conditions. Despite this knowledge the problem of tobacco-related disease has increased in many parts of the world. In Europe at the present time tobacco smoking is a major cause of premature death. Throughout Europe, in 1990 tobacco smoking caused three quarters of a million deaths in middle-aged individuals (between 35 and 69 years of age). In the Member States of the European Union in 1990 there were over one quarter of a million deaths in middle age directly caused by tobacco smoking: 219,700 in men and 31,900 in women. There were many more deaths caused by tobacco at older ages. In countries of central and eastern Europe, including the former USSR, there were 441,200 deaths in middle age in men and 42,100 deaths in women.[39] There is a need for urgent action to help contain this important and unnecessary loss of life: half of regular smokers die directly as a result of their habit.[38]

Tobacco research has turned to the association between exposure to environmental tobacco smoke and a diversity of adverse health events, including lung cancer.[40] On the basis of 30 epidemiologic studies, the United States Environmental Protection Agency (EPA) concluded that environmental tobacco smoke (ETS) was a human lung carcinogen. It has been estimated that each year in the United States, 434,000 deaths are attributable to tobacco use, in particular cigarette smoking[41]; 112,000 of these were from lung cancer.[42] There are an estimated 1500 deaths in nonsmoking women due to passive smoke inhalation and 500 deaths in nonsmoking men annually.

The focus on passive smoke inhalation in epidemiologic research and health policy in Western countries cannot be allowed to divert attention from the major public health issue of active cigarette smoking: smokers are at much higher risk of cancer than those who involuntarily inhale some of their cigarette smoke. It could be that the low levels of smoking now prevalent among physicians and research scientists has led them unconsciously to overlook smoking as still being an important cause of cancer. The situation in women worldwide is alarming,[10] with the numbers of women who smoke increasing and with lung cancer rates now rising sharply in women as well as men in many countries.[43,44] In Japan, since 1950 lung cancer mortality has increased 10-fold in men and 8-fold in women. There is a major buildup of tobacco-related disease in China, where the effects of increasing prevalence of cigarette smoking in the 1950s and 1960s are being translated into increases in the incidence and mortality of smoking related cancers. In central and eastern Europe where some data are available to follow the mortality patterns, currently more than 400,000 premature deaths each year are caused by tobacco smoking.[38] The rates of lung cancer in younger men (35 to 64) in Poland, Hungary, and Czechoslovakia in the coming years are expected to exceed the highest rates ever recorded elsewhere internationally (in Scotland between 1960 and 1964) with no end to the rise yet in sight.[43] In Poland, life expectancy at age 45 in men has been declining for over a decade due to the increasing premature death rates from cancer and smoking-related vascular disease.[6] In contrast to western Europe and North America, cigarette consumption in central and eastern Europe and China is still rising. Action must be taken both to monitor the evolution of this epidemic and to promote smoking prevention and hence disease prevention.

There are a number of agreed upon elements to the core strategies of a comprehensive tobacco control strategy that have the support of the International Union Against Cancer (UICC), the World Health Organization (WHO), the "Europe Against Cancer" program of the European Community, and the European Institute of Oncology. These include: (1) a ban on all advertising and promotion of tobacco products; (2) effective government health warnings on all tobacco products; (3) a low tar/ nicotine policy; (4) tax and pricing policies; (5) alternative economic policies; (6) policies to protect young people from tobacco promotion and sales to prevent the onset of tobacco use; (7) policies to protect the rights of nonsmokers and establish in law the right to smoke-free environments, including the workplace; (8) policies to control smokeless tobacco and prohibit other new methods of nicotine delivery;

and (9) policies to ensure the wide availability of help for tobacco users who wish to stop.

In any program of cancer control, top priority should be given to control of tobacco; this is likely to have the greatest impact on reducing cancer incidence, and cancer mortality, than any other strategy currently known. A series of recommendations for tobacco control have been made by the *European Cancer Experts Committee*[12] that deserve the active support of the international scientific community.

Diet   Diet and nutritional factors became the focus of serious attention in the etiology of cancer from the 1940s onwards.[45] Initially dealing with the effect of feeding specific diets to animals receiving chemical carcinogens, research turned to the potential of associations with human cancer risk. Initially this was conducted through international comparisons of estimated national per capita food intake data with cancer mortality rates. It was consistently found that there were very strong correlations in these data, particularly with dietary fat intake and breast cancer.[46] As dietary assessment methods improved, and certain methodologic difficulties were identified and overcome, the science of *nutritional epidemiology* emerged.[47]

Focus of attention in human studies has largely been centered around associations with fat intake and the intake of vitamins in the diet. A summary of the epidemiologic situation is likely to be quite contentious, particularly in a subject area that appears to attract more reviews than original articles. Present evidence indicates that an increased intake of fat, and also red meat, in the diet is associated with an increased risk of colorectal cancer and probably prostate cancer. High consumption of fruits and vegetables is associated with a reduced risk of a number of forms of cancer including lung, oral, pancreatic, laryngeal, esophageal, bladder, and gastric cancer; the major exceptions have been the lack of strong association with hormonally related forms of cancer such as that of the prostate, breast, ovary, and endometrium.[48] The relationship appears to be a general effect and consistently found with many different groups of fruits and vegetables. Although many candidate mechanisms (and molecules) have been put forward, there is little real evidence to suggest that it is one particular component of diet as opposed to another that is responsible.

It is difficult to imagine the successful implementation of a randomized trial of increased consumption of fruits and vegetables and the search continues for the molecule(s) in fruits and vegetables responsible for the apparent protection. The demonstration of a reduction in mortality in a randomized intervention trial in China is of considerable significance and gives hope for a potentially successful future for chemoprevention,[49] at least in certain circumstances. This is, of course, a special population with high cancer rates and a long history of low dietary intakes of several important micronutrients. The results from this population at a dietary extreme cannot be directly applied to most Western populations, who generally consume a diet much richer in essential micronutrients. Indeed, the failure of three recent major studies to demonstrate any beneficial effect of β-carotene supplementation on cancer risk[50–53] in populations with essentially normal intakes poses key strategic questions regarding future directions in chemoprevention studies.

Alcohol Consumption   Alcohol consumption is causally associated with cancers at a variety of sites but chiefly with cancers arising in the oral cavity, pharynx, larynx, and esophagus.[53] It appears that although there is an independent action of alcohol consumption, its main effect seems to arise in its joint effect with cigarette smoking where, in the sites mentioned above, the joint effect is multiplicative in many studies. Obviously, reduction of alcohol consumption would lower the incidence of these forms of cancer but so would cessation of tobacco smoking. Heavy consumers of alcohol should be advised to limit their intake and to stop smoking. The impact of this health advice could be quite important, as cancers of the upper respiratory tract are estimated to account for more than 850,000 new cases each year worldwide.[9]

Sunlight Exposure   Despite being the center of a great deal of attention in many developed countries, where the incidence is increasing quite quickly, it has been estimated that malignant melanoma accounted for a total of 92,000 incident cases in 1985 or 1.2% of the total cancer burden.[9] Personal characteristics of natural susceptibility to sunlight are associated with an increased risk of melanoma. These characteristics incorporate the number of nevi, the propensity to get a sunburn and the poor ability to develop a tan when in the sun, and fair hair color. However, these characteristics cannot explain the dramatic increase in melanoma observed during the second half of the century. The main factor responsible for that increase is generally held to be the increased levels of recreational sun exposure (as during sunbathing sessions or outdoor recreational activities) that has taken place as a result of the economic improvement of many white communities.[54] Currently, there is strong evidence from at least 24 epidemiologic (case-control) studies conducted in Europe, North America, and Australia that brutal, intermittent exposure of skin to the sun is the main environmental factor implicated in melanoma occurrence.[55] Sunburn experience is also associated with melanoma, but seems to be rather a marker of both excessive sun exposure and inherited susceptibility to ultraviolet radiation than a cause of melanoma per se. Finally, if a high nevi count is a strong predictor of melanoma, it is important to stress that in its turn, nevi development is fostered by sun exposure.

Since 1980, the suntanning fashion has fostered the large-scale marketing of sunbeds. In 1995, nearly half of Swedish women 15 to 35 years old reported regular exposure to sunbeds.[56] Repeated exposure to sunbeds is suspected to increase the risk of melanoma,[57] but further studies are needed to correctly assess the magnitude of melanoma risk associated with the so-called "UVA suntanning." The important message is to avoid overexposure to sunlight and, in particular, to avoid sunburns at all times and to be particularly careful to protect children.[58] There have been several very effective campaigns, especially in Australia and New Zealand. The widespread use of sunbeds among young women, as well as men, in many countries is of considerable concern. This habit has been associated with an increased risk of melanoma, particularly following several years of use, and the current levels of use may greatly influence future melanoma rates among younger individuals.

Occupational Exposures   There are a number of clearly defined occupational risk factors for cancer and a number of chemicals have been shown to be carcinogenic to man.[59] The list is long and reflects considerable work by scientific researchers in a number of disciplines including toxicology, carcinogenesis, and epidemiology. Today, with an improved safety profile in the workforce apparent in many developed countries, it is important to ensure that exposure to known carcinogenic hazards in the workplace is not transferred to the developing countries. The standards of protection in place in developed countries should be maintained in the developing countries. Included in the list of demonstrated carcinogenic exposures would be ionizing radiation, asbestos, and several other commonly used substances. However, for identified carcinogens there is generally legislation in place to define exposure restrictions and dose limits. Ensuring that these are followed would lead to further reductions in occupational cancers.

Infective Processes   There is now strong evidence that human papilloma virus (HPV) is associated with an increased risk of cervix cancer in women,[60] that Epstein-Barr virus (EBV) is associated with an increased risk of nasopharyngeal cancer,[61] that hepatitis B is associated with an increased risk of primary liver cancer,[62] and that HIV infection is associated with Kaposi's sarcoma[63] and some forms of lymphoma.[64] In 1985 it was estimated that there were 315,000 new cases of liver cancer, and 437,000 incident cases of cervix cancer. With a "guestimated" 100,000 incidences of nasopharyngeal cancer, it would appear that there are at least 850,000 cases each year in which infective processes play an important determining role; this represents about 11% of the global cancer burden.

Obviously, successful vaccination programs against these viral infections would have a considerable impact on reducing the burden of these forms of cancer and the global burden. This impact would obviously vary in different parts of the world. The effects would be greatest in the developing world, where over three quarters of the world's cases of liver cancer are diagnosed: it has been estimated that 44% of the total of cases of liver cancer worldwide are to be found in China alone. Because of the timing of the infection in developing and developed countries, it has been estimated that two thirds of all cases could be prevented by the introduction of vaccination against hepatitis B into the primary vaccination schedule for infants.[65]

Endogenous Hormones   A large number of studies have investigated the role of oral contraceptive usage in breast cancer risk.[66] Initially, there appeared to be consistent evidence supporting an increased risk of breast cancer in "young" women associated with current prolonged use (over 5 years) of oral contraceptives; "young" is certainly less than 35 years and perhaps less than 45.[66] The risk appears to level off after use of oral contraceptives has stopped. A recent important meta-analysis was undertaken to help clarify this situation. All available epidemiologic data collected on this association was undertaken by the ICRF Cancer Epidemiology Group at Oxford, United Kingdom. The Collaborative Group on Hormonal Factors in Breast Cancer[67] brought together and reanalyzed the entire epidemiologic database avail-

able regarding the relationship between breast cancer risk and use of hormonal contraceptives. The objective was to obtain a clearer picture of the quantitative nature of
the putative relationship between patterns of use of hormonal contraceptives and the
subsequent risk of breast cancer in users.

The findings from this study provide strong support for two main conclusions.
First, while women are taking combined oral contraceptives and in the 10 years after stopping, there is a small increase in the relative risk of breast cancer (relative
risk [RR] in current users 1.24, 95% confidence interval [CI] [1.15, 1.33]; 1 to 4
years after stopping use RR = 1.16 [1.08, 1.23]; 5 to 9 years after stopping use RR
= 1.07 [1.02, 1.13]) (Fig. 6.2). Second, there is no significant excess risk of breast
cancer 10 or more years after stopping use (RR = 1.01 [0.96, 1.05]). Breast cancers
diagnosed in women who had used combined oral contraceptives were less advanced
clinically than those diagnosed in women who had never used these contraceptives:
for long-term users compared to women who never used contraceptives the relative
risk for tumors that had spread beyond the breast compared to localized tumors was
0.88 [0.81, 0.95]. There was no obvious association in the results for recency of use
between women with different background risks of breast cancer, including women
from different countries and ethnic groups, women with different reproductive histories, and those with or without a family history of breast cancer. Other features of
hormonal contraceptive use such as duration of use, age at first use, and the dose and
type of the hormone within the contraceptives had little additional effect on breast
cancer risk once recency of use had been taken into account.

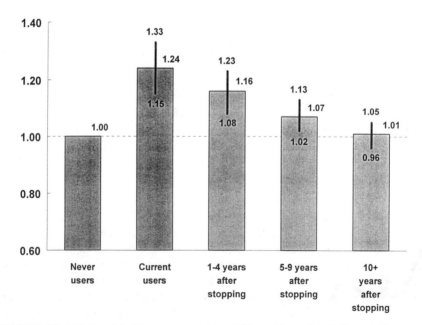

FIGURE 6.2. Relative risk of breast cancer (plus 95% confidence interval) according to use
of oral contraceptives.

The relationship between breast cancer risk and hormonal contraceptive use is unusual and it is not possible to infer from these data whether it is due to an earlier diagnosis of breast cancer in long-term users, the biologic effects of breast cancer in long-term users, or a combination of reasons. Women who are currently using combined oral contraceptives or have used them in the past 10 years are at a slightly increased risk of breast cancer, although the additional cancers diagnosed tend to be localized to the breast. There is no evidence of an increase in the risk of breast cancer 10 or more years after cessation of use, and the cancers diagnosed then appear to be less advanced clinically than the breast cancers diagnosed in women who had never used contraceptives. Further reassuring news is that the relative risks are small and the period-at-risk appears confined to times of life when the incidence of breast cancer, although not negligible, has not reached the highest levels attained in the latter part of the sixth and seventh decades of life.

The other important, and increasingly common, source of exogenous hormones in hormonal replacement therapy (HRT). There have been several important recent studies of breast cancer risk and hormonal replacement therapy use. To quantify the relationship between the use of hormones in postmenopausal women and the risk of breast cancer, the follow-up in the Nurse's Health Study was extended to 1992. There were 1935 cases of invasive breast cancer recorded during 725,550 woman-years of follow-up among postmenopausal women.[68] The risk of breast cancer was significantly increased among women who were currently using estrogen alone (RR = 1.32, 95% CI [1.14, 1.54]) as compared to postmenopausal women who had never used hormones. The risk of breast cancer was significantly increased among women who were currently using estrogen plus progestin (RR = 1.41, 95% CI [1.15, 1.74]).[68]

Women currently taking hormones and who had used such therapy for 5 to 9 years had an adjusted relative risk of breast cancer of 1.46 (95% CI [1.22, 1.74]). Women currently taking hormones and who had used such therapy for 10 years or more had an adjusted relative risk of breast cancer of 1.46 (95% CI [1.20, 1.76]). Breast cancer associated with 5 or more years of postmenopausal hormone therapy was greater among older women (RR for women aged 60 to 64 1.71 (95% CI [1.34, 2.18]). The relative risk of death from breast cancer was 1.45 (1.01, 2.09) among women who had taken estrogen for 5 or more years.[68]

Recent meta-analyses of the available studies on HRT use and breast cancer agree that little excess risk is associated with long-term use or short-term use of estrogen replacement.[69] A small increase in relative risk has a large impact on the number of women developing breast cancer because of the high baseline rates. For women in the United States aged 65, the baseline rate is 210 new cases per 100,000 women per year. A relative risk as small as 1.2 increases a woman's chances of developing breast cancer each year from 1 in 250 to 1 in 200.[70]

There is some evidence of an association between use of HRT and an increased risk of breast cancer: that was the conclusion of the Collaborative Group on Hormonal Factors in Breast Cancer,[69] based on a pooled analysis of individual data on 52,705 women with breast cancer and 108,411 women without breast cancer. Among current users of HRT or those who ceased use 1 to 4 years previously, the relative risk of breast cancer increased by a factor of 1.023 for each year of use: the relative risk was 1.35 (95% CI [1.21, 1.49]) for women who had used HRT for 5 years or longer. Five or more years after use of HRT ceased, there was no significant excess of breast cancer overall or in relation to duration of use. The cumulative excess numbers of breast cancers diagnosed between ages 50 and 70 years per 1000 women who began using HRT at age 50 and used it for 5, 10, and 15 years respectively are estimated to be 2 (95% CI [1 to 3]), 6 (95% CI [3 to 9]), and 12 (95% CI [5 to 20]). It was noted that cancers diagnosed in women who had used HRT long term tended to be less advanced clinically than those diagnosed in women who had never used HRT, but the effects on mortality are an open question.[69]

Screening

Cancer can be detected earlier than usual either when an individual recognizes symptoms and then quickly consults and is diagnosed by a physician or through the application of a screening test, aimed at diagnosing precancerous changes or cancer itself in generally asymptomatic individuals. Public education can be used to increase awareness of symptoms and their importance but the effects of such strategies have not been consistently evaluated.[71] Even without detailed scientific evaluation, there are important reasons for improving public knowledge and awareness of abnormal signs and symptoms. However, issues in population screening are once more of critical concern to physicians and public health specialists at the present time.

Cervical Cancer Screening for cervical cancer by examination of a cervical smear is widely recognized as leading to a reduction in the mortality from cervical cancer.[72] It has also been demonstrated to be cost-effective in older women, particularly among those who have not been screened regularly.[73] The impact is greatest where organized screening programs exist with personal letters of invitation; this leads to an improved attendance, particularly among those women who are at high risk of cervical cancer.[29]

It has been shown, particularly from the Nordic countries, that a population-based and well-organized screening program with a valid target age range, the correct frequency of screening, and built-in quality assurance programs at each stage of the screening process is more successful than opportunistic screening and that it can be effective in reducing both the incidence and mortality from invasive cervical cancer. It would appear that the most successful program in terms of reduction in risk of cervical cancer is in Finland, with an official recommendation that a screening program be started at age 30 and that the smear be repeated every 5 years.[29]

If cytologic screening programs seem to be effective in preventing invasive cervical cancer and cervical cancer mortality, numerous reports have underscored that that method may fail to detect a certain number of cervical cancers, mainly of the glandular type.[74] For instance, screening histories were examined in a case-control study in which the cases were all women with invasive cervical cancer in 24 health districts of health boards of Scotland, England, and Wales in 1992. It was estimated that the number of cases of invasive cervical cancer would have been 57% greater if there had been no previous screening; in women under 70 years it would have been approximately 75%.[75] The study further estimated that full adherence to current screening guidelines could have prevented 1250 cases of invasive cervical cancer in the United Kingdom in the same year but that further steps would have to be sought to prevent some of the remaining 2300 cases in women under the age of 70. Most frequent reasons evoked to explain the lack of sensitivity of cytologic screening refer to inadequate cell sampling with the spatula and to errors in the reading of smear slides. However, even in the best hands, a certain number of false-negative cytologic tests cannot be explained by sampling or reading problems. Hence, there is a strong feeling in the medical community that besides searching to improve screening coverage, there is also a need for additional ways to improve screening methods for cervical cancer. The first type of improvement consists of the improvement of the spatula used for cell sampling (with current preference for instruments such as the extended tip spatula), and in the automatization of cytologic reading. It remains to be assessed, however, whether these improvements in the cytologic methods will solve all types of false-negative results.

Methods based on other approaches to cervical cancer screening are under investigation: some may eventually be employed as adjuncts to the Pap smear. One is cervicography, which is popular in the United States and in some screening clinics in Europe. Although numerous groups have published results on screening with cervicography, well-conducted studies to evaluate cervicography (as compared to cytology) have remained rare.[76] The principal findings of these studies is that cytology and cervicography detect different premalignant lesions of the cervix. Hence, cervicography represents an interesting adjunct test to cytology, able to reduce the false-negative results of the screening process. Cervicography is not, however, a simple technique as it requires a large reading experience, and that experience is essential to maintain as low as possible the unnecessary referrals to colposcopy–biopsy.

Several other new technologies have shown some early promise although their potential value in the early detection of cervix cancer is at an earlier stage of assessment. For example, the PolarProbe is an instrument that is based on a mathematical recognition algorithm for detecting anomalies in the cervix. An initial pilot study with a prototype of the PolarProbe instrument has shown false-positive and false-negative rates on the order of 10% for the detection of premalignant lesions of the cervix,[77] which is a strong incentive to develop studies to further examine the potential role of PolarProbe in the detection of high-grade cervical lesions. Speculoscopy was developed in the United States around 1992 as an attempt to increase the sensitivity of the Pap smear by using chemical luminescence. It is currently being assessed in the screening setting in a variety of studies.

While this latter is being investigated as a tool in assisting the collection of a cervical smear, the technology may also have a potentially important application to cervical cancer detection in developing countries, where it could be very useful in improving the quality of a visual inspection of the cervix. Any means to advance the detection of cervical cancer, or preinvasive cervical lesions in the developing world would be particularly important; it is in such regions that typically have the highest rates of invasive cervical cancer (Table 6.3).

Given the implication of HPV infection in cervical cancer, detecting HPV could represent an appealing screening method. A study of 2009 women having routine screening in England and Wales revealed that 44% of cervical intraepithelial neoplasia (CIN) lesions of grade 2 or 3 detected had a negative cytology and were found only by HPV testing (for types 16, 18, 31, and 33); a further 22% were positive for HPV but demonstrated only borderline or mild cytologic changes.[78] However, 25% of CIN grade 2 or 3 lesions were not detected by the four HPV tests. Hence, there is convergence between the results obtained when comparing HPV testing to cytology, and cervicography to cytology. However, although appealing, routine HPV testing for cervical cancer screening is still controversial as HPV infection is very common in women less than 30 years old, and it is more important to evaluate women over the age of 30 with an HPV infection that persists over a long period of time. As it is impossible currently to identify those women with an HPV infection who will develop cervical cancer, HPV testing is proposed to be used in various ways—for instance, as an adjunct to cytology for sorting out the cytologic results classified as AS-CUS, referring ASCUS lesions positive for an HPV infection for colposcopy–biopsy. Another proposal consists of testing all women 30 years old or older for HPV, and referring to cytology only those positive for HPV.[79] Hence HPV testing is still to be thoroughly evaluated to find the exact role it could play in cervical cancer screening.

In conclusion, near maximal effectiveness in reducing incidence and mortality from cervical cancer can be achieved by an organized program of cervical smear testing with high coverage, in which screening is initiated at the age of 25 and is repeated at 3- or 5-yearly intervals to the age of 60. Extension of this approach should be considered only if maximal coverage has been attained, the resources are available, and the marginal cost-effectiveness of the recommended changes has been evaluated. HPV testing and other new technologies have still to be thoroughly evaluated although some of these could potentially usefully augment conventional cytology.

Breast Cancer   There is considerable evidence that breast cancer screening with mammography is effective in reducing mortality from breast cancer, especially in circumstances where the quality of the mammography is high with good quality control. The best estimates from randomized trial are that the size of the reduction may be around 30% if takeup of screening in the population is good and quality control standards high. An overview of the Swedish trials reported relative risks of death of 0.71 in the group randomized to and offer of screening with 95% confidence interval 0.57 to 0.89 for women aged 50 to 59 at entry. Results for women ages 60 to 69 were almost identical. When applied to a population it could be expected that a well-organized program with a good compliance could lead to a reduction in breast cancer mortality of the order of 20% in women aged over 50.[80] There is as yet no clear evidence that screening benefits older women and it is certain that they are less willing to undergo screening.

More importantly, results for younger women (under 50 years) are ambiguous, with no trials having large enough statistical power to analyze these women separately. The great controversy at the present time revolves around what recommendations should be made for mammographic screening of women between 40 and 49 years of age. This is an important social problem: more than 40% of the years of life lost due to breast cancer diagnosed before the age of 80 years are attributable to cases presenting symptomatically at ages 35 to 49 years, frequently an age of maximal social responsibility for women. In 1993, it was considered that there are no statistically significant results for this age group reported but point estimates including both reductions and increases in breast cancer mortality in women offered mammographic screening whiles aged under 50 years.[80] Since then it has become clear that the natural history of breast cancer among women younger and older than 50 years may be different. Reanalysis of the Swedish Two-County Trial has shed considerable light on two important issues. First, the mean sojourn time is estimated to be between 3 and 4 years for women age 50 or older but only about 20 months for women under 50 years of age, after adjustment for tumor size and nodal status.[81] Further, dedifferentiation often occurs at an early stage for women under age 50 but later for women over 50 years. This implies that the poorer performance of mammographic screening in younger women might be due to rapid progression and failure to arrest dedifferentiation in this age group because the screening interval is too long.[81] It has also been demonstrated mathematically that the same benefit in terms of breast cancer mortality reduction could be expected among younger women if they were screened approximately every 18 months.[82]

A collaborative meeting was held in Falun, Sweden early in 1996, for which data were submitted from all randomized trials of breast screening that included women ages 40 to 49. Update results from the Swedish Overview indicated that relative mortality associated with invitation to screening was 0.77 (95% CI [0.59, 1.01]). Combining all population-based randomized trials produced a relative mortality of 0.76 (0.62, 0.93) and when all trials were combined, the relative mortality was 0.85 (0.71, 1.01). It was concluded that mammographic screening of women ages 40 to 49 could reduce subsequent mortality from breast cancer and that it was probably necessary to screen every 12 to 18 months in this age range, with two-view mammography and double reading of films, to obtain substantial benefits.[83]

This position was not accepted by the recent United States National Cancer Institute Consensus meeting held in January 1997, and which ended in controversy and some acrimony,[84] but was upheld as a basis for recommendations to women by the American Cancer Society in March, 1997. Clearly, there are some remaining uncertainties surrounding this issue but women, and their families, deserve better ways to receive reliable information and clear recommendations about such an important issue than are available at present.

With regard to other methods of breast cancer screening, a recent large trial demonstrated mortality reduction among women who had been trained in breast self-examination although the authors concluded that the study would continue and that more conclusive results may emerge as follow-up continues.[85] The effect of taught breast self-examination is also currently being evaluated in a randomized trial in Russia.[86]

Colorectal Cancer   Fecal occult blood (FOB) testing has been reported from case-control studies to reduce colorectal cancer mortality rates by 31%[87] and 57% in women.[88] In a nonrandomized study it was shown that annual rigid sigmoidoscopy and FOB testing, rather than sigmoidoscopy alone, was associated with a reduction in colorectal cancer mortality.[89] There are now three randomized trials of FOB testing, each demonstrating a reduction in colorectal cancer mortality. Mandel et al.[90] reported a reduction of 33% in colorectal cancer mortality after 13 years in subjects who were offered annual screening with FOB tests, but an insignificant reduction (of 6%) in those who were offered biennial screening. In two more recent studies, from Nottingham, United Kingdom[91] and Denmark,[92] the colorectal cancer mortality rates in the group offered biennial FOB testing were respectively 0.85 and 0.82 the rates in the control population. A combined analysis of these latter studies produces a (approximate) relative risk of colorectal cancer death of 0.84 (95% CI 0.75 to 0.94).[93]

There are now some extremely important issues to address in the area of colorectal cancer screening. *Should FOB testing now be recommended as a population screening method?* This decision depends on many factors including the value placed on the magnitude of the mortality reduction, the false-positive rate associated with hemoccult testing, the acceptance of the test to the general population, and the economic costs involved. *Should consideration be given to other screening modalities for colorectal cancer?* Screening with sigmoidoscopy has been demonstrated in case-control and nonrandomized studies to reduce the incidence and mortality from colorectal cancer by more than 50%.[94–96] FOB testing does not appear to reduce the incidence of colorectal cancer. *Because a large proportion of individuals tested for FOB have positive tests and are referred for colonoscopy, could it prove effective to bypass FOB testing and go directly to a screening colonoscopy? Or flexible sigmoidscopy?* This latter strategy is currently being assessed in a large, randomized trial and it is a clear reflection of the tremendous potential for early detection of colorectal cancer by screening, which is clearly outlined in detail elsewhere.[97] This should continue to be a priority research activity at present.

Screening for Other Forms of Cancer   Although there are proposed screening tests for a number of different forms of cancer, there are no randomized trial data to support screening at other sites as a public health measure. There has been apparent success in Japan with screening for stomach cancer but this has not been carefully evaluated.[72] Screening tests are available and being evaluated for ovarian cancer, lung cancer, oral cancer, nasopharyngeal cancer, and neuroblastoma.[72] The issues in screening have been well outlined in two recent monographs.[98,99]

At the present time there is great pressure to screen for prostate cancer although widespread implementation of screening programs for prostate cancer cannot be recommended based on the available evidence; little has changed since the most recent review of the topic by an expert committee of the UICC (International Union Against Cancer) that came to the same conclusion.[72] Unfortunately there are national practices that are at complete variance; in the United States "screening" with PSA is widespread[100] while in the United Kingdom there is a strong bias against "screening" with PSA,[101] essentially on evidence-based grounds. The main reason for this situation is that no results are available from randomized trials assessing screening for prostate cancer. These are the only methods of evaluation that avoid bias and, in consequence, it is not known whether screening by any of the available modalities or a combination of them is effective in reducing the mortality from prostate cancer. Obviously, this is a necessary prerequisite for embarking on population screening or even screening high-risk groups (even if such a group can be defined for prostate cancer). Screening for prostate cancer at a population level would be expensive and consume a large proportion of available healthcare resources; it is therefore essential to have some indication of effectiveness and efficacy before embarking on such programs. There is no evidence available at present to indicate that any lives will be saved by such screening although it is logical to suppose that early detection and effective treatment could be effective. The current situation in the United States in favor of PSA screening has been compared with the enthusiasm and the similarity of the arguments put forward in favor of lung cancer screening several years ago,[102] although this bright promise did not subsequently materialize.

VARIATIONS IN THE OUTCOME OF CANCER TREATMENT

Advances in the outcome of treatment for breast cancer are taking place gradually. It is becoming clear that there are large variations in survival throughout Europe. The EUROCARE Project included 30 Cancer Registries throughout Europe in this project to investigate variations in cancer survival. The final database contained information on approximately 800,000 cancer patients.[103] This is a remarkable dataset but the results need to be interpreted with some caution because (1) criteria for admission of patients was not standardized in the centers; (2) the date of diagnosis varied between the centers (diagnosis, registration, treatment); (3) the completeness of follow-up varied between national registries and regional registries; and (4) no allowance was made for case-mix.

For breast cancer, using data from 12 countries, the three highest age-standardized relative 5-year survival rates calculated were from Switzerland (76%), Finland (74%), and France (71%). The three lowest were from Poland (44%), Estonia (59%), and Scotland (62%) (Fig. 6.3).

There are limitations that constrain the straightforward interpretation of these results. However, these limitations are unlikely to explain all of the variation noted and it can be safely concluded that real differences exist in breast cancer outcomes in Europe.

There is also evidence emerging that the outcome in breast cancer varies according to whether treatment was conducted in a specialist unit and according to the socioeconomic status of the patient. There has been a remarkable audit study conducted in the Greater Glasgow Health Board. This study was based on 4411 breast cancer cases in women under 75 years of age in a geographically defined region. After simultaneous adjustment for treatment center and tumor prognostic factors, the 5-year survival rate by deprivation status was 58% for affluent (1, 2), 51% for the middle group (3, 4, 5), and only 48% in the most deprived group (6, 7).[104] If applied to national data, the potential improvement in survival is 6%.

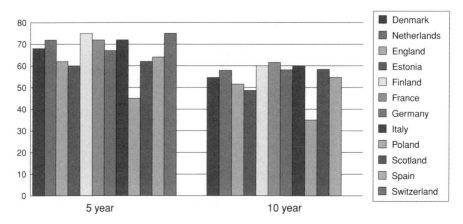

Figure 6.3. Five- and ten-year relative survival rate (%) from breast cancer in Europe.

Surgeons in GGHB were classified as specialist or nonspecialist breast cancer surgeons. The adjusted 5-year and 10-year survival rates among specialist surgeons were 66.8% and 49.1%, respectively. The corresponding survival figures for nonspecialist surgeons were 57.9% and 40.9%.[105] After adjustment for age, deprivation, tumor size, and nodal involvement, relative to nonspecialist surgeons (R R 1.0), the relative hazard ratio for specialist surgeons was 0.84 (95% CI [0.75, 0.94]). Specialist care could improve survival in the study population by 6.8 percentage points.

There is now some evidence emerging that ovarian cancer survival rates vary dramatically by stage and also by age within stage group.[106,107] The observation of differences in survival for patients with ovarian cancer throughout Scotland led to a detailed study to determine the potential role of suspected and unsuspected prognostic factors. After adjustment for age, stage, pathology, degree of differentiation, and presence of asctites, survival improved when patients (1) were first seen by a gynecologist ($p < 0.05$); (2) were operated on by a gynecologist ($p < 0.05$); (3) had residual disease of less than 2 cm postoperatively ($p < 0.0001$); (4) were prescribed platinum chemotherapy ($p < 0.05$); and (5) were referred to a joint clinic ($p < 0.001$). The improved survival from management by a multidisciplinary team was not solely due to the prescription of platinum chemotherapy.[108] These findings have recently been confirmed in large extent.[109]

By contrast, in a population-based study of 1588 patients with cervical cancer diagnosed and treated in western Scotland between 1980 and 1987, there was no difference in prognosis by age of treatment and socioeconomic status after controlling for stage, treatment type, and tumor grade.[110]

CONCLUDING REMARKS

There is strong evidence that cancer is, and will be for the immediate future, a major public health problem; that the majority of human cancers may be avoidable; and that several of the avoidable causes have already been identified. In global terms the greatest impact would be from the control of tobacco smoking and the control of breast cancer. While tobacco control could be achieved using a series of government and societal actions,[12] prospects for the prevention of breast cancer are more remote. In this regard, ongoing intervention trials of tamoxifen in healthy women have a unique role in being the only available intervention with a reasonable probability of success against this common condition. Other important reductions could be brought about by vaccination against hepatitis B and human papilloma virus. However, the results of the Gambia Hepatitis B Vaccination study are eagerly awaited as is the development of HPV vaccine for use against either in situ or invasive cervix cancer. Failing primary prevention, screening for breast and cervical cancer could have a significant effect on reducing mortality from these common diseases. Screening for other forms of cancer will emerge as public health strategies once there has been proper evaluation; the current situation with prostate cancer is salutary in this respect. With the expansion in the absolute numbers of cases of cancer set to continue into the next century, the role of prevention in cancer control strategies will increase in importance, as will the central role of epidemiology. This latter will also have to change; the time has come to deemphasize the search for risk factors and to refocus on the implementation of current knowledge in populations where many thousands, if not millions, of frequently premature deaths could be avoided.

Acknowledgments

This work was conducted within the framework of support from the Associazione Italiana per la Ricerca sul Cancro (Italian Association for Cancer Research).

FURTHER READING

1. Moodie RL (1918) Studies in paleopathology. *Ann Med Hist* 1:374–393.

2. Granville AB (1825) An essay on Egyptian mummies with observations on the art of embalming among the Ancient Egyptians. *Philos Trans R Soc* 115:269–279.

3. Pott P (1964) Chirurgical observations 1975. Reproduced in *J Natl Cancer Inst Monog* 10:7–13.

4. Redmond DE (1970) Tobacco and cancer: The first clinical report, 1761. *N Engl J Med* 282:18–23.

5. Ramazzini B (1743) *De Morbis Artificum*. Diatriba J Corona, Venezia.

6. Zatonski W, Boyle P (1996) Health transformations in Poland after 1988. *J Epidemiol Biostat* 1:123–126.

7. Parkin DM, Stjernsward J, Muir CS (1984) Estimates of the world-wide frequency of twelve major cancers. *Bull WHO* 62:163–182.

8. Parkin DM, Láára E, Muir CS (1988) Estimates of the worldwide frequency of sixteen major cancers in 1980. *Int J Cancer* 41:184–197.

9. Parkin DM, Ferlay J, Pisani P (1993) Estimates of the worldwide incidence of eighteen major cancers in 1985. *Int J Cancer* 54:594–606.

10. Chollat-Traquet C (1992) *Women and Tobacco*. World Health Organization, Geneva.

11. Brody J (1985) Prospects for an ageing population. *Nature* 315:463–466.

12. Boyle P (1997) Cancer, Cigarette smoking and premature death in Europe. A review including the Recommendations of European Cancer Experts Consensus Meeting, Helsinki, October 1996. *Lung Cancer* 17:1–60.

13. Clemmesen J (1965) *Statistical Studies in Malignant Neoplasms. I Review and Results.* Munksgaard, Copenhagen.

14. Macfarlane GJ, Boyle P, Evstifeeva TV, Robertson C, Scully C (1994) Rising trends of oral cancer mortality among males worldwide: The return of an old public health problem. *Cancer Causes Cont* 5:259–265.

15. Boyle P, Marfarlane GJ, Blot WJ, Chiesa F, Lefebvre JL, Mano Azul A, de Vries N, Scully C (1995) European School of Oncology Advisory Report to the European Commission for the Europe Against Cancer Programme: Oral carcinogenesis in Europe. *Oral Oncol* 31B:75–85.

16. Day NE, Munoz N (1982) Esophagus. In: Scottenfeld D, Fraumeni JF (eds). *Cancer Epidemiology and Prevention* WB Saunders, Philadelphia, pp. 596–622.

17. Lu JB, Yang WX, Liu JM, et al. (1985) Trends in morbidity and mortality for esophageal cancer in Linxian county, 1959–1983. *Int J Cancer* 36:643–645.

18. Muir CS, Waterhouse J, Mack T, Powell J, Whelan S (eds) (1987) *Cancer Incidence in Five Continents*, Vol. V. I ARC Scientific Publications no. 88, Lyon.

19. Kmet J, Mahboubi E (1972) Esophageal cancer in the caspian littoral of Iran: Initial studies. *Science* 175:846–853.

20. Smans M, Boyle P, Muir CS (eds) (1993) *Cancer Mortality Atlas of EEC*. IARC Scientific Publication no. 107, Lyon.

21. Napalkov NP, Tserkovy GF, Merabishuili VM, Parkin DN, Smans M, CS (eds) (1983) *Cancer Incidence in the USSR* (Supplement to *Cancer Incidence in Five Continents*, Vol. III) IARC Scientific Publication no. 48, Lyon.

22. Boyle P, Maisonneuve P, Levi F, Evstifeeva T, Zatonski W, Zaridze DG, La Vecchia C (1993) Cancer patterns in central and eastern Europe: Comparison with the rest of Europe. In: Bodmer W, Zaridze DG (eds) *Cancer Prevention in Central and Eastern Europe*. International Union Against Cancer (UICC), Geneva.

23. Srivatanakul S, Sontipong P, Chotiwan P, Parkin DM (1988) Liver cancer in Thailand: Temporal and geographic variations. *J Gastroenterol Hepatol* 3:413–420.

24. Parkin DM, Stiller CA, Bieber CA, Draper GJ, Terracini B, Young JL (eds) (1988) *International Incidence of Childhood Cancer*. IARC Scientific Publication no. 87, Lyon.

25. Ries LAG, Kosary CL, Hankey BF, Miller BA, Harras A, Edwards BK (eds) (1997) *SEER Cancer Statistics Review, 1973–1994*. National Cancer Institute. NIH Publication No. 97-2789, Bethesda, MD.

26. Balzi D, Carli P, Geddes M (1977) Malignant melanoma in Europe: Changes in mortality rates (1970–90) in European Community countries. *Cancer Causes Cont* 8:85–92.

27. Giles GG, Armstrong BK, Burton RC, Staples MP, Thursfield VJ (1996) Has mortality form melanoma stopped rising in Australia? Analysis of trends between 1931 and 1994. *Br Med J* 312:1121–1125.

28. Cuzick J, Boyle P (1988) Trends in cervix cancer mortality. *Cancer Surv* 7:417–439.

29. Hakama M, Magnus K, Petterson F, Storm H, Tulinius H (1991) Effect of organised screening on the risk of cervix cancer in the Nordic countries. In: Miller AB, Chamber-

lain J, Day NE, Hakama M, Prorock PC (eds) *Cancer Screening*. International Union Against Cancer, Geneva.

30. Muñoz N, Bosch FX, Jensen OM (eds) (1989) Human papillomavirus and cervical cancer. IARC Scientific Publications no. 94, Lyon.

31. Breslow N, Chan CE, Dhom G, Drury RAB, Franks LM, Gellei B, Lee YS, Lundberg S, Sparke B, Sternby NH, Tulinius H (1997) Latent carcinoma of prostate at autopsy in seven areas. *Int J Cancer* 20:680–688.

32. Schairer C, Hartge P, Hoover RN, Silverman DT (1988) Racial differences in bladder cancer risk: A case-control study. *Am J Epidemiol* 128:1027–1037.

33. Boyle P, Maisonneuve P (1996) Epidemiology of cancer in adolescents. In: Selby P, Bailey C (eds) *Cancer and the Adolescents*. BMJ, London, pp. 3–21.

34. McCredie M, Coates MS, Ford JM (1990) Cancer incidence in European migrants to New South Wales. *Ann Oncol* 1:219–225.

35. Higginson J, Muir CS (1979) Environmental carcinogenesis: Misconceptions and limitations to cancer control. A review. *J Natl Cancer Inst* 63:1291–1298.

36. Doll R, Peto R (1981) The causes of cancer: Quantitative estimates of avoidable risks of cancer in the United States today. *JNCI* 66:1191–1308.

37. Peto R, Lopez AD, Boreham J, Thun M, Heath C (1992) Mortality from tobacco in developed countries: Indirect estimation from national vital statistics. *Lancet* 39:1268–1278.

38. Peto R, Lopez AD, Boreham J, Thun M, Heath C, Doll R (1996) Mortality from smoking world-wide. *Br Med Bull* 52:12–21.

39. EPA (United States Environmental Protection Agency) (1992) Respiratory health effects of passive smoking: Lung cancer and other disorders. US Environmental Protection Agency, Washington, DC.

40. Centers for Disease Control (1991) Smoking-attributable mortality and years of potential life lost—United States, 1988. *MMWR* 40:62–71.

41. USDHHS (United States Department of Health and Human Services) (1989) Reducing the health consequences of smoking: 25 years of progress. A report of the Surgeon General. US Government Printing Office, Washington, DC.

42. La Vecchia C, Lucchini F, Negri E, Boyle, P, Maisonneuve P, Levi F (1992) Trends of cancer mortality in Europe, 1955–89. II Respiratory tract, bone, connective and soft tissue sarcomas, and skin. *Eur J Cancer* 28:514–599.

43. La Vecchia C, Lucchini F, Negri E, Boyle P, Levi F (1993) Trends in cancer mortality in the Americas, 1955–1989. *Eur J Cancer* 29A:431–470.

44. Tannenbaum A (1940) Relationship of body weight to cancer incidence. *Arch Pathol* 30:508–517.

45. Armstrong B, Doll R (1975) Environmental factors and cancer incidence and mortality in different countries, with special reference to dietary practices. *Int J Cancer* 15:617–631.

46. Willett WC (1990) *Nutritional Epidemiology*. Oxford University Press, Oxford.

47. Steinmetz KA, Potter JD (1991) Vegetable, fruit, and cancer I. Epidemiology. *Cancer Causes Contr* 2:325–358.

48. Blot WJ, Li J-Y, Taylor P, Guo W, Dawsey S, Wang G-Q, Yang CS, Zheng S-F, Gail M, Li G-Y, Yu Y, Liu B-q, Tangrea J, Sun Y-h, Liu F, Fraumeni JF, Zhang Y-H, Li B (1993) Nutrition intervention trials in Linxian, China: Supplementation with specific

vitamin/mineral combinations, cancer incidence, and disease-specific mortality in the general populaton. *J Natl Cancer Inst* 85:1483–1492.

49. Alpha-Tocopherol, Beta-Carotene Cancer Prevention Study Group (1994) The effect of vitamin E and beta carotene on the incidence of lung cancer and other cancers in male smokers. *N Engl J Med* 330:1029–1035.

50. Hennekens CH, Buring JE, Manson JE, Stampfer MJ, Rosner B, Cook NR, Belanger C, LaMotte F, Gaziano JM, Ridker PM, Willett WC, Peto R (1996) Lack of effect of long-term supplementation with beta-carotene on the incidence of malignant neoplasms and cardiovascular disease. *N Engl J Med* 334:1145–1149.

51. Omenn GS, Goodman GE, Thornquist MD, Balmes J, Cullen MR, Glass A, Keogh JP, Meyskens FL, Valanis B, Williams JH, Barnhart S, Hammar S (1996) Effects of combination of beta-carotene and vitamin A on lung cancer and cardiovascular disease. *N Engl J Med* 334:1150–1155.

52. IARC (International Agency for Research on Cancer) (1988) *Monographs on the Evaluation of Carcinogenic Risk of Chemicals to Humans*, Vol. 44. *Alcohol Drinking*. IARC, Lyon.

53. Autier P, Doré JF, Lejeune D, Koelmel KF, Geffeler O, Hille P, Cesarini JP, Liénard D, Liabeuf A, Joarlette M, Chemaly P, Hakim K, Koeln A, Kleeberg U (1994a) Recreational exposure to sunlight and lack of information as risk factors for cutaneous malignant melanoma. Results of a European Organisation for Research and Treatment of Cancer (EORTC) case-control study in Belgium, France and Germany. *Melanoma Res* 4:79–85.

54. Elwood M, Jopson J (1997) Melanoma and sun exposure: An overview of published studies. *Int J Cancer* 73:198–203.

55. Boldeman C, Beitner H, Jansson B, Nilsson B, Ullen H (1996) Sunbed use in relation to phenotype, erythema, sunscreen use and skin disease: A questionnaire survey among Swedish adolescents. *Br J Dermatol* 135:712–716.

56. Autier P, Doré JF, Lejeune F, Koelmel KF, Geffeler O, Hille P, Cesarini JP, Liénard D, Liabeuf A, Joarlette M, Chemaly P, Hakim K, Koeln A, Kleeberg U (1994b) Cutaneous malignant melanoma and exposure to sunlamps or sunbeds: An EORTC multicenter case-control study in Belgium, France and Germany. *Int J Cancer* 58:809–813.

57. Boyle P, Veronesi U, Tubiana M, Alexander FE, Calais da Silva F, Denis LJ, Freire JM, Hakama M, Hirsch A, Kroes R, La Vecchia C, Maisonneuve P, Martin-Moreno JM, Newton-Bishop J, Pinborg JJ, Saracci R, Scully C, Standaert B, Storm H, Blanco S, Malbois R, Bleehen N, Dicato M, Plesnicar S (1995) European School of Oncology Advisory Report to the European Commission for the "Europe Against Cancer Programme": European Code Against Cancer. *Eur J Cancer* 9:1395–1405.

58. Tomatis L, Day NE, Heseltine F, et al. (1990) *Cancer: Causes, Occurrence and Control*. International Agency for Research on Cancer, Scientific Publication no. 100, Lyon.

59. IARC (International Agency for Research on Cancer) (1996) *Monographs on the Evaluation of Carcinogens Risk of Chemicals to Humans*, Vol. 20. *Human Papilloma Viruses*. IARC, Lyon.

60. Epstein MA (1978) Epstein-Barr virus—discovery, properties and relationship to nasopharyngeal carcinoma. In: De Thé G, Ito Y (eds) *Nasopharyngeal Carcinoma: Etiology and Control*. IARC Scientific Publication No. 20, IARC, Lyon.

61. Beasley RP, Lin C, Hwang LY, Chien CS (1981) Hepatocellular carcinoma and hepatitis B virus. A prospective study of 22,707 men in Taiwan. *Lancet* ii:1129–1133.

62. Biggar RJ, Rosenberg PS, Cote T (1996) Kaposi's sarcoma and non-Hodgkin's lymphoma following the diagnosis of AIDS. Multistate AIDS/Cancer Match Study. *Int J Cancer* 68:754–758.

63. Pedersen C, Barton SE, Chiesi A, Skinhoj P, Katlama C, Johnson A, van Lunzen J, Hirschel B, Maayam S, Lundgren JD (1995) HIV-related non-Hodgkin's lymphoma among European AIDS patients. AIDS in Europe Study Group. *Eur J Haematol* 55:245–250.

64. Prentice RL, Thomas DB (1987) On the epidemiology of oral contraceptives and diseases. *Adv Cancer Res* 49:285–401.

65. Collaborative Group on Hormonal Factors in Breast Cancer (1996) Breast cancer and hormonal contraceptives: Collaborative reanalysis of individual data on 53,297 women with breast cancer and 100,239 women without breast cancer from 54 epidemiological studies. *Lancet* 347:1713–1727.

66. Colditz GA, Hankinson SE, Hunter DJ, Willet WC, Manson JE, Stampfer MJ, Hennekens C, Rosner B, Speizer FE (1995) The use of oestrogens and progestins and the risk of breast cancer in post-menopausal women. *N Engl J Med* 332:1589–1593.

67. Collaborative Group on Hormonal Factors in Breast Cancer (1997) Breast cancer and hormone replacement therapy. *Lancet* 350:1047–1059.

68. Hulka BS, Liu ET, Lininger RA (1994) Steroid hormones and risk of breast cancer. *Cancer* 74:1111–1124.

69. IARC Working Group on Cervical Cancer Screening (1986) Summary chapter. In: Hakama M, Miller AB, Day NE (eds) *Screening for Cancer of the Uterine Cervix*. IARC Scientific Publications No. 76, IARC, Lyon, pp. 133–142.

70. Miller AB, Chamberlain J, Day NE, Hakama M, Prorock PC (1991) *Cancer Screening*. International Union Against Cancer, Geneva.

71. Fahs MC, Mandelblatt J, Schechter C, Muller C (1992) Cost effectiveness of cervical cancer screening in the elderly. *Ann Intern Med* 117:520–527.

72. Koss LG (1989) The Papanicolaou test for cervical cancer detection: A triumph and a tragedy. *J Am Med Acad* 261:737–743.

73. Sasieni PD, Cuzick J, Lynch-Farmery E (1996) Estimating the efficacy of screening by auditing smear histories of women with and without cervical cancer. The National Coordinating Network for Cervical Screening Working Group. *Br J Cancer* 73:1001–1005.

74. Coibion M, Autier P, et al. (1994) Is there a role for cervicopgraphy in the detection of the pre-malignant lesions of the cervix uteri? *Br J Cancer* 70:125–128.

75. Coppleson et al. (1994) *Int J Gynecol Cancer* 4:79–83.

76. Cuzick J, Szarewski A, Terry G, Ho L, Hanby A, Maddox P, Anderson M, Kocjan G, Steele ST, Guillebaud J (1995) Human papillomavirus testing in primary cervical screening. *Lancet* 345:1533–1536.

77. Meijer CJ, van den Brulle AF, Snijders PJ, Helmerhorst T, Kenemans P, Walboomers JM (1992) In Munoz N, Bosch FX, Shah KV, Meheus A (eds) *The Epidemiology of Cervical Cancer and Human Papillomavirus*, IARC Scientific Publications no. 119, Lyon, pp. 271–281.

78. Wald NJ, Chamberlain J, Hackshaw A, Anderson T, Boyle P, Forrest P, Frischbier HJ, Hakama M, Rutqvist LE, Schaffer P, Seradour B, Tabar L, Rosselli Del Turco M, Van der Schueren E (1993) Report of the European Society of Mastology (EUSOMA) Breast Cancer Screening Evaluation Committee. *The Breast* 2:209–216.

79. Chen HH, Duffy SW, Tabar L, Day NE (1997) Markov chain models for progression of breast cancer. Part I: tumour attributes and the pre-clinical screen-detectable phase. *J Epidemiol Biol* 2:25–36.

80. Chen HH, Duffy SW, Tabar L, Day NE (1997) Markov chain models for progression of breast cancer. Part II: tumour attributes and the pre-clinical screen-detectable phase. *J Epidemiol Biol* 2:37–44.

81. Swedish Cancer Society and the Swedish National Board of Health and Welfare (1996) Breast-cancer screening with mammography in women aged 40–49 years. *Int J Cancer* 68:693–699.

82. News and Comments (1997) The breast-screening brawl. *Science* 275:1056–1059.

83. Thomas DB, Gao DL, Self SG, Allison CJ, Tao Y, Mahloch J, Ray R, Qin Q, Presley R, Porter P (1997) Randomized trial of breast examination in Shanghai: Methodology and preliminary results. *J Natl Cancer Inst* 89:355–365.

84. Semiglazov VF, Sagaidak VN, Moiseyenko VM, Mikhailov EA (1993) Study of the role of breast self-examination in the reduction of mortality from breast cancer. The Russian Federation/World Health Organisation Study. *Eur J Cancer* 29:2039–2046.

85. Selby JV, Friedman GD, Quesenberry CP, Weiss NS (1993) Effect of fecal occult blood testing on mortality from colorectal cancer: A case-control study. *Ann Intern Med* 118:1294–1297.

86. Wahrendorf J, Robra BP, Wiebelt H, Oberhausen R, Weiland M, Dhom G (1993) Effectiveness of colorectal cancer screening: A population-based case-control study in Saarland, Germany. *Eur J Cancer Prev* 1:221–227.

87. Winawer SJ, Flehinger BJ, Schottenfeld D, Miller DG (1993), Screening for colorectal cancer by screening with fecal occult blood testing and sigmoidoscopy. *J Natl Cancer Inst* 85:1311–1318.

88. Mandel JS, Bond JH, Church TR, et al. (1993) Reducing mortality from colorectal cancer by screening for fecal occult blood. *N Engl J Med* 328:1365–1371.

89. Hardcastle JD, Chamberlain JO, Robinson MHE, Moss SM, Amar SS, Balfour TW, James PD, Mangham CM (1996) Randomised controlled trial of faecal-occult-blood screening for colorectal cancer. *Lancet* 348:1472–1477.

90. Kronberg O, Fenger C, Olsen J, Jorgensen OD, Sondergaard O (1996) Randomised study of screening for colorectal cancer with faecal-occult-blood test. *Lancet* 348:1467–1471.

91. Hardcastle JD (1997) Screening for colorectal cancer. *Lancet* 349:358.

92. Selby JV, Friedman GD, Quesenbery CP, et al. (1992) A case-control study of screening sigmoidoscopy and mortality from colorectal cancer. *N Engl J Med* 26:653–657.

93. Greenberg R, Baron J (1993) Prospects for preventing colorectal cancer death. *J Natl Cancer Inst* 85:1182–1184.

94. Boyle P (1995) Progress in preventing death from colorectal cancer (Editorial). *Br J Cancer* 72:528–530.

95. Mandel J (1996) Colon and rectal cancer. In: Reintgen DS, Clark RA (eds) *Cancer Screening*. Mosby, St. Louis, pp. 55–96.

96. Chamberlain J, Moss S (eds) (1996) *Evaluation of Cancer Screening*. Springer-Verlag, Berlin.

97. Reintgen DS, Clark RA (eds) (1996) *Cancer Screening*. Mosby, St. Louis.

98. Catalona WJ (1996) Prostate cancer. In: Reintgen DS, Clark RA (eds) *Cancer Screening*. Mosby, St. Louis, pp. 97–117.

99. Chamberlain J, Melia J (1996) In: Chamberlain J, Moss S (eds) *Evaluation of Cancer Screening*. Springer-Verlag, Berlin, pp. 117–136.

100. Collins MM, Barry MJ (1996) Controversies in prostate cancer screening. Analogies to the early lung cancer screening debate. *JAMA* 276:1976–1979.

101. Berrino F, Sant M, Verdacchia A, Capocaccia R, Hakulinen T, Esteve J (1995) Survival of cancer patients in Europe: The EUROCARE Study. International Agency for Research on Cancer, IARC, Lyon.

102. Carnon AG, Ssemwogerere A, Lamont DW, Hole DJ, Mallon EA, George WD, Gillis GR (1994) Relation between socioeconomic deprivation and pathological prognostic factors in women with breast cancer. *Br Med J* 309:1054–1057.

103. Gillis CR, Hole DJ (1996) Survival outcome of care by specialist surgeons in breast cancer: A study of 3786 patients in the west of Scotland. *Br Med J* 312:145–148.

104. Ries LA (1993) Ovarian cancer. Survival and treatment differences by age. *Cancer* 71:524–529.

105. Markman M, Lewis JL, Saigo P, Hakes T, Rubin S, Jones W, Reichman B, Curtin J, Barakat R, Almadrones L, et al. (1993) Impact of age on survival of patients with ovarian cancer. *Gynecol Oncol* 49:236–239.

106. Junor EJ, Hole DJ, Gillis CR (1994) Management of ovarian cancer: Referral to a multidisciplinary team matters. *Br J Cancer* 70:363–370.

107. Woodman C, Baghdady A, Collins S, Clyma JA (1997) What changes in the organisation of cancer services will improve the outcome for women with ovarian cancer? *Br J Obstet Gynaecol* 104:135–139.

108. Lamont DW, Symonds RP, Brodie MM, Nwabineli NJ, Gilles CR (1993) Age, socioeconomic status and survival from cancer of cervix in the West of Scotland 1980–1987. *Br J Cancer* 67:351–357.

CHAPTER 7

THE CHEMOPREVENTION OF CANCER

FADLO R. KHURI, ANITA L. SABICHI, WAUN KI HONG, and SCOTT M. LIPPMAN

University of Texas M. D. Anderson Cancer Center
Houston, TX 77030, USA

Cancer chemoprevention is a highly promising, relatively young branch of the enormous field of cancer research. The term *chemoprevention* was coined in the mid-1970s by Dr. Michael B. Sporn, who also defined it as the pharmacologic intervention with natural or synthetic compounds to reverse or suppress carcinogenesis in its early or premalignant stages and so prevent the development of invasive cancer. Intensive worldwide interest in this emerging area of research derives largely from the inability of therapeutic advances over the last 30 or more years to effect any substantial improvements in survival of major invasive cancers of the lung, head and neck, colon, breast, and other sites. Cancers of these and other regions continue to account for hundreds of thousands of deaths annually in the United States alone. Many advances in epidemiologic, molecular biologic, and clinical research also have promoted chemoprevention to the forefront of new approaches for cancer control.

This chapter reviews several critical areas of chemoprevention research: the biology of chemoprevention, including the seminal biologic and molecular concepts of multistep carcinogenesis and field carcinogenesis; key design concepts of clinical and translational chemoprevention trials; major chemopreventive agents currently under development; and trials of various chemopreventive agents in several regions and sites, including, among others, the head and neck, lung, colorectal region, skin, cervix, breast, bladder, and prostate.

Manual of Clinical Oncology, 7th edition, Edited by Raphael E. Pollock
ISBN 0-471-23828-7, pages 163–179. Copyright © 1999 Wiley-Liss, Inc.

BIOLOGY OF CHEMOPREVENTION

Multistep Carcinogenesis and Premalignancy

The extraordinarily complex process of carcinogenesis can evolve over decades from the original mutagenic initiation through multiple stages before an endstage of invasive cancer is reached. This multistep process involves untold molecular and cellular alterations affected by several endogenous and exogenous factors that either enhance or retard the process. It was Sporn's proposal that this process we now call multistep carcinogenesis could be pharmacologically reversed or arrested that gave rise to the field of chemoprevention.

Two of the great dilemmas facing chemoprevention researchers are: (1) how to identify individuals most likely to develop cancer, as most people having endogenous and exogenous mutational burdens or even epithelial premalignant lesions do not develop cancer; and (2) how to identify truly efficacious preventive agents out of the thousands of apparently active compounds suggested by epidemiology and preclinical research. Continued advances in our limited understanding of multistep carcinogenesis are crucial to resolving these dilemmas by developing interventions for preventing cancers in the appropriate, or highest risk, populations.

The classic, somewhat oversimplified, model of cancer development involves the three distinct stages of initiation, promotion, and progression. Initiation is described as rapid and irreversible and involving direct carcinogen binding and damage to DNA. Promotion is described as the reversible stage between initiation and the appearance of a premalignant lesion and as involving primarily epigenetic mechanisms. Progression is irreversible and described as the stage between the appearance of the premalignant lesion and development of invasive cancer and as involving further alterations in genetic mechanisms.

Multiple genetic events within and affecting the multistep carcinogenic process have been identified in animal and human studies. These events involve gene mutations and gene-function alterations. Two gene types under intensive study are tumor suppressor genes and oncogenes. Tumor suppressor genes are thought to protect against cancer, whereas oncogenes are thought to promote cancer development. Disabling mutations of tumor suppressor genes can lead to cancer development. Conversion of a proto-oncogene to an oncogene via activating mutation (or gene overexpression) disrupts the normal regulatory function of the gene and also can lead to cancer development.

The three stages of the classic model apparently are clearly defined in animal studies. In humans, however, they can involve great overlap, occurring simultaneously or concurrently over several decades, and the concept of the model is evolving into a more complex understanding of carcinogenesis. A more recently identified class of genes, DNA-repair genes, also are helping reshape our concept of carcinogenesis. These genes function to correct inherited or acquired genetic alterations. Defects in or absence of these genes also can contribute to cancer development.

The extraordinary spectrum of cancer risk remains a mystery. After years of exposure to potent carcinogens, some people remain cancer free. After little or no known exposure, some people develop cancer. It may be that defects in the DNA-repair genes are a genetic condition, and this may partially explain differing profiles of cancer susceptibility of individuals. This is an intriguing aspect of the complex interactions between environmental and genetic factors leading to cancer that are only beginning to be understood by molecular biologists and epidemiologists.

Field Carcinogenesis

Coined by Slaughter in 1953, the term "field cancerization" (also called field carcinogenesis) describes Slaughter's findings that many heavy smokers had abnormal changes and premalignant areas throughout the aerodigestive tract (mouth, throat, and lungs). He theorized that diffuse carcinogenic exposure to cigarette smoke puts sites throughout the entire region at risk of cancer development. Auerbach, another important pioneer in this area, studied autopsy specimens and the airways of lung cancer patients to compare carcinogenic damage in heavy smokers versus light smokers versus nonsmokers. Auerbach's and Slaughter's findings of the late 1950s/early 1960s demonstrated that the degree of exposure to tobacco smoke is tightly linked to the degree of tissue damage in the airway.

The relatively frequent development of new cancers in cancer survivors was long thought to be exclusively a result of metastasis of the original cancer. The concept of field carcinogenesis, however, has led many researchers to believe that a portion of subsequent cancers are independent second primary cancers, not metastases. This concept, therefore, has very important implications for chemoprevention. Multiple independent premalignant lesions in the field of exposure may be vulnerable to suppression or reversal by chemopreventive agents before they can progress into invasive second primary cancers.

CHEMOPREVENTION TRIAL DESIGNS

Before the US Food and Drug Administration (FDA) approves a new chemopreventive agent, several steps of drug development must be taken, usually requiring several years. Following extensive testing in animal models, potentially safe and effective new chemopreventive drugs must pass through three major phases of human testing, called phases I, II, and III (briefly outlined in Table 7.1).

The first, or phase I, human trials are actually of two types: phase Ia (single dose application) and phase Ib (continuing dose application). Phase Ia trials are designed to assess the acute toxicity and pharmacokinetics (i.e., absorption, distribution, metabolism, elimination) of single administrations of various dose levels of an agent. Usually this is a dose-escalation design with the initial dose established by preclinical study. These trials generally involve 20 to 30 fasting and nonfasting subjects. The toxicity limit is that acceptable to generally healthy subjects ($\leq$ grade 2). Phase Ib trials are designed to assess the chronic toxicity and pharmacokinetics of repeated administrations of various dose levels of an agent. These trials may be randomized, even placebo-controlled, usually require 1 to 3 months in normal subjects

TABLE 7.1. Chemoprevention Trial Designs

Phase	Major Features
Ia	Single dose trial to characterize acute toxicity, pharmacokinetics
Ib	Repeated daily dose study to characterize chronic toxicity/pharmacokinetics/efficacy
IIa	Dose deescalation and fixed-dose single-arm trials; activity; surrogate endpoint biomarkers (SEBs)
IIb	Randomized, placebo-controlled, double-blind trials; definitive for SEBs
III	Definitive, cancer-incidence endpoint

(up to 12 months in higher cancer risk subjects), and have variable sample sizes. Phase Ib trials can include evaluations of potential surrogate endpoint biomarkers (SEBs).

Phase II trials also are divided into types IIa and IIb. Phase IIa trials are single-arm, fixed-dose trials to assess activity and possibly biomarkers or are dose-finding (deescalation) trials designed to define the optimal dose for further study and development. The optimal dose level is that which is maximally biologically active and has acceptable, or minimal, toxicity in the relatively healthy subject/patient population. Phase IIb trials are randomized, controlled trials designed to establish SEB modulation with the phase IIa-established optimal dose of an agent.

Phase III trials are large-scale, double-blind, placebo-controlled trials designed to definitively assess a chemopreventive agent's effectiveness. So far, the only definitive endpoint for these trials is cancer development. Because not everyone at apparent risk develops cancer, and because cancer requires many years to develop, phase III trials to assess reduced rates of cancer development can involve thousands of subjects and many years to complete. The obvious drawbacks to phase III chemoprevention trials are the time it takes to assess the drug and the enormous costs incurred by such long-term, large-scale trials. For this reason, there is intense interest in validating SEBs that could determine drug effectiveness via analysis of intermediate endpoints. SEBs are markers of cellular and molecular genetic changes associated with carcinogenesis and drug activity.

Potential SEBs are being assessed at every level of chemoprevention testing: preclinical and phases I, II, and III. So far, no SEBs have been validated for definitive chemoprevention trials, that is, markers that have been shown to be associated with carcinogenesis and to be modulatable by a chemopreventive agent have not yet been correlated with ultimate development of cancer. The intensive, ongoing effort to select and validate potential SEBs is designed to curtail the enormous time, sample size, and expense of definitive phase III trials.

A risk, and advantage, of currently designed phase III trials is that they will detect subtle or long-term adverse effects unseen in phase I and II testing. For example, the phase III α-tocopherol, β-carotene (ATBC) Trial and Carotene and Retinol Efficacy Trial (CARET) found that β-carotene, a well-known antioxidant found in many fruits and vegetables, was not only ineffective in preventing tobacco-related cancers but also increased risk of lung cancer. The epidemiologic finding that a diet of fruits and vegetables conferred lower cancer risk led to the hypothesis that β-carotene was one of the major active preventive components of those complex foods. This was supported by preclinical laboratory testing. The natural agent β-carotene had been thought to be virtually free of toxicity before surprising results of the ATBC trial and CARET were published. These trials pointed out the tremendous complexity of chemopreventive agent testing, not only in regard to long-term toxicity, but also in regard to confirming preliminary epidemiologic and preclinical laboratory findings. We are left with the valid epidemiologic knowledge that diets high in fruits and vegetables are beneficial, but we still do not know which specific constituents of these foods protect against cancer.

CHEMOPREVENTIVE AGENTS

Since coinage of the term *chemoprevention* by Sporn in the mid-1970s, several thousand agents have been identified through animal, epidemiologic, and clinical studies as potential cancer chemopreventive agents. Tables 7.2 and 7.3 list a wide sampling of agents currently undergoing preclinical and phase I testing (Table 7.2) or phase II/III testing (Table 7.3). This section highlights a few of the most active and intensively studied agents to date.

Retinoids

Retinoids is the name given a class of compounds that includes natural vitamin A and its synthetic and natural analogs. Retinoids are the best studied and among the most promising substances tested in chemopreventive research to date. Through activation of signal transduction pathways, retinoids are active in maintaining orderly

TABLE 7.2. Promising Chemopreventive Agents: Preclinical/Phase I Development

S-Allyl-l-cysteine	Plant monoterpenes
Curcumin	Limonene
DFMO combinations, e.g.	Perillyl alcohol
Plus 4-HPR	Polyphenolic compounds
Plus oltipraz	(e.g., tea/EGCG)
Flavonoids (e.g., genistein)	Retinoids
Fuasterone	CD437
Ibuprofen	Anti-AP-1 retinoids
Indole-3-carbinol	Sulindac sulfone
Lycopene	Ursodiol
PEITC	Vitamin D_3 analogs

TABLE 7.3. Promising Chemopreventive Agents: Phase II/III Development

Antiandrogens	Retinoids
Flutamide	All-*trans*-RA
Bicalutamide	9-*cis*-Retinoic acid (RA)
Aromatase inhibitors	Retinyl methyl ester
Examestane	Targretin (RXR-selective)
Letrozole	Vitamin A
Arimidex	13-*cis*-RA
Aspirin + calcium	4-HPR
Calcium	Selenium (Se)
COX-2 inhibitors	Selenomethioinine
DHEA	Selenate
DFMO	High-Se yeast
Finasteride (and other 5α-reductase	Se + vitamin E
inhibitors)	Selective antiestrogens
Folic acid	Triphenylethylene
Glutathione inducers	Raloxifene
N-Acetylcysteine (NAC)	Tamoxifen
Oltipraz	Vitamin D_3 analogs
NSAIDs	Vitamin E
Aspirin	
Piroxicam	
Sulindac	

growth, differentiation, and apoptosis of epithelial cells. Data from clinical and laboratory studies suggest that vitamin A and other retinoids have a preventive effect on epithelial cancer in a number of sites, including the skin, bladder, lung, breast, and oral cavity.

The synthetic retinoid 13-*cis*-retinoic acid (13cRA) has been shown to be effective in reversing oral premalignant lesions. Although significant toxicity was incurred in initial studies using high-dose 13cRA, subsequent studies defined effective drug regimens with acceptable toxicity profiles. Retinoids also have been used in preventing second primary tumors in subjects after definitive treatment for primary cancer of the lung or head and neck.

A very recent randomized placebo-controlled study of the natural compound retinol to prevent skin cancer found that a dose of 25,000 IU was effective in preventing new squamous cell carcinoma (SCC) but not basal cell carcinoma of the skin. This dose of retinol exceeds the common intake of most American adults and produced an approximately eightfold increase in serum retinyl palmitate in the treatment group. Results of this study corroborate positive results or previous studies of other retinoids, which prevented skin cancer in high-risk subjects (e.g., renal transplant and xeroderma pigmentosum patients).

Calcium

Studies done in both rats and humans suggest that calcium and several other micronutrients in the diet may have a preventive effect on colon carcinogenesis. Dietary calcium precipitates some of the cytotoxic agents that may promote colon cancer, such as fatty acids and secondary bile acids. Short-term (4 months) administration of 2000 to 3000 mg of calcium has been shown to favorably alter the bile acid profile in individuals with a history of resected adenocarcinoma of the colon.

Colon cancers arise in mucosa with abnormalities of increased proliferative rates and/or decreased rates of cell death (apoptosis) that lead eventually to formation of adenomas. Proliferation of the epithelial lining of the colon is altered in patients at risk for colon cancer and has been used in many human trials as a "marker" of the effects of calcium interventions on the colon. Five small, uncontrolled clinical trials have found that proliferation within the colonic epithelial layer was decreased by calcium administration. Three large, randomized, placebo-controlled trials of calcium effects on proliferation each produced a different result: no effect on, and a decrease and increase in the proportion of proliferating cells in the crypts of the colonic mucosa. A very recent randomized calcium trial reported a reduction in adenomas.

Data from prospective studies and multivariate analyses assessing the association between calcium intake and colon cancer appear to support the hypothesis that calcium intake is protective against colon cancer risk. Further studies are required, however, before calcium can be recommended for persons at risk of colon cancer, and calcium for prevention of colon cancer should be reserved for use in controlled clinical trials.

Aspirin/NSAIDs

A large body of epidemiologic and preclinical data suggests that the regular use of aspirin or other nonsteroidal antiinflammatory agents (NSAIDs) in humans reduces the risk of colon cancer and precursor adenomatous polyps. Data from women in the Nurses' Health Study indicate that regular aspirin use (at doses similar to those recommended for the prevention of cardiovascular disease) substantially reduces the risk of colorectal cancer. The data also indicate that this benefit may not be evident until after at least a decade of regular aspirin consumption. In this study, maximal reduction in risk was observed among women who took four to six tablets of aspirin per week. The US Physicians Study, employing a 2-by-2 factorial design to assess aspirin and β-carotene, did not show a reduction in colon polyps or cancer incidence in the aspirin-treated group.

Although promising for the prevention of human colorectal cancer, aspirin has not yet been fully evaluated for efficacy in prospective controlled trials. Also, the lowest effective dose of aspirin has not been determined, which should be a major objective of research with this agent. In one recent study, mucosal prostaglandins, which are thought to be involved in the pathogenesis of colon cancer, were significantly suppressed at a low dose of aspirin (81 mg/day).

Perhaps the most encouraging data for this class of agents have been achieved with the NSAID Sulindac. Sulindac was found to be significantly active in familial adenomatous polyposis syndrome, reversing existing adenomas and preventing new adenoma formation. Patients in their 20s who have this syndrome may develop thousands of precancerous colorectal adenomas, that, left untreated, almost invariably progress to cancer when these patients reach their 50s.

Side effects of chemopreventive agents are of particular importance because they are used in an asymptomatic population. Use of aspirin and other NSAIDS can be accompanied by considerable adverse effects. Serious complications of these agents have not been reported in chemoprevention studies conducted in Western countries. However, a recent report from Japan noted that four of six patients treated chemopreventively with the NSAID Sulindac (300 mg) for colonic polyps developed adverse side effects independent of the period of treatment that necessitated dose reduction or discontinuation of the drug. Until the results of definitive studies are available, a standard recommendation for the use of aspirin or other NSAID supplements as chemopreventive agents for people with predisposition to colon polyps or cancers, or healthy people at average risk of colon cancer, cannot be made.

Selenium

Perhaps one of the most promising substances identified as a potential chemopreventive is selenium. A number of epidemiologic studies have suggested an inverse correlation between estimated intake or blood and serum levels of selenium and the incidence of cancers including breast, colon, prostate, lung, and bladder. Selenium is an essential nonmetallic trace element that has potent antioxidant and antiproliferative properties. It can also induce apoptosis and promotes differentiation. Studies in animal models have shown that carcinogen-induced tumor formation can be inhibited with dietary supplementation with selenium. The chemopreventive potential of selenium in humans has been suggested by a trial conducted by Clark et al. in which 200 μg/day of selenium (high-selenium brewer's yeast tablet) significantly reduced overall cancer incidence and mortality. After 4.5 years of treatment and 6.4 years follow-up, Clark et al found that total cancer incidence was lower in the selenium-treated group than in the placebo group and that significant reductions in incidences of lung, prostate, and colorectal cancers occurred.

The Clark study was designed to test the hypothesis that selenium can prevent skin cancer. The results of this primary endpoint were completely negative, not even indicating a trend toward reduction in rate of skin cancer. Therefore, the statistical significance of the reduction of internal malignancies (lung, colorectal, prostate) must be viewed with caution, as these results derive from subset analyses of multiple secondary endpoints.

Tamoxifen and Raloxifene

Another successful chemopreventive agent is tamoxifen, a nonsteroidal triphenylene derivative that has been studied mostly in breast cancer. Tamoxifen has both pro- and antiestrogenic effects. In the breast, it acts as an antiestrogenic agent, and it has been shown to reduce the likelihood that postmenopausal women who have had breast cancer will develop a recurrence or a second primary cancer. In the uterus, however, tamoxifen acts as a proestrogenic agent, and it has been shown to slightly increase the risk of developing uterine cancer. Because of this increased risk, scientists are now evaluating a new agent called raloxifene, a compound similar to tamoxifen in its antiestrogenic activity in breast tissue, but without any evidence of proestrogenic activity in other tissue, such as that of the uterus.

Lycopene

Although the results of studies on β-carotene in prevention of lung cancer (discussed previously), were disappointing, trials using other carotenoids, such as α-carotene and lycopene, are generating encouraging results. The Health Professionals follow-up study assessed dietary intake for a 1-year period in a cohort of subjects and found that tomato-based foods (tomatoes, tomato sauce, and pizza) and strawberries were primary sources of lycopene (a non-provitamin-A carotenoid with potent antioxidant activity) and were associated with lower prostate cancer risk. Combined intake of greater than 10 servings versus fewer than 1.5 servings per week of tomatoes (fruit, sauce, juice, pizza) was inversely associated with risk of prostate cancer. This study also found that intake of more than 10 servings per week of lycopene-rich foods was inversely associated with advanced (stage C and D) prostate cancer. The authors concluded that their study suggests that intake of lycopene or other compounds in tomatoes may reduce prostate cancer risk. A follow-up study demonstrated that lycopene could be measured in the prostate at concentrations that were biologically active in laboratory studies. These findings support (1) the hypothesis that lycopene may contribute to reduced prostate cancer risk by direct effects within the prostate and (2) the need for a prospective intervention trial of lycopene to prevent prostate cancer.

Finasteride

Finasteride is a 5α-reductase inhibitor that inhibits conversion of testosterone to the active metabolite dihydrotestosterone, which is believed to play a crucial role in prostate cancer development. This agent has been used in the largest phase III trial ever conducted in the United States—the Prostate Cancer Prevention Trial (PCPT). This study was conducted through the Southwest Oncology Group, and its accrual was completed in 1997 (over 18,000 evaluable men). Results have not yet been reported.

Micronutrient Supplements

People in the Huixian and Linxian regions of China have low intake and blood levels of various micronutrients. Several large studies have shown that a strikingly high incidence of esophageal and gastric cancers exists in these regions. These observations led to several prevention trials. In one, subjects from Huixian were given supplements of retinol, riboflavin, and zinc for 13.5 months. There was no overall difference in the occurrence of premalignant lesions or prevalence or severity of dysplasia in the gastrointestinal tract between those who received the intervention and those who did not.

Another trial done in Linxian County tested the efficacy of four different nutrient combinations for inhibiting the development of esophageal and gastric cancers. The nutrient combinations included retinol + zinc, riboflavin + niacin, ascorbic acid + molybdenum, and β-carotene + selenium + α-tocopherol. There was a 13% reduction in total cancer deaths, 4% reduction in esophageal cancer deaths, and a 21% reduction in gastric cancer deaths in the group who received β-carotene + vitamin E + selenium. This finding has important public health implications for one of the major worldwide causes of mortality from cancer. None of the other nutrient combinations significantly reduced gastric or esophageal cancer deaths. It is not known which nutrient, or nutrients (β-carotene, vitamin E, or selenium), was/were responsible for the observed protection, and the applicability of these results to populations with adequate nutritional status and to other tumor sites may be limited.

A second trial in Linxian County was designed to determine whether a multivitamin/multimineral preparation plus β-carotene (15 mg/dl) could reduce esophageal and gastric cardia cancers in more than 3000 residents with esophageal dysplasia. After the 6-year intervention period, cumulative esophageal/gastric cardia cancer death rates were 8% lower, mortality from esophageal cancer was 16% lower, and total mortality from cancer was 4% lower in the supplemented group. Surprisingly, mortality from stomach cancer was 18% higher in the supplemented group. None of these results were statistically significant.

A study conducted in Basel, Switzerland, followed 2974 men prospectively and found that the overall mortality from cancer over a 17-year period was associated with low mean plasma levels of carotene and of vitamin C. Lung and stomach cancers were associated with low mean plasma carotene level (adjusted for cholesterol). Simultaneously low levels of plasma vitamin C and lipid-adjusted vitamin E also were associated with significantly increased risk for lung cancer. Low vitamin E levels in smokers were related to an increased risk for prostate cancer. The authors concluded that low plasma levels of the vitamins C and E, retinol, and β-carotene (a plant pigment and major precursor of vitamin A found in some fruits and in yellow, orange, and dark-green leafy vegetables) are related to increased risk of overall and lung cancer mortality, and that low levels of vitamin E in smokers are related to an increased risk of prostate cancer mortality.

These and a multitude of other experimental and epidemiologic data suggested that deficiencies of α-tocopherol (a prominent form of vitamin E found in nuts, grains, seeds, vegetable oils, and other foods) and β-carotene might increase risk of certain cancers, particularly lung cancer.

All the data mentioned in the preceding paragraph led to two large randomized double-blinded placebo-controlled chemoprevention trials (ATBC and CARET) involving β-carotene and α-tocopherol. To almost universal surprise and consternation, these studies found that administration of β-carotene or vitamin A to smokers not only had no chemopreventive benefit, but that β-carotene supplementation caused a modest increase in lung cancer incidence and mortality.

As in the case of β-carotene, positive epidemiologic data on other antioxidants (e.g., vitamins C and E) require rigorous follow-up testing before any recommendations can be made. The specific constituents or combinations of constituents in fruits and vegetables that might confer cancer protective effects have yet to identified.

MAJOR CHEMOPREVENTION CLINICAL TRIALS

More than 70 randomized chemoprevention trials have been reported to date, including phase II trials for the reversal of premalignancy in the head and neck, lung, colon, skin, esophagus, bladder, and cervix and phase III trials to prevent cancers of the head and neck, lung, colon, skin, breast, esophagus, and stomach.

Head and Neck Cancer Prevention

Oral Premalignancy   Oral leukoplakia is a premalignant condition that is manifested in the form of white patches found in the mouth or throat. These lesions are directly related to tobacco exposure (often in the form of chewing tobacco), and, depending upon their severity, have a 10% to 40% chance of transforming into cancer. Surgery and radiotherapy are not recommended for oral leukoplakia, as these lesions usually return after treatment. Oral leukoplakia is very responsive to chemopreventive treatment with various retinoids, including 13-*cis*-retinoic acid (13cRA) at high (induction) and low (maintenance) doses. The lesions relapse at a high rate, however, upon cessation of 13cRA treatment. In addition to trials of low-dose 13cRA for maintenance, newer trials of 4-hydroxyphenyl retinamide (4-HPR) in oral leukoplakia also have been conducted and achieved positive results. This agent is less toxic than is 13cRA and so is an especially attractive potential regimen for preventing oral cancer in relatively healthy oral leukoplakia patients.

Second primary cancers   Two large randomized phase III trials have been completed in the chemoprevention of second primary head and neck cancers. The first of these studies, high-dose 13cRA, acid achieved a marked decrease in the incidence of second primary cancers in patients after treatment for primary advanced head and neck cancer. Careful follow-up of the patients revealed a positive effect on incidence of second primary cancers, whereas the recurrence rate was unchanged. Serious side effects of the treatment included conjunctivitis, cheilitis, hypertriglyceridemia, and severe drying and cracking of the skin. In approximately 80% of the patients it was necessary to lower the dosage to complete the treatment.

The second phase III retinoid trial in preventing second primary cancers involved a different retinoid, etretinate, in patients treated for earlier stage head and neck cancer and was completed in 1993. This trial did not achieve a lower incidence of second primary cancers in the retinoid group. Ongoing studies are experimenting with newer retinoids and with lower doses of previously tested retinoids, such as 13cRA, in an effort to find the safest and most effective drug and drug dosage for head and neck second primary cancer chemoprevention.

Lung Cancer Prevention

Premalignancy   In contrast with positive studies in oral premalignant lesions and prevention of second primary cancers of the head and neck, lung cancer chemoprevention studies have been discouraging. Several such studies have been completed to date, producing no consensus on the activity of various retinoids, vitamin B_{12}, or β-carotene in this model. Strikingly positive studies of vitamin B_{12} and folic acid supplementation were significantly flawed, and therefore their results are doubtful. Studies of retinoids, including 13cRA, etretinate, and others, have failed to show a substantial effect in reversing premalignancy in people at risk of lung cancer.

Prevention of Second Primary Cancer   To date, only one study in the chemoprevention of second primary cancers of the lung has been reported. This was a phase III trial of the natural retinoid retinyl palmitate, which achieved a reduction in the development of second primary cancers. Completed in the early 1990s, this study led to a second, large, randomized phase III trial of 13cRA in approximately 1500 patients with stage I non-small-cell lung cancer. This second study was completed in early 1997, and the results are still being analyzed in preparation for publication.

Prevention of Initial Lung Cancers in Patients at High Risk   Four large primary lung cancer prevention studies have been completed to date. All four tested β-carotene; two also tested the retinoid retinol; and one tested β-carotene, retinol, and α-tocopherol (a natural form of vitamin E). These trials were conducted in subjects at high risk due to cigarette smoking or long exposure to asbestos. Two of these studies showed no difference in lung cancer development between the β-carotene and placebo groups. However, as mentioned previously in the Chemoprevention Trial Designs section, two of these studies, the ATBC trial and CARET, found that β-carotene not only did not decrease lung cancer incidence but actually increased it.

The ATBC and CARET β-carotene findings rigorously emphasize the need of confirmation of any epidemiologic data, which, in the case of β-carotene, strongly suggested that this substance could provide protection against cancer development.

The issue of smoking cessation remains paramount to prevention of lung and other tobacco-related cancers. Data indicate, however, that smoking cessation is not always sufficient to eliminate increased cancer risk. Many smokers remain at increased risk for 5 or 10 years after stopping the habit. Therefore, chemoprevention offers an approach for further decreasing former smokers' level of cancer risk.

Colorectal Cancer Prevention

Several colon and rectal cancer chemoprevention trials of various agents, including NSAIDs, calcium salts, and vitamin/micronutrient combinations, have been completed (see Chemopreventive Agent section). NSAIDs were suggested for colorectal chemoprevention by results of population-based analyses showing that long-term aspirin supplementation lowered the risk of colon cancer. Sulindac is the NSAID currently thought to show the most promise for preventing colorectal cancer. Extensive studies of calcium also have been conducted in this setting, producing encouraging results. Although two small early calcium studies were positive, calcium efficacy against colorectal cancer has not been confirmed in five subsequent larger, randomized studies. Current clinical trials are assessing the efficacy of more promising agents for preventing colorectal cancer, such as cyclo-oxygenase-2 (COX-2) inhibitors, selenium, DFMO, and oltipraz.

Skin Cancer Prevention

Retinoids have been used in chemoprevention of skin cancers. These agents have been particularly effective in reducing the incidence of skin cancers in patients at extremely high risk, such as those with xeroderma pigmentosum and renal transplant recipients. Xeroderma pigmentosum is a rare genetic disorder and the retinoid 13cRA can substantially reduce skin cancer incidence in these patients.

Based on these data, further studies were done in other patient populations. A placebo-controlled randomized trial of topical all-*trans* retinoic acid (ATRA) has successfully reversed actinic keratoses, which have a low rate of malignant transformation. Systemic retinoid therapy has also been studied in two randomized trials in which patients with actinic keratosis (AK) were treated with etretinate. Both studies showed significant regression of AK lesions in treated patients compared with those receiving placebo. Retinoids have not been as effective in other populations at high risk for developing skin cancers. One large phase III randomized study showed that oral retinol was effective in preventing squamous cell cancers, but not basal cell cancers, in patients with prior actinic keratoses. Three other agents—the retinoid 13cRA, β-carotene, and selenium—were tested in three separate phase III trials, and did not achieve protective effects against development of skin cancers.

Breast Cancer Prevention

Second Primary Cancers The increased risk of second breast cancers in women who had an initial breast cancer has focused breast chemoprevention research on this group of women. As mentioned previously in the Chemopreventive Agents section, the efficacy of tamoxifen has been established: data from more than 30,000 women participating in 40 randomized adjuvant trials have shown that tamoxifen achieved a highly significant reduction of 39% in the development of second primary cancers. Tamoxifen was most effective in women receiving long-term treatment and in postmenopausal women.

The retinoid fenretinide (4-HPR), which has fewer side effects than many other studied retinoids, also has demonstrated potent chemopreventive activity in breast carcinogenesis. Although a recently completed chemoprevention trial of 4-HPR failed to show an overall benefit in the prevention of second primary breast cancers, a subset analysis indicated that premenopausal women on 4-HPR did have fewer second primary cancers. Also, a 4-HPR preventive effect against ovarian cancer was suggested by the result that six women of this trial receiving placebo developed ovarian cancer during the study, whereas none of the women receiving 4-HPR developed ovarian cancer. Promising results of 4-HPR in this setting have led to large random-ized trials of 4-HPR versus tamoxifen and also of combined 4-HPR and tamoxifen versus 4-HPR or tamoxifen alone.

Primary Breast Cancer   Although tamoxifen can substantially reduce the risk of second primary breast cancer, this agent has not yet demonstrated any benefit in women at high risk of primary breast cancer. One of the large primary breast cancer chemoprevention trials of single-agent tamoxifen currently underway in high-risk women is the Breast Cancer Prevention Trial (BCPT) of the National Surgical Adjuvant Breast and Bowel Project (NSABP), which enrolled approximately 13,000 women thought to be at higher than average risk of breast cancer. Recently having completed accrual, this trial will require several years of follow-up before impact on long-term cancer incidence can be determined.

Bladder Cancer Prevention

Clinical interest in retinoids for preventing bladder cancer was raised by positive retinoid studies in animals and population-based studies showing that vitamin A protects against bladder cancer. To date, a few small trials have been completed in this setting, showing some potential benefit of low-dose, long-term retinoids in preventing recurrence of superficial bladder tumors. In one informative study, very high doses of vitamins A, C, and E; zinc; and paradoxene supplements were more effective than the recommended dietary allowance of multivitamins in reducing the rate of superficial bladder tumor recurrence. Currently planned and ongoing clinical and translational studies of fenretinide (4-HPR) will establish whether or not this promising agent is effective in bladder carcinogenesis.

Esophageal and Stomach Cancer Prevention

Five large placebo-controlled chemoprevention trials in esophageal and gastric car-cinogenesis have been conducted in regions of China with unusually high rates of esophageal/gastric cancers. In four of these five trials, multiple natural compounds, including retinol, β-carotene, vitamin E, and selenium, were tested (see Chemopre-ventive Agents section). In one of the trials, a small reduction in gastric cancer rates was achieved, but all five trials suffered from problems of high dropout rates and poor study compliance. Therefore, the jury is still out on whether high multivitamin supplementation can effectively reduce the risk of gastric or esophageal cancer in high risk populations.

Cervical Cancer Prevention

Cervical carcinogenesis is a well-defined process: the premalignant lesion dysplasia develops and proceeds through mild, moderate, and severe stages before developing into invasive cancer. Seven of eight chemoprevention trials that have been conducted in cervical dysplasia produced negative results with several agents, including folic acid, β-carotene, and interferon. One of the eight trials was a recently completed positive phase IIb trial of the retinoid tretinoin in 301 women. Tretinoin was significantly active in moderate dysplasia but not in severe dysplasia. Other ongoing retinoid trials are designed to confirm the early, promising results with tretinoin in this setting.

Prostate Cancer Prevention

The Southwest Oncology Group (SWOG), a cooperative group consisting of cancer treatment and research institutions from across the United States and other parts of the world, recently completed accrual of over 24,000 men into its phase III Prostate Cancer Prevention Trial (PCPT) of finasteride, or Proscar. Finasteride currently is accepted treatment for benign prostatic hypertrophy. The PCPT met its accrual goal in very good time, establishing that a large-scale chemoprevention study can be conducted in the multiple-institution setting of a cooperative group. The primary endpoint question of the effect of finasteride on prostate cancer incidence will require several more years of follow-up to answer.

Subset analysis from the phase III trial of selenium in skin cancer prevention (discussed previously in the Chemopreventive Agents section) has made selenium a highly attractive agent for chemopreventive testing in the prostate. Vitamin E (α-tocopherol) also is attractive for chemoprevention in this site, based on a subset analysis of the phase III Alpha-Tocopheral and β-carotene Trial (ATBC) discussed previously in the Chemoprevention Trial Designs, Chemopreventive Agents, and Lung Cancer Prevention sections.

FURTHER READING

Albanes D, Heinonen OP, Taylor PR, et al. (1996) Alpha-tocopherol and beta-carotene supplements and lung cancer incidence in the alpha-tocopherol, beta-carotene cancer prevention study: Effects of base-line characteristics and study compliance. *J Natl Cancer Inst* 88:1560–1570.

Auerbach H, Hammond EC, Garfinkel L (1979) Changes in bronchial epithelium in relation to cigarette smoking, 1955–1960 vs. 1970–1977. *N Engl J Med* 300:381–386.

Blot WJ, Li J-Y, Taylor PR, et al. (1993) Nutrition intervention trials in Linxian, China: Supplementation with specific vitamin/mineral combinations, cancer incidence, and disease-specific mortality in the general population. *J Natl Cancer Inst* 85:1483.

Bostick RM (1997) Human studies of calcium supplementation and colorectal epithelial cell proliferation. *Cancer Epidemiol Biomark Prev* 6:971–980.

Clark LC, Combs Jr GF, Turnbull BW, et al. (1996) Effects of selenium supplementation for cancer prevention in patients with carcinoma of the skin. A randomized controlled trial. *JAMA* 276:1957–1963.

Clinton SK, Emenhiser C, Schwartz SJ, et al. (1996) *Cis-trans* lycopene isomers, carotenoids and retinol in the human prostate. *Cancer Epidemiol Biomark Prev* 5:823–833.

Giardiello FM, Hamilton SR, Krush AJ, et al. (1993) Treatment of colonic and rectal adenomas with sulindac in familial adenomatous polyposis. *N Engl J Med* 328:1313.

Giovannucci E, Egan KM, Hunter DJ, et al. (1995) Aspirin and the risk of colorectal cancer in women. *N Engl J Med* 333:609–614.

Greenberg ER, Baron JA, Stukel TA, et al. and the Skin Cancer Prevention Study Group (1990) A clinical trial of β carotene to prevent basal cell and squamous cell cancers of the skin. *N Engl J Med* 323:789.

Greenberg ER, Baron JA, Tosteson TD, et al. and the Polyp Prevention Study Group (1994) A clinical trial of antioxidant vitamins to prevent colorectal adenoma. *N Engl J Med* 331:141.

Hennekens CH, Burning JE, Manson JE, et al. (1996) Lack of effect of long-term supplementation with beta carotene on the incidence of malignant neoplasms and cardiovascular disease. *N Engl J Med* 334:1145–1149.

Hong WK, Endicott J, Itri LM, et al. (1986) 13-*Cis*-retinoic acid in the treatment of oral leukoplakia. *N Engl J Med* 315:1501–1505.

Hong WK, Lippman SM, Itri LM, et al. (1990) Prevention of second primary tumors with isotretinoin in squamous-cell carcinoma of the head and neck. *N Engl J Med* 323:795–801.

Hong WK, Sporn MB (1997) Recent advances in chemoprevention of cancer. *Science* 278:1073–1077.

Jordan VC (1997) Tamoxifen: The herald of a new era of preventive therapeutics. *J Natl Cancer Inst* 89:747–749.

Kelloff GJ, Hawk ET, Karp JE, et al. (1997) Progress in chemoprevention. *Semin Oncol* 24:241–253.

Kelloff GJ, Johnson JR, Crowell JA, et al. (1995) Approaches to the development and marketing approval of drugs that prevent cancer. *Cancer Epidemiol Biomark and Prev* 4:1–10.

Kraemer KH, Digiovanna JJ, Moshell AN, et al. (1988) Prevention of skin cancer in xeroderma pigmentosum with the use of oral isotretinoin. *N Engl J Med* 318:1633–1637.

Li J-Y, Taylor P, Li B, et al. (1993) Nutrition intervention trials in Linxian, China: Multiple vitamin/mineral supplementation, cancer incidence, and disease-specific mortality among adults with esophageal dysplasia. *J Natl Cancer Inst* 85:1492.

Lippman SM, Batsakis JG, Toth BB, et al. (1993) Comparison of low-dose isotretinoin with beta carotene to prevent oral carcinogenesis. *N Engl J Med* 328:15–20.

Lippman SM, Benner SE, Hong WK (1994) Cancer chemoprevention. *J Clin Oncol* 12:851–873.

Lotan R, Xu XC, Lippman SM, et al. (1995) Suppression of retinoic acid receptor-beta in premalignant oral lesions and its up-regulation by isotretinoin. *N Engl J Med* 332:1405–1410.

Mayne ST, Lippman SM (1997) Cancer prevention: Chemopreventive agents. In DeVita VT Jr, Hellman, S, Rosenberg SA (eds) *Cancer: Principles and Practice of Oncology*, 5th edition. Lippincott-Raven, Philadelphia.

Meyskens F, Surwit E, Moon TE, et al. (1994) Enhancement of regression of cervical intra-epithelia neoplasia II (moderate dysplasia) with topically applied all-trans retinoic acid: A randomized trial. *J Natl Cancer Inst* 86:539–543.

Mao L, Lee JS, Kurie JM, et al. (1997) Clonal genetic alterations in the lungs of current and former smokers. *JNCI* 89:857–862.

Moon TE, Levine N, Cartmel B, et al. (1997) Effect of retinol in preventing squamous cell skin cancer in moderate-risk subjects: A randomized, double-blind, controlled trial. *Cancer Epidemiol Biomark Prev* 6:949–956.

Muto Y, Moriwaki H, Ninomiya M, et al. (1996) Prevention of second primary tumors by an acyclic retinoid, polyprenoic acid, in patients with hepatocellular carcinoma. Hepatoma Prevention Study Group. *N Engl J Med* 334:1561–1567.

Omenn GS, Goodman GE, Thornquist MD, et al. (1996) Risk factors for lung cancer and for intervention effects in CARET, the beta-carotene and retinol efficacy trial. *J Natl Cancer Inst* 88:1550–1559.

Omenn GS, Goodman GE, Thornquist MD, et al. (1996) Effects of a combination of beta carotene and vitamin A on lung cancer and cardiovascular disease. *N Engl J Med* 334:1150–1155.

Pastorino U, Infante M, Maioli M, et al. (1993) Adjuvant treatment of stage I lung cancer with high dose vitamin A. *J Clin Oncol* 11:1216–1222.

Ruffin IV MT, Koyamangalath K, Rock CL, et al. (1997) Suppression of human colorectal prostaglandins: Determining the lowest effective aspirin dose. *J Natl Cancer Inst* 89:1152–1160.

Sandler RS (1997) Aspirin and other nonsteroidal anti-inflammatory agents in the prevention of colorectal cancer. *Princ Pract Oncol Updates* 11(6):1–14.

Slaughter DP, Southwick HW, Smejkal W (1953) "Field cancerization" in oral stratified squamous epithelium: Clinical implications of multicentric origin. *Cancer* 6:963–968.

The alpha-tocopherol, Beta Carotene Cancer Prevention Study Group (1994) The effect of vitamin E and beta carotene on the incidence of lung cancer and other cancers in male smokers. *N Engl J Med* 330:1029–1035.

Vokes EE, Weichselbaum RR, Lippman SM, Hong WK (1993) Head and neck cancer. *N Engl J Med* 328:184–194.

Xu X-C, Sneige N, Liu X, et al. (1997) Progressive decrease in nuclear retinoic acid receptor-β messenger RNA level during breast carcinogenesis. *Cancer Res* 57:4992–4996.

CHAPTER 8

SCREENING AND EARLY DETECTION

DAVID A. SLOAN

University of Kentucky
Lexington, KY USA

Cancer screening refers to the process by which a large number of people within a population undergo one or more tests designed to find occult cancer. The main reason for detecting preclinical disease is to initiate treatment at an earlier time point in the natural history of the cancer. Only if earlier treatment results in improved outcomes will the screening have been worthwhile. Different outcomes can be measured, although the most important is often the most difficult to achieve: namely, reduced cancer-specific mortality. Deciding whether to screen for a particular cancer involves consideration of the biology and natural history of the cancer, the prevalence of the cancer, and the degree of morbidity and mortality the cancer causes in a population. The decision to initiate screening is also dependent on the quality of the screening test or tests available. Finally, financial, ethical, and societal issues must be resolved.

Screening programs by definition are large-scale events that for the most part involve considerable expenditures. In view of the increasing competition for health care resources within society, compromises are invariably necessary. What is best for the individual in terms of screening for cancer is not always best for society as whole when the cost-effectiveness of the screening is rigorously examined.

Cancer screening is an important tool that can alleviate the pain and suffering caused by cancer within society. Screening programs for a few cancers such as those of the breast and cervix have been shown to be effective, but controversies surround screening issues for most cancers. Even with regard to breast and cervical cancer, unresolved and controversial issues remain.

The general principles of cancer screening are discussed in the first half of this chapter. These include the biologic basis for cancer screening, the determinants of a good cancer screening test, screening biases, the measurement of outcomes related to

Manual of Clinical Oncology, 7th edition, Edited by Raphael E. Pollock
ISBN 0-471-23828-7, pages 181–199. Copyright © 1999 Wiley-Liss, Inc.

screening, and finally societal and financial issues associated with screening. In the latter half of the chapter, four models for cancer screening are examined in detail. For cervical, breast, colorectal, and prostate cancer, the history and current status of screening are examined in light of the general principles of cancer screening. The status of screening for these four cancers in terms of efficacy is very different, but the discussion of each of these models should serve to reinforce the fundamental principles of cancer screening.

GENERAL PRINCIPLES OF CANCER SCREENING

Biologic Basis of Screening

Screening is not necessarily appropriate for a cancer even if a good screening test is available. For screening to be appropriate, the biology of the cancer must be such that there is a protracted preclinical stage in which distant metastasis is uncommon. Because the presence of distant metastasis is generally synonymous with incurability for almost all cancer types, it is important that cancers be detected early in their natural history before the cancer has spread beyond the site of the primary tumor. Therefore, tumors that tend not to metastasize until they have reached a certain size (e.g., breast or prostate tumors) are best suited for screening.

The longer the asymptomatic preclinical phase, the more opportunity there will be to detect asymptomatic cancer by screening. If a cancer is very slow growing, even if an initial screen test fails to detect it, a subsequent screen may find it and still permit a cure. Colon cancer, for example, is associated with a long preclinical phase, a prolonged process that progresses from hyperplasia through adenomatous neoplasia, dysplasia, carcinoma in situ, and ultimately to invasive cancer. This multistep progression probably takes as long as 10 to 15 years. The preclinical stage is further lengthened, then, if the cancer in question is associated with a recognizable precancerous condition (e.g., cervical cancer preceded by cervical dysplasia). If a diagnosis of cancer or even precancer can be made early, the biology of the cancer should be such that early treatment will decrease mortality. Treatment of early disease must therefore be effective if screening is to be worth the effort.

Another consideration is the prevalence of the cancer. If the cancer is rare, then it is unlikely that mass screening programs will be of value. It is not surprising then that the most widely studied cancers in terms of screening are among the most common (e.g., breast cancer, colon cancer, prostate cancer, and cervical cancer). It is estimated that one woman in eight will develop breast cancer in her lifetime and that one man in ten will develop prostate cancer. In the case of prostate cancer, autopsy studies have shown that as many as 30% of men 50 years of age or older have demonstrable evidence of prostate cancer. Most prostate cancers are probably of little biologic significance. This point underscores the fact that the mere prevalence of cancer may not reflect its true aggressiveness. Similarly, papillary carcinoma of the thyroid, which, although it is a very common finding at autopsy, is in fact a rare cause of death from cancer. Figure 8.1 summarizes the conditions that should be met in deciding whether to screen a population for a specific type of cancer.

Is the cancer appropriate for screening?

☐ common cancer

☐ a high prevalence in preclinical state

☐ associated with substantial morbidity and mortality

☐ long disease-detectable, nonmetastatic preclinical phase

☐ preclinical detection of cancer permits improved treatment outcomes

☐ effective screening test(s) available

FIGURE 8.1. Checklist of the important characteristics of a cancer that would make the cancer suitable for screening.

Screening Test Determinants

The screening test is the most critical component of a screening program. It may be a single test (e.g., the Pap smear for cervical cancer) or it may be a combination of tests (e.g., clinical breast examination and mammography for breast cancer). In contrast to diagnostic tests, which are generally employed when patients develop symptoms, screening tests are generally deployed before any symptomatology is manifested. Screening tests focus on the preclinical phase of cancer in a population. Different types of tests may focus on different time points in the natural history of the cancer. For example, screening clinical breast examination (CBE) is used to detect palpable tumors, whereas mammography usually identifies nonpalpable tumors. A molecular test (e.g., *BRCA-1* or *BRCA-2* gene determination for breast cancer or the c-K-*ras* test for colon cancer) will be positive at a much earlier time point. Figure 8.2 lists the criteria by which the quality of the screening test should be measured. A good screening test should first and foremost be associated with high sensitivity and high specificity. Sensitivity refers to the probability of obtaining positive results if cancer is truly present. Specificity is the probability of obtaining negative results if there is in fact no cancer present. The predictive value of a screening test is another important parameter. The positive predictive value (PPV) is a measure of the accuracy of a test in gauging the likelihood that disease or cancer is actually present when the test is positive. For example, a PPV of 10% means that there is a 1 in 10 chance that disease is present. On the other hand, negative predictive value (NPV) is the accuracy of test in determining the absence of disease. Figure 8.3 presents a hypothetical population of 100 people, two of whom have subclinical cancer. The results of the available hypothetical screening test are positive for five people, only one of whom actually has cancer. When these numbers are used, hypothetical values for sensitivity, specificity, PPV, and NPV can be generated.

Screening tests vary in nature (Fig. 8.4). Some, such as the CBE for breast cancer detection, the digital rectal examination (DRE) for prostate cancer, and the complete skin examination for skin cancer, are simply focused physical examinations. Such tests, although simple and "low-tech," are subjective but nonetheless have great

Is the screening test a good one?

☐ high sensitivity

☐ high specificity

☐ inexpensive

☐ risk-free

☐ simple

☐ easy to administer

☐ lends itself to mass implementation

☐ leads to early treatment and reduced cancer-specific mortality

☐ low psychological and financial costs attached to workup of false positives

FIGURE 8.2. Checklist of the important characteristics of a screening test that would make the test suitable for use in a cancer screening program.

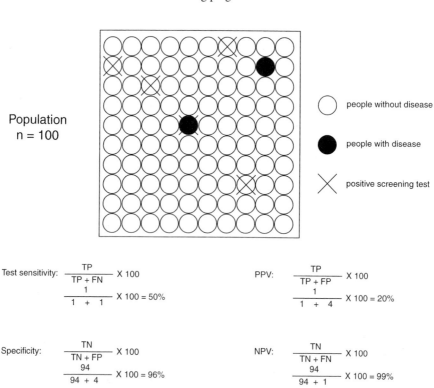

Population
n = 100

○ people without disease

● people with disease

✕ positive screening test

Test sensitivity: $\dfrac{TP}{TP + FN} \times 100$

$\dfrac{1}{1 + 1} \times 100 = 50\%$

PPV: $\dfrac{TP}{TP + FP} \times 100$

$\dfrac{1}{1 + 4} \times 100 = 20\%$

Specificity: $\dfrac{TN}{TN + FP} \times 100$

$\dfrac{94}{94 + 4} \times 100 = 96\%$

NPV: $\dfrac{TN}{TN + FN} \times 100$

$\dfrac{94}{94 + 1} \times 100 = 99\%$

FIGURE 8.3. Hypothetical population of 100 people, two of whom have preclinical cancer. A hypothetical screening test is positive for five individuals, only one of whom actually has cancer. The formulas for determining test sensitivity, specificity, positive predictive value (PPV), and negative predictive value (NPV) are provided along with the numbers applicable to the hypothetical example illustrated.

184

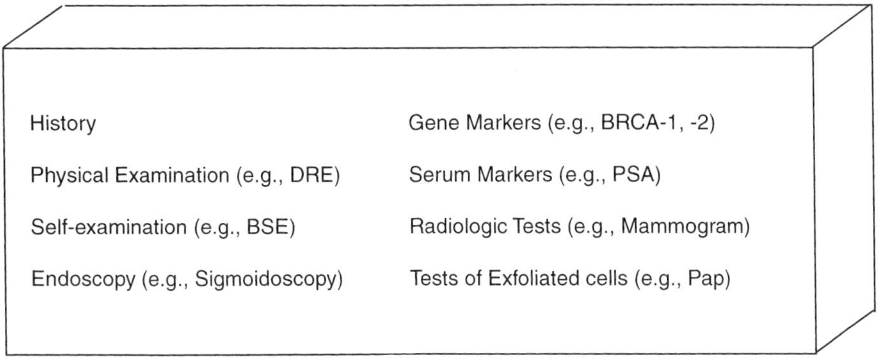

History	Gene Markers (e.g., BRCA-1, -2)
Physical Examination (e.g., DRE)	Serum Markers (e.g., PSA)
Self-examination (e.g., BSE)	Radiologic Tests (e.g., Mammogram)
Endoscopy (e.g., Sigmoidoscopy)	Tests of Exfoliated cells (e.g., Pap)

FIGURE 8.4. Various screening tools that are available for use by clinicians in screening people for occult cancer.

merit; however, the quality of physical examination can be quite variable. More objective are screening tests that consist of imaging studies such as chest radiograph, mammogram, or transrectal ultrasound (TRUS). Imaging tests such as these or screening cytologic tests such as the Pap smear are still subject to interpretation by specialists. The literature clearly shows that specialists never come close to 100% agreement when viewing images, be they mammograms, ultrasounds, or cytologic slides. Most objective are laboratory tests such as the prostate-specific antigen (PSA) or Hemoccult test. However, even though such laboratory tests are more objective, they are still fraught with problems of interpretation. For example, a "cutoff" point needs to be agreed upon at which "positives" are distinguished from "negatives." If Hemoccult specimens are rehydrated before the chemical testing is done, the likelihood of positive results will quadruple. The serum level for the "cutoff" point for the PSA test will affect the sensitivity and specificity of the test. For the four models of cancer screening that are discussed, the established screening tools are shown in Fig. 8.5.

How easy is the screening test to administer? How readily do healthy people submit to the screening test? There is a not surprising reluctance on the part of many people to provide stool samples for fecal occult blood testing (FOBT). Mammograms are associated with some discomfort and apprehension on the part of women. Some screening tests are associated with risks. Although the risk of radiation associated with screening mammography is minuscule, the risks associated with screening colonoscopy are significant (e.g., 0.1% incidence of bowel perforation). How difficult is it to ensure that a screening test is done well? Although it may be fairly easy to ensure the quality of a serum test, ensuring that a standard high level of quality accompanies every mammogram and Pap smear is much more difficult. The quality of mammography performed as part of the widely quoted Canadian breast screening studies has, for example, been harshly criticized.

A screening test needs to be incorporated into a sound administrative structure that ensures that the screening is carried out in a safe and orderly manner. Rigorous

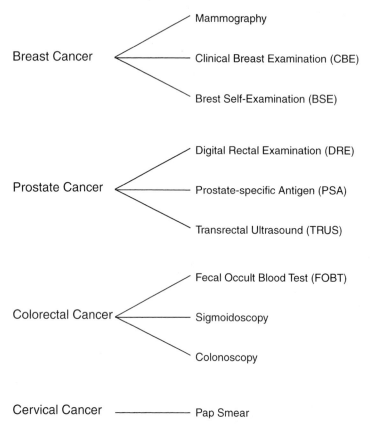

FIGURE 8.5. Commonly employed screening tests for breast, cervical, colorectal, and prostate cancer.

attention needs to be paid to the quality control of the particular test, the accurate recording of test results, and the notification of patients and physicians to make certain that all patients with positive test results are appropriately investigated.

Screening Biases

As screening programs are implemented and subsequently evaluated, a degree of caution needs to be exercised. Unfortunately, screening programs may appear more effective than they truly are because of one or more potential biases (Fig. 8.6). The first is a volunteer bias inserted into a screening program because of the characteristics of people volunteering for a screening study. Women volunteering for a mammography screening program might, for example, be more likely than matched controls to perform breast self-examination, which in turn might "contaminate" or overestimate the impact of mammography. Patients undergoing screening sigmoidoscopy in one case-control study had a 30% reduction in the risk of cancer of the rectum. The

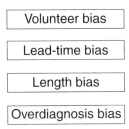

FIGURE 8.6. Typical biases encountered in the course of evaluating scientific studies for the purpose of determining the efficacy of cancer screening programs.

author observed a strong correlation between the number of sigmoidoscopies performed and the number of periodic health examinations undergone; people willing to be screened for rectal cancer appeared more likely to seek medical attention.

Lead-time bias refers to the "advantage" that a screened population has in having cancer detected at an earlier time point in the natural history of the cancer. If the cancer of patient A is diagnosed earlier than that of patient B because of screening but both die of cancer at the same time, patient A will appear to have had a longer survival time, but in fact the mortality data will be unchanged. Lead-time bias can be illustrated in a simple scenario in which two people get on the same bus, one passenger boarding the bus 20 minutes outside of the city center terminal and the other passenger 10 minutes from city center.

Length bias is not to be confused with lead-time bias. Length bias refers to the phenomenon that screening programs will tend to detect slower growing cancers and miss rapidly growing, more aggressive cancers. Many screening studies show that the screened population has a higher percentage of early tumors than the nonscreened population. An excellent example is colon cancer FOBT screening: many studies show significantly more early tumors and significantly fewer advanced tumors in FOBT-screened patients. Indolent cancers with a long preclinical phase (e.g., colon cancer) are ideal for screening detection from this standpoint. It follows that the survival rates of patients whose cancers are detected by screening may well be better than those of patients whose cancers are not detected by screening, thus artificially enhancing the benefit of screening to the observer.

Overdiagnosis bias refers to the danger of diagnosing cancer in a large percentage of the population when in fact the cancer is a significant cause of morbidity and mortality for only a small proportion of the population. The examples of prostate cancer and papillary thyroid cancer have already been provided. Another example may be the explosion in diagnosis precipitated by widespread mammography screening of ductal carcinoma in situ (DCIS), a cancer that exhibits a wide spectrum of biologic aggressiveness.

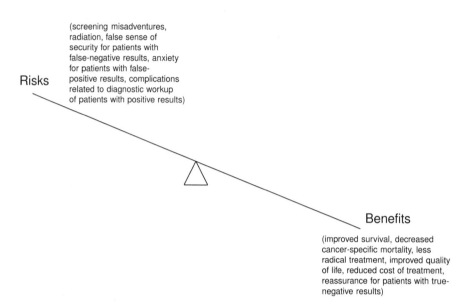

Risks
(screening misadventures, radiation, false sense of security for patients with false-negative results, anxiety for patients with false-positive results, complications related to diagnostic workup of patients with positive results)

Benefits
(improved survival, decreased cancer-specific mortality, less radical treatment, improved quality of life, reduced cost of treatment, reassurance for patients with true-negative results)

FIGURE 8.7. The benefits of cancer screening should outweigh the risks of screening if a cancer screening program is worthwhile.

Efficacy of Screening: Outcome Measurements

Screening programs are costly ventures that consume resources and require years of effort. It is crucial that the benefits of screening outweigh any "risks" or "negatives" associated with the screening program (Fig. 8.7). What sorts of risks might accompany a screening test? Radiologic studies such as chest radiographs or mammograms expose people to very small amounts of ionizing radiation. Much more important as a source of screening-related morbidity are the possible adverse effects related to the diagnostic workup of patients whose tests are positive. For example, although prostate screening tests such as DRE and PSA are associated with minimal morbidity, the potential morbidity of the many prostate biopsies necessitated by screening is much greater. Similarly, the colonoscopies performed as a result of positive FOBTs (up to 10% of screened people are FOBT positive) are associated with real risks (perforation, hemorrhage, risks related to sedation). If such complications occur among patients with false-positive results, the efficacy equation of the screening test is negatively affected. As many as 80% of breast biopsies performed because screening mammograms yielded positive results show the presence of benign disease, not cancer. Again, although biopsy-related complications are few, they do occur. Further, more than workup complications must be considered. Even if the procedures are complication free, they consume medical resources, occupy physician time, cause pain for patients, and keep patients away from work. It is also important not to overlook the psychological trauma inflicted on people who are told they have test results that are positive for cancer. Depending on the PPV of the screening test, varying numbers of people will ultimately be proved to be cancer free yet left with the emotional scars of the diagnostic testing procedures. With the previously mentioned problem of overdiagnosis bias, many patients suffer the trauma of being told that they have cancer even though the cancer may have little biologic significance. Nevertheless, the patients are forced to live with the diagnosis of cancer. Another "hidden" risk of screening is the false sense of security that some patients might receive as a result of negative test results. Colorectal screening studies have shown that only a minority of colon cancers actually result in detectable fecal blood at any given point in time. A person testing negative might not return for follow-up testing, a problem that plagues all screening programs.

What are the potential benefits of a screening test that would justify the previously discussed risks? One hopes to see patients with earlier diagnosed cancers treated with greater effect in terms of cancer cure. Improved survival is obviously sought, but one also hopes to see patients treated with less debilitating and less mutilating treatments. Small breast cancers that are diagnosed earlier, for example, are more likely to be amenable to breast-conserving treatments. Making an earlier diagnosis of breast cancer may also mean that adjuvant chemotherapy may be rendered unnecessary and that the patient may be spared the morbidity and inconvenience associated with such treatment. Improved quality of life for screened patients then might be enough to justify a screening program even if reduced mortality is not demonstrated.

It is apparent at this point in the discussion that the effectiveness of any screening program needs to be rigorously measured. What yardsticks are available? Most screening programs result in the diagnosis of an increased number of cancers among screened populations. However, simply diagnosing more cancers is not a satisfactory measure unless treatment leads to reduced mortality and, particularly, reduced cancer-specific mortality. Reduced cancer-specific mortality is the bottom line for any screening program. Screening programs can also be evaluated in terms of quality-of-life measures, as has already been alluded to in the discussion of breast cancer treatment. Finally, the costs associated with a screening test are easily measured.

As one reviews the cancer screening literature, three primary types of outcome studies are seen: historical studies, case-control studies, and prospective randomized trials (PRTs). A case-control study is a retrospective analysis comparing the outcomes of patients who have been screened with those of unscreened controls. Although the literature is replete with case-control studies, a much more satisfactory measure of screening effectiveness is the PRT. A PRT should negate the effects of volunteer, lead-time, and length bias as people are randomly assigned to screening and nonscreening groups. Both groups can then be evaluated in terms of the outcome measures already discussed: numbers of cancers diagnosed, survival, cancer-specific mortality, years of life saved, quality-of-life measures, and financial costs. PRTs unfortunately are hampered by various problems including compliance issues and the contamination of the control group by outside factors such as the availability of screening tests themselves. Although one might hope that a PRT would settle any debate about screening efficacy, this is often not the case, as the situation with breast cancer screening for younger women illustrates (Fig. 8.8).

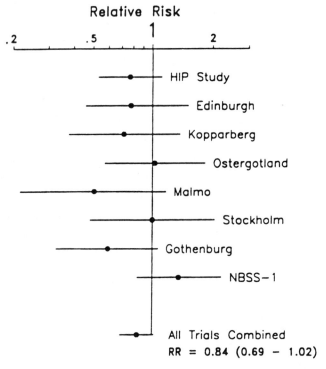

FIGURE 8.8. Relative risks and 95% confidence intervals from all breast cancer screening randomized clinical trials that have included women ages 40 to 49 years at entry. The last line shows meta-analysis results. (From Smart et al. *Cancer* 75:1619–1626, 1995.)

Cost and Societal Issues

The morbidity and mortality caused by cancer show little signs of diminishing despite substantial improvements in treatment regiments. For a society, the cost of cancer treatment is enormous in terms of health care resources, workplace losses, and individual suffering. Because the societal and financial costs of cancer treatment are greatest when disease is most advanced, there is a compelling reason to invest resources at the front end of cancer management. The essential purpose of screening programs is to make an early diagnosis of cancer in a large number of people, the goal being to reduce both cancer morbidity and cancer mortality. Unfortunately, there are many barriers to achieving this goal for the common cancers that plague society. These barriers are financial, educational, societal, and ethical.

There are formidable financial barriers to screening. Screening tests vary widely in cost. Although the test materials themselves may be inexpensive, the "downstream" costs, as one author has termed them, may be very high. A Hemoccult test may cost only a few dollars, but by the time one adds the associated costs bundled into a colorectal cancer screening program (administrative costs, diagnostic workup costs) the expenses are considerable. For people over the age of 50, current recommendations include flexible sigmoidoscopy every 3 to 5 years. If these guidelines were adhered to in the United States, the estimated cost would be well over $1 billion US per year. If the prostate cancer screening guidelines that some groups have recommended were implemented on a large scale, the cost would probably be staggering and health care facilities would be overwhelmed by patients. Such a scenario underscores the point that health care institutions need to have adequate infrastructures to support screening programs. Health care workers are needed to administer screening tests, interpret the tests, conduct the workups of those with positive results, and treat all patients who have newly diagnosed cancer. In the current climate of aggressive cost controls and judicious resource allocation, politicians, government departments, health care institutions, employers, physician organizations, and interested parties in society need to work together to prioritize screening-related issues. Cost-effectiveness analyses and benefit–cost analyses need to be looked at carefully. For example, by calculating the cost of a given screening program per year of life saved, public health authorities can compare the cost-effectiveness of various screening programs. One government agency has set as an arbitrary benchmark $40,000 per year of life saved by screening: if the cost of a screening program is below this figure, the screening is believed to be justified. Ideally, carefully designed multicenter PRTs measuring a number of endpoints should be carried out to determine the worthiness of a given screening program.

Education is a multilevel barrier to effective screening. Volunteers for screening programs tend to consist of people who are on the whole better educated and from higher socioeconomic groups. The poorly educated population may not recognize the importance of screening or of following physicians' recommendations if their test results are positive. The education pendulum can also swing the other way, however. One study showed that women under the age of 50 greatly overestimated both their risk of developing breast cancer and the effectiveness of breast cancer screening. If the education of the general population is a barrier, the education of health care professionals is an even greater one. A substantial majority of physicians do not adhere to recommended screening guidelines in their individual practices. Data show that physicians are inadequately trained in the area of cancer screening; they do not know when to order a mammogram or how to do a proper CBE. A number of authors have made pleas for the improved cancer education of physicians and other health care professionals.

SPECIFIC MODELS FOR CANCER SCREENING

Cervical Cancer

Cervical cancer is the second most common cancer among women worldwide. Four of every five new cases are diagnosed in the developing parts of the world. Cervical cancer is ideal for screening because it has a very long preclinical phase during which precancerous and early cancerous changes can be easily diagnosed with a simple test, the Papanicolaou (Pap) smear. The Pap test has been used in screening programs for half a century. Although the test is inexpensive, a number of problems are associated with it, including quality issues related to cervical sampling, slide preparation, and cytologic interpretation. In one study in which two institutions traded 20,000 slides, the rate of undercalling in situ or invasive cancer was 34% to 57%. False-negative rates for the Pap test are usually 5% to 10%, although they can exceed 50%. Screening intervals from 1 to 10 years have been used and there is good evidence that relatively long intervals of 3 to 5 years are associated with important reductions in cancer-specific mortality.

The evidence for the efficacy of Pap screening is based not on PRTs but on historic and case-control studies. Numerous studies have shown that the mortality rates associated with cervical cancer are up to 90% less for screened patients than for unscreened patients. The primary problem with cervical cancer screening has been to achieve high rates of screening in the population of women most at risk for the disease. Recent efforts to study the use of lay health advisors have been shown to significantly reduce barriers to understanding among women in low literacy level and poor populations. These strategies may greatly increase cancer screening among high-risk populations. Cervical cancer screening is a unique model for cancer screening that is built on a simple, low-tech test; it has been shown to be efficacious for all ages of women in both developed and undeveloped countries. Cervical cancer screening is without question not only the oldest cancer screening program but also the most solidly entrenched.

Breast Cancer

Breast cancer is common and the prevalence of premalignant breast disease and in situ cancer is high. Small preclinical tumors tend not to have metastasized; thus, patients can benefit from screening. Screening tests for breast cancer include breast self-examination (BSE), clinical breast examination (CBE), and mammography. Mammography as a screening tool has continued to evolve in terms of technical sophistication, but the most notable study demonstrating its efficacy is more than three decades old. The Greater New York Health Insurance Plan (HIP) study randomized 62,000 women between the ages of 40 and 64 to control or to yearly CBE and mammography for 4 years. Over a 10-year period, 30% fewer deaths occurred among the screened women. Almost 300,000 women were enrolled in the Breast Cancer Detection Demonstration Project. This nonrandomized but prospective study found that the incidence of breast cancer in the screened group was higher (1.34 times the expected incidence) and that the mortality rate was only 80% of that expected. Evidence has continued to accumulate for the efficacy of breast cancer screening. In contrast to prostate and cervical cancer screening, breast cancer screening has been demonstrated by a number of recent PRTs to be effective, particularly for women between the ages of 50 and 69. Screening generally means mammography (at 1- to 3-year intervals, depending on the study), sometimes with CBE. For women between 50 and 69 years of age, the PRTs indicate a reduction of mortality from 15% to 30% as a result of screening programs. Even the casual reader is aware of the controversy that has raged over the efficacy of screening for women between the ages of 40 and

49. Fig. 8.8 summarizes the PRTs for this age group. Meta-analysis of the available studies has shown a 16% reduction (not significant) in breast cancer mortality. If the first Canadian National Breast Screening Study (CNBSS) trial is excluded from the meta-analysis, the mortality reduction improves to 24%. Figure 8.8 shows that two of the PRTs showed no change in mortality at all, whereas the much-criticized Canadian study showed an increased risk of breast cancer in screened women. Screening mammography, although not particularly expensive, is associated with substantial "downstream" costs, including the cost of the large number of surgical consultations and biopsies that ensue (most of which are negative for cancer) and the anxiety caused for the numerous women with "false-positive" results from mammograms.

Although mammography is the dominant screening tool, the importance of CBE and BSE should not be overlooked. It has been estimated that most of the decrease in mortality in the screened population of the HIP study was because of CBE rather than mammography; in that study, 58% of the breast tumors were found with CBE alone. More recently, the second CNBSS trial randomized women between the ages of 50 and 59 to CBE and BSE or to mammography and BSE. The mammography group had significantly more node-negative small tumors, but there was no difference in the death rate from breast cancer at up to 7 years of follow-up. With regard to BSE and CBE, there is much room for improvement in terms of both patient and physician education. Greater efforts need to be devoted to improving physicians' understanding of the role of BSE, CBE, and mammography in breast cancer screening and in communicating positive clinical or mammographic findings to patients.

Colorectal Cancer

Colorectal cancer is an important cause of cancer deaths worldwide. Unfortunately, despite advances in adjuvant treatment, half of the patients with colorectal cancer die of the disease. Screening for colon cancer can be subdivided into screening for high-risk groups and screening for the general population. At-risk groups include patients with ulcerative colitis, patients with a history of polyps (including familial polyposis), and, to a lesser degree, patients with a history of colon cancer among first-degree family members. Because colorectal cancer largely affects older patients, screening programs have targeted those aged 50 and over. Current recommendations for screening the general population are best summarized with the following: yearly DRE and FOBT in association with flexible sigmoidoscopy every 3 to 5 years.

Colon cancer appears ideal for screening in that the disease is common and is associated with a long preclinical phase. The polyp-to-cancer sequence is an established tenet of oncology, because most cancers appear to arise from preexisting polyps. Patients with multiple polyps are at increased risk for colon cancer, and aggressive prospective extirpation of polyps results in a reduction of colon cancer.

Aside from the DRE, which should always be part of a general physical examination for adult patients, two other screening tests are available. The simplest test is the FOBT, which tests tiny amounts of stool for traces of blood. Popularized by Greegor, the FOBT is a simple screening test that is nonetheless beset with some important drawbacks. The first problem with the FOBT is patient compliance. One author commented that a great effort was expended to achieve a rather poor compliance rate of 68%. The second problem is that, because most colon tumors are not detectably bleeding at any given point in time, they will not be detected with a single screening FOBT. The third problem relates to the cutoff point of the test. Rehydration of the specimens results in a much higher positivity rate. Rehydration detects more cancers but on the other hand also results in a great many more false-positive results. There is evidence, however, for the efficacy of FOBT. In the Minnesota Colon Cancer Control Study, 46,551 people between the ages of 50 and 80 were randomized to one of three groups: annual FOBT screening, biennial screening, and control. With a study follow-up of 13 years, a significant reduction of 33% in colon cancer mortality was found in the group undergoing annual screening (Fig. 8.9). The mortality rates of the biennial group were almost identical, however, to those of the control group. The incidence of metastatic disease was twice as high for the control group than for the annual screening group. It should be noted, however, that most FOBT studies have not demonstrated an unequivocal benefit for FOBT screening.

Screening sigmoidoscopy (flexible preferable to rigid) has been advocated by many experts for people over the age of 50. Reductions of up to 30% in cancer-specific mortality have been suggested to result from periodic screening sigmoidoscopy, with intervals of up to 10 years. More complete colonic screening with colonoscopy is being actively studied. Some authorities have recommended a single colonoscopic screening at age 60. Endoscopic screening, although extremely sensitive and specific, is costly in terms of money and time and is associated with rare but significant complications. For the time being, flexible sigmoidoscopy every 3 to

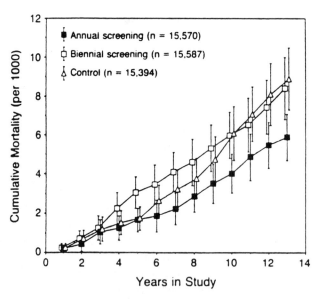

FIGURE 8.9. Cumulative mortality from colorectal cancer, according to FOBT screening group. (From Mandel et al. *N Engl J Med* 328:1366–1371, 1993.)

5 years is a reasonable approach. The ideal screening strategy for large populations must still be worked out.

Prostate Cancer

Prostate cancer is a leading cause of cancer death for men and its incidence continues to rise. The prostate cancer screening model is unique in that, although three effective and quite different screening tools are in use, the efficacy of screening for this cancer is far from established. As Fig. 8.10 shows, there is a spectrum for prostate cancer in terms of biologic aggressiveness. Prostate cancer is very commonly found at autopsy in men over the age of 50, but the mortality rates from prostate cancer are much lower than one would expect given the high prevalence of the disease. Most men with prostate cancer will not die of prostate cancer. On the other hand, though, for most men dying of prostate cancer the diagnosis was not made in time, when the disease was organ confined and curable. This dichotomy leads to the dilemma of prostate cancer treatment: how to make an early diagnosis for patients with potentially lethal prostate cancer, but how not to overdiagnose and overtreat cancer that is biologically indolent and nonlethal. This dilemma has resulted in much confusion about how to screen effectively for prostate cancer.

The long preclinical phase and high prevalence of prostate cancer among men over the age of 50 would appear to make prostate cancer an ideal tumor for screening. Three screening tests have been implemented in prostate cancer screening programs: physical examination (i.e., DRE); a serologic test (i.e., the determination of serum prostate-specific antigen [PSA] levels); and an imaging study (transrectal ultrasound

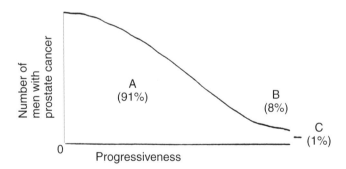

FIGURE 8.10. Latent, progressive, and rapidly progressive prostate cancers. **(A)** Non-progressive (latent): no need to screen-detect, as tumor will not progress. **(B)** Progressive: worthwhile to screen-detect as will eventually become symptomatic (and possibly fatal) and because screen-detection and early treatment can improve prognosis. **(C)** rapidly progressive: no need to try to screen-detect as tumor progresses so quickly that preclinical phase is very brief and death is likely outcome whether diagnosis is early or late. Percentages refer to relative weights of prostate cancer prevalence (27%), risk of diagnosis (2.31%), and risk of death (0.36%) for 65- to 69-year old white men. (From Waterbor et al. *Cancer Causes and Control* 6:267–274, 1995.)

[TRUS]). The DRE is a focused physical examination that, like the CBE, is simple yet is subjective and clearly operator dependent. The PPV of a DRE is 24% to 35%. Data from the American Cancer Society Prostate Cancer Detection Project showed a sensitivity of 50% and a specificity of 94% for DRE. The detection rate for DRE in prostate screening programs is less than 2%. Annual DREs are recommended for men more than 50 years of age (or younger if patients are high risk, e.g., positive family history, African-American), but not surprisingly compliance is a problem, and further there are real questions about how effective DRE alone is in detecting cancer early.

In contrast to tumor markers such as carcinoembryonic antigen (CEA), PSA is produced by only one organ, the prostate. PSA is not specific, however, for cancer, and elevated PSA levels are seen in a number of benign prostatic conditions such as prostatitis and benign prostatic hypertrophy. The higher the PSA, however, the more specific for prostate cancer it becomes. PSA determination illustrates the cutoff point principle: deciding at which level the test is positive affects both the sensitivity and the specificity of the test. For PSA levels greater than 10 ng/ml, the specificity exceeds 90%. The value of the PSA as a test can be increased further by looking at PSA density, age-specific reference ranges, the free-to-total PSA ratio, and the rate of change of the PSA level over time. The sensitivity and specificity of PSA are similar to that of the DRE, although the specificity of PSA tends to be lower. The two tests often do not detect the same cancers; thus, the combination of the two tests is superior to either test alone (Fig. 8.11). For this reason, some groups such as the American

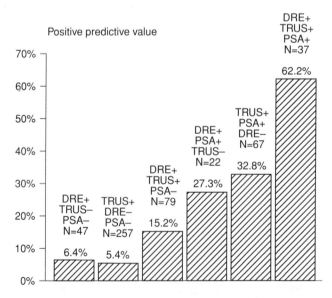

FIGURE 8.11. Positive predictive values according to combination of transrectal ultrasound (TRUS), digital rectal examination (DRE), and prostate-specific antigen (PSA) result. Positive PSA is defined as >4.0 ng/ml. (From Babaian et al. *Cancer* 69:1196–1200, 1992.)

Urological Association and the American Cancer Society have recommended that prostate cancer screening for men over the age of 50 (over the age of 40 if high risk) consist of a yearly DRE and PSA level determination.

The third screening test, TRUS, has been used for about 25 years. TRUS is an invasive test: an ultrasound probe placed into the rectum allows the user to detect areas of hypoechoicity within the prostate. In expert hands, TRUS can detect tumors much smaller than 1 cm. Because TRUS is invasive, expensive, and not reliable as a single-modality screening test, it is best reserved for prostate biopsy guidance for patients with abnormal PSA levels or DRE findings.

Prostate cancer screening detects many asymptomatic cancers, but does prostate cancer screening result in lowered mortality rates from prostate cancer? The answer to this bottom-line question is not available at this time. At least two ongoing longitudinal PRTs are currently underway. However, it will be several years before the results of these studies are known. In the absence of definitive outcome data, most cancer organizations have not supported large-scale prostate cancer screening. An important concern associated with prostate cancer screening is financial: the cost of the screening tests themselves, the cost of numerous prostate biopsies generated by the screening process, and the staggering cost of treating all of the cancers diagnosed. Because widespread screening with the tools currently available would result in the detection of huge numbers of new prostate cancers and could overwhelm health care facilities, it seems prudent to channel patients into available multiinstitutional PRTs.

CONCLUDING COMMENTS

The four models of cancer screening presented illustrate not only the general principles of screening but also the many problems that plague screening programs. Screening whole populations for a specific type of cancer, even if a simple screening test such as the FOBT exists, involves considerable expenditure. Thus, it behooves public health authorities to be certain of the efficacy of the particular screening program. That efficacy is best demonstrated by PRTs, although, as has been seen with breast cancer, PRTs do not necessarily quiet controversial issues in screening. As societies come to terms with controlling health care expenditures, cost–benefit analyses become an increasingly important part of decision making. As public health authorities increasingly take a bottom-line approach, controversial screening issues may ultimately be decided on the basis of cost–benefit analyses. For example, it can easily be demonstrated that with mammography a far greater amount of money must be spent to save 1 year of life for a woman between the ages of 40 and 49 than for a woman between the ages of 50 and 69. Other age-related issues arise. Patients at risk for cervical cancer and melanoma are younger than patients at risk for colon and prostate cancer. Should more of a society's resources be put into screening for cancers that afflict younger people? Do older patients who are near the ends of their lives and out of the work force have less of a right to cancer screening than younger patients? Other ethical issues also exist. For example, how much autonomy should individual practitioners have with regard to screening practices? A Health Maintenance Organization in the United States recently undertook a large-scale educational effort to dissuade their physicians from screening patients for prostate cancer.

The many issues operative in cancer screening do not lend themselves to easy solutions. Consensus conferences at which experts present data and then develop a strategic plan for screening can serve to inflame rather than quiet controversy, as illustrated by the recent discussions in the United States about breast cancer screening for younger women. To best serve their patients, individual practitioners should be aware of the general principles of screening, the risks and benefits associated with the different types of screening tests, the evidence for the efficacy of common screening tests, and the screening recommendations of national cancer organizations. Practitioners have a responsibility to their patients to select those individuals who are at risk; to be skilled in performing screening examinations such as CBE, DRE, pelvic examination, skin examination, and Pap smear; and to be at least aware of new screening strategies such as molecular testing. Above all, physicians need to help patients understand the importance of complying with screening recommendations, and they need to be able to communicate screening test results to patients in an understandable and compassionate manner.

FURTHER READING

Benoit RM, Naslund MJ (1997) The socioeconomic implications of prostate-specific antigen screening. *Urol Clin North Am* 24:451–458.

Catalona WJ, Smith DS, Ratliff TL, et al. (1991) Measurement of prostate-specific antigen in serum as a screening test for prostate cancer. *N Engl J Med* 324: 1156–1161.

Cupp MR, Oesterling JE (1993) Prostate-specific antigen, digital rectal examination, and transrectal ultrasonography: Their roles in diagnosing early prostate cancer. *Mayo Clin Proc* 68:297–306.

DeMay RM (1997) Common problems in Papanicolaou interpretation. *Arch Pathol Lab Med* 121:229–238.

Eckhardt S, Badellino F, Murphy GP (1994) UICC meeting on breast-cancer screening in pre-menopausal women in developed countries. *Int J Cancer* 56:2–5.

Eddy DM (1990) Screening for cervical cancer. *Ann Intern Med* 113:214–226.

Gohagan JK, Prorok PC, Kramer BS, et al. (1994) Prostate cancer screening in the prostate, lung, colorectal and ovarian cancer screening trial of the National Cancer Institute. *J Urol* 152:1905–1909.

Harris R, Leininger L (1995) Clinical strategies for breast cancer screening: Weighing and using the evidence. *Ann Intern Med* 122:539–547.

Jessup JM, Menck HR, Fremgen A, Winchester DP (1997) Diagnosing colorectal carcinoma: Clinical and molecular approaches. *CA Cancer J Clin* 47:70–92.

Mandel JS, Bond JH, Church TR, et al. (1993) Reducing mortality from colorectal cancer by screening for fecal occult blood. *N Engl J Med* 328:1365–71.

Miller AB, Chamberlain J, Day NE, et al. (1990) Report on a workshop of the UICC project on evaluation of screening for cancer. *Int J Cancer* 46:761–769.

Miller AB, Baines CJ, To T, et al. (1992) Canadian National Breast Screening Study: 1. Breast cancer detection and death rates among women aged 40 to 49 years. *Can Med Assoc J* 147:1459–1476.

Miller AB, Baines CJ, To T, et al. (1992) Canadian National Breast Screening Study: 2. Breast cancer detection and death rates among women aged 50 to 59 years. *Can Med Assoc J* 147:1477–1488.

Nelson RL (1997) Screening for colorectal cancer. *J Surg Oncol* 63:249–258.

Rimer BK, Schildkraut J (1997) Cancer Screening. In DeVita VT, Hellmann S, Rosenberg SA (eds) *Cancer: Principles and Practice of Oncology*, 5th edition. Lippincott–Raven, Philadelphia.

Toribara NW, Sleisenger MH (1995) Screening for colorectal cancer. *N Engl J Med* 332:861–867.

Winawer SJ, Flehinger BJ, Schottenfeld D, et al. (1993) Screening for colorectal cancer with fecal occult blood testing and sigmoidoscopy. *J Natl Cancer Inst* 85:1311–1318.

CHAPTER 9

CANCER DIAGNOSIS

JAMES G. GERAGHTY

Professorial Department of Surgery
City Hospital
Nottingham, England

ALBRECHT WOBST

European Institute of Oncology
Experimental Oncology
20141 Milan, Italy

History taking, physical examination, hypothesis forming, laboratory examinations, cancer localization, pathologic diagnosis, staging and evaluation of prognostic factors, and pretherapeutical examinations comprise steps in the diagnostic process in oncology. Awareness of cancer etiology, paraneoplastic symptoms, means of tumor localization, and histologic analysis guide cancer diagnosis. Understanding of clinical and pathologic prognostic factors on the one hand, and risk assessment on the other, are crucial in the decision making process.

HISTORY TAKING

A standard history covering acute symptoms, evaluation of the differing organ systems, and general physical condition is required. Assessment of cancer risk factors must be thorough. In many instances, history taking in the absence of physical examination can provide vital clues in the diagnosis of cancer.

Important diagnostic clues might be obtained if conditions predisposing to cancer development are found such as immunosuppression (iatrogenic in transplant patients or autoimmune diseases; infectious as in HIV); chronic infections (hepatitis, papil-

Manual of Clinical Oncology, 7th edition, Edited by Raphael E. Pollock
ISBN 0-471-23828-7, pages 201–214. Copyright © 1999 Wiley-Liss, Inc.

lomata, schistosomiasis); or autoimmune diseases (ulcerative colitis, Hashimoto's thyroiditis).

The drug history can reveal risk factors for specific cancer types (e.g., diethylstilbestrol and vaginal/cervical cancer) as well as known carcinogens (e.g., cigarette smoke) and thus help in making the diagnosis.[1–4]

A positive family history of cancer can lead to the identification of hereditary cancer syndromes. As a result of such information, careful attention can be directed in the physical examination to specific organs. Recent developments in genetic alterations in breast cancer, with risk determined by the strength of the familial situation, underpin the increasing importance of a well-taken, in-depth family history.

Occupational (e.g., dioxin) and environmental (e.g., sunlight) exposures to carcinogens need to be elucidated and suspected or established causal relationships (e.g., asbestos and pleuromesothelioma) clearly defined in the history.[5–9] A summary of these is outlined in Tables 9.1.

A history of autoimmune disease can provide useful clues as to potential sites of cancer. Such conditions include autoimmunegastritis (stomach cancer), Hashimoto's thyroiditis (thyroid cancer), myasthenia gravis (thymoma), primary biliary cirrhosis (hepatoma, bile duct neoplasms), and ulcerative colitis (rectal cancer). A history of specific infections can also point to individual cancers. Well-known associations include hepatitis B/C and liver cancer, human papilloma virus and cervical/larynx cancer, Epstein–Barr virus (EBV) and Burkitt's lymphoma, HTLV1 and leukemia, *Helicobacter pylori* and gastric cancer, schistosomiasis and bladder cancer, liver flukes and bile duct carcinoma, etc.[10,11]

Finally, neoplasms linked to drugs include anabolic steroids (hepatic neoplasms), phenacetine abuse (urothelial cancers) as well as chemotherapeutic agents themselves such as busulfan (bone marrow neoplasms) melphalan (bladder cancers), etc.[12]

PHYSICAL EXAMINATION

In addition to the routine physical examination, special attention should be dedicated to lymphatic, dermatologic, or neurologic symptoms of malignancy. A sound knowledge of the routes of lymphatic spread is a prerequisite in the detection of both locoregional and systemic spread. Meticulous dermatologic exam may reveal not only the primary tumor directly (melanoma, basal cell carcinoma) or indirectly by skin invasion (lymphoma, breast carcinoma), but also exhibit clues to tumor origin through paraneoplastic syndromes.

Paraneoplastic syndromes are defined as tumor-associated disorders of host organ function that occur at sites remote from the primary tumor and its metastases. Hormones, hormone precursors, or cytokines released by tumor cells are the major mediators of such syndromes. For diagnostic as well as therapeutic purposes, a working knowledge of paraneoplastic symptoms is very useful; these are outlined in Tables 9.2 and 9.3. It is important to keep in mind that some paraneoplastic symptoms can also be found with a variety of benign conditions.[13,14]

TABLE 9.1. **Hereditary Cancer Syndromes**

Cancer-Associated Syndrome	Gene Locus and Gene	Features	Genetic Testing
Cowdens's syndrome	10q22–10q23	Cutaneomucous tricholemmomas, breast cancer, colon and thyroid neoplasms	−
Familial breast and ovarian cancer	17q21 (*BRCA-1*) 13q12 (*BRCA-2*)	Elevated risk of breast and/or ovarian cancer in families with germline mutations	+
Familial melanoma	9p21 (CDKN2A) 12q13 (CDK 4)	Development of melanomas in nevi	+
Gorlin's syndrome	9q22–9q31	Basal cell carcinoma,odontogic keratocysts, medulloblastoma, ovarian fibroma, pits of the palms and/or soles,ectopic calcification, skeletal malformation	−
HNPCC (hereditary nonpolyposis colorectal cancer)	2p15–16(*MSH-2*) 3p21 (*MLH1*) 2q31–33 (*PMS-1*) 7p22 (*PMS-2*)	Colorectal cancer; cancer of endometrium, ovary, small bowel, and stomach, and transitional cell carcinomas can be associated sebaceous adenomas and carcinomas. Keratoacanthomas and basal cell epitheliomas associated in Muir-Torre syndrome	+
MEN 1	11q13 (*SCG-2*)	Hypophysial, pancreatic islet cell, parathyroid and thyroid adenomas, carcinoid tumors of intestine and bronchi	−
Men IIa	10q11 (C-*ret* proto-oncogene)	Medullary thyroid carcinoma, hyperparathyroidism, pheochromocytoma	+
Men IIb	10q11 (C-*ret* proto-oncogene)	Bilateral pheochromocytoma, neurofibromas	+
Neurofibromatosis	17q11	Neurofibromas, neurofibrosarcomas, acoustic neuromas, gliomas, meningiomas, juvenile myelogenous leukemia/juvenile myelomonocytogenic leukemia (café-au-lait skin pigmentation)	+
Peutz–Jehger's syndrome	19p (putative)	Gastrointestinal tumors, ovarian cysts, sex cord tumors (melanin spots of lips, buccal mucosa and digits)	−

(continued)

TABLE 9.1. Hereditary Cancer Syndromes (continued)

Cancer-Associated Syndrome	Gene Locus and Gene	Features	Genetic Testing
Polyposis coli	5q21–5q22 (APC gene)	Multiple adenomatous polyps in the colon and rectum with development of adenocarcinomas, association with epidermal cysts, lipomas, osteomas and lipomas in Gardner's syndrome, association with brain tumors in Turcot's syndrome	+
Retinoblastoma	13q14 (retino-blastoma gene)	Retinoblastoma, high risk for second primary tumors	+
Tuberous sclerosis	9q34 (C-*TSC-1*) 16p13 (TSC2)	Brain tumors, facial angiofibromas, renal angiomyolipomas (hypome-lanotic macules)	–
Von–Hippel Lindau syndrome	3p26	Angiomatosis of retina and cerebellum, renal adenocarcinoma, and pheo-chromocytoma	+

LABORATORY EXAMINATIONS

History taking followed by physical examination will result in a working differential diagnosis. Laboratory results serve first to evaluate the general status of the patient's health and also provide baseline values before therapy is commenced. They may uncover disease-related involvement of organ systems or unrelated pathologic conditions that have to be taken into consideration before treatment. Specific tests are used to substantiate the diagnosis, collect prognostic data that are important for the therapeutical decision making, and provide baseline values of tumor markers for follow-up reasons (Table 9.4).

Tumor Markers

Tumor markers are cellular products that are released into body fluids or exhibited on the cell surface. They may be produced by different types of normal and neoplastic cells but their excess, due to the monoclonal proliferation of a specific cell type, may lead to tumor diagnosis or aid in the monitoring of tumor load during therapy. It has to be kept in mind that tumor markers are often nonspecific and their levels may increase as a result of nonmalignant conditions as well. Table 9.5 includes some common tumor markers and their clinical uses.[15]

TABLE 9.2. **Paraneoplastic Syndromes of the Skin**

Disorder	Features	Associated neoplasms
Amyloidosis (amyloid light chain	Periorbital purpura, waxy nodules	Multiple myeloma
Acanthosis nigricans	Hyperkeratosis and darkened intertriginous areas	Gastric carcinoma, other intestinal adenocarcinoma
Bazex's syndrome	Papulosquamous lesions with pruritus, predominantly palms and soles	Squamous tumors of the upper aerodigestive tract
Dermatomyositis	Gottron's papules, heliotrope rash, and proximal myopathy	Gastrointestinal, various carcinomas
Digital clubbing	Loss of the nail bed angle	Small-cell lung carcinoma
Erythema gyratum repens	Concentric rings forming a wood-grain pattern	Lung and breast cancer
Florid cutaneous and papillomatosis	Disseminated wartlike lesions papillomavirus not found	Gastric carcinoma
Flush syndrome	Episodic head and neck flushes	Carcinoid
Hypertrichosis lanuginosa acquisita	Growth of lanuginous hair primarily on ears and face	Lung and colorectal cancer
Hypertrophic pulmonary osteoarthropathy	Periostitis of long bones with pain and swelling of joints	Lung cancer, lung metastasis
Generalized melanosis	Diffuse grayish skin darkening	Lymphoma, hepatoma, melanoma liver metastasis
Leser–Trelat	Rapid onset of a large number of seborrheic keratoses	Gastrointestinal, lymphoma
Necrolytic migratory erythema	Stomatits, circinate/gyrate rash with blistering and erosion	Glucagonoma
Paraneoplastic pemphigus	Painful blisters with involvement of mucosa	Lymphoma
Sweet's syndrome	Fever, neutrophilia, painful red plaques/nodules, dermal neutrophil infiltrates	Acute myelogenous leukemia, various carcinomas
Trousseau's syndrome	Migratory thrombophlebitis, vasculitis with septal panniculitis	Pancreatic cancer, lung cancer
Vasculitis (leukocytoclastic)	Without septal panniculitis, erythematous papules/nodules	Hairy cell leukemia, various other carcinomas

TABLE 9.3. Neurological Paraneoplastic Syndromes

Disorder	Features	Tumors and (Autoantibodies)
Subacute cerebellar degeneration	Bilateral cerebellar failure, ataxia, dysphagia, dysarthria, dementia	(Anti-Hu): SCLC, sarcoma, neuroblastoma (Anti-Yo): ovary, breast, SCLC (Anti-Tr): Hodgkin's lymphoma
Limbic encephalitis	Acute onset of mood changes, impairment of recent memory, hallucinations	SCLC, Hodgkin's lymphoma
Opsoclonus, myoclonus	Uncoordinated eye movements, myocloni	Neuroblastoma (predominantly children) (Anti-Ri): breast, gynecologic, SCLC, bladder
Encephalomyelitis	Variety of symptoms, can affect any part of the central nervous system	(Anti-Hu): SCLC, sarcoma, neuroblastoma
Cancer-associated retinopathy	Variety of visual symptoms	(Anti-retinal): SCLC, melanoma
Necrotizing myelopathy	Rapid ascending motor and sensory paralysis	Lung, kidney, Hodgkin's lymphoma
Dorsal root ganglionitis	Subacute onset of sensory loss	Lung
Sensorimotor peripheral neuropathy	Distal sensory loss, arreflexia, and wasting	Lung, gastrointestinal, breast
Autonomic neuropathy	Intestinal pseudoobstruction, neurogenic bladder, orthostatic hypotension	SCLC
Stiff-man syndrome	Rigidity of skeletal muscle with superimposed cramps	(Anti-amphiphisin): breast SCLC, thymona, Hodgkin's lymphoma
Lambert–Eaton syndrome	Proximally accentuated muscle	(Anti-VGCC): SCLC, thymoma, lymphoma

TUMOR LOCALIZATION

Tumor localization, pathologic analysis, and staging are the next consecutive steps in the patient's workup. The hypothetical diagnosis on the grounds of history, physical examination, and laboratory exams will guide the search for the primary tumor. Direct visualization with the chance to obtain tissue biopsies for pathologic analysis

TABLE 9.4. General Laboratory Examinations

Exam	Questions
CBC and differential	Hematology malignancies (diagnostic) Infection/anemia/leukopenia/thrombopenia (diagnostic, pretherapeutic, preoperative)
Liver panel	Cholestasis (pre-, intra-, posthepatic) Hepatitis (infectious/chemical) Alcoholism (preoperative)
Renal panel/electrolytes	Baseline values (pretherapeutic) Nutritional status (albumin/total protein) SIADH (paraneoplastic/drug induced) Hypercalcemia (paraneoplastic/metastases)
Coagulation exams	Hyper/hypocoagulation (preoperative, paraneoplastic platelet dysfunction, vitamin K deficiency or liver dysfunction, paraneoplastic hypercoagulability)
Urinalysis	Proteinuria, hematuria, urinary tract infection

is the well-recognized next stage in diagnosis. If the primary tumor or a metastasis is not easily accessible, imaging studies might help in localization, differential diagnosis, and eventual tissue diagnosis (Table 9.6).

SYSTEMIC METASTASES

For staging reasons and therapeutical considerations, the search for local and systemic metastases of a known primary tumor is crucial. Exact anatomic knowledge and awareness of preferred organ systems for metastases of specific tumors aid the search and help to avoid unnecessary total body screens. Table 9.7 gives an overview of the common methods currently used to detect metastatic disease.

PATHOLOGICAL ANALYSIS

A good pathological analysis is essential for decision making in cancer and a complete clinical profile provides essential background information. Pathologic material can now be used to detect underlying genetic alterations while evaluation of molecular (e.g., proliferation markers), cellular (dedifferentiation, polyploidy), prognostic factors, and pathologic tumor staging serve to estimate the tumor's malignant potential (Table 9.8).

The diagnosis of cancer must now also include pathologic tumor staging and histologic tumor grading as both are of high predictive value. Besides tumor stage and grade a number of other biologic markers have been associated and correlated with

TABLE 9.5. Direct Visualization and Biopsy of Suspicious Lesions

Method	Indication/advantages	Disadvantages/complications
Bronchoscopy	Diagnosis of pulmonary neoplasms, hilar neoplasms (transbronchial biopsy), possible bronchial involvement of esophageal neoplasm (if suspicious on CT)	Sedation, bleeding and pneumothorax (after transbronchial biopsy) peripheral infiltrates cannot be reached
Colonoscopy/ rectoscopy	Exact tumor localization and extent, possible discovery of multiple colon polyps, possible rectal endosonography with detection of infiltration depth and positive lymph nodes	Sedation, perforation, bleeding, limited information on lumen obstructing tumors
Cytoscopy	Urothelial tumors, possible bladder involvement of GI or GU tumor, endosonography	Anesthesia (rigid cytoscopy), urinary tract infections, urethral stricture, water intoxication
Esophagogastro- duodenoscopy	Laryngeal, esophageal, gastric, duodenal tumors, endosonography for staging and transgastric endosonography for pancreatic tumors	Sedation, cardiopulmonary complications, limited information on esophagus obstructing tumors
Hysteroscopy	Evaluation of postmenopausal uterine bleeding and endometrial hyperplasia, outpatient procedure	Pain, infection, possible intraperitoneal spread of endometrial or neoplastic cells
Laparoscopy	Exact staging and evaluation of operability	Anesthesia, hemorrhage from biopsy sites or abdominal varices, perforation, trocar injuries
Mediastinoscopy	Staging evaluation of mediastinal lesions, possible as an outpatient procedure	Scarring, not all lesions accessible, bleeding, laceration of trachea or endocard
Thorascopy	Evaluation of pleural effusion with negative cytology, evaluation of mediastinal lesions that cannot be reached by mediastinoscopy	Need for split ventilation and postoperative chest drainage, bleeding

survival prognosis. For some tumors (e.g., lymphomas) prognostic indexes have been established in which different factors enter with a defined value. Therapeutic decisions might then be guided by the prognostic index.[16]

Tumor grading classifies the malignant potential of a tumor according to its microscopic appearance. The histologic parameters used to categorize a tumor of low (grade I), intermediate (grade II), and high (grade III) malignancy include dedifferen-

TABLE 9.6. Diagnostic Imaging in Oncology

Method	Use in oncology
X-ray	Thorax (pulmonary/mediastinal lesions) Abdomen (suspected ileus or perforation) Bones (first choice for suspected lesions) Mammae (screening, diagnostic)
X − ray + contrast/ double contrast	Thorax (esophageal npl: longitudinal extent; thyroid npl: esophageal involvement) Abdomen (extent of gastric/intestinal neoplasms, possible second primary neoplasms and limited endoscopic accessibility, possible fistulas)
Angiography	Diagnostic: e.g., angiomas, angiosarcomas, neuroendocrine tumors Preoperative: e.g., variability in vascular anatomy, neoplastic infiltration of major vessels
ERCP	Bile duct, gallbladder, hepatic and pancreatic npl (diagnostic, preoperative)
Urography	Diagnostic: GU npl Preoperative: ureter/bladder involvement in GI npl, ureter anatomy, possible fistulas
CT (computerized tomography)	Diagnostic and preoperative: manifold indications with/without contrast (intravenous, angiographic, intrathecal), used to guide fine needle biopsies, good evaluation of enlarged lymph nodes limitations: discovery and staging of early tumors (e.g., GI or GU T1–T2 tumors), allergies to the contrast agent, cost, no sagittal or coronal planes
MRI (magnetic resonance imaging)	Diagnostic and preoperative: manifold indications especially CNS (no intrathecal contrast necessary, no bone artifacts in posterior fossa), musculoskeletal system and pelvis Advantages: multiplanar imaging, Limitations: poor lymph node visualization, no advantage in over CT thoracic/mediastinal diagnosis, long registration time with possible interfering patient movements, artifacts by steel implants, cost
PET (positron emission tomography)	Diagnostic, monitoring: Advantages: high sensitivity (picomolar), exact distinction between radiation necrosis, edema and tumor recurrence (e.g., brain tumors), measurements of physiologic activity (with possible estimation of malignant potential) Limitations: high cost limits clinical use; specific markers and antibodies yet to be developed

(continued)

TABLE 9.6. Diagnostic Imaging in Oncology (continued)

Method	Use in oncology
Scintigraphy	Diagnostic, staging, monitoring: bone tumors and metastases (^{99m}Tc-diphosphonate), thyroid cancer (^{123}I,^{131}I in NaI, and ^{99m}Tc-pertechnetat), neuroblastoma/pheochromocytoma/ medullary thyroid carcinoma (^{123}I-MIBG), neuroendocrine tumors (^{111}In-octreotide) Advantage: high sensitivity Limitations: costs, specificity, radioactivity
Ultrasonic scanning	Diagnostic, preoperative, intraoperative: external and internal, guiding of fine-needle biopsies Head: vessels, sinuses, lymph nodes Neck: lymph nodes, thyroid, parathyroid Mammae: distinguish palpable tumors (solid/cyst) Thorax/extremities: soft tissue tumors, lymph nodes, vessel involvement (Doppler), esophagus (endosono), heart (trans- and thoracic transesophageal echocardiography) Abdomen: liver, gallbladder, kidneys, spleen, stomach (endosono), ovaries, pancreas (transgastric or hydrosono), rectum (endosono), vessels Pelvis: bladder (endosono/hydrosono), prostate/seminal vesicles (transrectal), vagina/cervix/uterus (transvaginally) Extremities: soft tissue sarcomas, musculoskeletal tumors, lymph nodes, vessel involvement, cutaneous metastases Advantages: low cost, safe, good staging of infiltration depth and local lymph nodes in endosonography Disadvantages: limited use with gastrointestinal air

tiation, proliferative potential, and vascularization. They also include cellularity, matrix formation, margins, pleomorphism, mitotic activity, necrotic areas, hemorrhage, and inflammation. Because the consistency of a tumor is often very heterogeneous, various areas of the tumor have to evaluated. All of these factors are important in the diagnostic workup of the patient.

Molecular Markers

Molecular markers are cellular products (DNA, RNA, proteins) that can be detected immunohistochemically with in situ hybridization, PCR, or by blotting techniques. Molecular markers can be cellular hormone receptors (estrogen receptors) indicating possible responses to chemotherapy. Others are proteins that are produced in the synthesis phase and G_2 phase of the cell cycle (Ki-67, PCNA) and can thus be used to calculate the proliferative index of a given tissue. Others again are proteins involved in cell cycle checkpoint regulation (p21, p27, pRb, p53) or are oncogene products.

TABLE 9.7. Diagnosis of Tumor Metastases

Organ	Clinical setting	Diagnosis	Common primary tumors
Bone	Primary tumor still surgically curable and known to metastasize to bone	$99m$Tc-scintigraphy	Breast, lung, multiple myeloma, prostate, thyroid, sarcoma, Hodgkin's lymphoma
	Primary tumor still surgically curable but focal symptoms present	X-ray, CT, scintigraphy	
Bone marrow	Therapeutic decision changes in case of proven systemic metastases	Bone marrow biopsy (iliac crest, Jamshidi trocar)	Breast, lung (small cell), prostate, thyroid, lymphoma
Brain	Focal symptoms	CT, MRI	Lung, breast, melanoma
Liver	Staging before chemo/radiotherapy	Ultrasound/CT (for monitoring)	Colon, stomach, pancreas, breast, lung
	Preoperative, no symptoms without intent of hepatic reaction	Ultrasound	
	Sonographic evidence of possibly resectable liver metastases	CT + portal angiography (highest sensitivity)	
	Intraoperative suspicious liver lesions	Intraoperative ultrasound	
Lung	No symptoms, screening	X-ray	Lung, breast, colon stomach
	Resectable liver metastases present, suspicious X-ray	CT	
Lymphatic system	Localized primary tumor and clinically suspicious lymph nodes	Ultrasound, CT	Localized primaries: head and neck (upper and middle cervical), gastrointestinal (supraclavicular left), breast and lung (supraclavicular right), breast, melanoma, sarcoma (axilla), melanoma, sarcoma, vulva, anus, bladder, prostate (inguinal)
	Localized primary tumor and sentinel node biopsy	Lymphatic immunoscinti-graphy intraoperatively	
	Systemic disease	Lymphography (advantage over CT: even regular sized pathologic lymph nodes can be identified)	
Total body screen	Possible resectable metastases of scintigraphically detectable tumors	123I-MIBG scintigraphy, 111In-octreotide scintigraphy	Neural crest tumors, neuroendocrine tumors

211

TABLE 9.8. Diagnostic Means in athology

Tool	Use
Clinical information	Tumor localization, tumor size, macroscopic invasion, distant metastases
Resected material	Macroscopic appearance, texture, structural relation to surrounding tissue
Light microscopy (tissue staining)	Cellular phenotype, accompanying inflammatory reaction, tissue invasion (T-classification), metastatic seedlings (N-classification [lymph nodes] and M-classification [distant metastases]), tumor grading
Electron microscopy	Differentiate between carcinoma, melanoma, and sarcoma; identify neuroendocrine differentiation and histiocytosis X; aid the distinction of small round cell tumors and spindle cellular soft tissue tumors
Immunohistochemistry	Specific antibodies recognize surface antigens or intracellular proteins that lead to the identification of cellular origin
In situ hybridization	Identification and visualization of specific DNA/RNA sequences with probes
Blotting procedures	DNA (southern blot), RNA (northern blot) and proteins are extracted from tumor tissue (always including neoplastic and nonneoplastic cells) and visualized with probes or antibodies
PCR and in situ PCR	Identification of single copies of specific DNA/RNA sequences

The world of molecular markers is evolving rapidly and becoming an increasingly important part in cancer diagnosis. As soon as antibodies are available for cell surface receptors, proteins involved in cell cycle checkpoint regulation, signaling pathways, and DNA repair or apoptosis, they will be analyzed in human tumors and correlated with patient survival. The drawback of molecular markers is the diversity of spontaneous mutations in human tumors. Specific molecular markers might be valuable for a subset of human tumors, for example, p21 and gastric cancer,[17] while not showing prognostic significance in other subsets of human tumors, for example, p21 and gallbladder tumors.[18] Data for specific molecular tumor markers can thus not be generalized but have to be evaluated individually. Germline mutations identified with carcinogenesis can be used diagnostically (patient screening) and prognostically, and aid therapeutical decision making.

Genetic Testing

Germline mutations are passed on genetically, can be found in every cell of the carrier, and predispose to tumor development in specific tissues. These features enable diagnosis of the mutation in easily accessible cells (e.g., blood lymphocytes), surveillance or prophylactic treatment of gene carriers (e.g., proctocolectomy in familial polyposis), and screening of family members. As the oncogenic potential and penetrance of individual mutations differ, implications and consequences of genetic testing have to be carefully evaluated prior to its application.

Specific attention has been focused lately on commercially available tests for breast cancer susceptibility genes. General screening seems unjustified as women with a family history of breast cancer will have a negative test nine out of ten times. A negative test on the other hand does not exclude a hereditary risk from unknown genes and should not lead to a lessened vigilance or surveillance.[19,20] Once the relationship between genotype and phenotype becomes clearer, it is likely that, in future years, genetic profile will play a role in cancer diagnosis.

SUMMARY

A proper history and physical examination are the fundamentals in establishing a diagnosis of cancer. Advances in recent years have greatly facilitated the potential for diagnosing not just cancer, but also other characteristics such as subtype and aggressiveness, to mention but a few. The advent of molecular diagnostic laboratories and genetic testing has introduced new and exciting methods in cancer diagnosis. The ability of such new methods to facilitate early diagnosis of cancer is now one of the key areas in cancer diagnosis.

FURTHER READING

1. Mittendorf R (1995) Teratogen update: Carcinogenesis and teratogeneses associated with exposure to diethylstilbestrol (DES) in utero. *Teratology* 51:435–445.
2. Denissenko MF, Pao A, Tang M, Pfeifer GP (1996) Preferential formation of benzo[*a*]pyrene adducts at lung cancer mutational hotspots in p53. *Science* 274:430–432.
3. Phillips DH, Hewer A, Martin CN, Garner RC, King MM (1988) Correlation of DNA adduct levels in human lung with cigarette smoking. *Nature* 336:790–792.
4. Vineis P, Caporaso N (1995) Tobacco and cancer: Epidemiology and the laboratory. *Environ Health Perspect* 103:156–160.
5. Kogevinas M, Becher H, Benn T, et al. (1997) Cancer mortality in workers exposed to phenoxy herbicides, chlorophenols, and dioxins. An expanded and updated international cohort study. *Am J Epidemiol* 145:1061–1075.
6. Fingerhut MA, Halperin WE, Marlow DA, et al. (1991) Cancer mortality in workers exposed to 2,3,7,8-tetrachlorodibenzo-*p*-dioxin. *N Eng J Med* 324:212–218.
7. Higginson J, Muir CS, Munoz N (1992) Human cancer: Epidemiology and environmental causes. Cambridge University Press, Cambridge.

8. Ouhtit A, Ueda M, Nakazawa H, et al. (1997) Quantitative detection of untraviolet-specific *p53* mutations in normal skin from Japanese patients. *Cancer Epidemiol Biomark Prev* 6:433–438.

9. Ananthaswamy HN, Loughlin SM, Cox P, et al. (1997) Sunlight and skin cancer: Inhibition of *p53* mutations in UV-irradiated mouse skin by sunscreens. *Nat Med* 3:510–514.

10. Pisani P, Parkin DM, Munoz N, Ferlay J (1997) Cancer and infection: Estimates of the attributable fraction in 1990. *Cancer Epidemiol Biomark Prev* 6:387–400.

11. Schulz TF, Boshoff CH, Weiss RA (1996) HIV infection and neoplasia. *Lancet* 348:587–591.

12. Marselos M, Vainio H (1991) Carcinogenic properties of pharmaceutical agents evaluated in the IARC Monographs programme. *Carcinogenesis* 12:1751–1766.

13. Nathanson C, Hall TC (1997) Paraneoplastic syndromes. *Semin Oncol* 24.

14. Hall TC, Para S (1974) Paraneoplastic syndromes. *Ann NY Acad Sci* 230:1–577.

15. Ting SW, Chen JS, Schwartz MK (1987) Human tumor markers. Elsevier Science, Amsterdam.

16. The International Non-Hodkin's Lymphoma Prognostic Factors Project (1993) A predictive model for aggressive non-Hodgkin's lymphoma. *N Eng J Med* 329:987–994.

17. Gomyo Y, Ideda M, Osaki M, et al. (1997) Expression of *p21* (*waf1/cip1/sdi1*), but not *p53* protien, is a factor in the survival of patients with advanced gastric carcinoma. *Cancer* 79:2067–2072.

18. Lee CS (1997) Ras p21 protien immunoreactivity and its relationship to *p53* expression and prognosis in gallbladder and extrahepatic biliary carcinoma. *Eur J Surg* 23:233–237.

19. Couch FJ, DeShano ML, Blackwood MA, et al. (1997) *BRCA-1* mutations in women attending clinics that evaluate the risk of breast cancer. *N Eng J Med* 336:1409–1415.

20. Healy B (1997) BRCA genes—bookmaking, fortunetelling, and medical care. (editorial) *N Eng J Med* 336:1448–1449.

CHAPTER 10

THE ROLE OF CANCER STAGING IN EVIDENCE-BASED MEDICINE

WILLIAM J. MACKILLOP, PETER DIXON, MARY K. GOSPODAROWICZ
and BRIAN O'SULLIVAN

The Radiation Oncology Research Unit
Department of Oncology
Queen's University
Kingston Regional Cancer Centre
Kingston General Hospital
Kingston, Ontario
and
The Princess Margaret Hospital
Toronto, Ontario, Canada

A staging system is a system of classification of cancer based mainly on the anatomic extent of the disease. In this chapter we show how cancer staging contributes to the creation and dissemination of knowledge, and how staging can be used to guide the treatment of individual patients and the management of cancer control programs (Table 10.1). We begin by considering why staging is necessary and how a staging system is constructed, before going on to discuss how staging is used in practice.

THE CLASSIFICATION OF CANCER

The Problem of Diversity

Cancer is a diverse group of diseases characterized by uncontrolled cellular proliferation, genetic variability, invasion, and metastasis. The prognosis and the potential benefits of treatment vary widely from case to case. Some system of classification is required to identify groups of cases that share similarities in their clinical behavior. The classification of diseases may seem rather remote from clinical practice, but it is, in fact, at the heart of scientific medicine. Only when a specific clinical problem

Manual of Clinical Oncology, 7th edition, Edited by Raphael E. Pollock
ISBN 0-471-23828-7, pages 215–233. Copyright © 1999 Wiley-Liss, Inc.

TABLE 10.1. The Use of Staging in Oncology

In Creating Knowledge

- Permits clinical research to produce new information through the systematic observation of groups of similar patients.
- Permits integration of information about similar patients from diverse sources.

In Disseminating Knowledge

- Provides a common language for sharing information internationally.
- Facilitates the teaching of new health care workers, and the continued learning of those already in practice.

In Applying Knowledge to the Care of Individual Patients

- Permits the use of knowledge derived from past experience to guide medical decisions in the individual case.
- Fosters a disciplined, multidisciplinary approach to the evaluation of cancer patients.
- Facilitates communication with patients, and promotes their involvement in decisions about their care.

In Managing Programs of Cancer Control

- Permits projections of workload needed for strategic planning and resource allocation.
- Permits evaluation and improvement of cancer control programs.

has been recognized and defined can we start to accumulate the information about it that is needed to answer the fundamental questions that face doctors and patients in day-to-day practice: What will happen if the disease is left untreated, what treatments may help, and which is best?[1] In the physical sciences, new knowledge sometimes may be created by the process of deduction without reference to the external world, but biologic systems are not well enough understood to permit the valid use of deduction. Medical knowledge can only be created empirically by the process of induction, which allows us to infer what will happen in a specific set of circumstances in the future, based on what has been observed to happen in similar circumstances in the past.[2] The predictive value of inductive inference depends not only on how many observations have been made, but also on how uniform the outcome was in those cases, and that is determined by the effectiveness of the system of classification used to define the group.

The classification of cancers presents particular challenges because of the large number of sites and tissues that may be affected by neoplasia, and because of the genetic plasticity associated with neoplasia. Several complementary systems of classification are available. Cancers are usually classified by their site of origin,[3] and by their microscopic appearance,[4] but two cases that look alike from these aspects may prove to be very different when the phenotypic and/or genotypic characteristics of their tumor cells are studied in greater detail. Today, new techniques in immunology, biochemistry, and molecular genetics are beginning to provide a basis for refining the classification of some types of cancer. In the future, the measurement of cellular components that are directly involved in determining rates of proliferation, metastatic potential, and response to therapy, and/or the use of dynamic assays of tumor cell behavior, may hold the key to the development of clinically more useful classifications. Further, in defining similar groups of cases, the characteristics of the patient are as important as the characteristics of the cancer. Classification of patients based on their functional status is, therefore, also important.

Cancer Progression

Not only do cancers differ from one another, but each individual case also changes with the passage of time. During the progression of a cancer, both the volume of the tumor and its anatomic extent increase, and mutation and selection may lead to the evolution of new clones of cells with higher proliferative or metastatic potential.[5] The rate and pattern of progression of a cancer is partly determined by its primary site and its histology, but the course of a given disease varies widely from one patient to the next.[6]

The inherent cellular characteristics of the tumor in part determine how far it will progress before it is detected; cancers with faster growth rates and higher metastatic potential are less likely to be diagnosed at an early stage because there is a shorter window of opportunity to detect them before they spread. On the other hand, random events are involved in clonal evolution and metastasis, and the precise point in time at which a cancer first spreads may depend on chance alone.[5] Other factors entirely unrelated to cancer biology may determine when a cancer will be detected in a specific case. Some tumors are detected by deliberate screening, or are found incidentally by diagnostic tests done for other purposes, whereas others progress until symptoms develop. Many different factors determine how long symptoms persist before the diagnosis is made; patients' awareness of the potential significance of early symptoms varies, as does their willingness to get medical advice, and socioeconomic factors influence patients' access to medical care. Thus, many nonbiologic factors are involved in determining the extent of a cancer at presentation, and no system of classification based solely on the cellular characteristics of the tumor can be expected to produce groups of cases that are uniform in their anatomic extent at the time of diagnosis.

Cancer Staging

In general, as the anatomic extent of a cancer increases, the prognosis becomes worse, the range of treatment options becomes more restricted, and the potential benefits of treatment diminish. A system of classification based on the extent of the disease is, therefore, required to create groups of clinically similar cases. *Staging* is the term used to describe the classification of cancers based on their anatomic extent. Staging complements, rather than competes with, classifications based on inherent cellular characteristics.[7]

THE DESIGN OF A STAGING SYSTEM

In creating a staging system, certain attributes of the tumor are coded to become ranked variables.[8] Like any other system of measurement a good staging system must be valid, reliable, and practical.[9]

A clinically valid staging system will create groups of cases requiring similar management, and/or groups of cases that experience similar outcomes. To achieve this, the system should reflect the clinical findings that identify important subgroups. This requires a site-specific system tailored to the relevant anatomy, to the character-istic behavior of the specific cancer, and to the treatment options available. A valid system is exhaustive, that is, it should be capable of reflecting the full range of pos-sible presentations of each type of cancer. To retain its validity over time, the system also needs to be flexible enough to permit it to adapt to important changes in medical practice or medical knowledge.

A reliable staging system will, as far as possible, ensure that identical cases will always be assigned to the same category. To achieve this, it should be based on ob-jective assessment of measurable quantities. The system should be unambiguous and clearly written, and it should be accompanied by explicit rules for its application. To permit reliable comparisons over time, the system should not be subject to fre-quent changes. Reliability is discussed further in the section on potential barriers to communication.

A practical staging system is suitable for day-to-day use in a wide range of clin-ical settings. To meet this requirement, the whole system needs to be easy to com-prehend. This means it must be simple in concept and based on common principles that are applicable to all sites. It should not rely on extraordinary expertise or on diagnostic procedures that are not generally available. The system and the rules for its use should be readily accessible; it should be available in all major languages both in print and in electronic form, and the necessary documentation should not be expensive to buy. It should permit different users to apply it with different levels of precision; it should be capable of creating the small subgroups that are important to experts involved in the direct care of patients, and at the same time should be capable of creating the larger groups that may be required for statistical analysis.

In practice, the attributes listed above may sometimes conflict with one another, and compromises may be required. Attempts to make the system unambiguous and exhaustive should not be taken so far that it loses its simplicity. The requirement for stability over time should not exclude the flexibility to adapt to changes in medi-cal practice. A staging system has to be site specific to provide a valid description of cancers that differ in their natural history and response to therapy, but common principles are required to keep the system coherent and comprehensible to the user. A good system is precise enough to allow specialists to record important differences among cases, but it should not be so complicated as to become impractical for day-to-day use. A good system should be sufficiently reliable that results can be compared among observers, but it has to do this without the help of sophisticated technology to remain feasible for use in routine practice in a wide variety of settings.

To maximize the value of staging in communication, the same system should be used universally. Widespread acceptance is facilitated if the system is valid, reliable, and practical, but a solid administrative infrastructure is also required to maintain, promote, and disseminate it. Good governance is important. In directing the evolution of a staging system, every effort should be made to make it converge with competing systems, with a view to merging whenever possible.

THE TNM CLASSIFICATION

The TNM System and Its Relationship to Other Staging Systems

The TNM classification of malignant tumors is a mature system of anatomic staging that meets most of the criteria outlined in the preceding section. The TNM system evolved from the work of Pierre Denoix in the early 1940s.[10] The first TNM classification for cancers of the breast and larynx was published in 1958,[11] and the first comprehensive *livre de poche*, which included classifications for 23 sites, was published in 1968.[12] A great effort has been made over the years to reconcile differences between the TNM system and other systems. Today, the TNM classification is used both by the International Union Against Cancer (UICC), and by the American Joint Committee for Cancer Staging (AJCC), and their systems are now identical.[13,14] The TNM classifications for the gynecologic malignancies are essentially identical to those of the International Federation of Gynecology and Obstetrics (FIGO).[13,15] The TNM classification of colorectal cancer is compatible with the Dukes system and its modifications,[13,16,17] and the TNM classification for the lymphomas is identical to the Ann Arbor system.[13,18] The TNM classification is published today in a dozen languages, and is kept under continuous review by an international expert committee that makes occasional changes as necessary to meet the needs of the clinician based on recommendations from the international community. For example, in the fifth edition of the TNM Classification, which was published in 1997, the classification of nasopharyngeal cancer was revised to make it more clinically relevant to radiation oncologists.[13] Whenever possible, changes to the TNM system are made by creating new subgroups within the existing framework, thus preserving the ability to compare outcomes over time.

The Elements of the TNM System

The TNM system is based on a set of general rules that have been modified for application to specific primary sites.[12] The system requires that the primary site be defined and the diagnosis confirmed microscopically before stage is assigned. As well as providing a vocabulary for describing most of the common cancers, the TNM system provides the syntax, or rules of grammar, required to ensure that the language of stage is used correctly.[12]

The system is based on the assessment of three components:

TABLE 10.2. The TNM Classification

T—Primary tumor	
TX	Primary tumor cannot be assessed.
T0	No evidence of primary tumor
Tis	Carcinoma in situ
T1, T2, T3, T4	Increasing size and/or local extent of the primary tumor
N—Regional lymph nodes	
NX	Regional lymph nodes cannot be assessed.
N0	No regional lymph node metastasis
N1, N2, N3	Increasing involvement of regional lymph nodes
M—Distant metastasis	
MX	Distant metastasis cannot be assessed.
M0	No distant metastasis
M1	Distant metastasis

The category M1 may be further specified according to the following notation:

Pulmonary	PUL	Bone marrow	MAR
Osseous	OSS	Pleura	PLE
Peritoneum	PER	Hepatic	HEP
Brain	BRA	Adrenals	ADR
Lymph nodes	LYM	Skin	SKI
Others	OTH		

In some sites, further subdivisions of the main categories are available to permit a greater degree of precision (e.g., T1a, 1b, or N2a, 2b). For details of site specific classifications, see Refs. 13 and 14.

T—the extent of the primary tumor
N—the absence or presence and extent of regional lymph node metastases.
M—the absence or presence of distant metastases

As shown in Table 10.2, the addition of numbers to these three components indicates the extent of the cancer. If there is doubt about which T, N, or M category to assign to a case, then the lower, or less advanced category, should be chosen. After assigning T, N, and M categories, cases may be collected into stage groups. The TNM system provides rules for doing this, but acknowledges that other groupings may be better for the some specific purposes, and that clinicians may sometimes wish to create their own groups based on the T, N, and M categories.

Although the system is simple in principle, the details vary from site to site, and no clinician is likely to retain all of this information in memory. In fact, not relying on memory is the hallmark of the professional oncologist; the UICC *livre de poche* is carried and used daily by the most expert clinicians. Site-specific staging sheets are widely available, and should be included in every cancer patient's clinical record. User-friendly software for use in staging is also becoming available.

The Clinical and Pathologic TNM Classifications

There are, in fact, two TNM classifications described for each site.[12]

The first is a *clinical classification* that is based on evidence arising from physical examination, imaging, endoscopy, biopsy, surgical exploration, and whatever other pretreatment examinations are relevant to that specific site. This classification is used in making initial treatment decisions, and provides some information about the prognosis. This type of classification can be applied in every case and provides a level playing field for comparisons of outcome between treatment strategies that involve surgery and those that do not.

The second is a *pathologic classification*, designated pTMN. This is based on the evidence obtained before treatment, supplemented or modified by the additional evidence acquired from surgery and from pathologic examination. The pTNM classification does not replace the TNM classification in operated cases; the preoperative TNM stage remains unaltered, and the pTNM stage is recorded separately. pTNM is used to guide decisions relating to postoperative treatment, and provides additional information about the prognosis. Pathologic staging contributes to our understanding of how well clinical stage reflects the true anatomic extent of the cancer, and may be useful in assessing the value of new diagnostic techniques.

The TNM system is primarily intended for use in classifying newly diagnosed cases, but the same nomenclature can be employed in modified form in other circumstances. The TNM classification may be applied to recurrent tumors, but the TNM and pTNM categories are then to be identified by the prefix r, and recorded separately from the record of stage at diagnosis which should not be changed. The extent of disease may also be assessed after chemotherapy or radiotherapy, but the TNM or pTNM categories assigned in this context are to be identified by the prefix y.

THE ROLE OF STAGING IN RESEARCH

Staging plays a key role in studies of the effectiveness of cancer treatment, and in studies of the effectiveness of cancer control programs. It is also important in studies of the epidemiology and natural history of cancer.

Studies of the Effectiveness of Cancer Treatment

Experimental Studies   The prospective, randomized controlled trial (RCT) is accepted today as the standard method of comparing the effectiveness of different treatment strategies.[19] In RCTs in oncology, stage is almost always one of the entry criteria used to create uniform groups of cases for study. Stage may also serve as a basis for stratification to ensure an even balance of prognostic factors between the arms of a trial. Routine recording of stage at a cancer treatment center permits estimation of the number of cases eligible to participate in proposed trials, and also provides a way of monitoring accrual to trials in progress. Information about the stage mix in the community reveals how well the sample in a trial represents the overall population, and this is useful in estimating the generalizability of its results.

Observational Studies   Much of our knowledge about the results of cancer treatment still comes from retrospective, observational studies of the experience of individual institutions. Reviews of institutional experience are inferior to RCTs as a means of comparing the effectiveness of different treatments, but they are a means of learning from clinical experience, and are often the source of hypotheses that can later be tested in formal clinical trials. In the rarer malignancies, retrospective reviews may be the only source of information about the effectiveness of treatment, and their importance in that context cannot be overstated.[20] However, the problem with such observational studies is that comparisons of outcomes between treatment groups in the same institution are usually confounded by selection bias, and comparisons of outcome among institutions are often further confounded by the problem of referral bias. The ability to control for stage goes some way toward reducing these problems and permits a more valid comparison of the results of competing treatment strategies. Reporting results by stage also gives a clearer idea of the subgroup(s) of patients most likely to benefit from specific treatments.

Integrating Information About the Effectiveness of Treatment   Review articles and book chapters are the traditional way of bringing together information from diverse sources. In compiling these reports, stage is used to identify comparable groups, and to describe and compare outcomes achieved by different treatment strategies. There is, however, growing dissatisfaction with unstructured literature reviews because of (1) the potential for bias in the choice of information to be included, and (2) the lack of a valid process for combining data from different sources. This has led to a more structured approach known as the "systematic review" which is now promoted worldwide by the Cochrane collaboration.[21] Here the reviewer is forced to be explicit about the search process used to identify relevant material, and about criteria used to select the information to be included in the analysis. The results of different RCTs are combined by the formal process of meta-analysis.

It is crucial to the validity of the process of meta-analysis that the trials combined should have involved similar groups of patients. Information about stage is, therefore, necessary to select groups of cases for inclusion in a meta-analysis. Patient groups that have been created using different staging systems cannot usually be combined for the purpose of meta-analysis. Thus, the use of different staging systems may create separate streams of knowledge that cannot be combined or compared directly.[22] The universal use of a single staging system is, therefore, necessary to avoid the development of separate and potentially irreconcilable schools of thought about the management of one disease.

Studies of the Effectiveness of Cancer Control Programs

Population-based cancer registries were originally established to study the epidemiology of cancer, but they can also be used to study the epidemiology of cancer treatment. Like cancer incidence and mortality, patterns of cancer treatment and survival can be compared among communities, across socioeconomic strata, and over time. Registry-Based Observational Studies (RBOs) of the management and outcome of cancer deal with unselected cohorts of cases and are, therefore, free of the problems of referral bias and selection bias that confound institution-based observational studies.[23] RBOs and RCTs are complementary, rather than competing, methodologies; RCTs tell us how patients should be managed, whereas RBOs tell us what really happens in practice. RBOs have the potential to describe the impact of the results of RCTs, meta-analysis, and treatment guidelines on the management and outcome of cancer in the population. These are important questions, but they have to be addressed in the context of specific patient groups. Information about stage is required to define those groups. At present, not all cancer registries routinely capture stage, and this still limits the scope of this type of research in many communities.

Studies of Economic Aspects of Cancer Care

It is increasingly recognized that key decisions about the allocation of resources in the future will be determined not only by what health programs achieve, but by what they achieve per dollar.[24] This type of information is important in decisions at many levels. It may be used to decide how much public money to spend on health programs as opposed to other publicly funded programs, how much to spend on cancer care as opposed to other health programs, how much to spend on early detection as opposed to treatment, and how much to spend on palliative care as opposed to active treatment. In an economic analysis, it is just as important to define the patient group studied in terms of site and stage as it is in any other type of cancer research. Economic analyses are now being built into some RCTs, but RBOs may be the ultimate way of addressing economic questions. In either case, information about stage is essential.

Studies of the Epidemiology and Natural History of Cancer

Gathering information about stage mix at the population level extends the scope of conventional epidemiologic research in oncology by permitting the investigation of factors that are associated with advanced stage at presentation. Staging also contributes to studies of the natural history of cancer. In the evaluation of putative markers of metastatic potential and putative predictors of response to therapy, it is important to control for stage to ensure that the study indicator really does provide more prognostic information than was provided by conventional approaches.

THE ROLE OF STAGING IN DISSEMINATING KNOWLEDGE

Stage as a Language

Stage provides a common language of communication among doctors worldwide. In day-to-day practice, doctors use the language of stage to communicate with one another and with their patients. Stage provides a framework for teaching and learning in undergraduate, postgraduate, and continuing medical education. Journal articles, textbooks, and treatment guidelines all rely on the language of stage in summarizing their management recommendations, as do electronic sources of information.

Potential Barriers to Communication

Because stage is used in creating, integrating, and disseminating the knowledge that guides the practice of oncology, the fidelity of information transfer along this path is very important. This depends on how consistently the language of stage is used from one observer to the next, from one clinical trial to the next, and from one country to the next. Even when reliability has been given a high priority in designing a staging system, some inconsistency in its use is inevitable. It has been shown experimentally that the same clinician cannot always be relied upon to assign the same stage to identical cases on two separate occasions (intra-observer variation), and that there is a greater degree of variation in stage recorded by different clinicians observing the same cases (inter-observer variation).[25] Errors in staging may be random or systematic. Although both are equally important in the management of the individual case, systemic error is the more serious problem in the analysis and interpretation of collective experience.

Stage Migration

One particular type of systematic error deserves special mention. Figure 10.1 illustrates a curious phenomenon that arises when staging investigations change over time, or vary from one place to another. It was described more than half a century ago by Bradford Hill, who called it "the problem of attributes,"[1] but it is now more widely known as "stage migration."[26] The figure shows how this problem might affect reports of the outcome of a cancer with an overall 5-year survival of 50%, which is classified using a very simple two-stage system. On the basis of conventional investigations, half of the patients are assigned to a good prognosis group, stage I, which has a 5-year survival of 70%, and the other half to a poor prognosis group, stage II, which has a 5-year survival of 30% (Fig. 10.1a). Suppose that a new radiologic technique is adopted that has a higher resolution than conventional techniques, and this reveals that 20% of the former stage I cases are more extensive than was thought, and actually belong to stage II. Let us assume, as seems reasonable, that this subgroup has a worse prognosis than the rest of the stage I patients, but a better prognosis than the stage II patients, say 50% survival at 5 years. When the information provided by the new radiologic technique is used in assigning stage, this intermediate group is transferred from stage I to stage II. This leads to an "improvement" in survival in stage I, from 70% to 75%, and an "improvement" in survival in stage II from 30% to 33.3%, but the overall survival, of course, remains unchanged at 50% (Fig. 10.1b). It is a general truth that changes in investigations that lead to systematic upstaging improve results in each stage. It is also true that changes in practice that lead to systematic downstaging produce worse results in each stage, but this is a less frequent problem. The phenomenon of stage migration makes it hazardous to compare

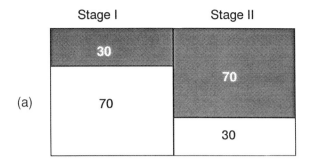

Stage I (n=100), 5 year survival=70/100=70%
Stage II (n=100), 5 year survival=30/100=30%
Overall Group (n=200), 5 year survival=100/200=50%

Stage I (n=80), 5 year survival=60/80=75%
Stage II (n=120), 5 year survival=40/120=33.3%
Overall Group (n=200), 5 year survival=100/200=50%

FIGURE 10.1. The problem of attributes: The two diagrams describe the five-year survival reported by stage in an imaginary cancer with an overall five-year survival of 50%, that is classified using a simple two-stage system. The shaded areas of the diagrams indicate the patients who died of the disease, and the areas shown in white indicate survivors. Panel (**a**) illustrates the results observed when stage is assigned using conventional investigations. Panel (**b**) shows the results observed after the introduction of a new diagnostic test that "upstages" a subgroup of patients with an intermediate prognosis from stage I to stage II. Survival "improves" in both subgroups, while overall survival remains unchanged.[1,25]

outcomes by stage in different series of cases that have not been investigated in the same way. The reader should always be suspicious of improvements in the outcome of subgroups that are not accompanied by any improvement in the outcome of the overall group.

There has so far been insufficient effort directed toward ensuring the uniform use of the TNM system, and additional work is required in this area. It can be argued that the TNM system could be enhanced by gradually becoming more prescriptive with respect to the information that may, and may not, be used in assigning stage. One of the reasons why the FIGO system has been so widely accepted as a valid means of comparing the results of treatment of the gynecologic malignancies around the world is that it very clearly defines what information may *not* be used in assigning stage.[15]

THE ROLE OF STAGING IN CLINICAL PRACTICE

What Is Involved in "Staging" the Patient?

In practice, "staging" involves three separate steps: assessment, classification, and recording. Assessment involves the gathering of information about the extent of disease from the clinical history, the physical examination, endoscopy and/or radiologic investigation, and in the case of pathologic classification, also from surgical and histologic evaluation. Classification involves the analysis of this information, and may require the reconciliation of apparently conflicting data. It culminates in a conscious judgment about the T, N, and M categories to be assigned to the case. This is followed by the act of recording the stage as a permanent part of the patient's record. We see this as the responsibility of the attending physician, although the stage assigned may reflect the combined views of several consultants.

It is sometimes thought that a commitment to staging implies that all cases of a particular cancer must be submitted to a given series of investigations whether or not they serve the needs of the individual patient. This is incorrect. Consider a patient who presents with cough, hemoptysis, and widespread bone pain, and who is found to have a large opacity at the right hilum on chest X-ray, malignant squamous cells in his sputum, and multiple hot spots on bone scan that are consistent with metastases. This patient would not benefit from the additional investigations that would be necessary to delineate the extent of the primary tumor, or to ascertain the status of the mediastinal lymph nodes. The TNM system does not mandate these investigations. Rather, the TNM system provides the X categories for use when the medically appropriate investigations do not yield sufficient information to permit classification. This case would be classified as TX, NX, M1. If a diagnosis of cancer is made in a patient who is not fit for any active treatment regardless of the stage of the disease, then it is perfectly correct to stage the patient TX, NX, MX without any staging investigations at all.[13]

The Role of Stage in Guiding Treatment Decisions

The way that knowledge is created dictates the way it must be applied. Almost all the knowledge about cancer treatment that has been created by clinical research trials is knowledge about specific stages of specific diseases. It can, therefore, be used to guide the management of the individual patient only once the site and stage of the cancer have been established. The staging of cancer is necessary but not sufficient for the practice of evidence-based medicine. Other factors must also be considered including, for example, the histologic characteristics of the cancer, the patient's medical status, and his or her treatment preferences.

Staging influences several aspects of the treatment decision. First, the stage of the cancer often determines whether the intent of treatment should be curative or palliative. Consider a patient who presents with dysphagia and weight loss and is found to have a squamous carcinoma of the esophagus and multiple metastases in the liver. Because metastatic squamous cancer of the esophagus is not curable by surgery, radiotherapy, or chemotherapy, the goals of therapy should be palliative. One of the great benefits of staging is that it avoids exposing patients to the morbidity of aggressive interventions that offer no real chance of cure or long-term survival. Second, the clinical stage of the cancer often decides the choice of primary treatment in patients with potentially curable cancers. Many of the site-specific T and N classifications were designed to reflect the boundaries of resectability. The clinical stage of the cancer at presentation, therefore, often determines whether an attempt at radical surgery would be worthwhile. Similarly, in many operated cases, the pT and pN status of the cancer provides information about the potential value of adjuvant radiotherapy, and/or adjuvant systemic therapy. Third, the stage of the cancer may serve as a basis for planning the details of treatment once the modality has been chosen. The T and N categories may delineate the extent of the surgery required for complete resection, or may serve to define the anatomic volume that must be encompassed in a curative radiotherapy plan. pT and pN categories may help to define the volume to be treated with postoperative radiotherapy.

Of course, neither the clinical nor the pathologic stage can be equated with the true extent of the cancer. The subclinical extent of the disease often becomes apparent only when it is manifested later by the sites of progression or recurrence following treatment. However, stage provides a link with past experience that permits us to infer the true extent of the disease. This type of reasoning, in fact, led to the concept of adjuvant treatment that, in some situations, has proved to decrease failure rates and improve survival. It was the analysis of patterns of failure that showed that the pathologic involvement of the axillary lymph nodes in breast cancer (pN1) was strongly associated with a high risk of occult distant metastases in M0 cases. RCTs then showed that the risk of subsequent distant relapse was diminished when adjuvant systemic treatment was given to pN1 cases in the absence of any clinical evidence of distant metastasis.

The Role of Staging in Promoting Good Medical Practice

The process of staging itself fosters good medical decision making. It promotes a rational and disciplined approach to the evaluation of patients with cancer, and encourages the clinician to make a judgment about the extent of the disease before initiating treatment. It provides a means of summarizing the patient's status, which makes it easier to discuss the case with colleagues, either informally or in the setting of a multidisciplinary tumor conference. Routine staging readily identifies patients eligible for management according to clinical practice guidelines, or for participation in randomized trials. Staging also permits real-time audit of treatment decisions, and retrospective audit of the process and outcome of treatment.

The Role of Staging in Promoting Autonomous Decision Making

In recent years there has been a trend toward actively involving patients in decisions about their medical care. The ethical requirement for respect for the autonomy of the individual is now widely recognized, and is enshrined in the legal doctrine of informed consent in many jurisdictions. An autonomous decision is one that is made intentionally, without coercion, and with understanding. To help patients understand the decisions that they face, they not only need information, but also a conceptual framework in which to process it. The concept of stage is readily understood by the majority of patients, and provides a useful framework for discussion of the details of the individual case.[27] Many patients ask doctors about the stage of their disease. A clear answer helps the patient to understand the treatment options, and to participate actively in treatment choices. A knowledge of the stage of cancer also helps patients to distinguish information that is relevant to them from that which is not. This is important because patients recently diagnosed with cancer are often bombarded with information on the experiences of relatives and acquaintances, which are often entirely irrelevant to their own situation. Once patients know the stage of their disease, they are also empowered to seek additional information about it for themselves from other sources such as support groups, books, or the Internet.

Stage is an important determinant of the prognosis in almost every type of cancer. The prognosis may be important to patients not only in making treatment decisions, but also in making decisions about other aspects of their lives.[28] Many patients ask about their chances of cure or survival, and they need an honest answer, whether the prognosis is good or bad. For many people, uncertainty is more difficult to deal with than the harshest of realities, and the information about the prognosis provided by staging helps them to face their future.

THE ROLE OF STAGING IN MANAGING CANCER CONTROL PROGRAMS

Just as a knowledge of stage in the individual case guides the individual treatment decision, a knowledge of stage mix in a population can guide the management of cancer programs. This is true of national and regional programs of cancer control that may embrace prevention, early detection, active treatment, and supportive care, and that target the entire population of a geographic region. It is equally true of programs with a narrower focus and a narrower population base, such as the oncology service of a general hospital. In this final section, we show how the routine use of staging is valuable both in the strategic planning of cancer programs and in their day-to-day management.

Cancer Staging and Strategic Planning

By studying trends in cancer incidence over many years, cancer registries have been able to predict the future incidence of cancer very accurately. In publicly funded health care systems, this information is sometimes used as a basis for making long-term plans about the location and size of cancer treatment facilities, and for estimating future requirements for specialized equipment and personnel. However, a knowledge of incidence alone does not provide an optimal basis for this type of planning because the appropriate treatment of cancer is highly stage dependent.

Predictions should be based on projections of the incidence of cancer by stage, and whenever possible population-based cancer registries should, therefore, collect and compile information about stage. A knowledge of trends in caseload in terms of disease and stage mix can also help to anticipate the future workload of a specific treatment center. Projections of case load can be integrated with projections of treatment patterns to estimate future requirements for equipment, manpower, and resources. However, this is possible only if the institutional cancer registry routinely collects and compiles information about stage.

Cancer Staging and Resource Allocation

A knowledge of case mix in terms of stage provides a basis for the rational allocation of resources at many levels. In publicly funded health care systems, cancer control competes with other programs for limited health dollars. The more precisely societal needs for cancer treatment can be defined, the more likely it is that an appropriate slice of the available resources will be allocated to cancer treatment. Accurate descriptions of case mix in terms of site and stage may also serve as a rational basis for the division of resources within a publicly funded cancer system. Information about case mix is also useful as a basis for the rational deployment of resources within private facilities.

Cancer Staging and Quality Management

Managing any health care program involves setting goals, developing processes, implementing them, evaluating what has been achieved, and modifying the program accordingly. Formerly the planning and evaluation cycle was aimed at achieving static goals. It is now seen as more appropriate to strive for continuous quality improvement without setting fixed upper limits on achievement. The appropriate criteria for measuring the success of a cancer program depends on its purpose and on the target population, but no cancer program can be adequately evaluated without information about case-mix in terms of stage.

Programs of early detection, such as mammographic screening for breast cancer, are intended to reduce cancer mortality, but the first indication of their success is a decrease in the proportion of patients presenting with more advanced stages.[29] Stage mix can be seen as an intermediate outcome of the program that may predict its long-term benefits. Because screening programs operate at the population level rather than at the level of individual institutions, evaluation of screening programs requires stage to be recorded in population-based registries.

Evaluation of cancer treatment programs requires consideration of access to the service, the quality of the service, and the outcomes achieved in specific groups of cases defined by stage. Stage is not an outcome measure here, but a means of defining the target population.

The overall effectiveness of any cancer treatment program is limited by the proportion of people who might benefit from it, who actually have access to it. Publicly funded health care programs in many countries are designed to remove financial barriers to care. However, they do not guarantee access to care unless resources keep pace with demand for service, and if they do not, waiting lists may develop and operate as a form of implicit rationing. Monitoring of access is necessary to identify this type of problem.[30] Access to care must also be examined carefully whenever centralized facilities are expected to provide services for dispersed populations, as is often the case with radiotherapy and other specialized forms of cancer treatment. Regional cancer services often create outreach programs to overcome geographic access barriers, but these require ongoing evaluation to ensure their success.[31] Measuring access to care at the population level requires a knowledge of the number of cases eligible for the service as well as the number who actually receive it. Eligibility is almost always stage dependent, so monitoring access requires information about stage in the population. For example, variations in the proportion of incident cases of rectal cancer referred to radiation oncology may reflect important variations in access to this service, or they may merely reflect variations in case mix. Distinguishing between these two possibilities requires that stage be available in the corresponding population-based registry.

Monitoring access to service within cancer treatment centers is equally important. In any institution that manages cancer patients, it is appropriate to ask what proportion patients with stage II breast cancer get the opinion of a medical oncologist, what proportion of patients with stage I prostate cancer get the opinion of a radiation oncologist, and what proportion of patients with stage IV non-small-cell lung cancer are seen by a palliative care service. This type of question can be addressed only if stage is routinely recorded and compiled in the institutional registry.

It is known that there are large variations in the management of many different cancers, both within institutions, among institutions, and among societies. Wide variations in practice suggest that the management of cancer may often be suboptimal,[32] but the extent to which these variations are appropriate or inappropriate can be determined only if information about stage has been collected. If stage is available, medical practice in a given region or in a given institution can be compared to practice elsewhere and/or with some standard deemed to be appropriate based on the scientific evidence available in the literature. However, when external standards are used to evaluate medical practice using only summary data about site, stage, and treatment, it should not be assumed that noncompliance in an individual case represents inappropriate management. Medical contraindications or patient preferences may sometimes make the standard approach inappropriate. It seems more reasonable to try to set targets based on experience of what is achievable in the field, for example, that more than 80% of patients with stage II breast cancer should receive systemic adjuvant treatment, or that fewer than 10% of patients with stage I breast cancer should have a bone scan.[33]

There is currently great interest in the use of clinical practice guidelines to assist medical decision making, and reduce practice variations.[34] The extent to which this approach succeeds in changing the practice of oncology will be evaluable only if stage information is recorded in the appropriate registry. Evaluating treatment at the population level obviously requires capture of stage information in a population based registry. Evaluating treatment within an institution can be achieved by recording stage routinely within an institution based registry.

Individual consumers and particularly the sophisticated purchasers who operate on behalf of health insurance programs now expect institutions to be able to describe not only how they manage their patients, but also what results they achieve. Monitoring cancer outcomes is the ultimate way of evaluating the success of any cancer control program, but a long time has to elapse before the outcome of the curative treatment of cancer can be evaluated in most diseases. For this reason, audit of outcome cannot be relied upon to optimize cancer treatment programs, and much attention has to be directed toward audit of the treatment process. In the long term, survival achieved in a given region or institution can be compared to the outcome expected based on clinical trials and with outcomes achieved elsewhere, but fair comparisons require a knowledge of stage mix.

CONCLUSIONS

Cancer staging plays a central role in the scientific practice of oncology. The TNM system is a sophisticated tool for classifying cancer that provides a vital link between research and medical practice, and is appropriate for use in most cancers. Doctors who provide care for cancer patients should record the stage of the disease in every patient's records using the TNM system. Institutions that provide care for cancer patients should create processes to ensure that stage is routinely and accurately recorded, and should regularly compile and report the management and outcome of cancer by stage. Agencies that certify doctors who treat cancer and those that accredit institutions that provide care for cancer patients should recognize the use of the TNM system as a standard of care.

FURTHER READING

1. Hill B.A. (1937) *Principles of Medical Statistics*, 1st edition, The Lancet Limited, London.

2. Howson C, Urbach P (1989) *Scientific Reasoning*. Open Court, LaSalle, IL.

3. WHO (1975) *Manual of the International Classification of Diseases, Injuries, and Causes of Death*. Geneva, Switzerland.

4. Percy C, Van Hollen V, Muir C (eds) (1990) *International Classification of Diseases for Oncology (ICD O)*, 2nd edition. WHO, Geneva, Switzerland.

5. Tannock IF, Hill RP (eds) (1992) *The Basic Science of Oncology*, 2nd edition. McGraw-Hill, Toronto.

6. Fielding PL, Fenoglio-Preiser CM, Freedman LS (1992) The future of prognostic factors in outcome prediction for patients with cancer. *Cancer*, 70:2367–2377.

7. Gospodarowicz MK, O'Sullivan B, Berkel HJ, Beatty D (1994) Staging of cancer revisited. *CMAJ*, 150:663–665.
8. Sokal RR, Rohlf FJ (1969) Biometry: The principles and practice of statistics in biological research. In Emerson R, Kennedy D, Park RB, Beadle GW, Whitaker DM (eds). WH Freeman, San Francisco.
9. Feinstein AR (1985) *Clinical Epidemiology: The Architecture of Clinical Research*. WB Saunders, Philadelphia.
10. Denoix PF (1952) *Bull Inst Nat Hyg* (Paris), 1:1–69 (1994) and 5-82 (1944), *WHO Tech Rep Ser*, 55:47–48.
11. International Union Against Cancer (UICC), Committee on Clinical Stage Classification and Applied Statistics (1958) Clinical stage classification and presentation of results, malignant tumors of the breast and larynx. Paris.
12. International Union Against Cancer (UICC) (1968) *TNM Classification of Malignant Tumors*, Geneva, Switzerland.
13. Sobin LH, Wittekind CH (eds) (1997) *UICC TNM Classification of Malignant Tumours*, 5th edition. Wiley-Liss, New York.
14. Fleming ID, Cooper JS, Henson JS, Hutter RVP, Kennedy BJ, Murphy GP, O'Sullivan B, Yarbro JW (eds) (1997) *AJCC Cancer Staging Manual*. JB Lippincott, Philadelphia.
15. International Federation of Gynecology and Obstetrics (1991) Annual report on the results of treatment in gynecological cancer. *Int J Gynecol Obstet* 36:27.
16. Dukes CE (1940) Cancer of the rectum: An analysis of 1000 cases. *J Pathol Bacteriol* 50: 527–539.
17. Nathanson SD, Schultz L, Tilley B, Kambouris A (1986) Carcinoma of the colon and rectum. A comparison of staging classification. *Am Surg* 52:428–433.
18. Carbone PP, Kaplan HS, Musshoff K, Smithers DW, Tubania M (1971) Report of the Committee on Hodgkin's Disease Staging Classification. *Cancer Res* 31:1860–1861.
19. Sackett DL, Haynes RB, Guyatt GH, Tugwell P (1985) *Clinical Epidemiology: A Basic Science for Clinical Medicine*, 2nd edition, Little, Brown, Boston.
20. O'Sullivan B, Mackillop WJ (1986) An approach to the interpretation of the literature of head and neck cancer. *Clin Onc* 5:411–433.
21. Bero L, Rennie D (1995) The Cochrane Collaboration. Preparing, maintaining, and disseminating systematic reviews of the effects of health care. *JAMA* 274:1935–1938.
22. Brundage M, Mackillop WJ (1996) Locally advanced non-small cell lung cancer: Do we know the questions? *J Clin Epidemiol* 49:183–192.
23. Mackillop WJ (1996) Registry based observational studies of the management and outcome of cancer: A new way to look at old problems. Fourth International Cochrane Colloquium, Adelaide.
24. Hayman J, Weeks J, Mauch P (1996) Economic analysis in health care: An introduction to the methodology with an emphasis on radiation therapy. *Int J Radiat Oncol Biol Phys* 35:827–841.
25. Eapen L, Nair R, Lavigne B, Laewan A (1990) The TNM system for oral and oropharyngeal cancer—A study into the accuracy and reproducibility with which it is used. *Int J Radiat Oncol Biol Phys* 19:227.
26. Feinstein AR, Sosin DM, Wells CK (1985) The Will Rogers Phenomenon: Stage migration and new diagnostic techniques as a source of misleading statistics for survival in cancer. *N Engl J Med* 312:1604–1608.

27. Quirt CF, Mackillop WJ, Ginsburg AD, Sheldon L, Brundage M, Dixon P, Ginsburg L (1997) Do doctors know when their patients don't? A survey of doctor–patient communication in lung cancer. *Lung Cancer* 18:1–20.

28. Mackillop WJ, Quirt CF (1997) Measuring the accuracy of prognostic judgements in oncology. *J Clin Epidemiol* 50:21–29.

29. Winawer SJ, Fletcher RH, Miller L, Godlee F, Stolar MH, Multrow CD, Woolf SH, Glick SN, Ganaits TG, et al. (1997) Colorectal cancer screening: Clinical guidelines and rationale. *Gastroenterology* 112:594–642.

30. Mackillop WJ, Fu H, Quirt CF, Dixon P, Brundage M, Zhou Y (1994) Waiting for radiotherapy in Ontario. *Int J Radiat Oncol Biol Phys* 30:221–228.

31. Mackillop WJ, Groome PA, Zhou Y, Zhang-Salomons J, Holowaty EJ, Cummings B, Feldman-Stewart D, Paszat K, Dixon P (1997) Does a centralized radiotherapy system provide adequate access to care? *J Clin Oncol* 15:1261–1271.

32. Anderson TF, Mooney G (eds) (1990) *The Challenges of Medical Practice Variations.* The Macmillan Press, London.

33. Hillner BE, McDonald K, Desch CE, et al. (1997) Measuring standards of care for early breast cancer in an insured population. *J Clin Oncol* 15:1401–1408.

34. Browman GP, Levine MN, Mohide EA, Hayward RSA, Pritchard II, Gafni A, et al. (1995) The practice guidelines development cycle: A conceptual tool for practice guidelines development and implementation. *J Clin Oncol* 13:502–512.

CHAPTER 11

PRINCIPLES OF SURGICAL ONCOLOGY

MICHAEL J. EDWARDS

James Graham Brown Cancer Center
University of Louisville
Louisville, KY 40202, USA

Within the world of medicine, the collective personal commitment of surgeons to their patients, and even individual personalities, are considered by some to be characteristic. This commitment and the associated character traits do not reflect personality so much as an attitude toward illness. That attitude is perhaps best characterized by actions that result from a prompt evaluation of treatment alternatives, in the context of the biology of an individual patient's disease and overall general health, and culminate in an acute therapeutic intervention with obvious, inherent treatment risks, most often outweighed by a profound therapeutic impact. Such has been the history of surgery, the first effective treatment modality for cancer, and currently the most effective treatment modality for patients with solid tumors. To understand the state-of-the-art and the future of surgical oncology as a discipline, we begin with a historical perspective.

HISTORICAL PERSPECTIVE

Although history documents the surgical treatment of tumors as early as ancient times, the modern era of elective surgery for visceral tumors began in Kentucky in 1809 when Ephraim MacDowell removed a 22-pound ovarian tumor from Mrs. Jane Todd Crawford. Skeptical citizens gathered around the house on that Christmas Day in Danville, Kentucky. Convinced that Dr. MacDowell had embarked on a course of intervention more akin to assault than what we now know as surgery, they hung a rope from a tree threatening his hanging should his patient die.[1] Ms. Crawford lived some

Manual of Clinical Oncology, 7th edition, Edited by Raphael E. Pollock
ISBN 0-471-23828-7, pages 235–250. Copyright © 1999 Wiley-Liss, Inc.

30 years following this first spectacularly successful elective abdominal operation. MacDowell performed 13 other ovarian resections, documenting the feasibility of elective abdominal surgery. Realizing the full potential of the surgical intervention for the general populace, however, hinged on overcoming three hurdles: eliminating the pain associated with the operation, controlling infection, and developing quality surgical training programs.

Anesthesia

The inquisitive mind of Crawford Long at 27 years of age led to the first operation under inhalation sulfuric ether anesthesia in Jefferson, Georgia, on March 30, 1842. That day a small tumor was removed from the posterior neck area of a 20-year-old man named James Venable. Mr. Venable later stated he "did not experience the slightest degree of pain...." This, the primary event in the history of anesthesia, would not be recorded until 1848.[2] The first public demonstration of ether anesthesia by the dentist William Thomas Green Morton might have been viewed as a relatively insignificant sequel to Crawford Long's discovery had Long proceeded immediately with publication, and if it were not for Morton's surgical connections and relentless opportunism.

Morton was instructed in the art of dentistry in the early 1840s by Horace Wells. He subsequently learned that ether induced sufficient analgesia to make the practice of dentistry tolerable. Morton pursued animal experiments with ether anesthesia, and even experimented on himself. On September 30, 1846, a Boston merchant presented at Morton's office with a painful tooth. Morton painlessly removed the tooth, an event chronicled in the lay Boston press. Morton communicated his observations regarding his preclinical and clinical experiences to John Collins Warren, the Chief of the Surgical Service at the Massachusetts General Hospital. An invitation for a demonstration of "anesthesia" was extended. Morton, who like Crawford Long was also 27 years of age at this time, administered ether at the Massachusetts General Hospital in 1846 while Warren ligated a congenital vascular malformation. Witnessing the efficacy of ether anesthesia, and recognizing the seminal nature of the event, Warren exclaimed to his audience of colleagues, trainees, and students, "Gentlemen, this is no humbug." The limitation of pain as an obstacle to the evolution of surgery was resolved.[3,4]

Infection

If Crawford Long and William Morton can be credited with making surgery tolerable, Joseph Lister can be credited with making surgery safe. Before the application of Lister's principles of antisepsis, operative mortality was almost prohibitive; most patients died from complications of wound infections. After Lister developed and instituted his antiseptic methods of wound management, infection-related mortality reached acceptable levels, setting the stage for continued surgical progress.

Lister's achievement had its origin with the observations of Pasteur. Pasteur showed that fermentation did not occur in dust-free air. In developing his "germ theory," Pasteur showed that "organisms" were associated with alcoholic fermentation, but were distinct from other "organisms" associated with milk souring.[5] After reading Pasteur's papers, Lister believed that the germ theory could be applied to the prevention of surgical wound infections and began his search for a chemical antiseptic. After experimenting with several substances he finally decided to use carbolic acid, having learned of the foul-smelling fluid's use as a sewage disinfectant in the town of Carlisle in northern England. Lister finally achieved success in preventing infection by treating wounds with carbolic acid in 1865. He eventually developed an antiseptic gauze dressing. Lister retreated the wound, his hands, and the instruments with carbolic acid throughout the course of an operation, and eventually designed a device to spray carbolic acid into the air surrounding the operative field.[5,6]

German surgeons were the first to accept the antiseptic techniques of Lister, but by 1880 the antiseptic technique was practiced throughout Great Britain as well. German researchers were also the first to learn that surgeons could reduce wound infection rates by scrubbing their hands and instruments with soap and water prior to surgery, thus becoming the first to practice a combination of antiseptic and aseptic techniques. Although Lister's antiseptic methods were eventually supplanted by the aseptic technique, his principle of antisepsis was the fundamental basis of all modern efforts in preventing infection in surgical wounds.

SURGICAL TRAINING AND EDUCATION

The history of the subject of modern surgical training also originates in Germany. The German surgical education model was primarily based on the system founded by Bernhard Rudolf Konrad von Langenbeck (1810–1887). Langenbeck's scholarly contributions to the developing discipline of surgery were distinguished, but by consensus, his greatest and most longstanding contribution was his systematic method of training young surgeons, the forerunner of today's surgical residency system.[7] William S. Halsted recognized, and concluded in his famous address entitled "The Training of the Surgeon" delivered at Yale in 1904, that German surgeons were the first to adopt antisepsis in large part because of " the character of the scientific and practical training of surgeons in Germany."[8] The trainees, or "residents," in German programs of the time had access to quality research facilities, were exposed to a broad clinical experience, and served under the greatest surgical educators. The German surgical educators and their students were Halsted's models. Their mentorship was justifiably appropriate, for it was Theodor Billroth, one of von Langenbeck's students, who between the years 1850 and 1880 successfully performed the first gastrectomy, the first laryngectomy, and the first esophagectomy.[9,10]

Halsted sought to duplicate this German education model in the United States. He said, "We need a system, and we shall surely have it, which will produce not only surgeons, but surgeons of the highest type, men who will stimulate the first youths of our country to study surgery and to devote their energies and their lives to raising the standard of surgical science."[8] He committed to a system in which highly qualified trainees were selected for an extended course of study that included clinical, educational, and research experience. Trainees acquired graded levels of clinical responsibility as they advanced and were responsible for teaching the more junior house staff. Many of the surgeons trained by Halsted went on to leadership roles in surgery and disseminated Halsted's surgical and educational philosophy.[11]

Halsted propagated Joseph Lister's principles of antiseptic surgery, promoted the careful handling of tissues and the minimization of blood loss, pioneered the use of surgical gloves, addressed fundamental problems of surgical science, and developed successful operations including the radical mastectomy. In addition to the radical mastectomy for breast cancer, he made important contributions to thyroid and parathyroid surgery, hernia surgery, surgery of the gastrointestinal and biliary tracts, and to vascular surgery. His meticulous technique made surgery safer and paved the way for the increasingly complex procedures. But most importantly, Halsted created the educational platform for the dramatic progress of 20th century American surgery. By the end of his career Halsted had transformed surgery from a trade practiced by variably trained physicians to an academic specialty and profession characterized by prolonged and effective training and scholarship.

MILESTONES IN THE EVOLUTION OF SURGICAL ONCOLOGY

Although specific developments may be debated with regard to their relative significance and overall impact, certain "firsts" have signaled the beginning of new eras of improved therapeutic efficacy for particular malignancies. For example, the radical mastectomy became the treatment of choice for breast cancer just after 1900, when Halsted demonstrated the effective local control of chest wall disease for the first time. Other examples of initial resections for cancers of specific organs from the early 1900s include the radical prostatectomy by Hugh Young in 1904, the radical hysterectomy by Ernest Wertheim in 1906, and the abdominoperineal resection for rectal cancer by W. Ernest Miles in 1908.[4,12] During the period from 1910 to 1930 Harvey Cushing pioneered surgery for brain tumors. The first successful surgical resection for cancer of the esophagus was performed in 1913 by Franz Torek, even though we still face a considerable operative mortality relative to the probability of cure by esophagectomy today. The treatment of lung cancer began with Evarts Graham's first successful pneumonectomy in 1933; successful surgical resections of lung tumors were made possible by developments that included intrathoracic anesthesia, and effective methods of ligating the pulmonary artery and the bronchial stump. The treatment of pancreatic tumors began in 1935 when A. O. Whipple performed a two-stage pancreaticoduodenectomy.[12] Progress with the pancreaticoduodenectomy was, however, limited owing to an extraordinary complication rate that has been minimized only in the last 10 to 15 years as the procedure became increasingly refined and practiced by tertiary centers with a critical volume of experience. In the last 25 years, we have also witnessed the expansion of the field of reconstructive surgery as techniques of wound coverage and reconstruction evolved. Coupled with improvements in our ability to assess operative risk and manage postoperative complications, we now routinely schedule extirpative operative interventions not thought possible only a few years ago.

Although more complex procedures are now feasible, perhaps our most significant progress in recent years has been the development of approaches that minimize the magnitude of the associated surgical injury. The evolution of prospective randomized clinical trials has accelerated the refinement of operations and their integration with other treatment modalities by scientifically quantitating therapeutic impact. Consider the progress and history of the National Surgical Adjuvant Breast and Bowel Project under the leadership of Bernard Fisher beginning in the 1960s and persisting to the present.[12] The precision of our operations has also been more finely tuned by new technologies. Some of our recent advances include ultrasound and stereotactic guided surgery, precise staging through the use of lymphatic mapping, and limited access surgery by laproscopic, thorascopic, and increasingly complex endoscopic techniques. Such approaches pay the dividend of limited morbidity while preserving diagnostic and therapeutic efficacy. In perhaps no other surgical speciality or field of interest have these advances been as revolutionary as in the field of surgical oncology.

THE CURRENT STATUS AND FUTURE OF SURGICAL ONCOLOGY

The surgeon's current role in the field of oncology is multifaceted and can be identified as specific goals. These goals include cancer prevention, screening, diagnosis, staging, all aspects of treatment, monitoring for recurrence and the development of new diseases, and the pursuit and application of new knowledge from both basic scientific and clinical perspectives.

Cancer Prevention and Screening

The mission of the surgical oncologist is to minimize the morbidity and mortality related to cancer; prevention and early detection of malignancies are obvious top priorities. Certain tumors are more likely curable when detected and treated at an earlier, less advanced stage. Surgeons have historically initiated and supported educational programs for health professionals and public awareness programs to identify such patients. Surgeons must be knowledgeable of the natural history, etiology, and epidemiology of malignances if we are to reliably impact prevention and early detection.

"Screening" refers to the clinical application of simple tests to a selected population to segregate individuals who probably have the malignancy in question from those who most likely do not. It is important to recognize that screening programs are applied to an asymptomatic, apparently healthy population and must be evaluated to verify the magnitude of reduction of the morbidity and mortality of the targeted disease. Adherence to this principle often precipitates debate. Consider, for example, the proper age for screening women with mammography for breast cancer, a controversial screening issue in recent years. Although screening is clearly effective and precisely defined for many diseases such as cervical cancer, not all cancers are suitable for screening; the prevalence and duration of the asymptomatic but clinically detectable curable disease state in the screened population may be insufficient to justify testing costs, especially in an increasingly hostile economic health care environment.[13]

Unfortunately, albeit less frequently recognized by the legal profession and lay public, certain malignancies are governed by a biologic nature characterized by incurability from the earliest possible date of clinical detection. Apparent increases in survival rates afforded by screening programs using fixed endpoint survival measures are an illusion created by lead-time bias, with no real, long-term, overall survival impact. In the absence of effective therapy, it is hoped that this subset of cancers may eventually be prevented.

Two primary factors have limited the impact of preventive measures to date. First, our understanding of the process of malignant transformation for our most common cancers is currently, at best, a primitive science; we simply do not know the clinically relevant inciting event or factors for the origin of our most common tumors. Second, adapting patterns of human behavior, especially in the context of substance addiction, has proven difficult, even when we have precisely identified the malignancy inducing behavior or habit. Consider the roles of tobacco and/or alcohol in lung and head and neck cancers, the duration of our knowledge of the deleterious effects of cigarette smoking, and the simultaneous dissemination of death and destruction over the globe by the tobacco industry in spite of this understanding. Nevertheless, some prevention has been achieved, and there is significant potential for progress through our evolving understanding of the genetics of inheritable disease.

We are increasingly aware that many cancers have a genetic basis, prompting the appropriate scheduling of screening examinations or diagnostic genetic evaluations. Multiple genes have been implicated in a variety of organ specific malignancies. Take, for example, familial polyposis and other polyposis syndromes of the large bowel. Historically, we relied on serial screening colonoscopies in family members of affected kindred to screen and diagnose polyposis or adenocarcinoma. Genetic mutations of these diseases are now defined, and as genetic testing becomes widely available, definitive one-time diagnostic genetic testing will progressively supplant serial screening colonoscopic examinations. The issue then becomes one of appropriate monitoring or the proper timing of the "preventative" surgical intervention. Consider also the example of multiple endocrine neoplasia type IIA (MEN-IIA). In the recent past patients were screened with the cumbersome pentagastrin stimulation test for calcitonin release as the indication for prophylactic thyroidectomy to prevent medullary carcinoma of the thyroid. Through the work of the surgeon Samuel Wells, perhaps more than any one individual, polymerase chain reaction (PCR)-based DNA testing for mutations in the RET proto-oncogene has been developed, proven effective as a straightforward definitive test, and used as the indication for "preventative" surgery.[14] As the discipline most frequently involved in the diagnosis and definitive treatment of all solid tumors we must be intellectually prepared to contribute to the identification of these and all other genetically susceptible patients.

Cancer Diagnosis

The diagnosis of cancer requires histopathologic confirmation prior to initiating therapy for most clinical situations. Some malignancies are readily accessible for biopsy and may be diagnosed preoperatively. Others, such as small bowel and pancreatic lesions, are usually biopsied at the time of surgery with definitive resection following frozen section analysis. Multiple techniques of acquiring cells or tissue for diagnosis are available, and new methods of obtaining samples for analysis with less invasive approaches such as endoscopy and laproscopy have increased the role of biopsy procedures over recent years. Each approach has distinct advantages and disadvantages, but all originate in certain fundamental principles.

- Biopsied tissue should be representative of the lesion in question. Areas of hemorrhage, necrosis, and infection should be avoided when selecting biopsy sites. Multiple specimens are most often helpful. Clamping, tearing, crushing, and charring of tissue creates distortion and should be avoided.
- The choice of biopsy technique should satisfy the tissue sample needs of the pathologist. For some tumors, electron microscopy, flow cytometry, or other specialized techniques may be necessary; sufficient tissue must be obtained and properly submitted. If biopsy specimens are immediately placed in formalin, the opportunity to perform these specialized diagnostic tests may be lost.
- Needle punctures and incisions should be carefully placed for excision as part of the subsequent definitive surgical procedure. Incisions on the extremity should be placed in the direction of the underlying muscle, almost always longitudinally. Hematomas may increase the magnitude of subsequent surgery and enlarge required fields of radiation therapy—meticulous hemostasis is mandatory for optimum therapy. Drainage exit sites should also be carefully planned, for similar reasons.
- Close cooperation should exist between the surgeon and the pathologist. The pathologist should always be provided with relevant clinical information. The surgeon should orient, label, and when indicated, ink the specimen for the pathologist.[4,13]

Certain specifics of each biopsy technique must be considered in choosing the optimum approach. Fine-needle aspiration biopsy cytology involves the aspiration of cells through a small-caliber needle. The needle may be guided into the suspicious lesion by palpation or image-directed assistance. Cytologic analysis provides a tentative diagnosis of malignancy and allows the surgeon to proceed with the staging evaluation. However, major surgical resections should not be undertaken solely on the basis of the conclusions of fine-needle aspiration biopsy cytology. A small but significant risk of a false-positive diagnosis exists in the hands of even the most experienced cytopathologist. Fine-needle aspiration biopsy cytology diagnosis must be confirmed by definitive histologic studies of tissue.

Core needle biopsy refers to obtaining a tiny piece of tissue in the hollow of a specially designed needle. This tissue may be histologically evaluated for architecture, and if of adequate size and quality, usually provides definitive diagnosis. Some tumors, such as lymphomas, sarcomas, and other tumors of mesenchymal origin, are difficult to diagnose with small tissue cores. Incisional biopsy refers to the surgical removal of a larger portion of tissue and is often the preferred method of diagnosing tumors of mesenchymal origin.

Excisional surgical biopsy provides the pathologist with the entire lesion. As such, excisional biopsies are most useful if they can be performed without compromising the outcome of the definitive operation. It is important to note that a diagnostic excisional biopsy makes no effort to achieve a gross or histologic margin of normal tissue. This is an important point of concern—reexcisions of biopsy sites initially done with "diagnostic intent" identify residual carcinoma in up to 50% of cases, even when the pathologist reported the original diagnostic excision as having "negative margins." Definitive excisions must proceed with "therapeutic intent" on the part of the surgeon.

Preoperative Considerations and Staging

Cancer patients are often elderly and sometimes in poor nutritional status. The general condition of the patient must be thoroughly evaluated before treatment. Cardiac, pulmonary, renal, nutritional, and other assessments are necessary to prepare the patient for major surgery. Ensuring adequate preoperative hydration is increasingly important in this era of outpatient mechanical cleansing of the bowel and the obligatory preoperative fasting for general anesthesia.

A preoperative mechanical cleansing bowel prep should be used for colon surgery, as well as for all patients undergoing extensive abdominal procedures; an unexpected en bloc partial colectomy may occasionally be necessary. The recovery from ileus is also thought more tolerable by some if mechanical cleansing is accomplished preoperatively. Patients undergoing major liver resections also require preoperative bowel preparation to reduce the risk of postoperative encephalopathy.

Timing the surgical intervention in patients receiving chemotherapy or radiation is important to ensure that bone marrow suppression will not complicate the immediate postoperative period. Bleeding problems should be suspected by a history of suggestive symptoms, or of drug use including aspirin and preoperative chemotherapy. A screening complete blood cell count with differential is usually necessary. Baseline liver function tests and tumor markers should be obtained prior to surgery, as trends in these levels may be monitored during follow-up. A chest X-ray film is usually indicated as a baseline and to identify potential other new primary cancers, metastases, or other pulmonary pathology.

Sepsis is a special consideration as a potential complication in immunocompromised patients with metastatic diseases and in patients receiving chemotherapy. The source of infection can vary, but must be identified and is usually best eliminated by the four surgical Ds: drainage, debridement, diversion, and drugs (antibiotics).

Patients recently treated with steroids are another special consideration. They should receive steroid supplements to prevent an Addisonian crisis.

A detailed history and thorough physical examination is the key to minimizing the unnecessary costs associated with extensive radiographic testing in the staging evaluation. In recent years clinicians, especially those from primary care and medical oncology specialities, have increasingly relied on various scans and other expensive imaging to evaluate potential sides of metastases. In many cases, these studies have not altered the treatment approach and often unnecessarily duplicate the operative findings for indicated operations. Surgeons must endeavor to educate other physicians as to the accuracy of operative staging, and uniformly document these findings as a regular part of the operative record. All oncologists must have a thorough knowledge of the natural history of the disease and appropriately investigate potential sites of metastases if they are to practice cost-efficient medicine.

The surgeon must also be familiar with the natural history of the disease under consideration and likely patterns of metastasis to guide his or her operative exploration. As an example, the propensity for ovarian cancer to metastasize to peritoneal surfaces mandates the need for routine surface biopsies and washings. Staging the disease is the most important factor in establishing the prognosis; it must be diligently and accurately pursued.

Cancer Therapy

For most solid tumors there is no more effective treatment modality than the proper operation for the particular stage of malignancy. The surgical treatment of cancer has the goals of cure, prolongation of duration of life among uncured patients, the palliation of clearly defined symptoms, and the local control of disease as a prophylactic measure to prevent subsequent complications. The surgeon should clearly recognize that prophylactic surgery causes associated surgical morbidity in an often asymptomatic patient. If we are to reliably help more patients than we harm, we must proceed with prophylactic interventions only after thoughtful consideration of the natural history of the disease and the individual patient's operative risk.

The extent of the appropriate local excision varies with the individual cancer type and the site of involvement. For many malignancies, definitive surgical therapy requires only a wide local excision defined by a sufficient margin of normal tissue. The magnitude of the required surgical resection may be modified when surgery is integrated with adjuvant treatment modalities. In some instances, effective adjuvant modalities have led to a decrease in the magnitude of surgery and preservation of function not possible without multimodal therapy. Consider our success in preservation of limb function with sarcoma surgery as we integrated surgery and radiation therapy. Rationally integrating surgery with other treatments requires a careful consideration of all effective treatment options. It is a knowledge of this rapidly changing field that often distinguishes the differentiated surgical oncologist from more generally oriented surgeons.[13]

In some diseases, such as ovarian cancer, extensive local metastases preclude the surgical excision of all gross disease. The debulking or cytoreduction of selected cancers may lead to enhanced local disease control. However, for most solid tumors, any significant patient benefit has been offset by associated surgical morbidity. Cyto-reductive surgery is usually of significant benefit only for diseases that respond to other treatments to control small residual deposits of unresectable disease.[4,13]

Although "cure" is our most noble goal, about 70% of patients with solid tumors have regional or distant metastases when they present with their first symptoms.[4] Surgical resections designed to include regional lymphatic metastases can cure some patients. But lymph node metastases, depending on the specific organ site and disease, may be an indication of systemic disease. The impact of surgery on long-term survival, and even cured fraction, in patients with metastatic disease is underestimated by most physicians. Patients with a limited number of pulmonary, hepatic, or cerebral metastases can also enjoy an extended life with surgical resection. For example, the resection of pulmonary metastases in sarcoma patients may benefit as many as 30% of carefully selected patients. Similarly, hepatic resection of colorectal metastases enhances long-term survival; patients with solitary hepatic metastases from colorectal cancer have a long-term survival of about 30%, a magnitude of benefit dramatically exceeding the uniformly fatal result in untreated, age-matched cohorts.

Palliative surgery is defined as the surgical relief of intractable symptoms; it does not apply to the asymptomatic patient. Judicious use of surgery for the relief of pain can improve the quality of life for many. Palliative surgery also includes the removal of masses causing disfigurement, and operations for emergencies from complications related to hemorrhage, obstruction, or perforation. Perforations of an abdominal, pelvic, or thoracic viscus may result from direct tumor invasion or from tumor lysis with systemic chemotherapy as tumors respond and disintegrate. Decompression of the central nervous system is another emergency situation that must be promptly addressed to preserve neurologic function.

Urinary obstruction is another relatively frequent complication. Urinary diversion must be carefully considered; it may sometimes only prolong patient suffering from an intractable, incurable malignancy. However, it may sometimes palliate symptoms due to urinary fistulas or injuries resulting from bladder irradiation. Fecal stream diversion should be similarly considered, but palliation is often much more beneficial in terms of quality of life issues. Locally advanced tumors of the aerodigestive tract may be managed by fulguration or laser surgery to establish patency without the disadvantage of a diverting cutaneous intestinal stoma. Feeding gastrostomies are sometimes required for feeding advanced head and neck cancer patients, or for palliative decompression with peritoneal carcinomatosis in the terminally ill.

Follow-Up Monitoring

One goal of follow-up monitoring is early detection of local, regional, or distant metastases to extend life after surgery or other therapy. Unfortunately, the impact of such screening programs has historically been poorly studied. Most screening programs are organized by intention, but without definitive scientific basis. Some current patterns of follow-up practiced by some disciplines frankly defy logic. Consider the routine follow-up of pancreatic cancer patients with computerized tomograms of the abdomen and chest. What is the evidence to suggest that *any* treatment based on these findings offers significant therapeutic impact? Such patients are also frustrated by the anxiety of equivocal results and may suffer the unnecessary morbidity of invasive biopsies in an attempt to clarify diagnosis. Proper follow-up monitoring can only be prescribed in the context of a clear understanding of the natural history of the disease, and a realistic probability of therapeutic impact in the screened population.

During the last 25 years, long-term venous access for the administration of chemotherapy, nutritional support, and for blood drawing has been progressively refined with numerous technological advances. The first silicone rubber catheter was introduced by Broviac just over 25 years ago after proving less thrombogenic than conventional materials of the time. The Hickman catheter, with a larger internal diameter, was subsequently developed as a modification of the Broviac type. Numerous studies have confirmed reliability and acceptable complication rates for these devices. In recent years there has been a virtually continuous series of modifications of existing vascular access devices, often with little if any significant improvement, but often in association with exaggerated claims and marketing fanfare on the part of the technology industry. Fundamentally, long-term vascular access devices take the form of external catheter devices such as the Broviac, Hickman, Lenonard, or Groshong, and a variety of totally implantable venous access reservoirs or ports. An intensive educational program for patients, families, and caregivers of meticulous catheter maintenance is essential to achieve extended catheter function in the absence of complications.[15] For further details of catheter selection, choice of site for venous access, and other aspects of management the reader is encouraged to review the details of the recent book by Alexander, a most comprehensive and excellent review of the state-of-the-art of long-term venous access.[16]

Research

We have witnessed no previous time in the history of cancer treatment with as much breakthrough potential as the era in which we now live. Surgeons, although acknowledged for their clinical contributions in providing the most effective treatment modality for patients with solid tumors, have historically pursued and greatly contributed to the advancement of our understanding of the basic molecular and biologic nature of cancer. Surgeons, and surgical trainees, now, as in Halsted's day, are committed to a depth of knowledge and exploration vital to answering basic, translational, and clinical questions. Increasingly, answers to these questions support the concept of cancer as a disease caused by mutation in genes that regulate cell division. It has been just over 10 years since the cloning of the first tumor suppressor gene. Significant progress continues with a human genome project and novel technologies fuel the gradual elucidation of the genetic nature of malignancy. The molecular regulation of tumor growth and malignant transformation has been a consistent research theme of surgeons for several years. Increasingly, molecular mechanisms of both cancer growth and mestatases are gradually being elucidated.

Efforts to realize the potential of gene therapy encompass a variety of approaches. Increasingly, clinical trials of gene-based therapies for cancer have their origin in strategies to augment immunotherapy or chemotherapy. These include exploiting unique synergies between gene-based agents and other cancer therapeutics, drug sensitization with genes regulating drug delivery, and the use of drug-resistant genes for organ protection from high doses of chemotherapy. Ex vivo and in vivo gene transfer, the regulation of gene expression, the inactivation of oncogene expression, and gene replacement of tumor suppressor genes are other strategies that surgeons have utilized to target underlying genetic lesions unique to the cancer cell. Significant effort has also been directed toward optimizing delivery systems and constructs for gene therapy; important areas of research include modifying viral vectors to reduce toxicity and immunogenicity, increasing transduction efficiency, and enhancing vector targeting and specificity. Early results with these gene therapy strategies are encouraging with regard to the possibility of mediating tumor regression with acceptable toxicity.[17]

Surgeons also continue contributing to our understanding of tumor immunology. Hope grows that the cycle of scientific discovery, renewed enthusiasm, and heightened expectation historically followed by disappointment will finally be overcome by a critical mass of knowledge resulting in clinical relevance. Strategies that incorporate genetic and molecular approaches to the activation of the immune system are gradually evolving. Other efforts in the field of angiogenesis have also yielded some early encouraging results as a number of antiangiogenic agents have been identified, and a variety of strategies targeting angiogenic factors have been postulated.

Novel Technologies

Technological advances in the last 5 or so years have had dramatic impact. Lymphatic mapping has become clinically reliable and enhanced the accuracy of the operative staging of melanoma. The validity of this approach for staging breast cancer has also recently been supported by reports from several institutions. Three separate reports document the accuracy of the technique. In a consecutive series of 163 women with operable breast carcinoma, Veronesi and associates used a handheld γ-ray detector probe to localize the sentinel lymph node for removal through a small axillary incision. A high degree of accuracy for sentinel lymph node mapping for breast cancer was achieved with concordance between sentinel nodes and axillary nodes in 75 of 79 cases with histologically negative sentinel lymph nodes.[18] Albertini and associates and Giuliano and co-workers reported series of 62 and 107 patients, respectively, with sensitivity and specificity of 100% for breast cancer sentinel node biopsy.[19,20] Our collective experience suggests that women with negative sentinel lymph nodes will routinely be spared axillary dissection and the associated morbidity in the near future.

Efforts to extend the staging accuracy of pathologic lymph node analysis have recently focused on the use of specific molecular diagnostic tools. Goydos and associates recently evaluated the efficacy and feasibility of the intraoperative liquid nitrogen preservation of lymph node biopsy specimens and rapid reverse transcriptase polymerase chain reaction (RT-PCR) analysis to detect the enzyme tyrosinase, and MART-1, a melanoma-specific antigen.[21] This early study suggests that both tyrosinase and MART-1 are more sensitive than routine histologic examination in detecting occult melanoma lymph node metastases. In a similar approach, Lockett and associates designed a multiple-gene panel to test for axillary lymph node metastases in patients with breast cancer. Of 29 pathologically negative patients, 14 were found to have evidence of micrometastases by RT-PCR analysis.[22] Studies of patients who are determined to have metastatic disease based on PCR technology alone, such as these from these two studies, require long-term follow-up to confirm clinical relevance. If confirmed, this improved diagnostic efficacy and enhanced staging discrimination will require proper stratification in future prospective comparisons to eliminate the Will Rogers phenomenon.

The importance of defining outcomes based on treatment decisions directed by more accurate staging is a current issue in melanoma management. Adjuvant therapy with recombinant interferon α-2B improves both disease-free and overall survival among a group of patients with a high risk of recurrence.[23] It may be that adjuvant therapy with interferon α-2B has the greatest benefit for patients with early nodal metastatic disease; however, it is not possible to extrapolate firm conclusions regarding the efficacy of interferon α-2B in patients with significant tumor volume, to the dissimilar population of patients with minimal metastatic disease in regional lymph nodes. In the past year the Sunbelt Melanoma Trial was organized to determine whether regional lymphadenectomy with adjuvant high dose interferon α-2B improves disease-free and overall survival for melanoma patients with early (sentinel lymph node-only) nodal metastases. In this study patients with malignant sentinel lymph nodes detected by histology and immunohistochemistry are separately analyzed from patients whose malignant nodal metastasis are detected by RT-PCR analysis for tyrosinase, GP100, MART-1, MAGE-3, and mRNA. Patients with histologically identified metastases in a single lymph node are stratified by tumor thickness and randomized to receive lymphadenectomy alone, or lymphadenectomy plus interferon α-2B therapy. Patients who have metastases to regional lymph nodes detected by RT-PCR analysis only are randomized to observation, lymphadenectomy alone, or lymphadenectomy and interferon α-2B therapy. All patients undergo RT-PCR analysis of peripheral blood cells to detect circulating melanoma cells to determine the predictive value of this molecular staging test. This study, involving participants from both the community and the academic setting, is also significant in that it demonstrates a surgeon-led initiative in the translation of molecular diagnostics to the clinical setting. The recent development of image-guided core needle breast biopsy, by both stereotactic and ultrasound technologies, has provoked a major change in the diagnosis of mammographically detected abnormalities. A rapid transition from conventional needle directed excisional biopsy to this less invasive alternative is underway. Recent reports, including several by surgeons, document accuracy equivalent to needle directed excisional breast biopsy and verify the validity of this approach; it is also more economically efficient. As a result the next decade will likely witness the demise of the diagnostic surgical breast biopsy. Issues related to the credentialling and privileging processes, and the respective roles of surgeons and radiologists remain controversial.[24] Incorporating the skills required of imaging, clinical management, and pathologic interpretation are significant concerns for patient safety. Necessary modifications in resident training are being implemented in several surgical training programs. Practicing surgeons with limited imaging skills must endeavor to extend these skills if they wish to become significantly involved.

The Future

What, then, is the future of the surgeon's role in the field of oncology? Some have suggested that the discipline has reached a peak and will be limited in future contributions; such thinking has been consistently erroneous in the past, and remains so. As quickly as one surgical intervention becomes antiquated, technological and conceptual advances spur the application of new ideas and technologies in areas previously thought beyond surgical endeavor.

Surgeons have historically provided a leadership role in the care of patients with cancer. The scope of surgery's future leadership role, relative to the other oncologic disciplines, will be defined by the extent to which individual surgeons persist in acquiring a comprehensive and differentiated knowledge of specific malignancies. In this regard, individual surgeons are increasingly faced with a fundamental choice: Do we narrow our individual interests and scope of clinical expertise to more effectively contribute to promising research and the clinical implementation of technological advances? Or, do we maintain a broader surgical practice and delegate these responsibilities to other tangentially related specialties? Perhaps too often in the past we pursued strategies that precipitated the involution of whole areas of clinical interest previously recognized within the purview of surgery. The resulting obligatory fragmentation of patient care has proven inconvenient for patients, and unnecessarily costly. In a world of tremendous economic pressures for the practice of medicine to conform to the efficiencies of business, we must increasingly pursue strategies that eliminate redundancies. In some cases, the fragmentation of patient care in recent years occurred because surgeons failed to expand the scope of their discipline through their commitment to the implementation of novel technologies. Other decisions, such as the indication for adjuvant therapy, have sometimes been referred as a matter of convenience for the surgeon, resulting in inconvenience for the patient, and increased costs for the payor. Surgeons should be sophisticated concerning decisions regarding adjuvant therapy and the treatment of metastatic cancer. Such treatment may involve significant expense and morbidity for marginal benefit. One of the prime goals of the discipline of surgical oncology is the education of all physicians and surgeons in the comprehensive management of cancer.[25] This is not to suggest that surgeons, or any other single discipline, should dominate the decision-making of oncologic management. It rather suggests that the surgical discipline must continue to occupy a central role in the treatment of solid tumors, and strong surgical representation is vital to ensure appropriate planned cancer care coordinated by multidisciplinary cancer teams. A successful cancer program is usually approved by the American College of Surgeons Commission on Cancer, certifying that such programs pass certain milestones in their care of their cancer patients.[24]

The traditional role of surgery is being transformed. For many years, there has been an ongoing debate regarding the role of the surgical oncologist relative to the general surgeon. The recent past has been characterized by a trend toward less "onco-logical surgery" and more "surgical oncology."[13] The surgical operation is only one intervention in an increasingly integrated therapeutic process requiring specialized physicians. This does not mean that the role of the general surgeon is necessarily diminished. It does mean that surgeons must commit to an expanded and specialized knowledge if they are to continue to participate and lead the integration of care.

Transforming growth and a redefinition of the scope and nature of surgical oncol-ogy is at hand. In this, an era of considerable transition and upheaval, we are encour-aged by young surgeons increasingly dedicated to quality research, the application of novel technologies, and a comprehensive disease specific fund of knowledge.

FURTHER READING

1. Flexner JT (1969) *Doctors on Horseback*. Dover Publications, New York, p. 10.

2. Long CW (1849) An account of the first use of sulphuric ether by inhalation as an anaes-thetic in surgical operations. *South Med Surg J* 6:705–713.

3. Meade RH (1968) An introduction to the history of general surgery. WB Saunders, Philadelphia.

4. Rosenberg SA (1997) Principles of cancer management: Surgical oncology. In *Cancer: Principles & Practice of Oncology*, 5th edition. Lippencott–Raven, Philadelphia.

5. Fisher RB (1977) *Joseph Lister, 1827–1912*. Stein and Day, New York.

6. Guthrie D (1949) *Lord Lister, His Life and Doctrine*. E & S Livingstone, Edinburgh.

7. Billroth T (1924) *The Medical Sciences in the German Universities*. Macmillan, New York.

8. Halsted WS (1904) The training of the surgeon. *Bull Johns Hopkins Hosp* 15:267.

9. Heuer GW (1952) Dr. Halsted. *Bull Johns Hopkins Hosp* (Suppl), 90:1.

10. Nunn DB (1989) William Stewart Halsted: A profile of courage, dedication, and scientific search for truth. *J Vasc Surg* 10:221–229.

11. Harvey AM (1981) The influence of William Stewart Halsted's concept of surgical train-ing. *Johns Hopkins Med J* 148:215–236.

12. Olson JS (1984) The history of cancer. (An annotated bibliography.) Greenwood Publish-ing Group, Westport, Connecticut.

13. Arnesjo B, Burn I, Denis L, Mazzeo F (1989) *Surgical Oncology (A European Hand-book)*. Springer-Verlag, Berlin.

14. Wells SA, Chi DD, Toshima K, et al. (1994) Predictive DNA testing and prophylactic thyroidectomy in patients at risk for multiple endocrine neoplasia type 2A. *Ann Surg* 220:237.

15. Broadwater JR, Henderson MA, Bell JL, Edwards MJ, Smith GJ, McCready DR, Swan-son RS, Hardy ME, Shenk RR, Lawson M, Ota DM, Balch CM (1991) Percutaneous subclavian catheterization for cancer outpatients. *Am J Surg* 60:676–680.

16. Alexander HR (ed) (1994) Vascular access in the cancer patient. Devices, insertion techniques, maintenance, and prevention and management of complications. JB Lippincott, Philadelphia.

17. Roth JA, Cristiano RJ (1997) Gene therapy for cancer: What have we done and where are we going? *J Natl Cancer Inst* 89:21–39.

18. Veronesi U, Paganelli G, Galimberti V, Vitale G, Zurrida S, Bedoni M, Costa A, de Cicco C, Geeraghty JG, Lini A, Sacchini V, Paolo V (1997) Sentinel-node biopsy to avoid axillary dissection in breast cancer with clinically negative lymph-nodes. *Lancet* 349:1864–1867.

19. Albertini JJ, Lyman GH, Cox C, et al. (1996) Lymphatic mapping and sentinel node biopsy in the patient with breast cancer. *JAMA* 276:1818–1822.

20. Giuliano AE, Jones RC, Brennan M, et al. (1997) Sentinel lymphadenectomy in breast cancer. *J Clin Oncol* 15:2345–2350.

21. Goydos JS, Borao F, Gartner M, Yudd A, Bancila E, Germino FJ (1997) Improved diagnosis of occult melanoma in sentinel nodes: RT–PCR studies of the tyrosinase and MART-1 genes. *Surg Forum* 48:823–825.

22. Lockett MA, Baron PL, O'Brien PH, Elliot BM, Robison JG, Metcalf JS, Cole DJ (1997) Occult breast cancer micrometastases: Detection in axillary lymph nodes using a multimarker RT-PCR panel. *Surg Forum* 48:861–863.

23. Kirkwood JM, Strawderman MH, Ernstoff MS, Smith TJ, Borden EC, Blum RH (1996) Interferon alpha-2b adjuvant therapy of high-risk resected cutaneous melanoma: The Eastern Cooperative Oncology Group Trial EST 1684. *J Clin Oncol* 14:7–17.

24. Edwards MJ, Israel PA (1997) Beyond the credentialling and privileging controversy for image-guided breast biopsy. *Bull Am Coll Surg* 82:20–23.

25. Cady B (1997) Basic principles in surgical oncology. *Arch Surg* 132:338–346.

CHAPTER 12

PRINCIPLES OF RADIATION ONCOLOGY

JOHN N. WALDRON and BRIAN O'SULLIVAN

Department of Radiation Oncology
University of Toronto
Princess Margaret Hospital
Toronto, Ontario M5G 2M9, Canada

The discovery of X-rays by Wilhelm Conrad Roentgen in 1895 was one of the most important events in the evolution of modern medicine. It was soon after this that X-rays were first used for both diagnostic and therapeutic purposes. Radiation therapy is one of the major therapeutic modalities for the treatment of malignant disease. It is estimated that 50% of cancer patients will require radiation therapy at some point in their illness,[1] which emphasizes the need for all physicians to be familiar with this form of treatment.

Radiation oncology represents the branch of medicine concerned with the application of radiation for the treatment of neoplastic disease. This application requires not only a sound knowledge of medicine and oncology but also expertise in the principles of radiation physics and radiation biology.[2] In most countries certification for the practice of radiation oncology requires 3 to 5 years of postgraduate training following medical school and internship. This training generally occurs in university-affiliated departments with emphasis not only on the clinical aspects of radiation oncology but also on research and teaching.

This chapter is a summary of the general principles of the clinical practice of radiation oncology and the physical and biologic concepts on which these are based. Tumor specific treatment issues are discussed elsewhere in this volume and historical summaries are also available.[2]

Manual of Clinical Oncology, 7th edition, Edited by Raphael E. Pollock
ISBN 0-471-23828-7, pages 251–274. Copyright © 1999 Wiley-Liss, Inc.

RADIATION PHYSICS—THE BASICS

The Nature of Radiation

Radiation is energy.[3,4] The term *radiation* applies to the emission, propagation, and absorption of energy through space or a material medium in either wave or particle form. All radiation travels at the speed of light (3×10^8 m/s in a vacuum) but the energy of radiation varies along a continuous spectrum defined as the electromagnetic spectrum (Fig. 12.1). The energy of radiation is measured in units termed electron-volts (eV). The position of a particular radiation within this energy spectrum is designated using common terms including radiowaves, microwaves, infrared (heat), visible light, ultraviolet light, X-rays, and γ-rays.

Radiation is propagated in two forms: photons or particles. Photons are "packages" of energy without mass or charge that behave as either particles or waves in terms of their interaction with each other or matter. Both X-rays and γ-rays comprise photons differing only in their method of production. Particle radiation is propagated by units of mass. The most commonly used forms of particle radiation are electrons, protons, and neutrons.

Interaction of Radiation with Matter

When radiation is absorbed energy is transferred to matter. The final effect depends on the nature and energy of the radiation as well as the quality of the matter. If the energy of the incident radiation is sufficiently high it causes ejection of orbital

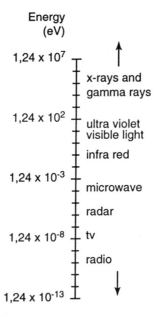

Figure 12.1. The electromagnetic energy spectrum. Ranges are approximate.

electrons from the atoms of the matter, resulting in a net deficit of charge termed ionization. Such radiation is called *ionizing radiation*. It is this process of ionization of atoms and further effects produced by the ejected electrons that leads to the molecular damage manifesting the biologic effects of radiation. The energy of ionizing radiation required for useful clinical effect ranges from 50 kV to 25 MV.

Production of Therapeutic Radiation

Photon radiation utilized clinically originates from one of two sources: the decay of radioactive elements to produce γ-rays or from the result of accelerated electrons bombarding a heavy metal target to produce X-rays. The most commonly used γ-rays originate from a cobalt-60 source that continuously decays releasing photons. X-rays are generated by two means: an X-ray generator or a linear accelerator. The X-ray generator uses an X-ray tube similar to that used to produce diagnostic X-rays to produce low-energy X-rays for superficial therapy (50 to 150 kV) or orthovoltage therapy (150 to 500 kV). Higher energy X-rays are produced in linear accelerators, which utilize high-energy microwaves to accelerate electrons toward a metal target; the resultant collision produces photons in a similar fashion to the X-ray tube. Because the electrons are accelerated to much higher speeds the X-rays produced are of much higher energy (4 to 25 MV). Further, by removing the metal target from the electron path the linear accelerator can be used to produce electron beams that can also be used clinically.

Measurement of Radiation Dose

Because radiation is essentially energy, the measure of the transfer of this energy to a given mass of material is the measure of radiation dose. Radiation dose was originally measured as the amount of ionization produced in a given volume of air. The unit assigned to this measurement was the roentgen. This system, however, did not strictly measure transfer of energy, and dose became impractical to measure with the advent of high-energy (mega electron-volt) machines. The roentgen was therefore replaced by the rad (radiation absorbed dose), defined as the dose of radiation resulting in an energy deposition of 100 ergs per gram. The rad has now been replaced by the SI unit the Gray (Gy), which is equivalent to a 1 joule per kilogram energy deposition. One Gray equals 100 rads. Even though the official SI unit is the Gray, dose is frequently quoted in centiGray (cGy) . Although the centiGray is incorrect nomenclature, and should be abandoned, it does allow the convenience of a 1:1 ratio with the older unit rad.

Dose Distribution

The distribution of radiation dose within irradiated tissues is dependent on the energy and type of radiation (photon versus electron versus other particles), the volume and composition of tissue irradiated, and the distance from the source of radiation.

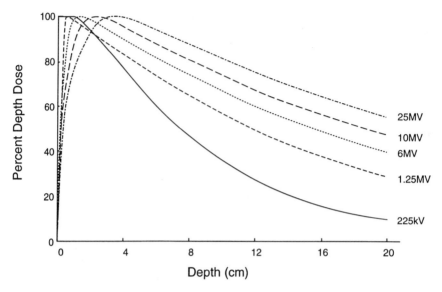

Figure 12.2. Depth-dose curves for some photon energies used to deliver radiation therapy.

The distribution of radiation dose within tissue can be graphically illustrated using a *depth-dose curve*, which plots the relative dose (% depth-dose) as a function of depth from the irradiated surface. Figure 12.2 illustrates such a plot for photon beams of increasing energies. As beam energy increases so does the depth of maximum dose deposition while the rate of dose falloff at depth decreases. Therefore, a low-energy beam, 225 kV for example, would be used to treat a superficial skin carcinoma and a high-energy beam, 25 MV, to treat a deep lesion, such as prostate cancer, while sparing the overlying skin.

The type of radiation used can influence the distribution of dose within tissue as illustrated in Fig. 12.3. This figure contrasts the depth-dose curves of beams comprised of photons, electrons, or protons. In contrast to photons, electrons provide a relatively flat "plateau" of dose to a given depth that then drops off rapidly. This allows relative sparing of deep structures, for example, spinal cord when treatment is given to the neck. Protons on the other hand tend to transfer most of their energy late in their passage through tissue, resulting in a dose peak (termed the Bragg peak) at depth. This serves to advantage when treating well-defined deep tumors such as clival chordomas.

Isodose Distributions

Although depth-dose curves serve to illustrate the distribution of dose in one dimension (depth) a more clinically practical method of depicting the distribution of dose within an irradiated volume of tissue is required. One such method is the *isodose distribution*. An isodose distribution represents a two-dimensional representation of

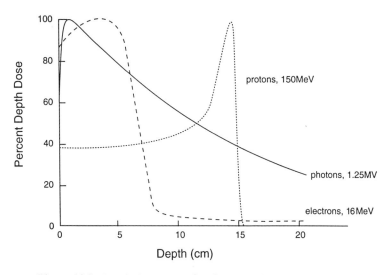

Figure 12.3. Depth-dose curves for electrons, photons, and protons.

dose within a plane through an irradiated volume by generating lines that connect points of equal dose (isodose curves). Three such distributions are illustrated in Fig. 12.4. By knowing the location of tumor and normal tissues within an isodose distribution the radiation oncologist can then determine the dose of radiation these structures will receive.

RADIATION PHYSICS—CLINICAL APPLICATION

The clinical application of radiation for the treatment of malignant disease requires an appreciation of not only the methods of delivery of radiation but also the principles of planning treatment including definition of the volume to be treated and treatment simulation.[3,4]

Delivery of Radiation

There are three main methods by which radiation therapy is delivered clinically: teletherapy, brachytherapy, and isotope therapy.

Teletherapy, more commonly known as external beam therapy, involves the delivery of radiation from a source located external to the body. This is the most common type of radiation therapy and utilizes the delivery systems previously described (X-ray generator, cobalt-60 unit, and linear accelerator).

Brachytherapy involves placement of the radiation source(s) in contact with the body whether the source(s) be physically implanted into the tissues (*interstitial therapy*), into existing cavities (*intracavitary therapy*), or approximated to the body surface (*surface or contact therapy*). Brachytherapy radiation sources consist of a

12 MeV Electrons   6 MV Photons   25 MV Photons

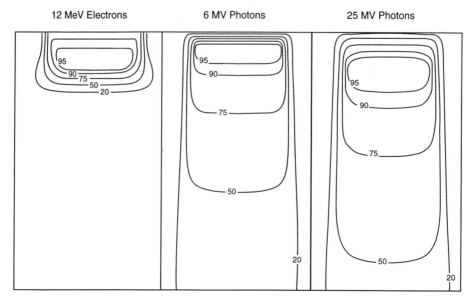

FIGURE 12.4. Isodose curves for 10×10 cm beams of 12 MeV electrons, 6 and 25 MV photons.

variety radionuclides similar in principle to cobalt-60 that release radiation as they decay. The process of brachytherapy is described in more detail later.

Isotope therapy consists of the administration, by either intravenous or oral routes, of radioactive isotopes that are selectively taken up by specific tumor bearing tissue. The subsequent decay and release of radiation by these isotopes produces the desired clinical effect. The most common examples of isotope therapy include intravenous strontium-89 for the treatment of bone metastasis from carcinoma of the prostate and oral iodine-131 for the treatment of certain thyroid carcinomas.

Treatment Planning for External Beam Therapy

A wide variety of tumors are treated using external beam therapy, from superficial skin lesions to deep-seated tumors. To be able to plan such treatments the radiation oncologist requires a sound knowledge of not only the tumor and its adjacent normal anatomy but also the capabilities and constraints of the equipment with which he or she works.

The process of treatment planning is that which ensures a homogeneous dose of radiation is reproducibly delivered to a defined volume to achieve tumor control with minimum effect on the surrounding normal tissues. This process requires the input and expertise of a team of individuals, that includes the radiation oncologist, pathologist, radiologist, surgeon, radiation therapist, and clinical physicist.

Volume Treated

The first step in planning radiation therapy requires a decision as to the volume of tissue to be treated. The radiation oncologist makes this decision based on the known extent and biologic behavior of the tumor in question. This information is provided by a careful physical exam and supplemented by information from appropriate radiologic exam. Review of the available pathology is essential to determine and confirm not only the histopathologic subtype of the tumor but also the completeness of resection if an operation was performed. Finally, communication with the surgeon is essential to ascertain the nature and extent of surgery performed and/or a detailed description of tumor location as seen at examination under anesthetic. The radiation oncologist then determines three separate and sequential volumes as defined by the International Commission on Radiation Units and Measurements[5] (Fig. 12.5). The first is the *gross tumor volume* (GTV), defined as the gross palpable or visible/demonstrable extent and location of malignant growth. The GTV is then expanded to define the *clinical target volume* (CTV) which contains the GTV plus areas at risk of harboring subclinical microscopic disease. The last is the *planning target volume* (PTV) which contains the CTV and is a geometric concept used to select appropriate beam sizes and energies to deliver the prescribed dose to the entire CTV given variations in day-to-day delivery of radiation due to both organ and patient movement.

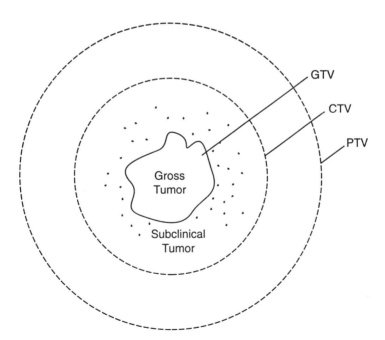

FIGURE 12.5. Schematic representation of the ICRU volumes used for treatment planning. See text for details.

Treatment Simulation

Once the CTV has been defined an arrangement of separate radiation beams can be designed to encompass it while minimizing the volume of uninvolved normal tissue irradiated. This may require the use of single or, more commonly, multiple beams. The orientation of these beams is defined with the patient in a fixed treatment position, which may involve the use of certain supports or immobilization devices such as masks to ensure reproducibility. Beams are then simulated using a fluoroscopic device called a *simulator* that reproduces the geometric relationship that will exist between the patient and the actual treatment machine. Using the simulator the relationship between the various beams and the bone and tissue structure can be defined. The use of metal or wire markers placed on the patient can aid in defining the position of tumor and/or critical structures. Similarly, the use of barium or contrast at the time of simulation can define the position of visceral structures such as the bowel or bladder. The use of computed tomography (CT) can be incorporated into the planning of treatment to deep or complex volumes in a process known as CT planning. This is performed by scanning the patient in the treatment position and the CT data entered into a computerized planning system that allows the position and resultant dose distribution of radiation beams to be displayed on the individual CT slices. Alternatively isodose distributions can be generated on contours taken through the simulated volume and critical structures located by reference to X-ray films. Three such isodose distributions for the treatment of breast, tonsil, and prostate cancer are illustrated in Fig. 12.6. The program is designed to take into account variation in patient external contour and tissue density when calculating isodose distributions. Once the number and orientation of beams is determined the patient is then simulated on a standard simulator to reproduce these beams.

At the time of simulation films are taken of each beam. This serves as a permanent record of the field treated and allows the radiation oncologist to define areas that are to be shielded during treatment (Fig. 12.7). The center and borders of each field are marked on the patient or immobilization device to allow reproduction at the treatment machine.

Treatment Delivery

The patient attends the treatment unit for delivery of radiation. These can be any one of a variety of machines described above and are operated by radiation therapists. The planned treatment field(s) are reproduced on the treatment machine with reference to small tattoos or marks placed on the patient or immobilization device at the time of simulation. The field is defined by collimation within the treatment machine and further modified with shielding, wedge filters, or missing tissue compensators

---

FIGURE 12.6. Axial contours and isodose distributions illustrating three typical radiation treatment plans with beam arrangement and resultant dose distribution. (**A**) Chest wall tangential beams for postoperative breast irradiation with 6 MV photons. (**B**) A four-field technique for the treatment of prostate cancer with 18 MV photons. (**C**) A perpendicular pair of beams for the treatment of a lateralized tonsil cancer with 6 MV photons.

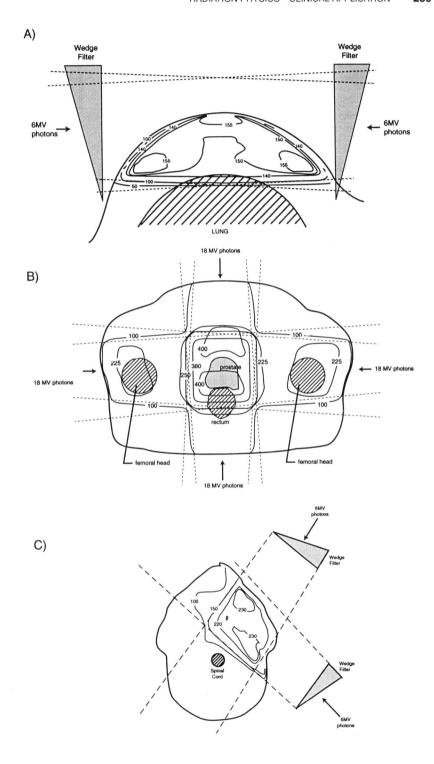

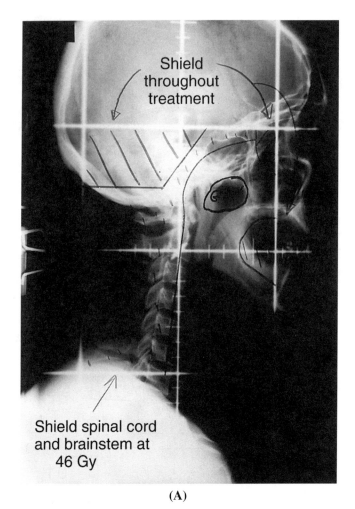

(A)

FIGURE 12.7. Radiographs taken for simulation of treatment for **(A)** nasopharynx cancer and **(B)** lung cancer. The white grid marks outline the treatment field. The gross tumor volume (GTV) and placement of shielding has been indicated by the radiation oncologist in wax pencil. **(B)**, wire has been placed around a palpable lymph node to permit it to be visualized at simulation.

placed in the path of the beam as needed to achieve the desired distribution of dose. The treatment machine is turned on for a length of time necessary to deliver the prescribed dose defined by the total dose, number of fractions, number and size of fields treated, and the known output of a given machine. Generally this is no longer than a minute or two for each beam in a multibeam plan. The majority of patients are treated as outpatients and receive once or twice daily treatments Monday to Friday for a period of 1 to 7 weeks. To ensure accuracy in treatment delivery X-ray films are exposed with the beams from the treatment unit with the first treatment and as needed thereafter. These X-ray films are compared with the simulator films taken

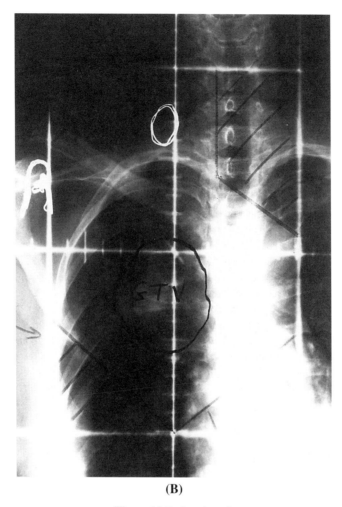

(B)

Figure 12.7. (continued)

during planning to ensure the CTV is being adequately treated and critical normal tissues are spared. Alternatively this can be done with the use of a portal imager that electronically captures the treatment image of the relevant beams for review.

RADIATION BIOLOGY

Our understanding of the biology of radiation has expanded rapidly over the last 50 years.[6-8] Many insights have been gained by the careful isolation and study of a variety of radiation-sensitive cell lines from normal tissues and tumors of both humans and animals. Initial studies documented the effects of radiation at the cellular level and described the radiation survival curve on which many of the principles of contemporary clinical radiation fractionation regimens are based. In recent decades, with the emergence of molecular biology attention has turned toward study of the effects of radiation at the molecular level. This has led to the description of critical molecular targets damaged by radiation and the complex responses of the cell to this damage resulting in cell survival or death. Other clinical and laboratory research is describing the important influence of the cellular microenvironment on outcome following radiation. Altogether progress in the field of radiation biology continues to lead to a variety of strategies for both the prediction and modification of outcome following cellular exposure to ionizing radiation.

Radiation Effects at the Cellular Level

Ionizing radiation produces a variety of effects at the cellular level. The irradiated cell can continue to reproduce (apparently unharmed), display a temporary or permanent delay in growth, or die either immediately or after several cell divisions. These outcomes can be measured with a variety of in vivo and in vitro techniques. The most common laboratory endpoint used to measure cellular outcome following exposure to ionizing radiation is clonogenic survival. This represents the ability of a cell to retain its reproductive capacity as measured by the formation of macroscopic colonies of cells arising from single parent cells following irradiation. Clonogenic survival for a population of cells is best illustrated by the *radiation survival curve* generated when the proportion of clonogenic survivors is plotted for a variety of single radiation doses (Fig. 12.8). Increasing dose results in increased cell kill; however, this relationship is not consistently linear, with a shallow curved shoulder region

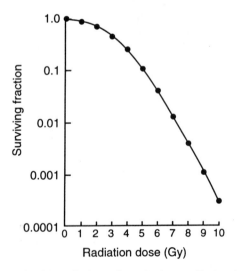

FIGURE 12.8. A typical in vitro radiation cell survival curve. Each point represents the surviving fraction of cells (plotted on the log scale y-axis) following a single acute exposure to the dose indicated on the x-axis.

followed by a steeper linear region at higher doses. This has been interpreted as illustrating both the capacity of the cell to repair damaged sustained at lower doses and the need to saturate such a repair system with damage before survival begins to drop off more steeply at higher doses.

Radiation Effects at the Molecular Level

Irradiated cellular atoms and molecules can be altered by direct interaction with photons or ejected orbital electrons (*direct effects*). However, the majority of the radiation effect is thought to be due to the generation of *free radicals* (unstable atoms and molecules containing an unpaired electron) that then interact with and damage cellular macromolecules (*indirect effects*). Although any atom within a cell can be ionized by radiation, it is likely that the vast majority of these ionizations have no consequence and rather it is damage to certain critical targets that determines cell survival. DNA is one of these critical targets and evidence is now emerging that damage to other structures such as cellular microtubules or membrane systems may play a role. Ionizing radiation activates a wide variety of cellular biochemical pathways (Fig. 12.9) and it is likely that it is damage to these critical targets that serves as the triggering event. In general these biochemical pathways involve the interaction of numerous cellular proteins in a complex and sequential fashion leading to a multitude of endpoints including altered gene expression. Some of these genes are involved with *DNA repair*, which requires the interaction of a host of nuclear proteins that recognize, excise, align, and ligate the damaged strands. Other genes are involved with the progression of cells through their normal reproductive cycle (the cell cycle). Ionizing radiation induces *cell cycle arrest* at specific checkpoints with the hypothetical function to provide the cells both the time and environment in which to repair DNA damage before proceeding with replication. Irreparably damaged cells may be diverted into an autodestructive process known as *apoptosis*, which is an orderly and highly regulated process involving specific proteins that essentially results in the dismantling of the cell. Although it is known that apoptosis represents one mechanism of cell death following exposure to ionizing radiation its relative importance versus clonogenic cell death has yet to be established.

Tumor Radiobiology

The response of a tumor to radiation is complex. Tumor control requires the eradication of every malignant cell capable of reproduction. Some of the main factors that influence this outcome include: (1) the number of clonogenic cells that need to be eradicated (how big is the tumor?), (2) the rate at which these cells are reproducing during treatment (how fast is the tumor growing?), and (3) how sensitive these cells are to ionizing radiation. For any given tumor the outcome is very likely determined by a unique balance of these factors. For example, a large tumor comprised of relatively radiation-sensitive cells (e.g., a bulky mediastinal lymphoma) may be controlled with radiation whereas a small carcinoma may not. Nevertheless some

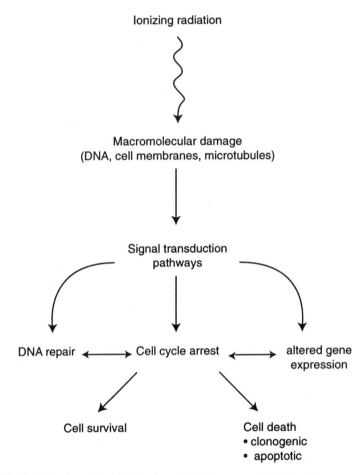

Ionizing radiation

Macromolecular damage
(DNA, cell membranes, microtubules)

Signal transduction
pathways

DNA repair ←——→ Cell cycle arrest ←——→ altered gene
expression

Cell survival

Cell death
• clonogenic
• apoptotic

FIGURE 12.9. A schematic simplification of cellular events following exposure to ionizing radiation culminating in either cell survival or death.

general conclusions can be made and for a given histology larger tumors are less likely to be controlled by radiation.

Tumors can respond to cell loss with accelerated cellular reproduction. Such a process is thought to occur during a prolonged course of radiation treatment and could unfavorably shift the balance of cell killing to reproduction such that the tumor is not controlled. It has been demonstrated for several human tumors that, for a constant radiation dose, an overall prolongation in treatment time (allowing tumor repopulation during treatment) results in decreased tumor control.

The radiation sensitivity of the cells comprising a tumor is influenced by a multitude of factors. Microenvironmental factors such as the oxygen level in which individual tumor cells exist can influence response to radiation in a profound manner. Because hypoxic cells are more resistant to radiation the proportion of such cells within a tumor can influence outcome. Clinical studies using polarographic electrodes to measure intratumoral oxygen have clearly demonstrated significant variations in oxygen pressures within and between tumors and have correlated tumor hypoxia with an adverse outcome following radiation therapy[9] (Fig. 12.10). Cells exposed to ionizing radiation can produce a variety of cytokines that could potentially influence tumor response to radiation. Cytokines are proteins secreted by cells that regulate cell behavior in an autocrine and/or paracrine manner by binding to cell surface receptors and initiating signal transduction pathways. The position of cells within the cell cycle is known to affect their radiation sensitivity; therefore, the proportion of cells actively cycling and the distribution of these cells within the cell cycle could affect outcome of a tumor.

The influence of microenvironment and cell cycle effects can be controlled for by studying cultures of cell lines established from human tumors growing in vitro under controlled conditions. Radiation survival curves of such cultures demonstrate considerable variation in radiation sensitivity both between different tumor types and within a given type of tumor. This variation is thought to be due to differences in the *intrinsic radiation sensitivity* of the cells themselves. A convenient way of expressing the intrinsic radiation sensitivity of a line of cells is the surviving fraction after a dose of 2 Gy (the SF2). Radiation sensitivities of cervix cancer cell lines established from individual patients and measured in such a way have been correlated with clinical outcome following treatment with radiation therapy.[10] Factors that determine cellular intrinsic radiation sensitivity are likely genetic in origin and include those influencing signal transduction pathways resulting in cell cycle arrest, DNA repair, and apoptotic cell death.

Normal Tissue Radiobiology—Acute and Late Effects

Normal tissue injury due to radiation is a consequence of cell loss and resultant structural and functional impairment. Therefore, for any given normal tissue, the rate and extent of cell killing dictate the pattern of radiation injury. The time course and severity of injury are dependent on total radiation dose, the daily fraction size, the overall time of radiation, and the volume and type of tissue irradiated. Tissues containing a large population of rapidly proliferating cells manifest injury within days or weeks of being irradiated. These tissues include mucosa, skin, and bone marrow in which injury is in part due to the loss of proliferating cells leading to the inability to replace the normal day-to-day cell loss. Such normal tissue injuries, occurring during or up to 3 months from completion of radiation, are termed *acute effects*. Some acute effects of radiation injury are noted in Table 12.1. It should be kept in mind, however, that not all acute effects of radiation therapy are due to cell loss. For example, patients will experience nausea and vomiting within hours of irradiation to a significant volume of the upper abdomen; somnolence can occur soon after cranial irradiation; and acute edema and erythema can occur within an irradiated volume. The exact etiology of these acute radiation effects is poorly understood but may be related to radiation-induced cytokine release.

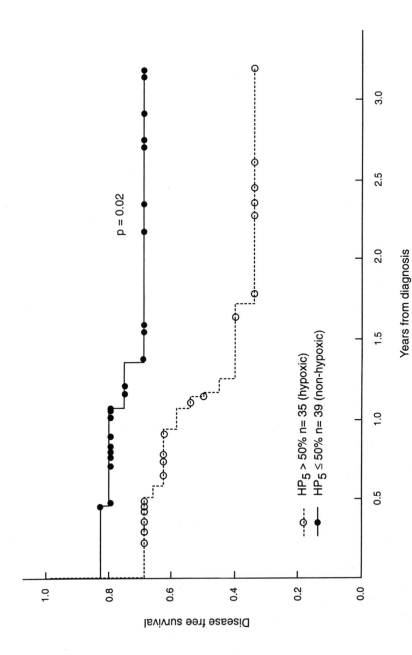

FIGURE 12.10. The influence of tumor hypoxia, as measured with an Eppendorf polarographic electrode, on disease free survival for 74 cervix cancer patients treated with radiation alone. Patient groups are divided based on the fraction of measurements with partial pressure of oxygen 5 mm Hg or less (HP_5). (Reprinted with permission from Fyles et al. 1998.)

TABLE 12.1. Acute Effects of Radiation Therapy

Normal Tissue Irradiated	Acute Effect(s)	Symptoms and Signs	Management
Skin	Erythema, dry and moist desquamation, epilation	Warmth, pruritus, pain	Drying agents, topical steroids, topical antibiotics for superinfection
Oropharyngeal mucosa	Mucositis	Dysphagia, odynophagia, thick secretions, halitosis with super infection	Oral hygiene, viscous xylocaine, analgesics, antibiotics for super-infection
Esophagus	Esophagitis	Dysphagia, odynophagia	Viscous xylocaine, analgesics, antibiotics for superinfection
Lung	Pneumonitis	Cough, pleuritic chest pain, dyspnea	Observation if mild, systemic cortico-steroids in severe cases, rule out pneumonia
Bowel	Gastroenteritis	Nausea, vomiting, cramping, diarrhea	Antiemetics if a significant volume of bowel included in the high dose volume, anti-diarrheal agents, diet modification
Bladder	Cystitis	Frequency, dysuria, urgency	Urinary analgesic (pyridium), rule out infection
Rectum	Proctitis	Tenesmus	Stool softeners, analgesics
Bone marrow	Cytopenia	Fatigue, bleeding, febrile neutro-penia	Transfusion, alteration in treatment time or volume if severe, ? role of cytokines

Normal tissue damage by radiation can manifest itself gradually over many months or years from the completion of treatment. The exact etiology of these *late effects* of radiation therapy is not known. They are likely the consequence of gradual loss of small vessel vasculature, parenchymal cell dysfunction, and fibrosis. The ability of a given normal tissue to withstand the effects of radiation is termed its *tolerance* and is dependent on a number of factors including total dose, fraction size, and the volume of tissue irradiated. Radiation tolerance has been documented for

TABLE 12.2. The Late Effects of Radiation Therapy

Normal Tissue	Late Effect	Tolerance Dose (Gy)
Brain	Necrosis	50
Eye (lens)	Cataract	10
Eye (retina)	Retinopathy	50
Salivary gland	Xerostomia	32
Mandible	Osteoradionecrosis	60
Spinal cord (5 cm segment)	Paralysis	50
Lung	Pneumonitis/fibrosis	17
Heart	Pericarditis	45
Esophagus	Stricture	55
Liver	Hepatitis	30
Kidney	Nephritis	25
Small bowel	Stricture	45

Tolerance dose represents the dose (delivered in 2-Gy fractions once daily, Monday to Friday) known to produce a 5% incidence of the late effect within 5 years of completion of treatment. Unless otherwise stated dose volumes are to whole organ.

a variety of normal tissues by careful clinical observation of large populations of individuals treated over many years.[11] The tolerance limit of a tissue is defined as the radiation dose, delivered in a standard fashion of 2 Gy once per day five days a week, that produces a 5% chance of a severe late effect over the subsequent 5 years. Some tolerance doses for late effects are listed in Table 12.2. The consequence of normal tissue radiation injury depends on the clinical importance of the tissues irradiated, the extent of injury, and the reserve capacity of the remaining unirradiated tissues. These factors in turn can be influenced by the age of the patient and comorbid disease.

CLINICAL USE OF RADIATION THERAPY

Indications

Radiation therapy can be given as the sole curative modality or in combination with surgery or chemotherapy for the treatment of malignant disease (Table 12.3). Although certain generalizations can be made, there is considerable variability in the use of radiation therapy throughout the world. Alternate approaches exist for a variety of cancers such that the patient could be treated with radiation alone with surgery reserved for salvage, or the initial treatment could be surgery alone with radiation given either pre- or postoperatively in selected cases. In many instances the treatment approach chosen is often based on specific local patterns of practice and the availability of expertise rather than evidence based.[12]

TABLE 12.3. Some Tumor Sites for Which Radiation Therapy Can Be Used as a Sole Curative Modality or in Combination with Surgery and/or Chemotherapy

Radiation Alone	Radiation in Combination with Surgery and/or Chemotherapy
Head and neck cancer	Breast cancer
Lymphoma	Rectal cancer
Cervix cancer	Lung cancer
Lung cancer	Head and neck cancer
Esophageal cancer	Sarcoma
Anal cancer	Brain cancer
Prostate cancer	Lymphoma
Bladder cancer	Endometrial cancer
Skin cancer	Thyroid cancer

Principles of Dose and Fractionation

The goal of treatment is to achieve an optimum balance between the probability of tumor cure and normal tissue damage (*the therapeutic ratio*). The dose of radiation required to achieve an optimum therapeutic ratio depends on the tumor being treated and the nature of the normal tissues within the volume to be irradiated. Our appreciation of these optimal doses has evolved empirically by careful clinical observation. One such observation was that a higher total dose could be delivered with similar normal tissue effects if it was divided into smaller fractions separate in time and that by delivering this higher dose the likelihood of controlling the tumor increased. This phenomenon is thought to be due to a differential ability of tumor and normal tissue to repair the damage induced by radiation between fractions given.

While there is considerable variation in dose and fractionation regimens in clinical use throughout the world, a useful standard for comparison would deliver a 2 Gy fraction once a day Monday to Friday. Using this convention the total dose required for cure depends on the tumor being treated. For example, a lymphoma or seminoma may require only 35 to 45 Gy for a high likelihood of cure whereas a carcinoma or sarcoma would require 60 to 70 Gy to achieve any chance of cure, with dose often being limited by normal tissue tolerance. Similarly the bulk of tumor to be treated often dictates the dose required. For example, 45 to 50 Gy is considered sufficient dose to eradicate subclinical disease that may exist within lymphatics draining a tumor site, whereas a higher dose is required for gross palpable or radiologically visible tumor.

It is important to realize that once daily, 5-day a week treatment regimens were developed more for logistic than biologic reasons. Attempts to optimize the therapeutic ratio based on our understanding of radiobiology have led to a variety of alternate fractionation strategies. One such strategy is *hyperfractionation*, which involves the delivery of two or more small daily fractions to a larger total dose over approximately the same time as a conventional regimen. Hyperfractionation regimens use small fraction size, usually <1.5 Gy, with an interfraction interval of at least 6 h. This exploits the fact that most normal tissues are less sensitive to the late effects of a given total dose of radiation if it is delivered in small fractions with a sufficient interfraction interval for repair. In this way the total dose delivered can be increased without increasing the risk of normal tissue damage. Clinical trials are underway comparing various hyperfractionation regimens to standard once daily treatment for a variety of tumor sites. Preliminary results have been encouraging and many centers now consider hyperfractionation their standard treatment regimen for some tumors. Another fractionation strategy is *accelerated fractionation* in which the overall treatment time is reduced while the number of fractions, fraction size, or total dose remain similar. This is accomplished by treating more than once a day and/or treating on the weekends. This strategy attempts to counteract accelerated tumor repopulation during treatment.

Combining Radiation and Surgery

Radiation or surgery can be used alone for the treatment of selected cancers while the other is reserved for the salvage of persistent or recurrent cancer. However, many tumors require a combination of radiation and surgery. Usually this involves the use of radiation following surgery to eradicate any residual disease. This approach has resulted in improved rates of organ preservation (e.g., breast cancer, rectal cancer, and sarcomas) by permitting less radical resections to be performed without compromising cure rates. Alternatively, preoperative radiation may sterilize the periphery of larger tumors, possibly allowing a more limited resection or even rendering an inoperable tumor operable. These two approaches have advantages and disadvantages and it often remains unclear which approach is superior for a given tumor (Table 12.4).

Combining Radiation and Chemotherapy

Radiation and cytotoxic chemotherapy are often combined in the treatment of tumors. In most cases chemotherapy is given with the intention of eradicating distant micrometastasis while the radiation treatment addresses local control of the primary tumor. Such examples would be the treatment of node positive breast cancer or rectal carcinoma with postoperative radiation to the primary site to improve local control and systemic chemotherapy to reduce the risk of distant relapse.

Concurrent chemotherapy and radiation has been used for a number of different tumors (Table 12.5). The goal of concurrent chemotherapy is to enhance local tumor control, as the doses given are too low to have a noticeable systemic effect. Concurrent chemotherapy may provide an advantage in terms of local tumor control; however, it can also produce increased local toxicity (within the irradiated tissues) such that it is unclear whether the same result could not have been achieved without simply increasing the dose of radiation. Nevertheless there are theoretical advantages from the concurrent approach and this remains an important area of active clinical research.

TABLE 12.4. Advantages and Disadvantages of Preoperative Radiation versus Postoperative Radiation

Timing of Radiation	Advantage	Disadvantage
Preoperative	Smaller volume irradiated Reduced contamination of the surgical field with viable tumor cells Possibly allows more limited resection Lower radiation dose	Impaired wound healing in irradiated tissue Delay in resection Surgical pathology not available to guide planning
Postoperative	Surgical pathology available to guide planning A large proportion of the viable tumor already removed surgically	Larger volume needs to be irradiated to include operative bed Interruption of vascular supply may lead to hypoxic residual tumor Delay in radiation due to postop complications

Chemical Modifiers of Radiation Sensitivity

Therapeutic advantage can be obtained by one of two strategies: protection of normal tissues from the deleterious effects of radiation or selective sensitization of tumors to radiation. Both of these concepts have been studied clinically and serve as the focus of ongoing research including the development of compounds to protect normal tissues from the effects of ionizing radiation or to sensitize hypoxic tumor cells. The compound that has received the most attention for radiation protection has been amifostine (WR-2721). Clinical trials are presently underway to address its role as a radioprotective agent. Trials in lung, cervix, and head and neck cancer patients have shown positive results using hyperbaric oxygen to sensitize hypoxic cells. However, given the logistical difficulties of treating patients in hyperbaric chambers, the unorthodox fractionation schemes this required, and some increased normal tissue toxicity these approaches have not been repeated and perhaps abandoned prematurely. Clinical studies using hypoxic cell radiosensitizers mimicking the radiosensitizing

TABLE 12.5. Concurrent Chemotherapy Given During Radiation of Selected Tumors

Primary Tumor	Concurrent Chemotherapy
Nasopharynx	Cisplatinum
Esophagus	Cisplatinum or 5-fluorouracil and mitomycin C
Bladder	Cisplatinum
Cervix cancer	Cisplatinum or 5-fluorouracil and mitomycin C
Anal cancer	5-Fluorouracil and mitomycin-C

properties of oxygen (metronidazole, misonidazole, etanidazole, and nimorazole) have shown some improvement in outcome for selected subgroups of patients; however, toxicity has limited their use. In addition compounds that are specifically toxic to hypoxic cells (tirapazamine and mitomycin-c) show promise.

The Palliative Role of Radiation Therapy

Approximately 50% of patients diagnosed with malignant disease will succumb to their illness. For these patients attention should be given to palliation of the symptoms of progressive disease. Every doctor should be familiar with the general principles of palliative medicine including pain management. Differences exist between radiation treatment with palliative versus curative intent. Palliative treatments are of lower dose and shorter duration than curative treatments to minimize side effects and patient inconvenience (Table 12.6.). In selected cases when the patient has minimal or slowly progressive disease a more prolonged course of treatment to a higher dose may be justified.

Radiation therapy can provide effective palliation of a variety of symptoms including pain, bleeding, and compression produced by expanding tumor. Palliative radiation therapy is most frequently employed for painful bone metastasis, and the cough or hemoptysis resulting from lung tumors. A short course of treatment (one to ten fractions) can produce clinical improvement in at least 70% of patients. Similarly short courses of treatment can produce benefit for other palliative indications including compression of airways, viscera, or nervous system (nerves, brain, or spinal cord).

Clinical Brachytherapy

Brachytherapy involves placement of a radioactive source in physical contact with the patient. The major advantage of this approach is that the radiation dose delivered close to the source is very high and drops off as an inverse square of the distance from the source, thus sparing tissues distant from the source. The most common use

TABLE 12.6. Contrast Between Radiation Treatments of Palliative versus Curative Intent

	Palliative Intent	Curative Intent
Goal of therapy	Reduction of some disease	Eradication of all disease
Clinical endpoint	Symptom control	Cure
Length of treatment	1 day to 2 weeks	4–7 weeks
Total dose	8–30 Gy	Greater than 50 Gy
Fraction size	Large (3–10 Gy) to reduce overall treatment time	Small (2.5 Gy or less) to reduce late effects
Volume treated	Gross symptomatic disease only	All tumor and potential areas of microscopic spread

of brachytherapy involves the temporary placement of a source (usually cesium-137 or iridium-192) into an existing body cavity. This is termed intracavitary therapy and is most often used in the treatment of cervix cancer to provide a boost dose to the cervix following external beam treatment to the pelvis. Because of the rapid dose dropoff with distance from the source the cervix will receive a high dose while the bladder and rectum will be relatively spared. Intracavitary therapy can also be used in the treatment of esophageal, tracheobronchial, and nasopharyngeal tumors.

The placement of sources involves the positioning and fixation of hollow metal or plastic stems under local or general anesthesia. The patient is then transported to the treatment room, which is usually a specially shielded hospital room, and the stem(s) attached to a remote afterloading device that automatically loads the radioactive source(s) once the hospital personnel have left the room. Doses delivered with such techniques are in the range of 10 to 20 Gy at a rate of 100 to 200 cGy per hour requiring treatment times of 10 to 20 hours. Brachytherapy sources may be implanted into tissues (interstitial therapy) using catheters with remote afterloading to boost the operative bed in the treatment of breast and head and neck cancers as well as sarcomas and as an adjunct to external beam therapy in the treatment of cancers of the tongue. Permanent implants with gold seeds are used by some centers for the treatment of carcinoma of the prostate.

ADVANCED TECHNOLOGIES AND RADIATION ONCOLOGY

Radiation oncology has recently seen rapid technological advances that include information systems and treatment, planning and delivery systems. This is largely a result of rapidly expanding computer capabilities. Information systems contain electronic records of demographics, staging, treatment, and outcome for research and audit. The Internet has also expanded our ability to educate ourselves and our patients about all aspects of radiation oncology.

The introduction of advanced treatment planning and delivery systems will have a major impact on the delivery of radiation therapy as we enter the next millenium. Linkage between dosimetry software, linear accelerator operating systems (including mulitleaf collimators and dynamic wedges), and CT and MRI data has allowed the development of a variety of treatment approaches. Among these is *stereotactic radiation therapy* whereby small volumes (typically isolated brain lesions) can be treated within an accuracy of millimeters to very high doses with little dose to surrounding tissues. The development of *conformal radiation therapy* utilizing multiple often noncoplanar beams shaped to conform to irregular target volumes may allow dose escalation without a significant increased risk of late complications. Computed tomography has been more closely linked to the simulation and planning of radiation therapy by a process termed *CT simulation*. Powerful software is now allowing the simultaneous modulation of beam orientation, shape, and intensity during treatment to optimize dose distribution by a process known as *intensity modulated radiation therapy*.

QUALITY ASSURANCE

An active continuous quality assurance program serves to ensure the provision and maintenance of high-quality care. This begins with a careful review of all clinical and laboratory findings. Ideally the prescribed radiation therapy is validated by case presentation at a multidisciplinary tumor conference to ensure compliance with established treatment guidelines. Next a review of the treatment plan and dosimetry by the radiation oncologist, therapist, and medical physicist is necessary prior to the initiation of treatment. Every patient must have verification films performed periodically during treatment. All elements of planning and delivery should be discussed at a regular quality review meeting to minimize errors in treatment, including verification of the irradiated volume. The radiation oncologist should personally assess every patient on a weekly basis for acute toxicity and tumor response if feasible. Equipment calibration and evaluation should take place on a regular basis. Every department should regularly review its results and compare these to established benchmarks to ensure that any adverse systematic anomalies in clinical outcome are detected and appropriately investigated.

FURTHER READING

1. Mackillop W, et al. (1997) Does a centralized radiotherapy system provide adequate access to care? *J Clin Oncol* 15:1261–1271.
2. Perez C, Brady L (eds) (1998) *The Principles and Practice of Radiation Oncology*. Lippincott–Raven, Philidelphia.
3. Johns H, Cunningham J (1983) *The Physics of Radiology*. Charles C. Thomas, Springfield, IL.
4. Kahn F (1984). *The Physics of Radiation Therapy*. Williams & Wilkins, Baltimore.
5. International Commission on Radiation Units and Measurements (ICRU) (1993) Prescribing, recording, and reporting photon beam therapy. Bethesda, MD.
6. Hall E (1994) *Radiobiology for the Radiologist*. JB Lippincott, Philadelphia.
7. Steel G (ed) (1993) *Basic Clinical Radiobiology*. Edward Arnold, London.
8. Tannock I, Hill R (eds) (1998) *The Basic Science of Oncology*. McGraw-Hill, Toronto.
9. Fyles A, et al. (1998) Hypoxia measured with a polarographic electrode correlates with radiation response in cervix cancer. *Radiother Oncol* (in press).
10. West C (1995) Invited review: Intrinsic radiosensitivity as a predictor of patient response in radiotherapy. *Br J Radiol* 68:827–837.
11. Emami B, et al. (1991) Tolerance of normal tissue to therapeutic irradiation. *Int J Radiat Oncol Biol Phys* 21:109–122.
12. O'Sullivan B, et al. (1994) Controversies in the management of laryngeal cancer: Results of an international patterns of care survey. *Radiother Oncol* 31:23–32.

CHAPTER 13

PRINCIPLES OF MEDICAL ONCOLOGY

JAMES H. DOROSHOW

City of Hope National Medical Center
Duarte, CA 91010, USA

The first successful systemic therapies for cancer in humans were the use of oophorectomy by Beatson for the treatment of advanced breast cancer in 1895, and, very much later, the application of folate antagonist antimetabolites by Farber and alkylating agents by Gilman, Goodman, and Karnofsky in the mid-1940s. Systemic cancer therapy with cytotoxic drugs, hormonal agents, or biologic response modifiers is now capable of providing curative treatment for advanced Hodgkin's disease and certain types of non-Hodgkin's lymphoma, acute myelogenous and lymphoblastic leukemia, testicular cancer, gestational trophoblastic disease, and a variety of childhood leukemias. Systemic therapies have also been clearly shown to improve the survival of patients with breast, ovarian, and colorectal cancer as well as osteosarcoma when utilized as postoperative adjunctive treatment. For patients with all forms of lung cancer, and metastatic cancers of the breast, bladder, prostate, head and neck, and gastrointestinal tract, systemic treatment with palliative intent can frequently improve quality of life and reduce the symptoms of advanced disease.

Over the past half-century, several critical concepts in tumor biology and pharmacology important in determining the effectiveness of systemic therapy for cancer have been established. These include the role(s) of tumor burden and cellular heterogeneity; drug resistance; drug delivery and dose intensity; host factors; and multimodality treatment in the success of chemo-, hormonal, or biologic therapies. These concepts provide the background for a more specific understanding of the mechanism(s) by which systemic agents alter the growth of tumor cells.

Manual of Clinical Oncology, 7th edition, Edited by Raphael E. Pollock
ISBN 0-471-23828-7, pages 275–292. Copyright © 1999 Wiley-Liss, Inc.

PRINCIPLES OF TUMOR BIOLOGY AND PHARMACOLOGY UNDERLYING SYSTEMIC CANCER TREATMENT

Tumor Burden and Tumor Cell Heterogeneity

Initial experimental therapeutic studies in murine leukemia models established the ability of many classes of antineoplastic agents to kill tumor cells according to first-order kinetics; that is, a given concentration of drug utilized for a particular time period will kill a fixed number of tumor cells. If each treatment course at a given dose is cytotoxic for a constant fraction of cells, the curability of the particular therapy depends on the number of courses delivered, the drug concentration applied, and the initial tumor burden. Although this concept has been unequivocally verified in many animal tumor models that undergo logarithmic tumor cell expansion, it is not clear how well it applies to much more slowly growing and genetically heterogeneous solid tumors in man. However, the model does, in part, form the basis for the rational use of postsurgical adjuvant chemotherapy that is employed to destroy microscopic residual disease after surgical excision or irradiation has removed or destroyed most or all macroscopically detectable tumor cells. It is assumed that the decreased tumor burden that follows surgery (which would assist fractional cell kill) as well as the potential for stimulation of cell cycle progression in the residual tumor cells will increase the cytotoxic potential of systemic treatments that frequently are more effective during active tumor cell proliferation.

A major factor that underlies the efficacy of all systemic cancer treatment is the genetic heterogeneity of human tumors. Although most cancers may develop initially from a single malignant clone, all malignancies demonstrate genetic instability that leads to a remarkable degree of biochemical heterogeneity that can be observed not only from metastatic site to metastatic site but from cell to cell in a single tumor mass. Thus, the enormous inherent variation in the expression of any one of the wide range of proteins that establish the innate sensitivity of malignant cells to systemic agents is probably responsible for both the unpredictability of the efficacy of treatment (from patient to patient but not in populations of patients) in the common solid tumors as well as the regrowth of clones of malignant cells after an initial response to treatment. Regrowth, thus, may represent the expansion of tumor cells that, prior to any systemic drug exposure, already expressed gene products capable of providing a growth advantage under the selective pressure of treatment with a cytotoxin.

The demonstration of heterogeneous populations of tumor cells in humans has provided a critical rationale for the use of combinations of systemic agents with different sites of action that might circumvent at least some mechanisms of inherent drug insensitivity and for the use of surgical or radiotherapeutic tumor "debulking." In the latter instance, it has been predicted by Goldie and Coldman that the probability of a tumor possessing random mutations leading to insensitivity to systemic treatment is a function of the tumor cell burden. Thus, removal of tumor mass prior to systemic treatment may decrease not only the total body burden of cancer but also the percentage of tumor cells inherently resistant to treatment.

Tumor cell heterogeneity also plays a critical role in establishing the genetic makeup of the tumor cell with respect to growth regulation. Normal tissues undergo a regular process of growth and decay governed by the highly regulated expression of several critical cell cycle control genes including *p53* and the cyclin genes, as well as the genes that regulate apoptosis (programmed cell death) such as the *bcl-2* and *bax* gene families. In many human tumors, alterations in the expression of these genes, which occur as a regular feature of genetic instability, are intimately related to both their unregulated growth as well as their resistance to systemic treatment.

Drug Resistance

Antineoplastic chemotherapy is not uniformly successful because, as noted previously, many types of cancer in humans are either intrinsically resistant to treatment, acquire resistance during therapy, or because the chemotherapy cannot be successfully delivered in cytotoxic concentrations to the tumor. Mechanisms by which drug resistance can develop are, at least in part, specific to the mechanism of action of the class of agents being utilized. However, a wide variety of biochemical and physiologic phenomena have been observed either in vitro or in vivo that can modulate the effectiveness of several different antineoplastic drug classes. These include reduced drug uptake by the tumor cell; enhanced drug efflux; increased repair of drug-induced damage to DNA or other critical tumor cell targets; development of alternative routes for the synthesis of biologically important molecules when the primary synthetic pathway is blocked by a given drug; overexpression of the target gene product for a specific drug; production of an aberrant drug target that does not interact with a given agent, yet retains biochemical function sufficient to support tumor cell growth; enhanced intracellular metabolism or detoxification of the chemotherapeutic agent that limits tumor cell toxicity; overexpression or modification of cytoprotective gene products that alter tumor cell sensitivity to the anticancer agent; variations in the oxygenation state or blood supply of the tumor that can blunt the effectiveness of the drug directly or the delivery of the drug to the tumor itself; and factors in the normal tissues of the host that can significantly change the concentration of drug delivered to the tumor (such as alterations in renal or hepatic drug metabolism or variations in the tolerance of hematopoietic tissues to cytotoxic drug exposure).

Although the clinical relevance of each of these mechanisms is uncertain, samples of human tumors have been shown to express one or more of these phenotypic markers of drug resistance. As noted previously, the mutations that lead to expression of these characteristics occur *prior* to the recognition of a tumor and may become more prominent under the selective pressure of therapy. A tumor cell does not "begin" to express a resistance phenotype in the presence of a given drug; instead, cells with a particular phenotype emerge by a process of mutation/evolution and then are "selected" during therapy because cells lacking this phenotype are killed.

Drug Delivery and Dose Intensity

Certain characteristics of tumor masses can impede delivery of effective concentrations of drug to the entire tumor. A major impediment is size. Large tumor masses often contain areas of poorly vascularized tissue. Consequently, delivery of cytotoxic drugs to these areas of tumor via the blood will also be poor. The problem can be partially addressed by preferential administration of a drug to a region of the body involved by tumor. For example, infusion of agents metabolized by the liver directly into the hepatic artery permits the delivery of large concentrations of drug to the liver and tumors in the liver with limited exposure of the rest of the body to this same drug. Fluoropyrimidines (5-fluorouracil and 5-fluorodeoxyuridine) are the prototypical drugs that have a great pharmacologic advantage with hepatic artery infusion. Similarly, administration of drug directly into the peritoneum (cisplatin) or directly into the bladder (mitomycin C) allows for considerable local concentration of cytotoxic drug to tumors confined to those areas, with a much lower systemic exposure. Although the clinical utility of such regional approaches in curing cancer continues to be investigated, the pharmacologic advantage presented by this approach holds promise.

A corollary to the general problem of drug delivery is the issue of tumor sanctuaries. There are pharmacologically privileged sites in the body where tumor cells can lodge, but to which antineoplastic drugs cannot gain access. The blood–brain and the less well characterized blood–testis barriers are two clinically relevant examples. The blood–tissue barriers are constituted by components of vascular endothelium and basement membranes. The blood–brain barrier prevents large molecules and biologic agents from penetrating into the substance and supporting membranes of the brain. However, tumor can invade the blood–brain barrier and then spread within the substance of the brain or in the cerebrospinal fluid. This accounts for examples of central nervous system relapse of diseases such as acute lymphoid leukemia or small cell lung cancer despite complete suppression of systemic tumor growth by chemotherapy.

To the degree that first-order kinetics apply in humans, or at least that a dose–response relationship exists for many of the systemic agents in common clinical practice, the efficacy of treatment is likely to be enhanced if a higher dose of drug is administered. Considerable preclinical data and clinical experience support the hypothesis that maximally effective therapy is achieved if maximally tolerated or even supralethal doses of chemotherapy are administered. The most striking example of this concept is the success of very high doses of chemotherapy for acute myeloid leukemia and lymphomas, with subsequent reinfusion of allogeneic or autologous bone marrow cells to avert or reduce infectious complications of prolonged marrow aplasia. The hematopoietic growth factors further enhance the ability to give high-dose chemotherapy with a reduction in the time required for recovery of bone marrow function. With improvements in supportive care techniques and the development of hematopoietic growth factors, it is now possible to administer doses of cytotoxic drugs heretofore considered lethal. With this approach, tumor regression and long-term tumor-free survival may be seen in refractory hematopoietic malignancies and even some epithelial tumors. Although the optimal dose intensity for each human tumor and each clinical situation is not defined, it is clear that administration of maximally tolerated dose intensity is an important concept in cancer chemotherapy.

Host Factors

The success of systemic therapies for cancers is clearly linked to a number of factors specific to the host organism bearing the tumor. Among these factors are nutritional status, functional capabilities, and integrity of major organ systems. The effects of some of these factors on the success of chemotherapy are easily understood. For example, the ability of an individual to withstand the toxic side effects of a drug is linked to the reserve in the organ systems that might be targets of the toxicity of that drug. Patients with dysfunction of an organ necessary for the metabolism or excretion of a cytotoxic are likely to suffer more toxicity from that drug. The folate antagonist methotrexate is dependent on the kidney for excretion. Individuals with abnormal renal function suffer considerably more toxicity with methotrexate than do individuals with normal renal function. This toxicity is directly related to enhanced systemic exposure to methotrexate because of diminished clearance. Algorithms for adjusting dose to achieve a "normal" exposure in patients with abnormal renal or hepatic function are not generally available; however, as described later, knowledge of the pharmacokinetics and routes of metabolism and excretion of every antineoplastic is required so that dosages can be appropriately adjusted for each agent in patients with abnormal organ function who require therapy.

Less clear, but nonetheless important, are generalized host factors. The functional capability or performance status of a patient has been repeatedly shown to be of great prognostic importance in determining the outcome of systemic cancer treatment. Performance status is presumably a reflection of overall organ function integrity. Patients with poor performance status suffer greater toxicity with almost all forms of cancer therapy; they have shorter survival even when reasonable doses of therapy are administered and optimal supportive care is provided.

Multimodality Therapy

Over the past decade, it has become increasingly clear for the common solid tumors in humans that tumor destruction can be improved by the application of a number of modalities of therapy and that the judicious use of more than one modality is often important. The first clinical examples of this were obtained in pediatric oncology, where it was shown that the use of combination chemotherapy, surgical tumor removal, and local tumor site irradiation enhanced the cure of tumors such as Wilms' tumor, Ewing's sarcoma, and neuroblastoma. Application of these concepts in adult malignancies have been somewhat slower to develop but are now well established. The best example of the advantage of multimodality treatment in the treatment of adult malignancies is the clear demonstration of the importance of systemic therapy administered in concert with optimal local therapy for clinically localized breast cancer. For many years, it was known that women with breast tumors could be cured with surgical removal of the breast. However, it was also known that many women died despite removal of all visible tumor because of the presence of micrometastatic disease at the time of primary tumor treatment. The use of cytotoxic chemotherapy, hormonal therapy, or combinations of cytotoxic and hormonal therapy increases the cure rate in women with clinically localized breast cancer when such therapy is administered together with optimal local treatment of the primary tumor (irradiation or surgery). Such adjuvant chemotherapy has also now been demonstrated to increase cures in colorectal and ovarian cancers and lymphoma.

CHEMOTHERAPEUTIC DRUGS

Based on the fundamental principles of tumor cell biology and clinical pharmacology that form the basis for the rational use of systemic anticancer therapies, the choice of an appropriate chemotherapeutic agent is related to the inherent sensitivity of a specific disease to the various classes of drugs that are currently available and on the ability to administer these drugs either as single agents or in combination based on their combined toxicity for critical organ systems. The major classes of chemotherapeutic agents can be grouped by their underlying antineoplastic mechanism of action or source.

Alkylating Agents and Platinum Coordination Compounds

The first nonhormonal agents to be successfully utilized in the treatment of cancer were the alkylating agents, a large group of drugs with the ability to covalently bond DNA and other biologically significant molecules through an alkyl group consisting of one or more saturated carbon atoms. The common features of these compounds is that they are composed of mono- or bifunctional alkyl groups linked to a core structure that confers pharmacologic and toxicologic differences on the alkylating moieties. The simplest backbone for a bifunctional alkylating agent is that of nitrogen mustard (HN_2, mechlorethamine) which consists of a nitrogen atom (as NCH_3) linked to two chloroethyl groups. By contrast, L-phenylalanine mustard (LPAM; melphalan) consists of the same bifunctional alkylating groups attached to the L-phenylalanine molecule; chlorambucil, cyclophosphamide, and ifosfamide are three other clinically useful alkylating agents in which other side chains have been substituted for the methyl group in HN_2. These four drugs have replaced nitrogen mustard in common clinical practice; cyclophosphamide and ifosfamide are distinct among this class of drugs because they require activation by hepatic microsomal enzyme systems to specific, short-lived metabolites that produce their cytotoxic action.

The common mechanistic feature of the alkylating agents is that, upon entering cells, the alkyl groups bind to electrophilic sites in DNA and other biologically active molecules; bifunctional alkylation of DNA can result in crosslinks between strands of DNA, which impedes replication. Other biochemically important molecules are also alkylated by such agents, but the dominant effect seems to be DNA crosslinking.

Both cyclophosphamide and chlorambucil are orally bioavailable and are used both intravenously and by mouth; melphalan and HN_2 because of either variable bioavailability or chemical reactivity are best utilized by the intravenous route. Except for the requirement for hepatic metabolism of cyclophosphamide, which prolongs its primary elimination as well as the disappearance of its metabolites ($\approx$ 8 h), the elimination of the alkylating agents is rapid ($<$ 2 hours) in the blood owing to chemical decomposition.

The toxicity of alkylating agents is primarily hematopoietic. Some alkylating agents have more prominent effects on granulocytes (HN_2); with other agents, platelet toxicity may be more pronounced (melphalan) although granulocytopenia occurs often; hematologic toxicity is most frequently observed 8 to 14 days after drug administration. In addition to hematologic toxicity, the cyclophosphamide metabolite acrolein can irritate the bladder mucosa, requiring strict attention to hydration and urine flow for its safe use; and ifosfamide metabolites, in addition to irritating the bladder, may produce renal tubular injury. All of the alkylating agents can produce alopecia, nausea, and vomiting, as well as gastrointestinal mucosal damage, gonadal dysfunction, and infertility. These agents are also those most closely associated with treatment-related second malignancies. Clear-cut evidence connects alkylating agents with the development of secondary leukemias, the frequency of which is related to the amount of alkylating agent received. The presumed mechanism of this effect is damage to normal bone marrow stem cells resulting in mutagenic changes.

Alkylating agents are among the most widely used antineoplastics and form an important part of curative therapy regimens for Hodgkin's disease and non-Hodgkin's lymphoma as well as important surgical adjuvant regimens for breast cancer. Alkylating agents are also the class of drugs whose doses can be most readily escalated, as well as the class with the steepest dose–response curves in vitro. Thus, these drugs are frequently employed as part of high-dose chemotherapy regimens administered with autologous or allogeneic bone marrow support.

There are several other families of alkylating drugs in which the classic nitrogen mustard backbone has been altered. The nitrosoureas are bifunctional alkylating agents linked to a nitrosourea moiety. Nitrosoureas are lipid soluble and appear to be among the most effective agents for use in central nervous system (CNS) tumors. It is believed that their lipid solubility enhances penetration through the blood–brain barrier and hence delivery into the CNS. These agents have a unique pattern of toxicity for normal tissues, although their mechanism of tumor cell killing seems to be DNA crosslinking like the more classic alkylating agents. Nitrosoureas tend to exert their most pronounced toxic effects on the hematopoietic system at a later time than do classic alkylating agents. Following nitrosourea therapy with carmustine (bis-chloroethylnitrosourea, BCNU) for example, the nadir of myelosuppression occurs at day 30 to 36 although drug disappearance from the circulation is rapid; further, nitrosoureas appear to have the ability to damage bone marrow stem cells more effectively than other classic alkylating agents. Nitrosoureas are also associated with pulmonary interstitial fibrosis more commonly than other alkylating agents and can produce cumulative renal injury. Other alkylating species in clinical practice include busulfan, an alkane sulfonate widely used for the treatment of chronic myelogenous leukemia; and dacarbazine (DTIC), which methylates as well as binds to DNA and is used to treat soft tissue sarcomas and malignant melanoma.

The serendipitous finding that platinum salts were toxic to bacteria led to the discovery that such salts are also quite effective antineoplastic agents. The prototype platinum coordination complex is the drug cisplatin (*cis*-diamminedichloroplatinum II). This rather simple molecule exerts effects similar to those of the alkylating agents. The chloride groups on cisplatin are labile and, in biologic systems, the sites on the platinum atom previously occupied by the chloride groups can be covalently linked to biologically important macromolecules. The primary target for cisplatin damage in proliferating cells is DNA. "Platinated" DNA contains intra- and interstrand crosslinks that disrupt DNA function and replication. The clearance of cisplatin is primarily through endogenous inactivation via binding to biologic macromolecules, including protein sulfhydryls and the half-life of the unchanged parent molecule in the plasma is short; hepatic metabolism and renal excretion play little role in the drug's elimination. The toxicity of cisplatin can be significant; severe nausea and vomiting, renal tubular impairment, damage to cochlear hair cells with high-frequency hearing loss, and peripheral nerve damage resulting in a sensorimotor neuropathy can accompany treatment. However, careful attention to enhanced intravenous hydration and urine output can largely ameliorate the nephrotoxicity of cisplatin; and the recent development of improved antiemetic regimens has dramatically reduced the emetogenic side effects of cisplatin administration. On the other hand, the myelotoxicity of cisplatin is modest. The introduction of cisplatin into oncologic therapeutics has led to a remarkable change in the therapy of disseminated testicular germ cell cancer (significantly increasing the curability of this disease), as well as the management of advanced ovarian, small cell and non-small-cell lung cancers, and squamous cancers of the head and neck.

Carboplatin (diammine 1,1-cyclobutanedicarboxylatoplatinum II) is an analogue of cisplatin in which the two chloride ligands are replaced by the carboxylate moiety. The DNA crosslinking species formed by carboplatin are identical to those formed with cisplatin, but the pharmacokinetics and spectrum of toxicity of this analogue are markedly different. The half-life of carboplatin is more prolonged (4 to 6 hours) than cisplatin, and the disposition of carboplatin is determined primarily by renal excretion. Carboplatin is substantially less toxic to the kidneys and has a lesser propensity for causing nausea and vomiting. Similarly, no neurotoxicity is seen except at high doses of carboplatin. Unlike cisplatin, carboplatin is a potent bone-marrow-suppressing agent. Platelets are more affected than are granulocytes. Generally speaking, carboplatin appears equivalent to cisplatin in terms of antitumor activity, except for the treatment of germ cell malignancies. The precise dose equivalents of these two drugs are uncertain, however. Further, in combination chemotherapy, carboplatin presents the problem of myelosuppression, generally requiring dose reduction of both carboplatin and other myelosuppressive agents used at the same time.

Antimetabolites

A substantial group of highly effective chemotherapeutic drugs disrupt the intermediary metabolism of malignant cells. These compounds can inhibit important enzyme targets or serve as psuedosubstrates, resulting in the incorporation of a "fraudulent" component into biologically active molecules. Several antimetabolites are widely used as part of curative chemotherapeutic regimens for the treatment of childhood malignancies, the acute leukemias and lymphomas, and for the palliation of patients with common solid tumors.

Methotrexate   Methotrexate is the most widely used folate antagonist and was the prototype of the antimetabolite class, first developed for the treatment of childhood leukemias in the late 1940s as structural analogues of folic acid. Methotrexate binds to and inhibits the enzyme dihydrofolate reductase (DHFR). DHFR is necessary for the genesis of reduced folates that serve as sources of methyl groups for the synthesis of thymidine and other biologically important molecules critical for DNA replication. Methotrexate is water soluble and is cleared by glomerular filtration with a terminal half-life of 8 h. Impaired renal function can considerably alter the pharmacokinetics and toxicity of methotrexate. Because methotrexate impairs the genesis of reduced folates, methotrexate toxicity and efficacy can, in part, be inhibited by the concomitant administration of exogenous reduced folates, such as leucovorin (citrovorum factor). However, when the toxic effects of methotrexate such as renal dysfunction, myelosuppression, or mucositis have become clinically evident, reduced folates play little role in their resolution. Methotrexate is a drug with broad activity in the treatment of acute lymphocytic leukemia (ALL), breast cancer, and head and neck cancer.

Fluoropyrimidines   The fluoropyrimidines 5-fluorouracil (5-FU) and 5-fluorodeoxyuridine (FUdR), after metabolic conversion and in the presence of reduced folates, bind to the DNA synthetic enzyme thymidylate synthase in the place of the normal substrate, uracil. Formation of a covalent complex between the fluoropyrimidine metabolite, fluorodeoxyuridylate, reduced folate, and thymidylate synthase inactivates the enzyme. Fluoropyrimidines can also be directly incorporated into RNA in place of uracil, leading to impaired RNA processing. Fluoropyrimidines are cleared rapidly by hepatic metabolism, principally by the enzyme dihydropyrimidine dehydrogenase (DPD) with a half-life in the plasma of 10 to 15 min; the large capacity of the liver to detoxify these drugs provides a pharmacologic advantage when they are infused directly into the liver (high local drug concentration with modest or no systemic drug exposure and toxicity). Hepatic artery infusion of fluoropyrimidines is modestly successful in the treatment of hepatic metastases from colorectal cancer. Recently, patients with partial or complete deficiencies of DPD have been described; these individuals are at markedly increased risk of developing severe side effects after treatment with a fluoropyrimidine. The toxicity of the fluoropyrimidines is manifested as reversible, usually mild myelosuppression, and potentially more severe diarrhea and stomatitis, with very occasional cerebellar dysfunction and minimal alopecia, principally occurring 8 to 14 days after completion of therapy. Fluoropyrimidines are important components of combination regimens utilized for breast cancer and are the most active compounds for the treatment of a wide variety of gastrointestinal malignancies. Because the binding of fluoropyrimidines to thymidylate synthase can be enhanced by increasing intracellular concentrations of reduced folates, the combination of 5-FU and leucovorin was evaluated and has been shown to be one of the most active regimens for the treatment of colorectal cancer in both the advanced disease and adjuvant settings. Treatment with this combination, however, is associated with an increased risk of severe mucositis or diarrhea.

Cytosine Arabinoside   Cytosine arabinoside (Ara-C) is a "fraudulent" nucleoside consisting of the purine cytosine linked to the sugar arabinose; arabinose does not occur normally in man. Cytosine arabinoside is metabolized by enzymes necessary for the synthesis of cytosine triphosphate (CTP), which is incorporated into DNA. Incorporation of the fraudulent base Ara-CTP inhibits DNA replication and repair, and leads to impaired cellular proliferation, in part through the induction of apoptosis. The efficacy of Ara-C is directly related to the rate of formation of Ara-CTP, a process that can be enhanced by administering the drug in a high dose. Cytosine arabinoside is rapidly catabolized in the liver, peripheral tissues, and serum by the enzyme cytidine deaminase with a terminal half-life of 2 h. The major toxicities of Ara-C are bone marrow suppression, stomatitis, and intrahepatic cholestasis. At high doses of Ara-C, CNS toxicity consisting of disorientation, cerebellar dysfunction, and coma may result. The primary use of Ara-C is in the treatment of acute myelogenous leukemia (AML).

Gemcitabine   Gemcitabine (2′ 2′-difluorodeoxycytidine; dFdC) is a new cytidine analogue that, like Ara-C, is activated by deoxycytidine kinase and detoxified by cytidine deaminase. The mechanism of action of gemcitabine also depends on incorporation of its major intracellular metabolite into DNA. However, gemcitabine is also a potent inhibitor of ribonucleotide reductase, which leads to a decrease in all intracellular deoxynucleotide triphosphates, and, unlike Ara-C, an inhibitor of deoxycitidine deaminase that decreases the breakdown of its intracellular metabolites. Despite these known differences, a clear explanation for the different antineoplastic spectrum of action of gemcitabine, compared to Ara-C, remains to be determined. The dose-limiting toxicity of gemcitabine is myelosuppression with neutropenia occurring more frequently than thrombocytopenia. Fever, skin rash, and flulike symptoms may occur. Gemcitabine has been shown to improve the quality of life of patients with advanced pancreatic cancer and has a palliative benefit in the treatment of non-small-cell lung cancer, ovarian cancer, and breast cancer.

Antitumor Antibiotics

Actinomycin D   Actinomycin D is a byproduct of a species of *Streptomyces*; it is actively used for the treatment of childhood malignancies, particularly soft tissue sarcomas and neuroblastoma. The mechanism of action of actinomycin D is inhibition of RNA and protein synthesis that occurs after DNA intercalation, RNA chain elongation being principally affected. The drug is excreted in part by the kidney and into the bile as the unchanged parent molecule with a long terminal half-life of over 30 h. The major toxicities of actinomycin D are myelosuppression, which may be severe; alopecia; nausea and vomiting; diarrhea and mucositis; and the potential for extravasation injury if the drug leaks from a vein into the surrounding soft tissues.

Mitomycin C   Mitomycin C was also isolated from a species of *Streptomyces* yeast. It is a unique molecule that combines quinone and aziridine moieties that both play important roles in its reductive intracellular activation to a potent alkylating species, as well as in the generation of reactive oxygen molecules. Under hypoxic conditions, reductive alkylation appears to be responsible for tumor cell killing. Mitomycin C is metabolized by the liver, and excreted in part by the kidney with a terminal half-life of 30 to 60 min. Its major toxicities include myelosuppression (which may be delayed up to 4 to 5 weeks after treatment), alopecia and stomatitis, hemolytic-uremic syndrome, extravasation injury, and the exacerbation of anthracycline cardiac toxicity. The major therapeutic role of mitomycin C is in the treatment of superficial bladder cancer where it is administered by direct instillation, and for the palliative therapy of gastrointestinal, breast, and non-small-cell lung cancers.

Bleomycin   Bleomycin is a complex mixture of peptides isolated from the *Streptomyces verticillus* fungus that plays an important role in the treatment of testicular germ cell neoplasms and non-Hodgkin's lymphoma. Bleomycin has a unique mechanism of tumor cell killing that involves the formation of a metal–bleomycin complex, which rapidly binds oxygen; the activated metal (usually ferrous iron)–oxygen–bleomycin complex is stabilized by and actively cleaves DNA, producing both single- and double-strand breaks. The drug is metabolized by a hydrolase that is found in both normal and malignant cells but in low concentration in skin and in the lung, two organs that are particularly sensitive to bleomycin. Bleomycin is excreted in the urine with an elimination half-life in plasma of approximately 3 h; the pharmacokinetics of the drug are markedly altered in patients with abnormal renal function. Bleomycin produces little myelosuppression, but its administration is frequently associated with fever and occasionally with an acute allergic reaction. The major side effect of bleomycin is a cumulative pulmonary toxicity the etiology of which remains unclear; however, the clinical picture of bleomycin-induced lung damage is well known and is characterized by nonproductive cough and shortness of breath, with minimal findings on physical examination, and occasionally a patchy interstitial infiltrate on chest X-ray film. Pulmonary function studies demonstrate a reduced diffusion capacity especially in patients with a total dose of more than 240 mg. Discontinuation of the drug may lead to complete resolution of signs and symptoms of respiratory compromise over a period of months to years; however, all patients previously exposed to bleomycin are at risk of developing acute respiratory failure postoperatively if exposed to high oxygen tensions during the induction of anesthesia.

Topoisomerase Inhibitors and Agents with Pleiotropic Mechanisms of Action

Anthracyclines   The anthracyclines doxorubicin and daunorubicin were also isolated from *Streptomyces* species and thus are antitumor antibiotics. However, these drugs interact significantly with a wide range of biochemical systems in tumor cells; many of these interactions contribute to their broad antineoplastic activity. Anthracyclines appear to exert their antiproliferative activity, at least in part, by the following mechanisms: binding to the nuclear enzyme topoisomerase II to form a "cleavable complex" that interferes with the ability of the enzyme to reduce torsional strain in DNA; the generation of reactive oxygen species that interfere with mitochondrial function and that of other critical macromolecules; and activation of signal transduction pathways ultimately leading to the stimulation of apoptosis. The pharmacokinetics of doxorubicin and daunorubicin, as well as epirubicin, the anthracycline analogue most frequently used in Europe, demonstrate triexponential decay with a long terminal half-life in plasma of approximately 10 h. All of the anthracyclines are metabolized primarily by the liver and excreted, in part, into the bile; individuals with liver dysfunction may exhibit considerably enhanced anthracycline toxicity because of delayed drug clearance. The toxicity profile of anthracyclines includes myelosuppression and damage to oral and gastrointestinal mucosa, resulting in stomatitis and diarrhea. Alopecia is a universal accompaniment of anthracycline administration. The anthracycline antibiotics are also potent vesicants; extravasation of these agents into soft tissues results in extensive necrosis and soft tissue damage. Consequently, great care must be exercised when anthracyclines are administered intravenously. Continuous infusion must be done through indwelling central venous catheters. A unique toxicity of the anthracyclines is cumulative, dose-dependent myocardial damage. Recent studies that have employed either gated cardiac blood pool scanning or endomyocardial biopsy as endpoints for functional or histologic confirmation of doxorubicin cardiac toxicity have demonstrated that the incidence of measurable heart damage begins to climb precipitously above a cumulative dose of 350 to 400 mg/m^2 if the drug has been administered by short intravenous infusion. Thus, in patients who begin therapy with normal cardiac function, several months of anthracycline can be administered with low risk of myocardial dysfunction. However, in individuals who have a history of hypertensive heart disease or prior left chest wall irradiation, the maximum safe dose of doxorubicin may be substantially lower. Data indicate that infusional therapy with anthracyclines (e.g., 96-h continuous infusion) allows a higher cumulative dose to be administered with diminished risk of cardiac toxicity. A novel agent that appears to significantly ameliorate doxorubicin cardiac toxicity, dexrazoxane, has recently come into clinical practice. Anthracyclines have a broad range of antineoplastic activity and form an important component of combination therapies for non-Hodgkin's lymphoma and Hodgkin's disease, breast cancer, osteogenic sarcoma, and a variety of pediatric solid tumors. Daunorubicin and doxorubicin are also among the most active drugs for the treatment of lymphoid and myeloid leukemias.

Podophyllotoxins   Podophyllotoxin derivatives have been known for many years to possess antiproliferative effects. Etoposide (VP 16) and teniposide (VM 26) are the two podophyllotoxin derivatives now commonly used in clinical oncologic practice. These agents exert their anticancer activity through interaction with the enzyme topoisomerase II (topo II), which facilitates the uncoiling of DNA prior to DNA replication. VP 16 and VM 26 are metabolized by the liver; about 40% of a dose of etoposide is excreted by the kidney. The terminal half-lives of both drugs are from 8 to 10 h in plasma after intravenous administration. VP 16 is the most frequently used podophyllotoxin and can be administered either intravenously or orally. Recent data suggest that continuous low-dose oral VP-16 might be active when intermittent schedules have failed. The toxicity of these agents is primarily leukopenia and thrombocytopenia, as well as mild to moderate alopecia; at high doses stomatitis occurs. Because the primary toxicity of VP 16 is hematopoietic, it has frequently been used in high-dose regimens requiring bone marrow reconstitution. A recently recognized late effect of VP 16 is the development of secondary leukemia. VP 16 is active in germ cell tumors, small cell and non-small-cell carcinoma of the lung, Hodgkin's and non-Hodgkin's lymphoma, and myeloid and lymphoid leukemia.

Camptothecins   Camptothecin and its derivatives are active cytotoxics that kill tumor cells through inhibition of the nuclear enzyme topoisomerase I, a distinct 100-kDa protein that, like topoisomerase II, plays a critical role in relieving torsional strain in DNA during replication; however, unlike topoisomerase II, the nuclear content of topoisomerase I does not vary significantly with the cell cycle. It has been postulated that this difference is important for explaining the activity of the topoisomerase I inhibitors in tumors with low growth fractions. The camptothecin derivatives topotecan and irinotecan (CPT-11) have now been introduced into clinical practice for the treatment of advanced ovarian and colorectal cancer, respectively. Topotecan is metabolized by a nonenzymatic process that produces a carboxylated derivative that is less active; about one third of the drug is excreted into the urine. The major toxicity of topotecan is myelosuppression, especially neutropenia, which occurs approximately 10 days after administration. Topotecan has demonstrated moderate activity in patients with platinum-refractory ovarian cancer. Irinotecan is a prodrug that requires side chain cleavage by an esterase to produce its active metabolite SN-38; like topotecan, both irinotecan and SN-38 undergo hydrolysis of the lactone to produce a carboxylate metabolite. Whereas the excretion of the irinotecan parent drug is into the urine and bile, SN-38 is excreted by several mechanisms into the bile. In addition to neutropenia, treatment with irinotecan can produce two forms of diarrhea that may be dose-limiting. The early type of diarrhea, which occurs within hours of drug administration, is probably cholinergic, and is associated with cramping and diaphoresis; it can be prevented by pretreatment with atropine. A more difficult to control, late-onset diarrhea is frequently seen after the second or third weekly dose of irinotecan; it can produce dehydration if not aggressively managed with loperamide and fluid replacement. Irinotecan clearly can produce objective remissions in patients with fluoropyrimidine-refractory colorectal cancer.

Antimicrotubule Agents

Vinca Alkaloids   Derivatives of the periwinkle plant (*Vinca rosea*) were among the earliest antineoplastics discovered. The two most commonly utilized vinca alkaloids are vincristine and vinblastine. These drugs are complex molecules whose mechanism of action is based on disruption of microtubular function through microtubular aggregation. This results in disruption of the formation of the mitotic spindle and inhibition of cells progressing through the cell cycle at the stage of mitosis. Vinca alkaloids are metabolized primarily by the liver and their toxicity is considerably enhanced in individuals with severe hepatic dysfunction. The primary toxicity of vincristine is neurologic. Vincristine administration results in peripheral neuropathy and ileus. Ileus is thought to be due to damage to autonomic nerves supplying the gastrointestinal tract; peripheral neuropathies are related to nerve damage associated with microtubular disruption. Vinca alkaloids are components of effective combination therapies for a wide variety of tumors. They are most active in hematologic malignancies and germ cell tumors. Activity in breast cancer, small cell lung cancer, and non-small-cell lung cancer is limited but real. The primary toxicity of vinblastine is myelosuppression affecting both granulocytes and platelets. Neuropathy is an uncommon side effect of vinblastine administration.

Taxanes   Paclitaxel is the lead compound in the taxane class of antimicrotubule agents; it was originally isolated from the bark of the Pacific yew, *Taxus brevifolia*, but is now available from semisynthetic approaches. This agent has a wide spectrum of antineoplastic activity and a unique mechanism of cytotoxicity. Paclitaxel interacts with microtubules, but rather than inhibiting their formation as the vinca alkaloids do, paclitaxel stabilizes microtubules and inhibits their dissolution, upsetting the dynamic balance between microtubular formation and dissolution upon which many intracellular processes are dependent. The most obviously affected process is mitosis. Although both paclitaxel and vinca alkaloids inhibit microtubular function, cells resistant to one class of drugs are not always resistant to the other. Paclitaxel is cleared primarily by the liver; dose adjustment is required for patients with moderate elevations of hepatic enzymes. The primary toxicities of paclitaxel are myelosuppression and peripheral neuropathy. Toxicities of paclitaxel that complicated its development are hypotension and anaphylactoid reactions, which appear to be related to the vehicle (Cremophor-EL) in which paclitaxel is prepared; the hypersensitivity reactions have been averted by pretreatment with antihistamines and corticosteroids. Paclitaxel is active in refractory ovarian cancer and in small cell and non-small-cell lung cancer and breast cancer.

The taxane analogue docetaxel is a product of semisynthetic approaches to synthesis. Docetaxel shares the hepatic metabolism of paclitaxel but interacts differently with cells based on their level of *bcl-2* phosphorylation; this may explain the partial lack of cross-reactivity of docetaxel and paclitaxel. Docetaxel is very active in the treatment of breast, lung, and ovarian cancer. Because of its enhanced solubility, it is not prepared in the same vehicle as paclitaxel and thus does not produce the same incidence of immediate hypersensitivity reactions although they do occur; however, unlike paclitaxel, docetaxel can produce a capillary leak syndrome characterized by peripheral edema, ascites or pleural effusion, and weight gain observed in patients treated with cumulative doses >400 mg/m^2. Premedication with dexamethasone can decrease the severity and delay the onset of this syndrome.

Hormonal Agents

Beatson demonstrated in 1895 that oophorectomy would slow the progression of breast cancer. Since that observation, a variety of hormonal agents have been proven to be useful in the therapy of human cancers. The mechanisms by which hormonal therapy can favorably affect the growth of cancers may depend upon withdrawal or inhibition of secretion of endogenous hormones necessary for the sustenance of the growth of the cancer (e.g., estrogens, androgens), or by direct interference with the biochemical effects of endogenous hormones.

Estrogens, progestins, and androgens derived from the ovaries have been shown to be important in the progression of breast cancer and endometrial cancer. Removal of the ovaries or suppression of their function through the administration of gonadotropin-releasing hormone (GNRH) agonists play a role in the suppression of those cancers. Prostate cancer and breast cancer in the male are dependent upon the secretion of androgens from the testes. Orchiectomy or inhibition of testicular antigen synthesis through the use of luteinizing hormone-releasing hormone (LH-RH) analogues play an important role in the control of those cancers.

Adrenal-derived androgens and estrogens appear to be important in supporting the growth of prostate cancer and breast cancer. A number of agents such as aminoglutethimide (AG) and ketoconazole have been shown to inhibit enzymes necessary for the synthesis of adrenal androgens and estrogens. In addition, AG and other newer aromatase inhibitors such as anastrazole alter the peripheral conversion of androgens to estrogens (aromatization); because of the enhanced tolerance of the newer aromatase inhibitors, they have become important additions to the hormonal management of advanced breast cancer.

Another class of hormonal agents were originally classified as "antihormones." Tamoxifen, which is a nonsteroidal antiestrogen, and flutamide, a nonsteroidal antiandrogen, are the prototypes of this class of compounds. They exert their antiproliferative effects by a variety of mechanisms including, in the case of tamoxifen, alterations in the activation of the estrogen receptor gene, blockade of estrogen-stimulated progesterone receptor synthesis, and stimulation of other growth-regulating gene products such as transforming growth factor beta. Tamoxifen has been proven to be safe and beneficial in both the surgical adjuvant therapy of breast cancer and in the treatment of advanced disease. It is currently being evaluated as a chemopreventive agent for women at high risk for developing breast cancer. Tamoxifen, however, possesses both agonist and antagonist effects; while blocking the effects of estrogen on the breast, it is an estrogen mimic with respect to the uterus. This can lead to hyperplasia and an increased risk of endometrial cancer after long-term tamoxifen exposure. Other side effects include weight gain, hot flashes, and an increased risk of deep venous thrombosis. Flutamide competes with natural androgen for binding to the androgen receptor. Flutamide is a modestly active agent in advanced prostate cancer; it is sometimes used in combination with either orchiectomy or LH-RH analogues in a so-called total androgen deprivation approach to the treatment of prostate cancer. The superiority of this approach over orchiectomy alone for advanced prostate cancer remains unclear.

Progestational agents are also effective in some forms of cancer. Endometrial cancer is suppressed in 40% to 50% of cases by exogenous administration of progesterone or progesterone analogues. Progestational agents are also effective in advanced breast cancer, particularly in women whose tumors have previously responded to hormonal manipulation; these agents also have some activity in advanced prostate cancer. Although the cytotoxic mechanism of action of progestins is unclear, these drugs produce a characteristic spectrum of toxicity including weight gain, fluid retention, hot flashes, cholestasis, and an increased risk of thromboembolic events.

BIOLOGIC RESPONSE MODIFIERS

As our understanding of the immune system has advanced, the use of molecules with the ability to modulate activities based on immune function has become a reality. In the last decade, two classes of compounds have emerged that have been clearly shown to play a role in the therapy of some human tumors.

Interferons

The interferons are a class of compounds produced normally by human cells. Their major role was initially thought to be in the defense of cells against viral infections. There are three major types of interferons (INF-α, -β, and -γ). These compounds are biochemically and biologically different; the spectrum of their biologic effects is enormous including a complex array of immunologic effects, antiangiogenesis, and cell cycle regulation. INF-α is the most widely tested and has clear activity in hairy cell leukemia, chronic myelogenous leukemia (CML), multiple myeloma, and certain non-Hodgkin's lymphomas. INF-α also has limited but real activity in renal cell carcinoma, melanoma, Kaposi's sarcoma, and carcinoid tumors. The side effects of treatment with INF-α include fever, chills, and myalgias acutely, and anorexia and fatigue with chronic administration.

Interleukins

Interleukin 2 (IL-2) is the second biologic response modifier to clearly show clinical anticancer activity. The major biologic effects of IL-2, originally identified as a T cell growth factor, appear to be dependent upon the support of T cell proliferation. When administered alone or in combination with autologous T cells expanded in vitro, IL-2 has considerable antiproliferative activity in a number of preclinical systems. IL-2 has limited but real activity against renal cell carcinoma and is the only agent capable of producing long-lived remissions of disseminated metastases in that disease. IL-2 also can produce clinical remissions in patients with malignant melanoma. However, when administered in an intermittent high-dose schedule as originally developed, IL-2 produces significant side effects including hypotension, oliguria, dermatitis, and a potentially severe capillary leak syndrome. Even at lower doses, IL-2 therapy must be administered under careful supervision.

Hematopoietic Growth Factors

A group of substances normally secreted by lymphocytes and macrophages has proven to be useful in reducing side effects of cytotoxic chemotherapy. These substances are the hematopoietic growth factors. Granulocyte–macrophage colony-stimulating factor (GM-CSF), granulocyte colony-stimulating factor (G-CSF), and erythropoietin (EPO) are normally produced by cells of the macrophage–lymphocyte system (especially G-CSF) or renal tubular cells (especially EPO). These compounds are critical for the stimulation of granulocyte and macrophage maturation (G-CSF, GM-CSF) or erythrocyte formation. It is clearly demonstrable that G-CSF and GM-CSF will hasten recovery of granulocyte suppression following cytotoxic chemotherapy. These drugs permit more rapid hematologic reconstitution following high-dose chemotherapy and bone marrow transplantation; their use with more standard doses of chemotherapy has also been shown to reduce duration of neutropenia and hospitalization. Administration of EPO, for example, which is effective in stimulating red cell production, will raise hemoglobin concentrations suppressed by cytotoxic chemotherapy. This may reduce the need for blood transfusion and may be a useful addition to the agents available for the support of patients undergoing cancer therapy. A major continuing problem is thrombocytopenia that occurs following cytotoxic therapy. Recombinant human thrombopoietin is currently undergoing active clinical investigation for the amelioration of chemotherapy-induced thrombocytopenia.

SUMMARY

The use of systemic cancer treatment includes drugs that are directly cytotoxic to tumor cells by a wide variety of different mechanisms, compounds that may affect the hormonal milieu in which the tumor proliferates, or biologic agents that enhance the patient's immunologic response to the tumor. The use of each of these classes of systemic therapies provides curative treatment options for patients with several forms of disseminated hematologic malignancies as well as postsurgical adjunctive therapy that improves the cure rate for early stages of breast, ovarian, and colorectal cancer; and effective palliative treatment for all of the common solid tumors in humans. Systemic cancer treatments can best be understood through an appreciation of several critical concepts in tumor biology that form the foundation of Medical Oncology as well as an understanding of the clinical and molecular pharmacology of the specific drugs currently in use.

FURTHER READING

Chabner BA, Longo DL (eds.) (1996) *Cancer Chemotherapy and Biotherapy: Principles and Practice*. Lippincott–Raven, Philadelphia.

Goldie JH, Coldman AJ, Gudanskas GA (1982) Rationale for the use of alternating non-cross-resistant chemotherapy. *Cancer Treat Rep* 66(3): 439–449.

Hryniuk W, Bush H (1984) The importance of dose intensity in chemotherapy of metastatic breast cancer. *J Clin Oncol* 2: 1281–1288.

Lowe SW, Ruley HE, Jacks T, Housman DE (1993) p53-dependent apoptosis modulates the cytotoxicity of anticancer agents. *Cell* 74: 957–967.

Moscow JA, Cowan KH (1988) Multidrug resistance. *J Natl Cancer Inst* 80: 14–20.

Pommier Y (1993) DNA topoisomerase I and II in cancer chemotherapy: update and perspectives. *Cancer Chemother Pharmacol* 32: 103–108.

Ratain MJ, Schilsky RL, Conley BA, Egorin MJ (1990) Pharmacodynamics in cancer therapy. *J Clin Oncol* 8: 1739–1753.

Schilsky RL, Ratain MJ, Milano GA (eds.) (1996) *Principles of Antineoplastic Drug Development and Pharmacology*, Marcel Dekker, New York.

Schnipper LE (1986) Clinical implications of tumor-cell heterogeneity. *N Engl J Med* 314: 1423–1431.

CHAPTER 14

BONE MARROW TRANSPLANTATION

GEORGE SOMLO

Medical Oncology Department
City of Hope National Medical Center
Duarte, CA 91010

Bone marrow transplantation (BMT) is a therapeutic procedure consisting of procurement of approximately 500 to 1000 ml (2 to 3×10^8 nucleated marrow cells/kg of recipient body weight) of bone marrow followed by intravenous reinfusion into the recipient. Bone marrow is aspirated from the posterior iliac crests either under general or epidural anesthesia. The marrow suspension contains hematopoietic progenitor cells characterized by the presence of the CD34 surface antigen, as well as their committed progeny, stromal supportive elements, and other regulatory/facilitating components such as the T lymphocytes. Following procurement the marrow is placed in a container of tissue culture medium and heparin and is filtered through stainless steel screens. The bone marrow is usually reinfused shortly after procurement although it can be frozen for future use.

Allogeneic BMT most frequently involves removal of bone marrow from a human leukocyte antigen (HLA) matched sibling donor. Two sets of HLA antigens of class I (A and B loci) and II (HLA DR) group (three loci each inherited on chromosome 6 from each parent, totaling six loci) need to be identical in the donor and recipient for a perfect 6/6 histocompatible match. Serologic testing, and more recently, molecular methods such as PCR amplification of HLA genes and the use of allele-specific or sequence specific oligonucleotides, are available to define the suitability of an allogeneic donor.

Syngeneic BMT implies BMT between an identical twin donor and recipient; partially matched (5/6, one HLA antigen mismatch) donor marrow from a parent or other family members can also be used as the source of stem cells for BMT. The probability of finding a matched related sibling donor within one's family depends

Manual of Clinical Oncology, 7th edition, Edited by Raphael E. Pollock
ISBN 0-471-23828-7, pages 293–305. Copyright © 1999 Wiley-Liss, Inc.

on the number of siblings and may be as low as 25% (in the case of two siblings) and greater than 90% in families with five or more siblings.

With the availability of millions of potential volunteer donors in the International Donor Registry, candidates for BMT may find a suitable donor by searching the registry computer files. The feasibility of BMT from an unrelated donor is then verified by serologic and molecular confirmation of a histocompatible 6/6 or 5/6 HLA-A, B, and DR match. At present, the timely availability of a suitable unrelated donor depends greatly on the ethnicity and social background of the recipient. Efforts to expand the pool by including previously underrepresented categories of donors are ongoing worldwide.

Hematopoietic progenitor cells are also present in peripheral blood, although their number is relatively low at 1%, compared to the 3% to 5% estimate in the bone marrow. The population of CD34 antigen positive progenitors contains the very early hematopoietic progenitor cells (stem cells) capable of repopulating the ablated bone marrow as well as generating and maintaining long-term hematopoiesis. These peripheral blood progenitor stem cells (PBPC) can be collected by a cell separator. The procedure (leukapheresis, or apheresis) usually takes 3 to 4 hours and is repeated daily until the targeted number of cells (the recommended minimum is $\geq 2 \times 10^6$ CD34$^+$ cells/kg of recipient body weight) have been procured and cryopreserved. To improve the yield and quality of the PBPC product, the donor undergoes "priming" or "mobilization" by receiving subcutaneous or intravenous injections of the cytokines G-CSF or GM-CSF for several days prior to, and during, the days of PBPC collection. The efficacy and safety of allogeneic PBPC in comparison to BMT from either related or unrelated donors are at present the subject of ongoing randomized trials.

Another promising and relatively rich source of allogeneic hematopoietic stem cells is umbilical cord blood. Cryopreserved cord blood from a fully or partially matched, related, or unrelated donor provides a potentially unlimited source of transplantable cells. At present, the relatively small volume of cord blood makes this source available mostly for pediatric recipients. Ex vivo expansion may render this type of transplant more universally available in the future.

Autologous BMT and PBPC Transplant

During this procedure the patient's own bone marrow and /or PBPC are procured and are cryopreserved for future use. The target number of nucleated and CD34$^+$ cells/kg of patient body weight are the same as for patients undergoing allogeneic BM or PBPC transplants. Priming/mobilization with the hematopoietic growth factors G-CSF or GM-CSF improves the quality of PBPC products dramatically and accelerates granulocyte and platelet recovery following PBPC reinfusion in comparison to autologous BMT. To avoid reinfusion of potentially tumor-contaminated BM or PBPC grafts, several methods of positive and/or negative selection have been undergoing clinical testing. Negative selection via chemical, and immunologic (removal of CD8 and or CD4 antigen positive T lymphocytes by lectins covalently bound to the surface of a plastic chamber) methods, or positive selection of CD34 antigen bearing hematopoietic progenitor cells by means of flow cytometric sorting, or by applying magnetic bead-bound, or avidin/biotin-bound anti-CD34 antibodies are directed toward decreasing the percentage of potentially clonogenic tumor cells and increasing the CD34 antigen positive progenitor cell content in the graft.

INDICATIONS FOR BMT AND PBPC TRANSPLANT

Allogeneic BMT/PBPC Transplant

Allogeneic BMT can potentially benefit and possibly cure patients suffering from diseases of the following categories: The first class includes either genetically determined or secondarily diminished hematopoiesis of single- or multiple-cell lineages. Diseases include aplastic anemia, the thalassemias and other red cell disorders, as well as the myelodysplastic syndromes. Because the pathology is inherently due to a malfunction in the patient's own hematopoietic system, at present only replacement of the patient's bone marrow by an allogeneic transplant can be considered effective except for very special circumstances where immunosuppressive therapy alone may be sufficient (e.g., aplastic anemia).

The second category includes diseases consisting of predominantly genetically predetermined deficiencies of specific enzymatic functions such as the severe combined immune deficiency syndrome due to adenosine deaminase deficiency, or Gaucher's disease. An allogeneic source of replacement is curative in such conditions.

The third category of diseases includes development and expansion of malignant clones within the bone marrow. The bone marrow is either the primary source of disease such as in the case of chronic myelogenous leukemia, acute myeloid and lymphocytic leukemias, and multiple myeloma, or is a site involved in an otherwise systemic process as in the case of non-Hodgkin's lymphomas and Hodgkin's disease. Hence, chemoradiotherapeutic elimination of malignant clones with the concurrent ablation of normal bone marrow necessitates hematopoietic rescue, that is, transplant.

An allogeneic transplant provides not only the means of replacing malfunctioning or ablated bone marrow but it may also (through the graft versus tumor phenomena) produce direct cytotoxic damage on the targeted malignant elements.

The following hematologic malignancies should be considered for treatment by allogeneic BMT in patients under age 60 or younger who are otherwise in good general condition. (For patients ≤ 55 years without the availability of a matched, related donor, BMT from an unrelated donor can also be considered for the same indications).

Acute Myeloid Leukemia (AML)   Patients in first remission with poor risk cytogenetic features at diagnosis (-5, -7, $+8$, 11q23), or with multiple chromosomal abnormalities and those with intermediate risk leukemia with normal karyotype, or solitary, nonmyelodysplasia associated, cytogenetic abnormalities are candidates for allogeneic BMT. Patients in early relapse or in second remission can also benefit from BMT.

In two randomized trials of allogeneic BMT versus autologous BMT versus intensive chemotherapy of patients in first remission AML, allogeneic BMT resulted in the longest projected relapse-free survivals at 66% and 55% at 3 and 4 years, respectively. Relapse-free survival following autologous BMT was identical to that following intensive chemotherapy in the first trial and slightly better (48% versus 30%) in the second trial. Overall survival was similar in the three groups, primarily due to BMT-related complications. Relapse-free survival is 20% to 30% in patients transplanted in second remission.

Acute Lymphocytic Leukemia (ALL)   Patients in first remission with white cell counts $> 30,000/\mu l$ at diagnosis or with the presence of Philadelphia chromosome, translocations (8,14), (4,11), (1,19), extramedullary disease, L3 phenotype and those requiring > 4 weeks of induction therapy to achieve remission should be considered for BMT. Early relapse or second remission are additional indications.

The probabilities of relapse-free and overall survival for high-risk patients at 5 years are 39% and 44% in first remission and approximately 20% to 30% in second remission.

Chronic Myeloid Leukemia (CML)   Patients under age 55 in chronic phase should undergo BMT from a matched, sibling donor preferably within 1 year from diagnosis, as this is the only proven curative treatment for CML. Older patients should undergo a trial of α-interferon and could be considered for allogeneic BMT up to age 60 should they fail to achieve cytogenetic remission. Relapse-free survival rates following BMT are estimated at 60% to 70%.

For patients with CML in accelerated phase or in blast crisis, allogeneic BMT, or BMT from an unrelated donor yield relapse-free survival rates of 40% and 15%, respectively. The risk of severe graft-versus-host disease (GVHD) and graft failure is significantly higher after unrelated BMT than following allogeneic BMT from a sibling donor.

Non-Hodgkin's Lymphoma (NHL)   Carefully selected patients with high-grade lymphomas with evidence for BM and peripheral blood involvement and patients with low-grade, therapy-resistant or relapsed disease are considered candidates for allogeneic BMT.

Multiple Myeloma (MM)   Patients with a suitable sibling donor can be considered candidates for allogeneic BMT. The projected progression-free survival is 30% to 40% at 3 years from BMT. The mortality rate following BMT is relatively high, approximately 30% in the first 12 to 16 months.

THE THREE PHASES OF ALLOGENEIC BMT/PBPC TRANSPLANT

Pretransplant Phase

Patients with minimal residual neoplastic disease benefit the most from a transplant. To optimally utilize the allogeneic BMT/PBPC procedure patients undergo treatment with a preparatory regimen, first. The ideal preparatory regimen would eradicate all residual malignant elements and would provide sufficient immunosuppression to prevent graft rejection, in addition to inflicting only mild and reversible toxicities. The following preparatory regimens have been used most frequently in the largest series of allogeneic BMT: cyclophosphamide 120 mg/kg and fractionated total body irradiation (FTBI) with 8 to 14 Gy; etoposide 60 mg/kg and FTBI 12 to 13.2 Gy; melphalan 110 mg/m^2 and FTBI 9.5 to 14 Gy; cyclophosphamide 120 mg/kg with busulfan 14 to 16 mg/kg; BCNU 300 to 600 mg/m^2, cyclophosphamide 6 gm/m^2 and etoposide 600 to 2400 mg/m^2. Newer regimens adding a third therapeutic drug to well-tested two-drug combinations, or incorporating radioactive iodine or yttrium chelated antitumor antibodies against a variety of target antigens such as the myeloid marker CD33, and the B lymphoid marker CD20 are at present being evaluated in the preclinical and clinical setting.

Regimen-related toxicities (RRTs) vary depending on the specific and potentially additive side effects of the individual therapeutic agents. Acute and subacute toxicities include nausea; vomiting; mucositis; diarrhea (cyclophosphamide, etoposide, FTBI); seizure; mental status changes; headaches (busulfan, BCNU); rash; facial and salivary gland swelling; acidosis; hypotension (etoposide); hemorrhagic cystitis (cyclophosphamide); rash (FTBI); cardiac toxicity (cyclophosphamide); and venoocclusive disease consisting of hepatomegaly, jaundice, and weight gain starting 10 to 25 days following administration of the preparatory regimen (busulfan, FTBI?). Prophylactic use of antiemetics, intense hydration, and antiseizure medications aimed to prevent or ameliorate the specific side effects associated with the given preparatory regimen are necessary. Long-term toxicities include sterility, cataracts, osteoporosis, renal, pulmonary, cardiac, hepatic, and central and peripheral nervous system abnormalities. Potentially fatal long-term side effects include the development of secondary malignancies, both solid tumors and hematologic malignancies.

Transplant Phase

ABO incompatibility between the donor and recipient could be the source of life-threatening hemolytic complications in up to 30% of allogeneic BMT provided that no necessary steps are taken. Incompatibility is not a contraindication in an otherwise well-matched transplant setting. In case of a major ABO mismatch the recipient's plasma contains isoagglutinins against the donor red cell antigens (for instance, the recipient's blood type: O; donor type: B). The solution is removal of red cells from the donor graft prior to BMT via a variety of methods (for instance, by continuous flow cell separators) and plasma exchange from the recipient in case of high titers ($\geq$ 1:256). The management of minor mismatch (for instance, group 0 donor, group B recipient) includes red cell exchange from the recipient and removal of plasma from the donor marrow if the isoagglutinine titer is ≥ 128.

To decrease the incidence of potentially life-threatening grade II-IV graft versus host disease (GVHD), several methods to deplete the number of T lymphocytes in the graft (cells thought to be primarily responsible for the development and severity of GVHD) have been applied prior to transplant. Methods of T cell depletion include exposure of the graft to monoclonal antibodies and to complementary physicochemical techniques of cell separation. The result is a decrease in the incidence and severity of GVHD. T cell depletion, unfortunately, has been associated with an increased incidence of relapse owing to the loss of the graft versus tumor effect thought to be caused by subsets of T lymphocytes. Additional complications include the development of Epstein–Barr virus-associated B cell lymphoproliferative disorders and increased incidence of graft failure. Therefore, shortly prior to BMT, instead of T cell depletion of the graft, most transplant teams initiate administration of an immunosuppressant combination in order to prevent severe acute GVHD.

The actual reinfusion of BM or PBPC product usually takes place 1 to 3 days after completion of the preparatory phase to avoid any potential damage to the graft caused by circulating chemotherapeutic drug metabolites or parent compounds from the preparatory regimen.

Transfusion

Recipients with defective cell-mediated immunity are at risk of T-lymphocyte mediated GVHD. Therefore, all products should be irradiated with 1.5 to 2 Gy to avoid engraftment of lymphocytes contained in the transfusion product. Transfusion products are also filtered to decrease the chance of febrile reactions due to agglutinins. Patients who become refractory to random platelet transfusions may require single pheresis units, ABO matched products, HLA matched products, and occasionally intravenous IgG and plasma exchange to maintain acceptable levels of platelets > 5 to $10,000/\mu l$ in a nonbleeding situation without severe mucositis.

GVHD   At least 50% of posttransplant (both related and unrelated) mortality is due to GVHD. Therefore, all patients (except recipients of syngeneic BMT) receive GVHD prophylaxis for 6 to 12 months consisting of combinations of cyclosporin A and/or methotrexate, and/or prednisone.

GVHD is caused by transplanted lymphocytes targeting HLA-related antigens in the recipient. T cell depletion of BM by a variety of methods will decrease the incidence and severity of GVHD but at the price of an increased incidence of graft failure and relapse in the case of leukemias. Owing to the ablative effects of the preparatory regimens, host-versus-graft reaction and the resulting graft rejection are quite rare.

Acute GVHD is a syndrome occurring within the first 100 days post allogeneic BMT. HLA mismatch, unrelated donor BMT, sex mismatch between the donor and recipient, donor with multiple prior pregnancies, and older age of the recipient are all factors predicting higher incidence and possibly greater severity of GVHD. The incidence of GVHD varies from 20% in a recipient with fully matched BMT and no other adverse factors to a probability of greater than 80% for developing grade II-IV GVHD in a case of two or three loci mismatched BMT. Biopsy confirmation is recommended since a variety of pathologic conditions arising in the post-BMT period need to be distinguished in the differential diagnosis. The primary manifestations of GVHD include at least one and possibly all three entities of dermatitis, enteritis, and hepatitis. The overall grade of acute GVHD predicts the final outcome. Additional adverse prognostic features include thrombocytopenia and anemia. Patients suffering from grades III-IV GVHD have a greater than 80% probability of dying. Treatment options are limited and include increased doses of corticosteroids, antithymocyte globulin (ATG), and ultraviolet irradiation. Response to treatment is also a predictor of outcome.

Chronic GVHD can develop as the continuation of acute GVHD, or could manifest de novo. Under the second scenario the clinical features are similar to certain autoimmune diseases. The incidence of chronic GVHD varies depending on the age of the recipient and the type of BMT; in younger patients following fully matched BMT the incidence is under 20%; in recipients of unrelated donor BMT the incidence is closer to 60%. The primary manifestations include scleroderma-like skin changes and oral GVHD, keratoconjunctivitis sicca, liver dysfunction, bronchiolitis obliterans, myositis, and occasionally cerebral and peripheral nervous system involvement. Treatment options include immunosuppression with corticosteroids, cyclosporine and azathioprine, thalidomide, and total lymphoid irradiation. Patients with de novo chronic GVHD, without preexisting liver dysfunction and thrombocytopenia and with limited skin and liver function abnormalities, have a far better prognosis then those with extensive GVHD evolving from acute GVHD. The clinical staging system of acute GVHD is illustrated in Table 14.1.

TABLE 14.1. Clinical Staging of Acute GVHD

Stage	Skin	Liver	Gastrointestinal Tract
1	Maculopapular rash on < 25% of body surface	Bilirubin 2-3 mg/dl	Diarrhea 500–1,000 ml/day
2	Maculopapular rash on 25%–50% of body surface	Bilirubin > 3–6 mg/dl	Diarrhea >1000–1500 ml/day
3	Generalized erythroderma	Bilirubin > 6–15 mg/dl	Diarrhea > 1500 ml/day
4	Desquamation and bullae	Bilirubin >15 mg/dl	Severe pain or ileus

	Stage		
Grade	Skin	Liver	Gut
I	1–2	0	0
II	1–3	1	1
III	2–3	2–3	2–3
IV	2–4	2–4	2–4

SECONDARY MALIGNANCIES

The incidence of secondary malignancies (lymphoproliferative disorders, squamous-cell carcinomas, and tumors of the aerodigestive system) depends to a large extent on the underlying disease condition and preparatory regimen and is estimated at 6% 15 years from BMT. Patients treated with an FTBI-containing preparatory regimen are at a higher risk.

AUTOLOGOUS BMT/PBPC TRANSPLANT

Of the three disease categories listed as indications for allogeneic BMT, treatment of genetically diminished/dysplastic hematopoiesis is not possible by autologous BMT at the present time, as the problem is inherent to the malfunction of the patient's own bone marrow. Hereditary deficiencies of specific enzymatic functions might be suitable targets for gene transfer. An autologous BMT/PBPC transplant of gene-transfected progenitor cells has the potential to supplement missing enzymatic functions and is an attractive and possibly the only option in view of the scarcity of suitable allogeneic donors. The feasibility of such approaches applying a variety of gene transfer methods/factors is at present being tested.

Inadequate hematopoiesis secondary to the effects of high-dose chemo/radio-therapy can be supplemented/supported by autologous bone marrow, or by growth factor primed/mobilized PBPC transplant, procured prior to therapy. Autologous BMT has been almost completely replaced by the use of growth factor (G-CSF or GM-CSF) primed/mobilized PBPC transplant in the treatment acute myeloid leukemia, multiple myeloma, and the lymphomas. However, the greatest increase in the number of autologous PBPC transplants has occurred in the treatment of solid tumors, especially breast, ovarian, and testicular carcinomas. The role of autologous PBPC transplant in these settings is primarily supportive following high-dose chemo-/radiotherapeutic consolidation at a time when the tumor load in the hematopoietic system is felt to be reduced, hence the risk of reinfusion of clonogenic tumor cells is thought to be the lowest.

Patients with the following hematologic and solid neoplasms should be considered candidates for autologous BMT/PBPC transplants.

AML

Earlier randomized trials in patients in first remission demonstrated only border-line benefits when comparing autologous BMT to intense chemotherapy consolidation/maintenance. With the advance of PBPC transplants the mortality rate associated with autologous BMT decreased from the previous 15% to approximately 5%. Accordingly, projected event-free and overall survival is approaching that of patients undergoing allogeneic BMT for intermediate risk AML, although randomized trials are necessary to confirm this trend. Although methods to "purge" the harvested BM especially by chemotherapeutic means have been utilized in clinical trials, no clear benefit has been demonstrated in comparison to more intense in vivo depletion of potential tumor contamination by intravenous chemotherapy prior to procurement of the BM or PBPC graft.

Non-Hodgkin's Lymphoma (NHL)

Patients in first remission, in sensitive and resistant relapse, or with primary resistant NHL are candidates for transplant. Patients with high-risk disease (age < 60, elevated LDH, poor performance status, more than one extranodal site and slow response to induction chemotherapy) and relapsed high-grade and intermediate grade lymphomas benefit from high-dose chemo-/radiation therapy and autologous PBPC transplant. Projected event-free survival for high-risk patients in first remission is 60% to 80% at 4 years. Patients with chemotherapy-sensitive relapse or resistant relapse experience event-free survival rates of 35% to 46% and 20%, respectively. In one randomized study of chemotherapy-sensitive NHL relapse-free and overall survival rates at 5 years were 46% and 53% in the transplant group compared to 12% and 32% in the cohort of patients treated with chemotherapy only.

Patients with low-grade lymphomas may also benefit from PBPC transplant, or alternatively from undergoing high-dose chemotherapy and monoclonal antibody purged BMT. However, owing to the long natural history of low-grade NHL prolonged periods of observation will be necessary to definitely prove the benefits of BMT.

Hodgkin's Disease

Patients with induction failure or in early—<12 months from induction therapy—relapse should be offered transplant. The projected event-free survival rates are 60% for patients failing only one prior therapy and approximately 20% for those failing more than 2 regimens.

Multiple Myeloma (MM)

Patients with stage I to III MM with minimal bone marrow involvement in response benefit from transplant. In a randomized trial of 200 patients treated first with induction chemotherapy the probabilities of event-free and overall survival at 5 years were 28% and 52% for patients undergoing consolidation with BMT and α-interferon. Event-free and overall survival were lower at 10% and 12% in the control group treated with chemotherapy/interferon only.

Breast Cancer

Several phase II trials suggest that high-dose chemotherapy and PBPC transplant may improve relapse and progression-free survival for patients with high-risk primary stage II ($\geq$ 10 axillary lymph nodes involved with metastasis) and IIIA and B (locally advanced and inflammatory) breast cancer in comparison to historical controls. Although relapse-free survival rates seem to be improved by 15% to 25%, definite conclusions regarding the efficacy of high-dose chemotherapy in this setting will be possible only following the completion and assessment of presently ongoing, prospective, randomized studies. The preparatory regimens include combinations of cyclophosphamide with either etoposide and cisplatin, cisplatin and carmustine, or carboplatin and thiotepa. Newer regimens have incorporated taxanes in combination with cisplatin and cyclophosphamide, or doxorubicin and cyclophosphamide.

In a prospective randomized trial of stage IV breast cancer progression-free survival was significantly longer for patients treated with two cycles of high-dose chemotherapy and stem cell transplant in comparison with a cohort treated with conventional dose chemotherapy. Pooled data from the international bone marrow registry project an approximately 35% 3-year survival, suggesting improved outcome in comparison to historical controls. Repeated cycles of primarily alkylator-based high-dose chemotherapeutic regimens are presently being tested in phase I to II clinical trials. Ongoing randomized trials compare conventional chemotherapy versus BMT both as first line of treatment and as consolidation following chemotherapy induction.

Other Solid Tumors

There are encouraging preliminary results with high-dose chemotherapy and BMT/PBPC transplant with phase II trials of ifosfamide, etoposide, and carboplatin, or cisplatin and cyclophosphamide based combinations for testicular carcinoma with an estimated 20% to 25% salvage rate in therapy resistant/relapsed patients.

Ovarian Carcinoma

Several phase II/pilot studies (with preparatory regimens including high-dose carboplatin, melphalan, anthracyclines) suggest an improved approximately 25% to 30% progression-free survival at 2 to 3 years from BMT.

Miscellaneous

Phase II trials in Ewing's sarcoma and other types of sarcoma are presently ongoing with high-dose ifosfamide and other alkylator based (melphalan, cisplatin, carboplatin) regimens.

THE THREE PHASES OF AUTOLOGOUS BMT/PBPC TRANSPLANT

Preparatory regimens similar to those used for allogeneic BMT need further improvement to increase efficacy. Although quite a few of the regimens are identical to those used in the allogeneic setting, owing to the variety of diseases targeted with autologous BMT the number of preparatory regimens are far greater. The toxicities associated with cyclophosphamide, etoposide, BCNU, FTBI, busulfan, and melphalan have been described earlier. Additional side effects include renal failure, electrolyte wasting, high-frequency hearing loss (cisplatin, carboplatin), confusion, seizure, hemorrhagic cystitis, myalgias, peripheral and central neuropathy (paclitaxel), and cerebellar toxicities (ARA-C).

Transplant Phase

The side effects associated with BMT are usually minimal and include nausea, potential fluid overload, shortness of breath and headache. Decreased oxygen saturation can be observed in up to 15% of patients due to fluid overload and the irritant effects of the cryopreservative dimethyl sulfoxide (DMSO).

Posttransplant Phase

General support is similar to that described under allogeneic BMT, but there is no need for Pneumocystis prophylaxis.

Graft Failure   Following G-CSF or GM-CSF primed PBPC transplant graft failure is extremely unusual. Application of negative selection techniques (purging) or positive selection of CD34 antigen positive progenitor cells, however, may deprive the graft of sufficient numbers of facilitator cells, resulting in delayed neutrophil and platelet recovery.

Bacterial Infections   The incidence and types of bacterial infections are similar to what has been observed following an allogeneic BMT but the period of absolute neutropenia (average duration: 10 days) is shorter. Similarly, although antifungal and antiherpetic prophylaxis are useful, the threat of fatal viral and fungal infections is relatively small.

Secondary Malignancies   MDS and secondary leukemias have been reported following autologous BMT/PBPC transplants. The reported incidence of clonal karyotypic abnormalities can be as high as 9% by 9 years following PBPC transplant, making vigorous follow-up mandatory.

SUMMARY

Bone marrow transplantation (BMT) includes harvesting hematopoietic progenitor cells able to establish short-term and long-term hematopoietic and immune function followed by intravenous reinfusion of the heparinized and filtered product into the recipient. Patients potentially benefitting from BMT include those suffering from diminished hematopoiesis and hematologic malignancies. In addition, BMT can be used to support and reestablish hematopoietic function following treatment with high-dose chemotherapy for most hematologic and solid neoplasms. The specific indications for patients with allogeneic and autologous BMT and the advantages of peripheral blood progenitor stem cell transplant have been outlined.

FUTURE DIRECTIONS

Allogeneic BMT

Improved preparatory regimens with the possible incorporation of radio-immuno-therapeutic agents, increased utilization of PBPC in order to accelerate engraftment, further expansion of the unrelated donor pool, and ex vivo expansion of cord blood are tools at varying levels of clinical development. Incorporation of new growth factors (e.g., thrombopoietin) in the therapeutic schema as mobilizers of PBPC, separation of GVHD from the graft versus tumor effect by T cell depletion, and subsequent selective reinfusion of tumor specific, and if necessary graft facilitating elements of the negatively selected lymphocyte population, are at present undergoing clinical testing. Incorporation of more efficient antiviral and antifungal agents into supportive care, and fast reconstitution of immune competence via T cell clone transfer from he recipient are likely to further decrease treatment-associated toxicities.

Autologous BMT

Improved preparatory regimens with the possible incorporation of radioimmunotherapeutic agents and novel therapeutic agents/combinations and multiple cycles of BMT are designed to enhance therapeutic efficacy. Incorporation of new growth factors (e.g., thrombopoietin) into the therapeutic schema as mobilizers of PBPC and as accelerators of posttransplant recovery and ex vivo expansion of purified hematopoietic progenitor cells may accelerate hematopoietic recovery. Ex vivo expansion of autologous cytolytic tumor-specific lymphocytes, adaptive immune therapy, and antisense and other gene therapeutic approaches against fusion targets (e.g., bcr–abl) are some of the potential modalities complementing cytoreductive therapy.

FURTHER READING

Forman SJ, Blume KG, Thomas ED (eds.) (1994) *Bone Marrow Tranplantation*, Blackwell, Boston.

Zittoun RA, Mandelli F, Willemze R, de Witte T, Labar B, Resegotti L, et al. (1995) *N Engl J Med* 332: 217.

Reiffers J, Stoppa AM, Attal M, Michallet M, Marit G, et al. (1996) Allogeneic vs. autologous stem cell transplantation vs. chemotherapy in patients with acute myeloid leukemia in first remission: the BGMT 87 study. *Leukemia* 10: 1974.

Sebban C, Lepage E, Vernant JP, Gluckman E, Attal M, Reiffers J (1994) Allogeneic bone marrow transplantation in adult acute lymphoblastic leukemia in first complete remission: a comparative study. French Group of Therapy of Adult Acute Lymphoblastic Leukemia. *J Clin Oncol* 12: 2580.

Snyder DS, Negrin RS, O'Donnell MR, Chao NJ, Amylon MD, Long GD, et al. (1994) Fractionated total-Body irradiation and high-dose etoposide as a preparatory regimen for bone marrow transplantation for 94 patients with chronic myelogenous leukemia in chronic phase. *Blood* 84: 1672.

McGlave P, Bartsch G, Anasetti C, Ash R, Beatty P, Gajewski J, Kernan NA (1993) Unrelated donor marrow transplantation therapy for chronic myelogenous leukemia: initial experience of the National Marrow Donor Program. *Blood* 81: 543.

Walter EA, Greenberg PD, Gilbert MJ, Finch RJ, Watanabe KS, Thomas ED, Riddell SR (1995) Reconstitution of cellular immunity against cytomegalovirus in recipients of allogeneic bone marrow by transfer of T-cell clones from the donor. *N Engl J Med* 333: 1038.

Armitage JO, Antman KH (eds.) (1995) *High-Dose Cancer Therapy: Pharmacology, Hematopoietins, Stem Cells*, Williams & Wilkins, Baltimore.

Philip T, Guglielmi C, Hagenbeek A, Somers R, Van der Lelie H, Bron D, et al. (1995) Autologous bone marrow transplantation as compared with salvage chemotherapy in relapses of chemotherapy-sensitve non-Hodgkin's lymphoma. *N Engl J Med* 333: 1540.

Freedman AS, Gribben JG, Neuberg D, Mauch P, Soiffer RJ, Anderson K, et al. (1996) High-dose therapy and autologous bone marrow transplantation in patients with follicular lymphoma during first remission. *Blood* 88: 2780.

Gribben JG, Schultze JL (1997) The detection of minimal residual disease: implications for bone marrow transplantation. *Cancer Treatment Res* 77: 99.

Matthews DC, Appelbaum FR, Press OW, Eary JF, Bernstein ID (1997) The use of radiolabeled antibodies in bone marrow transplantation for hematologic malignancies. *Cancer Treatment Res* 77: 121–139.

Attal M, Harousseau JL, Sotto JJ, Fuzibet JG, Rossi JF, Casassus P, et al. (1996) A prospective, randomized trial of autologous bone marrow transplantation and chemotherapy in multiple myeloma. *N Engl J Med* 335: 91.

Bezwoda WR, Seymour L, Dansy RD, et al. (1995) High-dose chemotherapy with hematopoietic rescue as primary treatment for metastatic breast cancer: a randomized trial. *J Clin Oncol* 13: 1483.

Somlo G, Sniecinski I, Odom-Marion T, et al. (1997) Effect of CD34$^+$ Selection and various schedules of stem cell reinfusion and granulocyte colony-stimulating factor priming on hematopoietic recovery after high-dose chemotherapy for breast cancer. *Blood* 89: 1521.

Somlo G, Doroshow JH, Forman SJ, Odom-Marion T, Lee J, Chow W, et al. (1997) *J Clin Oncol* 15: 2882.

Traweek ST, Slovak ML, Nademanee AP, Brynes RK, Niland JC, Forman SJ (1994) Clonal karyotypic hematopoietic cell abnormalities ocurring after autologous bone marrow transplantation for Hodgkin's disease and non-Hodgkin's lymphoma. *Blood* 84: 957.

CHAPTER 15

BIOSTATISTICS AND CLINICAL TRIALS

RICHARD SYLVESTER, PATRICK THERASSE, MARTINE VAN GLABBEKE, and FRANÇOISE MEUNIER

EORTC Data Center/Central Office
83 avenue E Mounier, Bte 11
1200 Brussels, Belgium

Medical practice and medical research, including basic research, clinical research, and teaching, all depend on each other. Clinical research in cancer is not a luxury, but is essential to rapidly develop and identify new state of the art treatments and to invalidate ineffective ones. To decrease the time needed to evaluate new therapeutic modalities and transfer laboratory discoveries into routine clinical practice, various partners in clinical research such as industry, academic centers, international research organizations, and regulatory affairs agencies must all work together. A multinational, multicenter, and multidisciplinary team effort allows complex therapies to be evaluated even in rare cancers.

To have the most impact on day-to-day clinical practice, simple, large-scale, multicenter, randomized, phase III clinical trials with key endpoints are required. The role of biostatistics in the field of cancer research, clinical trials in particular, has undergone enormous changes since the first randomized clinical trial in acute lymphocytic leukemia, which was organized in 1954 by the US National Cancer Institute (NCI). It is just within these past 40 years that the ground rules for conducting clinical trials on a scientific basis have been worked out and the appropriate statistical methodology developed. A number of authorities have been actively involved in the development of statistical guidelines. Within the European Union, in 1990 the Committee for Proprietary Medicinal Products (CPMP) published an EEC Note for Guidance[1] dealing with the subject of Good Clinical Practice. In 1994, the CPMP adopted a Note for Guidance dealing with biostatistical methodology in clinical trials[2] that has been followed up by a Note for Guidance on the Eval-

Manual of Clinical Oncology, 7th edition, Edited by Raphael E. Pollock
ISBN 0-471-23828-7, pages 307–324. Copyright © 1999 Wiley-Liss, Inc.

uation of Anticancer Medicinal Products in Man.[3] The International Conference on Harmonization (ICH), a joint effort of the United States, European Union, and Japan, has recently developed the draft ICH Harmonized Tripartite Guideline E8 entitled General Considerations for Clinical Trials[4] and the ICH Harmonized Tripartite Guideline E9 entitled Statistical Principles for Clinical Trials.[5] This chapter will review some of the basic concepts dealing with the design, conduct, analysis, and reporting of clinical trials.

WHAT IS A CLINICAL TRIAL?

A clinical trial may be defined as a carefully designed, prospective medical study that attempts to answer a precisely defined set of questions with respect to the effects of a particular treatment or treatments.[6] The results of a clinical trial, which are based on a limited sample of patients, are then used to make decisions about how a given patient population should be treated in the future.

A prerequisite for any clinical trial is a good idea that is worth testing. A clinical trial should attempt to answer the most important questions concerning the disease under study, obtain reliable results, and be able to convince others of the validity of the results. A clinical trial is a major undertaking that requires considerable money, personnel, facilities, time, and effort. Thus the need for the study, its value, and its potential impact on the medical community must all be carefully considered to ensure that the interest of the question justifies the time and expense necessary to carry it out.

THE PROTOCOL

The most important document pertaining to any clinical trial is the protocol, a self-contained description of the rationale, objectives, and logistics of the study.[6] The success or failure of the trial may depend on how well the protocol was written because a poorly designed, ambiguous, or incompletely documented protocol will result in a trial that may not be able to answer the questions of interest. The protocol must be detailed and precisely worded so that the study is uniformly carried out by all participants.

In phase III trials a committee of researchers representing each of the different disciplines involved in the study should be appointed to plan, design, and write the protocol. Sufficient time must be allowed for the protocol to be designed, written, revised (one or more times), and eventually reviewed by external review boards before its implementation and the start of patient enrollment.

TYPES OF STUDIES

The testing of a new therapy is a long-term project, involving different types of trials during its development. The first step in planning a new trial is to precisely define its objectives and to determine the type of study to be carried out. Studies generally fall into one of three categories: phase I, phase I, and phase III, whereas trials within the pharmaceutical industry also go through phase IV or post-marketing surveillance studies. Phase IV trials are not considered in this chapter.

Phase I Trials

Phase I trials are the first studies in humans after the completion of preclinical studies.[7] They screen for toxicity as the dose is gradually escalated. The usual aims of a phase I study are to:

- Establish the maximum tolerated dose (MTD) for the new drug for a given schedule via a given route of administration and propose a safe dose for phase II evaluation in humans
- Identify the dose-limiting toxicity (DLT) and determine the qualitative (which organ system is involved) toxicity as well as the quantitative (predictability, extent, duration, and reversibility) toxicity of the drug
- Determine the pharmacokinetic and the pharmacodynamic profile of the drug
- Document possible antitumor activity in cancer patients.[8]

The following general eligibility criteria are applicable for phase I trials of anti-cancer drugs:

- All patients must have microscopically confirmed advanced disease that is no longer amenable to established forms of treatment.
- Their life expectancy should be at least 8 weeks.
- In general, they should not have received chemo-, immuno-, or radiotherapy within the last 4 weeks prior to entry in the trial.
- They should have a normal bone marrow function and no major impairment of hepatic, renal, and cardiac functions.
- All patients must give their written informed consent.

Further eligibility criteria will depend on the drug under study.

Various methods for selecting a safe starting dose are used. For example, in European Organization for Research and Treament of Cancer (EORTC) studies, one tenth of the LD_{10} (lethal dose) in mice, expressed as mg/m^2, is used as the starting dose for phase I trials, provided that this dose is not toxic in a second species (normally the rat).

The classic method for dose escalation in phase I trials utilizes the modified Fibonacci search scheme: the first cohort of patients is treated with the recommended starting dose for phase I trials and subsequent cohorts of patients are treated with a dose level increased by a certain percentage ($100, 67, 50, 40, 33, 33, 33\ldots$) above the preceding dose level.

An initial cohort of three patients is given the new compound at the starting dose level and the toxic effects are carefully observed. If no acute toxicity is observed after a predetermined period of observation, or if toxicity is mild to moderate and reversible before the start of the next treatment course, the dose is escalated in another cohort of three patients and toxicity is again documented. The dose escalation procedure is successively repeated, using proportionately smaller dose increments as the dose is increased and toxicity is observed until the maximum tolerated dose (MTD) is reached. The latter is defined as the highest dose that can be safely given to patients, producing significant, but yet manageable and reversible toxicity in at least one third of the patients. The definition of "significant, but yet manageable and reversible toxicity" depends on the type of toxicity and the organ involved.

The recommended dose for phase II will usually be the dose level just below the MTD. It is therefore desirable that when the MTD has been reached, at least three more patients are entered at the dose level just below the MTD and kept on treatment to determine chronic or cumulative toxicity.

In general, phase I studies based on the modified Fibonacci scheme require a median of five or six dose escalation steps.

Besides the modified Fibonacci scheme, other designs have been proposed[7,9] to consider particular situations such as phase I trials of combinations of well-known agents (fixed intervals, doubling the dose until toxicity) or to speed up the process and minimize the number of patients treated with inactive doses of anticancer agents (continual reassessment method, pharmacokinetically guided dose escalation.) So far none of these methods have really been preferred to the modified Fibonacci approach. However, more recently, the US NCI has opened new perspectives for phase I trials with the accelerated titration method,[10] which permits a rapid dose escalation early in the trial with intrapatient dose escalation in successive cohorts of single patients. This method has also the advantage of providing more information on cumulative toxicity.

Phase II Trials

Phase II trials are carried out following the phase I assessment of a new agent, but before large-scale comparative studies are launched in the framework of randomized phase III trials.

The term *phase II* encompasses clinical studies of widely differing intentions. A major distinction should be made between single-agent phase II trials, assessing the activity and toxicity of a new agent in a defined tumor type, and phase II feasibility studies, exploring the therapeutic effect of a new agent or of an established active agent in combination with other drugs or other treatment modalities.[11]

Single-Agent Phase II Trials   Within the category of single-agent phase II trials, a further distinction should be made between "early phase II trials" and "late phase II trials," which differ in both their goals and the need for intensive monitoring.

Objectives   Early (single-agent) phase II trials are designed to identify antitumor activity in a representative sample of tumor types, usually selected on the basis of the targets used for drug development and the results of both preclinical studies and phase I trials. A further aim of early phase II trials is to obtain a more detailed description of the drug's toxicity, particularly cumulative toxicity (which is easier to study in a phase II patient population than in phase I) and to study ways to manage toxicity (e.g., by preventive measures, concomitant medication, etc.). Early phase II trials may also study the pharmacokinetics/pharmacodynamics relationship, if possible. At the conclusion of an early phase II trial a decision is made whether to stop the further research and development of a new agent or to continue its clinical development.

Once early phase II trials have been successfully conducted in an initial sample of patients, late (single-agent) phase II trials may be conducted to document antitumor activity in other types of tumors. Further documentation of the toxicity profile is also a goal in late phase II trials, but at this stage the principal toxicities have generally already been identified. At the conclusion of a late phase II trial a decision is made whether to further evaluate the drug in a specific tumor type.

Endpoints   The primary endpoints for both early and late single-agent phase II trials are:

- Antitumor activity, expressed in terms of "response to therapy"
- Toxicity

Response to therapy is assessed on the basis of objective criteria that measure the decrease in size of prospectively selected "target lesions." International standards are available for measuring response in phase II trials, the most common being that proposed by the WHO in 1979.[12] A new set of criteria is, however, currently in preparation. It should be underlined that response to therapy is not an appropriate surrogate for therapeutic benefit but only an indicator of antitumor activity.

Toxicity is graded according to standard scales based on objective parameters. The "Common Toxicity Criteria" (CTC) defined by the NCI (US) are the most widely used criteria. More recently the NCIC (Canada) has provided additional toxicity scales not defined in the CTC. The US NCI is currently in the process of revising the CTC in cooperation with several other groups. In single-drug phase II studies, toxicity should be separately assessed for each cycle of therapy to evaluate potential cumulative side effects.

Pharmacokinetic parameters are generally secondary endpoints in early phase II trials.

Patient Selection Criteria   Essential patient selection criteria for both types of single-agent phase II trials are:

- Histologic confirmation of the tumor type specified in the trial
- Presence of objectively measurable disease

Further, patients selected for these studies should have a reasonable potential for responding to an active compound and should not have any extra risk of experiencing toxicity. The remaining selection criteria therefore concern the prior therapy that the patient has received and ensure that the patient is fit to receive an investigational drug:

- Patients should not be candidates for standard therapy or they should have progressed under those therapies.
- Patients should have a reasonable performance status (WHO ≤ 2).
- Bone marrow, hepatic, renal, and cardiac function must be normal (impaired hepatic or renal function may result in abnormally elevated serum drug levels that could induce unexpected or more severe side effects).
- Written informed consent must always be obtained from the patient.

Further specification of the targeted population for late phase II trials may require more restrictive patient selection criteria (i.e., in terms of histology and/or prior therapy)

Statistical Design Single-agent phase II trials enroll as few patients as possible and can only demonstrate whether a new agent has antitumor activity or not. They are generally nonrandomized, with all patients receiving the same treatment.

For ethical reasons some type of sequential approach is necessary so that inactive drugs and drugs for which the toxicity has been underestimated in phase I studies are rejected from further study as quickly as possible.

When deciding on the future of a new agent, two types of errors can be made: a false-positive or type I error (recommending an inactive agent for further study) and a false-negative or type II error (declaring an active agent to be inactive). The false-negative is the more serious error of the two because, once rejected, the drug will generally have no further chance to show its activity, whereas an inactive drug can still be rejected if its activity is not validated at a later stage. Thus most designs employed in this type of trial try to minimize the probability of a false-negative result.

A number of two-stage statistical designs have been developed (Simon,[13] Fleming,[14] and Gehan[15]) that allow the drug to be rejected at the end of the first stage if there is insufficient activity to warrant further testing. Otherwise, the second stage continues to the full sample size, allowing a more precise evaluation of the response rate (Gehan) and a decision rule for further investigation of the agent (Simon, Fleming).

The Gehan design[15] is generally preferred for early phase II trials because it minimizes the number of patients treated during the first stage if the drug is totally inactive. Its major drawback is that it does not provide a clear statistical decision rule concerning the further development of the drug. Therefore, the Simon[13] and the Fleming[14] design are generally preferred for late single agent phase II trials because they provide such a decision rule.[16]

Randomized phase II trials are of potential interest in the following situations:

- If different schedules of the same drug are to be tested
- If two or more drugs are ready for testing at the same time
- If an analogue of an active compound is to be screened.

A randomized phase II trial should be viewed as a simultaneous screening of several compounds and *not* as a comparative trial. The principal purpose of randomization is to eliminate conscious or unconscious bias on the part of the investigator in assigning treatments, that is, to balance the treatment groups with respect to all prognostic factors, both known and unknown, that may affect a patient's response to treatment.

When screening analogues it may be useful to carry out a randomized phase II trial including the parent compound as a control arm to reduce the incidence of false-negatives. That is, if the analogue is found to be inactive but the parent compound is also found to be inactive in a patient population for which it is normally active, then the negative results with the analogue may be due to the patient population studied and does not necessarily mean that the analogue is inactive.

In randomized phase II studies, the sample size for each arm is computed using one of the previously described classic phase II designs.

Phase II Feasibility Trials

Objectives   Although a phase II trial might demonstrate that a potential new therapy has some activity, it can never conclude that it would be of therapeutic benefit to patients. This is the goal of phase III trials. In most situations the information provided by phase I and single-agent phase II trials is not sufficient to justify the treatment of a large number of patients with the new drug in a randomized phase III trial. Particularly when a new agent is incorporated in a combined therapy, the feasibility of the new therapeutic approach is unknown.

Phase II feasibility studies aim at providing the justification for a subsequent large randomized phase III trial that will assess the potential therapeutic value of a new treatment. It must be underlined that a nonrandomized feasibility study will never provide evidence of a possible therapeutic benefit.

Endpoints   The choice of an appropriate endpoint(s) that reflects the feasibility of a new therapeutic approach is delicate. The toxicity profile of the complete projected plan of therapy is an obvious index of the treatment's feasibility. If possible it may also be desirable to study the treatment's long-term side effects. The proportion of patients completing therapy may also be used as an index of its feasibility.

Response to therapy is not necessarily an endpoint in these trials: indeed, antitumor activity of all agents should have been previously documented in single-agent trials and response to treatment is not an appropriate surrogate for therapeutic benefit. However, a minimum response rate is sometimes used as a criterion for continuing investigation of the treatment.

The interest of the investigators and the potential of the group to conduct the phase III trial may also need to be evaluated in the framework of a feasibility study. The recruitment rate may be used to assess these factors.

Patient Selection   Patients selected for a feasibility study should be those who would be included in the following randomized trial. Therefore, inclusion and exclusion criteria should be as close as possible to those that will be used in the future phase III trial.

Statistical Design   The diversity of possible endpoints explains the diversity of statistical designs proposed for feasibility studies.

For trials in which toxicity and response rate have been chosen as principal endpoints, Bryant and Day have proposed a two-stage design based on predefined "acceptable" and "unacceptable" levels of toxicity and response rate.[17] This design provides a decision rule based on the number of responses and the number of cases with unacceptable toxicity observed during the first and second stages of the trial.

If feasibility trials are not randomized, they will then provide the temptation of making conscious or unconscious comparisons based on "historical" controls. This attitude carries a high risk of the medical community adopting overly toxic or overly aggressive therapies despite the lack of scientific evidence of a real therapeutic benefit. In this situation, large-scale randomized trials may become extremely difficult to conduct.

It is therefore recommended in feasibility studies to randomize the new treatment versus the standard therapy that would serve as the control arm in the future phase III trial. Patients randomized in the feasibility trial might then be included in the phase III trial, reducing the total number of patients needed to complete both studies.

Therapeutic Approaches Other Than Cytotoxic Drugs

The methods described previously have been developed for the investigation of cytotoxic drugs. They are based on the assumption of an increasing dose–effect relationship, both for efficacy and adverse events. They should not be blindly applied in other situations, for example when investigating:

- A drug for which a maximum in its dose–response curve has been attained
- A drug designed to enhance the activity of another agent
- A drug designed to reduce the side effects of another agent
- An investigational radiotherapy schedule
- A radiosensitizer
- A biologic response modifier
- A cytostatic drug

In these cases the entire policy of early development may need to be redefined because standard guidelines are inadequate.

Phase III Trials

After a drug has been found to have at least some predefined minimal amount of activity in phase II trials, the next step is to determine its relative efficacy in a randomized phase III trial. Phase III trials are thus comparative in nature, that is, the experience of a group of patients receiving a new treatment is compared either to a group of patients receiving a standard treatment or to an untreated control group.

The possible goals of a phase III trial are:

- To determine the effectiveness of a treatment relative to the (treated) natural history of the disease. In this case the trial has a no treatment or a placebo control arm.
- To determine the effectiveness of the new treatment as compared to the best current standard therapy
- To determine if a new treatment is as effective as the standard therapy but is associated with less severe toxicity (equivalence study).

Phase III clinical trials should be planned to reliably detect small to moderate treatment differences, not to identify major breakthroughs. The minimum treatment benefit that is considered to be clinically worthwhile depends on the severity of the disease and on the undesirable side effects of the treatment. Although a large survival improvement may be demanded of an aggressive therapy for a fatal condition, it is self defeating to hope for more than a small survival improvement with an adjuvant therapy in good prognosis patients.

Preference should be given to large simple studies that compare two treatments that are as different as possible. Crossover trials are generally to be avoided because the underlying assumptions for carrying out such trials are almost never valid in cancer studies.

PROCEDURES

Patient Selection

In randomized trials the entry of patients should be guided by the uncertainty principle. That is, only if there is substantial uncertainty over the best treatment should the patient be randomized.

Two diverging attitudes may be adopted in defining eligibility criteria: they can be very precisely and narrowly defined so that only a small fraction of the available patients are eligible, or at the other extreme they can be left as loose as possible so that most available patients can be entered into the trial.

Narrow eligibility criteria make the patient sample as homogeneous as possible. This may be desirable to unequivocally identify treatment benefits in a subgroup of patients with well-defined prognostic features. All future patients in the same group may then be offered the treatment should it prove to be effective in the clinical trial. Narrow eligibility criteria are preferable to broad ones when there are good a priori reasons to believe that the treatment will be beneficial only to a subgroup of patients, an assumption that is rarely true in practice. Patient accrual may suffer, however, if the patient eligibility criteria are too restrictive.

Broad eligibility criteria result in a faster patient accrual into the trial, therefore reducing the total duration of the study. They also yield a sample of patients that is more closely representative of the total patient population. Their results can therefore be more readily extrapolated to all future patients outside the trial. Broad eligibility criteria are preferable to narrow ones when little is known at the time of designing the trial concerning the possible benefit that may be expected from the treatment under investigation in different subgroups of patients. In this (common) situation, the most plausible hypothesis is that the treatment effect will be similar in different subgroups of patients and that the best strategy is to then choose eligibility criteria that are as broad as possible.

Randomization and Stratification

Treatment allocation by a random process is the method of choice in phase III trials. Randomization ensures that the decision of treating a patient with one of the treatments being tested does not depend on the patient's characteristics. Therefore, if a difference in outcome is observed, it can reasonably be attributed to a difference in treatment effect and not to differences in the prognosis of the groups of patients being treated. Randomization is the single most important technique to prevent selection bias.

Randomization does not only guarantee the validity of the statistical tests used to compare treatments, but also balances, *on the average*, the distribution of both known and unknown prognostic factors in the treatment groups. To reduce the possibility of bias, a central randomization via an electronic network or telephone is recommended.

Especially in small to moderate size trials, random allocation does not ensure that an equal number of patients will receive each treatment or that all the prognostic factors will be equally distributed in the treatment groups. Consequently the randomization should be stratified for a small number of factors of known prognostic importance.

With stratified randomization, patients are stratified prospectively at the time of entry into the trial to obtain an approximately equal balance of patients and important prognostic factors in the treatment groups. Two different techniques may be used: static methods, for example based on randomized blocks, or dynamic methods such as the minimization technique.[18]

With the system of randomized blocks, a separate randomization list (set of treatment assignments) for each possible cross-classification of the prognostic factors to stratify for is required. Within each block the treatments are ordered at random. If there are only a few patients within a block, balance within the block and hence within the trial is not assured. Stratification by too many factors may, by chance, be worse than no stratification at all.

Dynamic methods use the actual treatment assignments and the baseline characteristics of patients who have already been entered to determine the treatment assignment for each new patient. The minimization technique's goal is to ensure a balance within each level of each stratification factor separately, but not necessarily within all the possible combinations of the different factors.

All multicenter trials should be stratified by institution. If the minimization technique is used to allocate treatments, a larger number of stratification factors may eventually be taken into account. It is recommended, however, that the randomization procedure be kept simple by stratifying only by the one or two most important prognostic variables in addition to institution.

Endpoints

Adjuvant Trials Adjuvant therapy is given to patients treated by a potentially curative primary therapy, but for whom there is a substantial risk of recurrence. The primary therapy is usually surgery, but may also include radiotherapy, chemotherapy, or a combination of these. Adjuvant trials thus study treatments given to patients who are clinically disease free after a "curative" primary treatment.

The goal of an adjuvant trial is generally to compare the duration of survival, disease-free survival, or disease-free interval in two or more treatment groups. Another characteristic of adjuvant trials is the necessity for large sample sizes and long-term follow-up. Large sample sizes are needed because the power to detect differences in survival and disease-free interval depends on the number of events (deaths or recurrences) in each group rather than on the total number of patients entered.

Advanced Disease Trials Advanced disease includes all patients for whom local treatment is no longer curative. There are two types of advanced disease: *recurrent* or *locally advanced disease* in which the disease is still confined to the region of the primary tumor as opposed to *metastatic disease* in which the disease has spread to distant sites.

When studying the effects of a new agent, the CPMP[3] recommends the following endpoints in order of relative importance: progression free survival, overall survival, and response rate.

Late side effects may also be important in phase III trials. The "time to event" approach is preferred for the analysis of these endpoints.

To assess the symptomatic effect of a treatment, an additional efficacy endpoint that may be used is symptom control, which is supported by quality of life data. In recent years much interest has focused on integrating both quality of life endpoints and economic evaluations in randomized phase III trials. In both adjuvant and advanced disease trials these may play an important role and be among the endpoints studied. Quality of life assessment is the subject of another chapter in this book.

Definition of Endpoints   The starting point in any time to event analysis is the date of randomization. Use of the date of surgery (or start of treatment) as the starting point may be biased if not all patients are operated on at the same point in time. If the event has not yet been observed at the time of the last available information, then the patient is censored at this date.

In the definitions that follow, disease "progression" is understood to mean progression, relapse, or recurrence as appropriate. Thus no distinction is made between progression, relapse, or recurrence when defining the following time intervals:

- Response to treatment: To be assessed in accordance with WHO recommendations.[12] As a general rule the denominator of the response rate must include all eligible patients.
- Duration of complete response (complete responders only): the time interval between the date of randomization and the date of disease progression after complete response
- Duration of response (complete and partial responders taken together): the time interval between the date of randomization and the date of disease progression
- Time to progression: the time interval between the date of randomization and the date of disease progression

Note: for these last three endpoints, in the case that progression has not yet been observed, the patient is censored at the date of the last examination.

- Disease-free interval (adjuvant trials): the time interval between the date of randomization and the date of first disease progression (the period during which there is no evidence of disease activity). For patients who die prior to progression (for any reason other than malignant disease), their follow-up is censored at the date of death. Otherwise it is censored at the date of the last follow-up examination if no progression has been observed.
- Disease-free survival (adjuvant trials): the time interval between the date of randomization and the date of disease progression or death, whichever comes first. If neither event has been observed, then the patient is censored at the date of the last follow-up examination.
- Duration of survival: the time interval between the date of randomization and the date of death. Patients who were still alive when last traced are censored at the date of last follow-up. Although a separate analysis of death due to malignant disease may be carried out (deaths due to other causes are censored at the date of death), the main analysis should include deaths due to any cause.
- Any other "time to event" endpoint should be precisely defined in the protocol and include the starting date (often the randomization date), an exhaustive list of events considered to be a failure and a definition of the date of censoring.

Number of Patients Required

To obtain the correct results and to be able to convince others of their validity, large randomized trials are required to have a high power to detect small but medically important differences: randomized to reduce the possibility of systematic bias and large to reduce the risk of random errors.

To ensure the feasibility of a phase III trial, the design should be kept as simple as possible. In most cases a simple randomization between just two treatments is recommended. Trials with more than two treatment arms require proportionately more patients and are generally more difficult to recruit because patients must agree to receive any of the possible treatments.

When a clinical trial is being planned, the size of the type I (false-positive) and II errors (false-negative) must be specified. It is customary to set the probability of a type I error, α, at 0.05 (5%), and the probability of a type II error, β, at 0.20 (20%) or less. The value $1 - \beta$ is called the power. The number of patients entered into a phase III trial (the sample size) is usually calculated to ensure a high power of detecting a postulated treatment difference at a pre-specified significance level (α).

A distinction should be made between trials attempting to show a difference in therapeutic effect and trials designed to show equivalence. In equivalence trials one considers a more conservative treatment to be equivalent to the standard when it is not worse than the standard by some given amount.

In both situations the null hypothesis is the "opposite" of what you are trying to prove. In trials attempting to show a difference, one attempts to reject the null hypothesis of no difference in treatment efficacy, whereas in trials attempting to show the equivalence in treatment efficacy of a new more conservative treatment, the null hypothesis is that the new treatment is less effective than the standard treatment by some given amount.[19]

Using the primary endpoint of interest, the determination of the sample size depends on the following factors:

- A realistic prior estimate for the endpoint of interest in the control group
- Realistic estimates of the size of the plausible treatment effect and the medically worthwhile treatment effect
- The size of the type I error α (≤ 0.05, generally two-sided except for equivalence trials) and type II error β (≤ 0.20)
- Realistic estimates of the expected accrual rate and duration of patient entry. In general the expected duration of patient entry should not exceed 5 years
- The duration of follow-up after closing the trial to patient entry

Based on this information the total number of events (in case of a time to event endpoint) and patients needed can be calculated.[20]

The number of patients sharply increases when the size of the treatment benefit of interest decreases. For example, the total number of *deaths* required in a phase III study may vary from 192 for a simple two-arm study trying to detect a 50% increase in the median duration of survival to more than 1500 trying to detect a 5% difference in absolute survival. Enough patients must be entered so that the required number of events can be observed within a given follow-up period.

To detect a difference in response rate, assuming a response rate of 50% in the control arm, the number of patients required on each arm for a two-sided test, with type I and type II errors of 5% and 20% respectively, is approximately:

Number of Patients Per Arm Difference

1400	5%
360	10%
160	15%
90	20%
60	25%

A 2×2 *factorial design* can often be employed to answer two questions for the price of one. An example of such a trial is a study with the following treatment groups:

1. Surgery
2. Surgery + radiotherapy
3. Surgery + chemotherapy
4. Surgery + radiotherapy + chemotherapy

Through the proper use of retrospective stratification, each treatment group can be used twice, once to study the benefit of radiotherapy and once to study the effect of chemotherapy. For example, the effect of radiotherapy is assessed by comparing radiotherapy to no radiotherapy (2 and 4 versus 1 and 3) with a retrospective stratification for whether or not patients received chemotherapy. The number of patients required for this study will be similar to that needed for a two-arm trial if there is no radiotherapy/chemotherapy interaction.

Statistical Analyses

The time to an event should be estimated using the Kaplan–Meier technique.[21] In general, univariate time to event comparisons are based on the logrank test,[21] whether testing for a difference (two-sided) or for equivalence (one-sided). For response data, chi-square tests are to be employed.

The main prognostic factors should be taken into account in a multivariate analysis. The Cox model[21] for time to event analyses and logistic regression[22] for binary endpoints are to be recommended. Retrospective stratification or multivariate models may be employed to adjust the treatment comparison for the possible effect of a prognostic factor.

As a general rule, no subgroup analyses (comparing treatments in only a subgroup of patients) should be performed unless they were specified a priori in the protocol. Any subgroup analyses that are carried out must be interpreted with extreme caution.

Interim Analyses

If one or more interim analyses are performed, the following information should be clearly stated in the protocol:

1. The intention to perform interim analyses, their number, and the timing of analyses
2. The statistical stopping guidelines that will be used, whether it be to prematurely close the trial to patient entry or to decide whether to publish the results of the trial before observing the required number of events. Stopping guidelines based on an α-spending function with an O'Brien–Fleming boundary are generally to be recommended for efficacy endpoints.

While a trial is still open to patient entry, the results of the interim analysis must not be presented to trial participants. The report should be submitted to an Independent Data Monitoring Committee (IDMC) composed of at least one statistician and two medical doctors who are not participating in the trial. The IDMC will take into account not only the statistical stopping guidelines but also all other available information, for example adverse events, quality of life, and results from other similar trials in making their recommendations.[23,24]

Inclusion/Exclusion of Patients from Analyses

Patient Eligibility   A patient is eligible if he or she satisfies all the patient inclusion criteria as defined in the protocol. Eligibility is based only on the patient's status at the time of entry into the trial and cannot be based on something that happens to the patient after registration or randomization.

All patients, including ineligible ones, should be treated and followed in accordance with the protocol whenever possible. If the cause of ineligibility is such that a patient cannot be kept in the protocol, then the patient must at least be followed for the duration of survival. Patients who are randomized and refuse all treatment and examinations should also be followed for the duration of survival. Thus all randomized patients, including ineligible ones, should be followed for survival.

Patients who do not meet the entry criteria based on histologic review (or the review of any other material that is taken prior to entry in the trial, but for which the conclusions are known only after the patient has been entered) should continue in the protocol whenever possible and at least be followed for the duration of survival.

Intent to Treat Principle   Patients should be analyzed according to the "intent to treat" principle (all conclusions are based on all randomized patients according to the treatment group assigned by randomization).

All randomized patients, including the ineligible patients, must be included in at least the survival comparisons. For practical reasons, additional analysis may be carried out which are restricted to the eligible patients.

Patients who are randomized to one treatment, and then for whatever reason receive one of the other protocol treatments, are analyzed as follows:

1. For analyses of treatment efficacy, the main analysis and all conclusions are based on keeping the patient in the treatment group assigned by randomization.
2. Toxicity analyses are based on the treatment the patient actually received.

Meta-Analyses

Probably the biggest flaw in most clinical trials is that too few patients have been entered and an insufficient number of events have been observed to have a high probability of detecting a medically plausible difference in treatment efficacy should it exist. Meta-analysis (overview)[25] is the process of using formal statistical methods to combine together the quantitative results of separate but similar studies in order to

1. Increase the statistical power to detect differences in treatment efficacy
2. Increase the precision of the estimated treatment effect

Although meta-analyses can play a very important role in the overall scientific assessment of a treatment's efficacy, they are not a panacea or a cure-all. In particular they should not be a replacement for large-scale randomized clinical trials.

QUALITY CONTROL

With clinical trials becoming more and more complex, necessary quality control procedures must be established to ensure that the trial is performed and the data are generated in compliance with good clinical practice. It is important that all observations and findings are verifiable. In multicenter trials quality control procedures may include:

- On-site monitoring of the participating institutions to ensure protocol compliance and data quality
- Verification of data transfer to a central data center
- Establishment of external review committees: treatment modality, response to treatment, pathology
- Review and quality control of data by a central data center

Quality control must be applied at each stage of the trial to ensure that all data are reliable and that they have been processed correctly.

REPORTING RESULTS

All patients entered in a trial must be accounted for when reporting results. The data presented per treatment group should include:

- Accrual per center
- Patient eligibility per treatment arm. The reasons for being ineligible should be presented in detail.
- Patient characteristics at randomization per treatment arm
- Treatment data based on all eligible patients who started their treatment. For chemotherapy this should include the number of cycles delivered, dose intensity, dose reductions and delays, premature interruption of treatment, reasons for the discontinuation of treatment, toxicity, and side effects. For other modalities, corresponding data should be presented. Special attention should be paid to serious adverse events. Detailed case descriptions should be provided for each toxic or early death. A standardized toxicity grading system such as the NCIC Common Toxicity Criteria should be used.
- Efficacy results, generally including data on the duration of survival, cause of death, time to progression, etc. While the trial is still open to patient entry, efficacy data MUST NOT be presented by treatment arm in to avoid premature conclusions. Rather than just reporting p values that give no information about the possible size of the treatment effect, it is important to provide an estimate of the size of the treatment effect along with its 95% confidence interval.

Guidelines[26] have recently been published in an attempt to standardize the format for the reporting of clinical trials and to improve the quality of published reports.

FURTHER READING

1. CPMP Working Party on Efficacy of Medicinal Products (1990) EEC note for guidance: Good clinical practice for trials on medicinal products in the European community. *Pharmacol Toxicol* 67: 361–372.
2. CPMP Working Party on Efficacy of Medicinal Products, Note for Guidance III/3630/92-EN (1995) Biostatistical methodology in clinical trials in applications for marketing authorizations for medicinal products. *Statist Med* 14:1659–1682.
3. CPMP Working Party on Efficacy of Medicinal Products (1997) Note for guidance on evaluation of anticancer medicinal products in man.
4. ICH Topic E8 (1997) Note for guidance on general considerations for clinical trials (CPMP/ICH/291/95).
5. ICH Harmonised Tripartite Guideline E9 (1997) Statistical principles for clinical trials.
6. Sylvester, R (1984) Planning Cancer Clinical Trials. In: *Cancer Clinical Trials, Methods and Practice*. Buyse M, Staquet M, Sylvester R (eds). Oxford University Press, Oxford, pp. 47–63.
7. Perry KT (1997) From mouse to man: The early clinical testings. *Drug Informat J* 31: 729–736.
8. American Society of Clinical Oncology (1997) Critical role of phase I clinical trials in cancer treatment. *J Clin Oncol* 15: 853–859.
9. Dent SF, Eisenhauer EA (1996) Phase I trial design: Are new methodologies being put into practice? *Ann Oncol* 7: 561–566

10. Simon R, Freidlin B, Rubinstein L, Arbuck S, Collins J, Christian M (1997) Accelerated titration designs for phase I clinical trials in oncology. *J Natl Cancer Inst* 89: 1138–1147.

11. The Protocol Review Committee, the Data Center, the Research and Treatment Division, and the New Drug Development Office (1997) Phase II trials in the EORTC. *Eur J Cancer* 33: 1361–1363.

12. WHO Handbook for Reporting Results of Cancer Treatment (1979) WHO Offset Publication No. 48, World Health Organization, Geneva.

13. Simon R (1989) Optimal two-stage designs for phase II clinical trials. *Controlled Clin Trials* 10: 1–10.

14. Fleming T (1982) One sample multiple testing procedure for phase II clinical trials. *Biometrics* 38: 143–151.

15. Gehan E (1961) The determination of the number of patients required in a preliminary and a follow-up trial of a new chemotherapeutic agent. *J Chron Dis* 13: 346–353.

16. Kramar A, Potvin D, Hill C (1996) Multistage designs for phase II clinical trials: Statistical issues in cancer research. *Br J Cancer* 74: 1317–1320.

17. Bryant J, Day R (1995) Incorporating toxicity considerations into the design of two-stage phase II clinical trials. *Biometrics* 51: 1372–1383.

18. Pocock S (1979) Allocation of patients to treatment in clinical trials. *Biometrics* 35: 183–197.

19. Blackwelder W (1982) Proving the null hypothesis in clinical trials. *Controlled Clin Trials* 3: 345–353.

20. Machin D, Campbell M, Fayers P, Pinol A (1997) *Sample Size Tables for Clinical Studies.* Blackwell Science, Oxford.

21. Parmar M, Machin D (1995) *Survival Analysis: a Practical Approach.* John Wiley, Chichester.

22. Collett D (1991) *Modelling Binary Data*, Chapman & Hall, London.

23. Fleming T, DeMets D (1993) Monitoring of clinical trials: issues and recommendations. *Controlled Clin Trials* 14: 183–197.

24. Smith MA, Ungerleider RS, Korn EL, Rubinstein L, Simon R (1997) Role of independent data-monitoring committees in randomized clinical trials sponsored by the National Cancer Institute. *J Clin Oncol* 15: 2736–2743.

25. Gelber R, Goldhirsch A (1991) Meta-analysis: The fashion of summing-up evidence. *Ann Oncol* 2: 461–468.

26. Begg C, Cho M, Eastwood S et al (1996) Improving the quality of reporting of randomized controlled trials: The CONSORT statement. *JAMA* 276: 637–639.

CHAPTER 16

SKIN AND MELANOMA CANCER

B.H. BURMEISTER, B.M. SMITHERS, M.G. POULSEN, D. KENNEDY,
and D.B. THOMSON

Queensland Radium Institute and Princess Alexandra Hospital,
South Brisbane, Queensland, Australia

Skin and melanoma cancers are common in Caucasian populations, especially within the tropics. True incidences of nonmelanomatous skin cancers are difficult to assess owing to poor reporting by physicians and patients. A large proportion of skin cancers are in fact never biopsied and therefore never registered. Melanomas, however, are carefully registered and incidences are known in most countries. Although cure rates are high, it is important to remember that deaths still occur despite widespread public awareness of the importance of early diagnosis. Clinicians practicing in tropical areas or where sun exposure is common should be able to identify both melanomatous and nonmelanomatous skin cancers. Education of the patient in identifying lesions is also extremely important. Management of skin cancer is extremely complex and in this chapter some basic guidelines regarding management are outlined.

EPIDEMIOLOGY AND ETIOLOGY

Skin cancers are diseases of fair skin populations. The incidences of skin cancer rises steadily the closer one gets to the equator. More than 90% of skin cancers develop in exposed areas such as the head, neck, and limbs. Basal cell carcinomas (BCCs) are the most commonly diagnosed nonmelanomatous skin cancers. Squamous cell carcinomas (SCCs) are less common and Merkel cell carcinomas are rare. The median age of onset of BCCs and SCCs is 68 years. It is, however, common to see nonmelanomatous skin cancers in young people as a result of both recreational and occupational

Manual of Clinical Oncology, 7th edition, Edited by Raphael E. Pollock
ISBN 0-471-23828-7, pages 325–340. Copyright © 1999 Wiley-Liss, Inc.

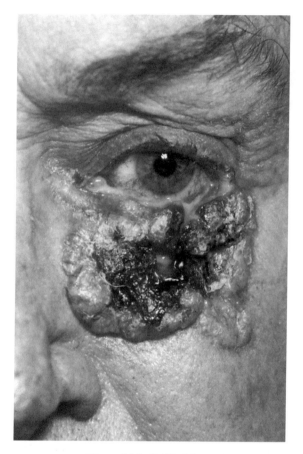

Figure 16.1. BCC of face.

exposures. The male-to-female ratio is 4 to 1. Factors other than sunlight that may be related to the incidence of skin cancer include some genetic conditions such as xeroderma pigmentosum and Gorlin's syndrome. Prolonged immunosuppression associated with organ transplantation or low-grade lymphomas may result in a 20-fold increase in nonmelanomatous skin cancer. Rarer predisposing factors include exposure to chemicals such as arsenic, tar, nitrogen mustard, and ionizing radiation. Sites of trauma from burns or smallpox vaccination scars may also be associated with skin cancers.

The incidence of melanoma varies but the annual increase is between 2% and 5% in the white populations worldwide. In Australia the mortality trends have stabilized recently but in general the mortality trends have increased. The incidence rises after 50 years of age. The incidence is similar between males and females within a population.

Pale skin, a tendency to sunburn, fair or red hair, large numbers of melanocytic nevi, and multiple dysplastic nevi have been shown to be independent risk factors

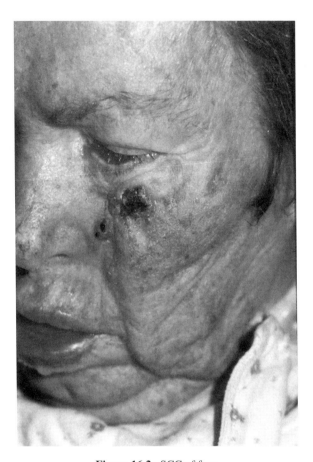

Figure 16.2. SCC of face.

for the development of melanoma. Melanoma is rare in black populations and has a lower frequency in populations with increased skin pigmentation, where the most common form of melanoma tends to be the subungual form and melanoma on the palms of the hands and soles of the feet.

SCREENING

Skin cancer prevention has consisted mainly of education programs aimed at altering attitudes about sunlight and suntans. In Australia this has resulted in increased wearing of hats, avoidance of the sun around the middle of the day, and the increased use of sunscreens. Recent data have suggested that the regular use of sunscreens certainly can prevent the development of new solar keratoses. The main purpose of screening is to detect tumors at an early stage, thus leading to reduced costs and morbidity of treatment. The American Academy of Dermatologists initiated a national melanoma/skin cancer prevention program in 1985 that has reached more than 600,000 people. As a result of this program more than 35,000 nonmalanomatous skin cancers were diagnosed and 3500 melanomas identified.

Screening high-risk individuals detects melanoma at an early stage. Population screening has not been proven cost effective. People with a strong family history, especially in first-degree relatives and those with more than 100 melanocytic nevi and multiple dysplastic nevi, should be monitored by general skin examination and given advice relating to the appropriate measures of sun protection. Prophylatic excision of dysplastic nevi and other benign nevi does not reduce the melanoma risk because a melanoma may develop as a new lesion rather than from preexisting nevus.

DIAGNOSTIC MEASURES INCLUDING PATHOLOGY

BCCs and SCCs commonly present on sun-exposed areas. BCCs usually present as a slow growing well circumscribed papule, often with a pearly surface and telangectasiae visible. Larger lesions may have central ulceration. Sometimes central regression may occur. SCCs may have a variety of clinical appearances and may appear as a hyperkeratosis, an ulcer, or a scaly patch that bleeds. Some may resemble a proliferative lesion such as a keratoacanthoma. Merkel cell carcinomas do not have a classic appearance and typically arise in the head and neck region of an elderly person. Commonly they present as a rapidly growing nodule that is painless and has a bluish red color. Many patients may present initially with nodal disease and no obvious primary.

Clinical evaluation of all sun-exposed areas in the patient with skin cancer is essential. Examination of regional lymph nodes close to a documented lesion should also be performed. Suspicious lesions may be biopsied with a shave excision or punch biopsy. Advanced lesions may require further investigations to establish their true extent. Lesions on the face and scalp may be associated with bone or neural invasion. CT scan or MRI in this setting may be indicated. Merkel cell tumors have a high metastatic potential and may require a routine systemic baseline workup.

The pathology of nonmelanomatous skin cancers is well recognized. BCCs are characterized by nests of palisading small basal type cells with relatively large, basophilic nuclei. Mitoses are common. Several morphologic types are known, the most common being solid, cystic, pigmented, and multifocal superficial varieties.

BCCs are generally not invasive during the first 5 to 10 years of the growth cycle. Once invasive, however, extensive local destruction can occur. Nodal spread is exceptionally rare. SCCs arise from epidermal keratinocytes and are typified by keratinization and horn pearl formation. They are commonly associated with solar keratoses from which they arise. SCCs are more aggressive than BCCs with a tendency to local recurrence and lymph node spread. Perineural invasion is also common, particularly around the face. Merkel cell carcinomas are of neuroendocrine origin and are composed of sheets of small cells that stain for neuron-specific enolase. They are highly malignant with a propensity for local recurrence, nodal spread, and distant metastases.

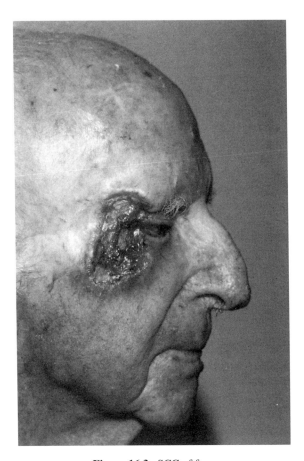

Figure 16.3. SCC of face.

The requirements to make the diagnosis of melanoma are understanding the variance of melanoma, the history relating to the lesion, a good light, and magnification. A melanotic melanoma is more difficult to diagnose but should be considered when there is any unusual nonpigmented lesion of the skin. The ABCDE mnemonic is useful:

A = Assymmetry in shape

B = Border notably irregular

C = Color variation often with a number of different shades of black, brown, blue, or progressive pallor within a pigmented lesion

D = Diameter often greater than 5 mm

E = Elevation

Recently the use of skin surface microscopy (dermatoscopy, dermoscopy, epiluminescence microscopy) has been advocated to improve the diagnosis of pigmented

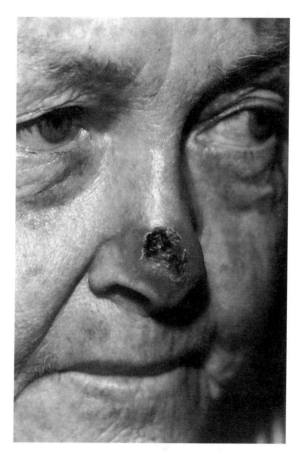

Figure 16.4. SCC of nose.

lesions. This technique uses a high-quality light with magnification in combination with immersion oil at the skin microscope interface, allowing improved recognition of pigment patterns by making the epidermis translucent.

Melanoma is a cancer of the melanocytes and thus arises in the basal layer of the epidermis. The potential for metastasis relates to the depth of invasion, in particular the thickness of the melanoma at the time of diagnosis. Four clinicopathologic types exist:

1. *Superficial spreading melanoma (50% to 60%):* Lateral growth phase predominates with subsequent vertical growth phase.
2. *Nodular melanoma (10% to 15%):* Vertical growth phase predominates and thus melanomas tend to be thicker at the time of diagnosis.
3. *Lentigomaligna melanoma (10% to 15%):* Slow growing and commonly found in UV-exposed regions, particularly the head and neck.

TABLE 16.1. Survival According to Depth of Invasion

Melanoma in situ	100%
≥ 0.75 mm	97%–98%
≥ 0.75–1.5 mm	90%
1.5–3.0 mm	75%
≥ 3.0 mm	55%

4. *Acral lentiginous melanoma (1% to 10%):* Occur on the palms, soles, and nail beds and are not related to sun exposure.

Desmoplastic or neurotropic melanomas are variants of nodular or superficial spreading melanomas having a propensity for local recurrence and spread along superficial nerves.

Increasing number of nodes involved is associated with decreasing survival. The presence of extracapsular invasion of a lymph node may be associated with higher rate of recurrence in a lymph node field following block dissection.

The prognosis of melanoma is dependent on the depth of invasion (Table 16.1). Other indicators of a poor prognosis include male gender, ulceration, and a high mitotic rate.

STAGING

The stage at presentation of skin cancer and particularly melanoma is the most important factor influencing outcome.

The following is the staging according to the UICC TNM pretreatment clinical classification.

T—Primary Tumor (Nonmelanomatous Skin Cancer)

Tis	Preinvasive carcinoma (carcinoma in situ)
T0	No evidence of primary tumor
T1	Tumor 2 cm or less in largest dimension
T2	Tumor more than 2 cm but not more than 5 cm in its largest dimension
T3	Tumor more than 5 cm in its largest dimension
T4	Tumor invades deep extradermal structure, for example, cartilage, skeletal, muscle, or bone.

N—Regional Lymph Nodes (Nonmelanomatous Skin Cancer)

N0	No evidence of regional node involvement
N1	Regional lymph node metastasis

pT—Primary Tumor (Melanoma)

pTis   Melanoma in situ (Clark level I) (atypical melanocytic hyperplasia, severe melanocytic dysplasia, not an invasive malignant lesion)

pT1   Tumor 0.75 mm or less in thickness and invades the papillary dermis (Clark level II)

pT2   Tumor more than 0.75 mm but not more than 1.5 mm in thickness and/or invades to the papillary–reticular dermal interface (Clark level III)

pT3   Tumor more than 1.5 mm but not more than 4.0 mm in thickness and/or invades the reticular dermis (Clark level IV)

N—Regional Lymph Nodes (Melanoma)

N0   No regional lymph node metastasis

N1   Metastasis 3 cm or less in greatest dimension in any regional lymph node(s)

N2   Metastasis more than 3 cm in greatest dimension in any regional lymph node(s) and/or in-transit metastasis.

SURGERY

Surgical excision offers a high rate of cure for BCC and SCC and produces a specimen that can be analyzed for completeness of excision and subtype. Histologic features are in turn predicative of the future behavior of the tumor where a recurrence would be destructive, for example, adjacent to an eyelid, lip, or nasal margin or endanger of becoming seriously invasive, for example, inner canthus, nasal base, or postauricular areas. Maximum information about the tumor behavior is desirable. Surgical excision of primary BCCs offers a 4.8% recurrence at 5 years and 2.9% recurrence if the lesion is less than 5 mm. Curettage and electrocautery (C & E) can be effectively and efficiently used to treat small, peripheral BCCs with a 9.5% recurrence rate at 5 years. Large lesions (> 1 cm) have a 22.7% 5-year recurrence rate and lesions on critical features such as nose, lip, eyelid, etc. can recur without any obvious surface signs after C & E, thus delaying appropriate treatment and allowing added destruction. C & E is not considered complete treatment for SCC. Special problems attend recurrent lesions, infiltrative lesions, and lesions showing invasion along nerves. Generally a wider margin of clearance and a more comprehensive pathology assessment is indicated. Recurrences are more likely with the infiltrative type of BCC, the poorly differentiated SCC, and certain positions. Clinically involved nodes should be treated at the time of surgery by means of a lymphadenectomy. In particular, mucocutaneous SCC, large SCCs, peripheral SCCs, and SCCs arising in burns scars will show a higher rate of metastasis.

With view to margins, BCCs can be cleared histologically with a 2 to 5 mm margin when of the solid or circumscribed variety. SCCs generally require a 5 to 10 mm margin depending on the size and aggressive nature of the tumor. Between 5 and 8 mm is required when BCCs are infiltrative. Incomplete deep margins involving

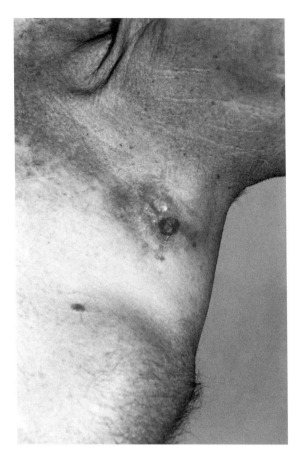

Figure 16.5. SCC of shoulder.

BCCs should be reexcised but incomplete lateral margins can be considered for observation. All incompletely excised SCCs should be reexcised where possible. Completeness of excision is enhanced by careful preoperative markings before the local anaesthesia is infiltrated. Adequate lighting and good surgical technique increase the rate of complete excision. Moh's micrographic surgery can produce a 98% cure rate for BCCs but is tedious and slow. It should be reserved for difficult BCCs in critical sites because the operator maps out the entire cut surface histologically.

Lesions suspicious of being melanoma should be treated by *complete* excisional biopsy. Punch biopsy or incisional biopsy should be reserved for large lesions where complete excision is not reasonable as the initial diagnostic maneuver. The margin of diagnostic excisional biopsies should be a minimum of 2 mm.

The minimum margin for definitive therapy of an invasive melanoma is 1 cm. For melanomas greater than 4 mm and desmoplastic variants the potential for local recurrence is greater and thus some experts would recommend margins of 2 to 3 cm. There is no evidence that this will offer a survival benefit and will only improve

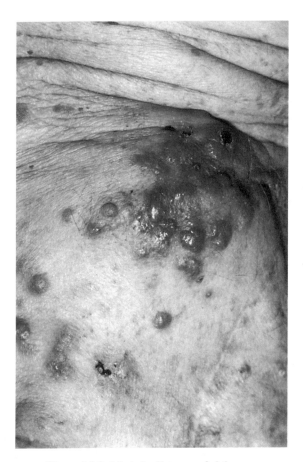

Figure 16.6. Merkel cell tumor of abdomen.

local control. The depth of excision should at least equal the excision margin. There is no need to excise the deep fascia. Reexcision is recommended if the margins of excisional biopsy were less than those recommended for a definitive lesion. At the time of definitive excision a primary melanoma should be manipulated minimally to decrease the potential for implantation of the wound. Flap repair or skin graft may be required at certain sites to obtain satisfactory skin coverage. Melanoma in situ (level I melanoma) should be excised with a minimum margin of 5 mm.

Subungual melanomas are removed by amputation, usually proximal to the interphalangeal joint of the thumb or the distal phalangeal joint of a finger or toe. Tumors of the sole of the foot should be excised appropriately but with an aim to preserve weight-bearing skin. The use of specialized plastic surgical flap repairs may assist in coverage over weight-bearing areas at this site.

Elective lymph node dissection is not recommended for the majority of patients with melanoma. There may be some subgroups who benefit but this is yet to be defined. The presence of lymphatic invasion within the primary lesion may be a marker

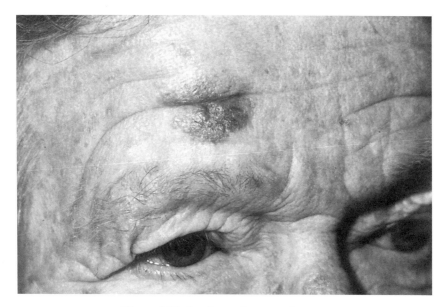

Figure 16.7. Lentigo malignant melanoma.

for lymph node metastasis and elective lymph node dissection may be considered in these patients. Clinical evidence of lymph node involvement should be confirmed with fine-needle aspiration cytology if this is available. If open biopsy is absolutely necessary the biopsy excision should be removed in continuity with the lymphatic field on block dissection. Confirmed lymph involvement indicates the need for a full therapeutic lymph node dissection. Removal of single nodes is not satisfactory because of the potential for multiple nodal involvement. There is a risk of local recurrence within a dissected lymph node field in patients who have positive lymph nodes, notably if multiple nodes are involved or if extracapsular invasion is present. If a single lymph node is involved the 10-year survival may be as high as 50%. The potential for survival is reduced as the number of nodes increases or in the presence of extracapsular invasion.

Recently lymphatic mapping, sentinel lymph node biopsy, and selective lymphadenectomy have been reported. At this stage these techniques are being evaluated in randomized trials and should be regarded as experimental.

Metastases localized to a limb may be treated using a technique of limb vascular isolation with chemotherapy. This technique is called isolated limb perfusion or isolated limb infusion. The latter technique has been more recently developed and is simpler and less morbid. Response rates of up to 80% have been reported, with 40% of those being complete responses. There is a significant incidence of recurrence following treatment both locally and with distant metastasis. Eventually 70% of these patients will fail because of the presence of distant metastases that were not evident at the initial presentation.

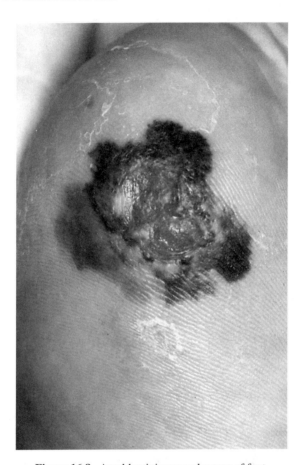

Figure 16.8. Acral lentiginous melanoma of foot.

Surgery offers the better course of action for patients with isolated distant metastases. A small percentage of these patients will have long-term survival. This is notably the case in solitary lung and cerebral metastases. Symptomatic metastatic disease may be managed by surgical excision to offer a better quality of palliation in selected patients.

RADIATION THERAPY

For early nonmelanomatous lesions radiation therapy offers cure rates approaching 100%. It offers the advantages of painless treatment that can be delivered on an outpatient basis. To maximize the effect on the tumor and minimize the effect on normal tissues, treatment is generally fractionated. For small lesions a dose such as 40 Gy in 10 fractions is often sufficient. Larger tumors require higher doses and more fractions. In some more elderly or frailer patients shorter schedules may be used but they do result in greater scarring. Radiation therapy does result in good preservation of function and cosmesis which may be an advantage on the face, particularly around the eyes, nose, and ears. Later changes of atrophy and telangectasiae may result; these are not very noticeable in elderly patients with extensive skin damage. Extensive infiltrating tumors are best managed in combination with surgery. Radiation combined with surgery may be used to minimize the morbidity of surgery and may limit the extent to which a radical surgical procedure needs to be performed. In some centers the use of radiation has declined in recent times as a result of the increasing awareness of late radiation effects. This has been accompanied by a proportional rise in the use of surgical and dermatological techniques. Radiation is still, however, recommended in the following situations:

1. Treatment in the elderly or frail
2. Where surgery will result in major deformity (lower eyelids, nose, and ears)
3. Postoperative treatment for advanced or recurrent lesions, positive margins, tumor spill, perineural spread, or lymphovascular invasion
4. Treatment of advanced inoperable lesions where relief from bleeding, infection, odor, and pain may be required

Radiation should be avoided in areas of poor blood supply or areas that would be exposed to friction, trauma, or excessive sunlight. A favorable response is less likely to occur with bone or cartilage infiltration. Elective nodal radiation is not required for BCCs and SCCs as the incidence of nodal spread is low. Clinically involved lymph nodes, however, should be therapeutically dissected after confirmation with cytology. Postoperative irradiation to the nodal bases is indicated if multiple nodes are involved, or if there is extracapsular extension or perineural spread. Metastatic involvement of the parotid nodes is not uncommon and is best managed with a superficial parotidectomy followed by postoperative irradiation to the parotid and ipsilateral neck.

Merkel cell tumors should be resected if practical but gross tumor can be controlled with radiation alone. Surgery should, however, always be followed by wide field radiation therapy to the primary site and relevant nodal areas with the coverage of intransit tissue. A dose of 50 Gy given in 25 fractions is usually adequate.

Radiation for primary melanoma has been used on the face but most melanomas are treated by primary excision. It may, however, be considered where a melanoma is close to an eye in an elderly frail patient. The major role of radiation therapy for melanomas is metastic disease, where, contrary to popular belief, significant responses occur. Radiation may be used as an adjuvant following dissection, although this area remains controversial. The policy at the Queensland Melanoma Project at Princess Alexandra Hospital in Queensland is to offer all patients adjuvant radiation therapy for the following situations:

1. Multiple nodal involvement
2. Extracapsular spread of disease
3. Tumor spill at surgery
4. Recurrences

Patients having these criteria are at high risk of local recurrence and radiation would appear to reduce this risk. There is, however, no proven benefit in overall survival. Typical doses used are 48 Gy in 20 fractions or 30 Gy in five or six fractions. Contrary to popular belief, there is only a very slight increase in the incidence of major side effects following surgery with lymphedema of a breast or limb being the most common effect. In many instances, however, the lymphedema is of low grade and not particularly troublesome. Bulky inoperable nodal disease in the absence of metastases is also amenable to high-dose radiation treatment. Doses of the order of 50 Gy in 20 fractions may be used although hypofractionated regimens such as 21 Gy in three fractions or 30 Gy in six fractions may be used if the tumor is not close to the spinal cord or a major nerve. Although it is widely believed that radiation in large fractions is more effective in controlling bulky disease, there are no randomized trials to confirm this. Radiation may also be used extensively the palliation of metastatic disease. Melanoma commonly spreads to the brain, bone, and subcutaneous tissues. In these sites it can cause troublesome symptoms that may be rapidly relieved with the use of radiation therapy. For brain metastases a dose of 30 Gy in 10 fractions is appropriate although at other sites such as bone and subcutaneous tissues hypofractionated regimens may again be used.

CHEMOTHERAPY/IMMUNOTHERAPY

Topical 5-fluorouracil is useful for the management of solar keratoses and basal cell carcinomas but may allow deep progression of underlying BCC while the surface clinically regresses. Intralesional recombinant interferon-α can control local BCCs but surgical approaches are preferred. Photodynamic therapy is associated with a significant risk of any sun exposure for many days, a problem in warm climates. There is no standard chemotherapy for metastatic BCC or SCC of the skin and literature is sparse. However, drugs such as cisplatin, 5-fluorouracil, methotrexate, and bleomycin have recorded activity although there are no large-scale trials. One of the more commonly used regimens is one of cisplatin and infusional 5-fluorouracil similar to that used in head and neck cancer. It is well tolerated and has a reasonable response rate. Toxicity of such treatments must be balanced against clinical improvement. There are major difficulties in managing metastatic skin cancer in transplant recipients with renal impairment. Merkel cell carcinomas respond well to a number of drugs including regimens such as CHOP (cyclophosphamide, adriamycin, vincrstine, prednisone) or carboplatin and etoposide. Response rates are variable but complete responses regularly occur.

With melanoma it is now recognized that patients with positive lymph nodes (microscopic or clinical) may have a survival benefit when treated with 12 months of therapy of high-dose adjuvant recombinant interferon-α. This is based on a recent study by the Eastern Cooperative Oncology Group. Toxicity is severe, with more than 50% of patients requiring significant dose reductions both during the first month of induction and subsequent 11 months of maintenance. The results of this trial, however, have yet to be confirmed. There are no randomized data reported as yet to support the use of other adjuvant immunotherapy strategies such as melanoma vaccines or BCG. For metastatic disease there is no standard therapy. Systemic chemotherapy has a low activity with regular agents such as dacarbazine, lomustine, and cisplatin all having response rates of less than 17%. The duration of response is usually less than 6 months and complete responses are in less than 5% of cases. Systemic recombinant interferon-α also has a response rate of 17% but is, however, associated with significant toxicity. Most centers would employ a standard therapy dacarbazine given once every 3 weeks, either as a single dose or over 5 days. With the use of 5-HT$_3$ inhibitors and dexamethasone, nausea and vomiting are uncommonly seen. Other immunotherapy strategies for systemic disease such as interleukin-2, gene transfection with granulacyte, macrophage colony-stimulating factor (GM-CSF), and tumor necrosis factor or dendritic cell therapies remain experimental.

FOLLOW-UP

Patients with both nonmelanomatous and melanomatous skin cancers require extremely close follow-up by the treating physician. It is extremely common for patient with skin cancers to develop second malignancies of both types, particularly in sun-exposed areas. Recurrences of the primary tumor may also occur. Most recurrences for BCCs and SCCs occur within the first 2 years. Patients with advanced nonmelanomatous tumors and melanomas may develop spread to the lymph nodes. Examination of regional lymph node areas is mandatory at follow up examination. It is recommended that a 3-month follow-up visit be conducted during the first 2 years and every 6 months after that period. Patients with melanoma having unusual symptoms such as headache, vomiting, abdominal pain, bone pain, or breathlessness should be investigated for the presence of metastases in the brain, abdomen, liver, or lungs respectively.

REHABILITATION

Surgery or radiation therapy for skin cancers seldom requires extensive rehabilitation. After nodal dissection with or without postoperative irradiation some rehabilitation may be required to maximize movement at a specific joint, for example, shoulder. Patients having cosmetic surgery around the face area with removal or reconstruction of an important anatomic part may require appropriate rehabilitation in accordance with their outlook.

PREVENTION

In most instances skin cancer is preventable. Caucasians living in climates of high sun exposure should wear protective sunscreens with minimum sun protection factor (SPF) of 15 on all sun-exposed areas. Where possible, parts of the body such as the head should be shielded with the use of hats and light clothing should be worn to cover other areas. Where possible, activities outdoors should be restricted to the early and late parts of the day with avoidance of full sun between 10 a.m. and 2 p.m. Patients with a family history of melanoma or with the dysplastic nevus syndrome should be closely followed by clinicians with the object of detecting early melanomatous change of an existing nevus.

FURTHER READING

Ashby MA, McEwan L (1990) Treatment of non-melanomatous skin cancer: A review of recent trends with special reference to the Australian scene. *Clin Oncol* 2:284–289.

Australian Cancer Network (1997) *Guidelines for the Management of Cutaneous Melanoma.* The Stone Press, Sydney.

Boyle F, Pendlebury S, Bell D (1995) Further insight into the natural history and management of primary cutaneous neuroendocrine (Merkel cell) carcinoma. *Int J Radiat Oncol Biol Phys* 31:315–232.

Balch CM, Urist MM, Karakousis CP, et al. (1993) Efficacy of 2cm surgical margins for intermediate thickness melanomas 1–4 mm—results of a multi-institutional randomised surgical trial. *Ann Surg* 218:262–269.

Burmeister BH, Smithers BM, Poulsen M, et al. (1995) Radiation therapy for nodal disease in malignant melanoma. *World J Surg* 19:369–371.

Calabro A, Singletary SE, Balch CM (1989) Patterns of relapse in 1001 consecutive patients with melanoma nodal metastases. *Arch Surg* 124:1051–1055.

Emmett AJJ (1990) Surgical analysis and biological behaviour of 2277 basal cell carcinomas. *Aust NZ J Surg* 60:855–863.

Emmett AJ, O'Rourke MG (1991) *Malignant Skin Tumours.* Churchill Livingstone.

Fleming ID, Amonette R, Monaghan T, Fleming MD (1995). Principles of management of basal and squamous cell carcinoma of the skin. *Cancer* 75:699–704.

Giles G, Armstrong B, Burton R, et al. 1996) Has mortality from melanoma stopped rising in Australia? Analysis of trends between 1931 and 1994. *Br Med J* 312:121–125.

Kirkwood JM, Strawderman MH, Ernstoff MS, et al. Interferon alfa-2b adjuvant therapy of high-risk resected cutaneous melanoma: The Eastern Cooperative Oncology Group Trial EST 1684. *J Clin Oncol* 14:7–17.

Marks R (1995) An overview of skin cancer. *Cancer* 75:607–612.

McDonald C (1995) Status of screening for skin cancer. *Cancer* 72:1066–1070.

Morton DL, Wen DR, Cochran AJ (1992) Management of early-stage melanoma by intra-operative lymphatic mapping and selective lymphadenectomy. *Surg Oncol Clin North Am* 1:247–259.

Tompson JF, Waugh RC, Saw RPM, et. al. (1994) Isolated limb infusion with melphalan for recurrent limb melanoma: A simple alternative to isolated limb perfusion. *Regional Cancer Treat* 7:188–192.

CHAPTER 17

HEAD AND NECK CANCER

BRIAN O'SULLIVAN

Department of Radiation Oncology
Princess Margaret Hospital
University of Toronto
Toronto, Canada

JONATHAN IRISH

Department of Surgical Oncology
Princess Margaret Hospital
University of Toronto
Toronto, Canada

LILLIAN SIU

Cancer Therapy and Research Center
The University of Texas Science Center at San Antonio
San Antonio, TX

ANNE LEE

Department of Radiation Oncology
Pamela Youde Nethersole Eastern Hospital
3 Lok Man Road, Hong Kong

The rubric "head and neck cancer" covers a wide variety of cancers arising from the mucosal lining of the upper aerodigestive tract. In this chapter, most sites are dealt with generically but where distinctions exist, these will be acknowledged. Experience in the treatment of this group of cancers has emphasized the need for multidisciplinary care in treatment and rehabilitation. Local and regional failure remain the paramount concern although distant failure rates may increase as local and regional control rates improve. The challenge in the treatment is compounded by the fact that

Manual of Clinical Oncology, 7th edition, Edited by Raphael E. Pollock
ISBN 0-471-23828-7, pages 341–358. Copyright © 1999 Wiley-Liss, Inc.

this patient population carries a significant risk of medical comorbidity and of development of second primary cancers, with both risks related to chronic exposure to tobacco and alcohol.

ETIOLOGY AND EPIDEMIOLOGY

Cancers of the head and neck comprise approximately 5% of all new cancer diagnoses. With the exception of the postcricoid subsite in hypopharyngeal carcinoma, in which the male-to-female ratio is nearly equal, this is predominantly a disease of men. However, increased tobacco use by women during the last 20 years has led to an increase in incidence among women. Patients have usually attained their sixth decade of life by the time of diagnosis.

The major etiologic factor in the development of mucosal head and neck cancer is the use of tobacco, which imparts a relative risk of cancer occurrence of two- to three-fold. Tobacco reacts synergistically with alcohol, leading to a 10- to 15-fold increase in head and cancer risk. Human papillomavirus (HPV) has been identified in squamous cell carcinomas of the oral cavity and larynx but direct causation remains unconfirmed. Lip cancer is associated with sun exposure, whereas nasal and sinus squamous cell carcinomas have been linked to nickel exposure and to woodworking. Dietary deficiency of some vitamins (A, E, and C), elements (iron), and foods (fruit, vegetables, dairy products) has also been implicated. In particular, the iron deficiency found in Plummer–Vinson syndrome is associated with cancer of the postcricoid hypopharynx and proximal esophagus. Poor oral hygiene and chronic mucosal inflammatory conditions such as lichen planus could also be etiologic factors in oral cancer.

Two regions of the world merit special comment. In India, the custom of inverse smoking and the prevalence of areca nut ("betel" nut) chewing has resulted in one third of all cancers originating in the head and neck, with a high predilection to the oral cavity. There is also a high incidence of oral submucous fibrosis of the oral cavity in the Indian population that is related to areca nut chewing and considered a premalignant condition.

Nasopharyngeal carcinoma (NPC) also manifests a particular geographic and ethnic distribution. The annual incidence varies from 19 per 100,000 Chinese population in Southeast Asia to 0.2 per 100,000 Caucasian population. Study of Chinese who had emigrated to the United States showed that subsequent generations had progressively lower incidence, but their risk was still substantially higher than that of other races born in the same locality. Other risk groups include the Greenland Eskimos and Maghrebin Arabs in North Africa. Etiology is likely to be multifactorial: both genetic predisposition (HLA subtype susceptibility) and environmental factors are important. Epstein–Barr Virus (EBV) is strongly associated with this malignancy, particularly in endemic areas, but its exact role has yet to be defined. Further support for an environmental etiology is an association seen in endemic areas with a dietary intake high in salt-cured fish and vegetable products.

SCREENING

Because head and neck cancer predominantly affects population groups that can be easily identified there is a significant opportunity for early detection of precancerous lesions and conditions and cancerous lesions. Despite this, in many parts of the world patients present with advanced disease. Patient awareness about the adverse effects of tobacco use and the inability to access rural populations in many parts of the world probably contribute to this. In India, implementation of sentinel screening has yielded much of our knowledge of oral cancer and its premalignant conditions and illustrates the merits of such programs in the developing world

Similarly, NPC affects a large population at risk in the developing world. Screening has been attempted in endemic areas, but the cost-effectiveness has yet to be assessed. However, with the strong tendency of familial aggregation, regular monitoring of immunoglobulin A (IgA) against viral capsid antigen of EBV together with nasopharyngeal examination is advisable for high-risk populations with positive family history.

Populations at risk for head and neck cancer must be taught the early warning signs or symptoms of possible malignancy so that early presentation is possible. The typical symptoms are described by the common sites of origin (Table 17.1).

DIAGNOSIS

Pathology

The epithelial-lined tract of the upper aerodigestive tract gives rise to most of the malignancies of the head and neck, in particular squamous cell carcinoma, which is

TABLE 17.1. Typical Symptoms by Common Sites of Origin in Head and Neck

Site of Origin	Symptoms
Nasopharynx	Early: Hearing loss, tinnitus, epistaxis, nasal obstruction, single lymph node involved
	Late: Headache, cranial nerve abnormalities, trismus, multiple lymph nodes involved, weight loss
Oral cavity	Early: Superficial mucosal pain, denture malposition, mouth bleeding
	Late: Pain from bone invasion, cranial nerve abnormalities, tongue tethering, trismus, palpable lymph nodes, weight loss, skin infiltration
Glottic larynx	Early: Hoarseness (glottic)
	Late: Dyspnea (airway obstruction), cartilage penetration (neck mass)
Supraglottis/oropharynx/ Hypopharynx	Early: Dysphagia or otalgia (supraglottic)
	Late: Dyspnea (airway obstruction), odynophagia, palpable lymph nodes, weight loss

the most common and, therefore, the focus of this chapter. Tumors may also arise from other tissue including connective tissues (sarcomas of bone and soft tissue); lymphoid tissue (lymphoma and plasmacytoma); skin (melanoma, squamous, and basal cell carcinoma); and major (parotid, submandibular, and sublingual) and minor salivary glands. The latter are distributed throughout the mucous membranes of the oral cavity, paranasal sinuses, and nasal cavity. Mucoepidermoid and adenoid cystic carcinomas comprise the majority of salivary gland malignancies. Lymphomas in this region have a particular predilection to Waldeyer's ring.

The pathologic predictors of outcome for most typical squamous carcinomas include the presence of perineural spread (predictive of invasion along nerves), angiolymphatic invasion, grade of tumor, and the presence of ulceration.

In NPC, the WHO classification recognizes keratinizing squamous carcinoma (type 1), nonkeratinizing carcinoma (type 2), and undifferentiated carcinoma (type 3). Type 1 NPC is the least common among the Asian populations and is also the least radiosensitive of the three and carries the most unfavourable prognosis.

Natural History

The behavior of head and neck cancers is relevant to diagnosis because certain patterns exist and should be understood. Local spread is usually orderly to contiguous sites. However, submucosal spread is common and tumor may remain in the oral tongue and base of tongue until quite large with eventual ulceration, invasion of musculature, and fixation. Posterior pharyngeal wall lesions enlarge submucosally and may present as skip lesions. They tend to remain on the posterior wall and spread up and down with posterior tethering and painful ulceration when advanced. Extension into the nasopharynx superiorly, or inferiorly to the arytenoid region, may be unexpected in a lesion with its epicenter in the posterior oropharynx and should be looked for.

Tumors may penetrate potential spaces such as the preepiglottic space in the base of tongue or supraglottic cancers, or through the sinus of Morgagni, a defect in the muscular wall of the superior pharynx, to reach the parapharyngeal space in NPC. In NPC, erosion of the skull base and/or cranial nerves is common and relates to their proximity to the primary origin. In other sites the orderly infiltration provides common presentations for the different tumors at their various stages, for example, orbit and facial skin in advanced paranasal sinus disease, mandibular invasion in advanced floor of mouth disease, and pterygoid muscle invasion when tumors gain access to the pterygomaxillary region.

Lymphatic invasion to lymph nodes is also generally orderly and usually involves the upper and mid jugular chain (levels II and III; see definitions below). NPC not infrequently involves any part of level V although the upper portion is most common. In addition, retropharyngeal (nodes of Rouviere) are common in NPC and can be appreciated radiologically only when early, although grossly enlarged nodes can displace the soft palate inferomedially and be palpable. Anterior oral cavity characteristically may skip to levels III or IV in approximately 15% of cases without involvement of the upper neck. In general, lateral lesions of the tongue, tonsillar region, and floor of the mouth tend to spread to the ipsilateral neck, whereas in midline lesions, for example, in the larynx, hypopharynx, and nasopharynx, if treatment is required it should encompass both sides of the neck.

Distant metastases are uncommon, excepting NPC, and are usually associated with advanced N categories. The most common sites are the lungs, followed by liver and bone.

Diagnostic Work-up

Every head and neck cancer case requires a complete history and physical examination with particular attention to the primary and neck disease extent for staging purposes. Examination with the patient awake is essential for some sites (e.g., tongue tethering denoting deep muscle extension of an oral cancer or glottic fixation in a laryngeal cancer require dynamic assessment). Examination under anesthesia (nasopharyngoscopy, laryngoscopy, esophagoscopy, and bronchoscopy) is important to assess the extent of primary disease and to exclude the presence of a synchronous primary cancer (5 to 15% risk) in another head and neck site or the esophagus or lung. If the presentation is with a metastatic lymph node in the neck from an unknown primary tumor, the patient must also undergo endoscopy with guided biopsies of the nasopharynx, tongue base, and pyriform sinus and tonsillectomy to detect possible occult disease at these sites. If no primary disease is confirmed an open biopsy of the lymph node is recommended to confirm histopathology.

Radiologic investigations include a chest X-ray film to rule out metastatic disease or a second primary malignancy of the lung. Computerized tomography (CT) scan with its ability to assess bone involvement and soft tissue extent is particularly valuable for assessment of primary disease of the temporal bone, nasal and sinus cavity, hypopharynx, and larynx and is valuable for the assessment of regional lymphadenopathy. Magnetic resonance imaging (MRI) with its capability to delineate soft tissue anatomy is particularly helpful in assessing the nasopharynx (especially retropharyngeal lymph nodes and invasion of the parapharyngeal space), and in oral and base of tongue lesions. In many cases, MRI and CT are complementary, especially in the vicinity of the skull base or where inflammatory changes are present around tumor (e.g., nasal cavity and sinuses).

Panelipse and dental occlusive X-ray films can also assess mandible involvement in oral cancer. Coronal plane laryngeal tomograms in combination with CT imaging may facilitate assessment of subglottic involvement in laryngeal cancer. Although esophagoscopy is essential to assess proximal esophageal involvement in hypopharyngeal carcinoma and to rule out a second primary tumor of the esophagus some authors prefer a barium swallow screening test.

Fine-needle aspiration (FNA) for cytologic diagnosis may be useful in the investigation of patients with cervical lymphadenopathy or salivary gland tumors. Although the accuracy of cytology can vary from center to center, in the salivary gland it can reach 75%.

STAGING

The TNM staging system is the only widely accepted staging classification. Recently the TNM has been revised to its 5th edition to reflect relevant assessment and management strategies and knowledge about outcome (Tables 17.2 and 17.3). In the head and neck, a major change has included a revision of the nasopharyngeal classification. The T classifications differ in specific details for each site because of anatomic considerations. The N classification for cervical lymph node metastasis is uniform for all mucosal sites except the nasopharynx.

Any diagnostic information that contributes to overall accuracy of the pretreatment assessment should be considered in clinical staging and treatment planning. Cancer of the head and neck can be staged (pathologic stage: pTNM) using all information from the clinical assessment as well as from the pathologic study of the resected specimen. The pathologic stage does not replace the clinical stage, which must be reported because not every patient is treated with surgery. Thus valid comparisons between groups of patients must rely on the clinical stage which can be recorded in every patient.

TABLE 17.2. TNM Classification (5th Edition) for Head and Neck Cancers

T Category—Primary Tumor
ALL SITES
TX Primary tumor cannot be assessed.
T0 No evidence of primary tumor
Tis Carcinoma in situ

LIP, ORAL CAVITY, OROPHARYNX
T1 Tumor 2 cm or less in greatest dimension
T2 Tumor more than 2 cm but not more than 4 cm in greatest dimension
T3 Tumor more than 4 cm in greatest dimension
T4 Lip: Tumor invades adjacent structures (e.g., through cortical bone, inferior alveolar nerve, floor of mouth, skin of face).
    Oral cavity: Tumor invades adjacent structures (e.g., through cortical bone, into deep (extrinsic) muscle of tongue, maxillary sinus, skin. Superficial erosion alone of bone/tooth socket by gingival primary is not sufficient to classify as T4.)
    Oropharynx: Tumor invades adjacent structures [e.g., pterygoid muscle(s), mandible, hard palate,deep muscle of tongue, larynx].

NASOPHARYNX
T1 Tumor is confined to the nasopharynx.
T2 Tumor extends to soft tissues of oropharynx and/or nasal fossa.
    T2a Without parapharyngeal extension
    T2b With parapharyngeal extension
T3 Tumor invades bony structures and/or paranasal sinuses.
T4 Tumor with intracranial extension and/or involvement of cranial nerves, infratemporal fossa, hypopharynx, or orbit

(continued)

TABLE 17.2. TNM Classification (5th Edition) for Head and Neck Cancers (continued)

T Category—Primary Tumor

HYPOPHARYNX

T1 Tumor is limited to one subsite of hypopharynx and 2 cm or less in greatest dimension.
T2 Tumor involves more than one subsite of the hypopharynx or an adjacent site, or measures more than 2 cm but not more than 4 cm in greatest diameter without fixation of the hemilarynx.
T3 Tumor measures more than 4 cm in greatest dimension or with fixation of hemilarynx.
T4 Tumor invades adjacent structures (e.g., thyroid/cricoid cartilage, carotid artery, soft tissues of neck, prevertebral fascia/muscles, thyroid, and/or esophagus).

SUPRAGLOTTIC LARYNX

T1 Tumor is limited to one subsite of the supraglottis with normal vocal cord mobility.
T2 Tumor invades mucosa of more than one adjacent subsite of supraglottis (e.g. base of tongue, vallecula, medial wall of pyriform sinus) without fixation of the larynx.
T3 Tumor is limited to larynx with vocal cord fixation and/or invades any of the following: postcricoid area, preepiglottic tissues.
T4 Tumor extends through the thyroid cartilage, and/or extends into soft tissues of the neck, thyroid, and/or esophagus.

GLOTTIC LARYNX

T1 Tumor is limited to the vocal cord(s) (may involve anterior or posterior commissures) with normal mobility.
    T1a   Tumor is limited to one vocal cord.
    T1b   Tumor involves both vocal cords.
T2 Tumor extends to the supraglottis and/or subglottis, and/or with impaired vocal cord mobility.
T3 Tumor is limited to the larynx with vocal cord fixation.
T4 Tumor invades through the thyroid cartilage and/or to other tissues beyond the larynx (e.g., trachea, soft tissues of the neck, including thyroid, pharynx).

SUBGLOTTIC LARYNX

T1 Tumor is limited to the subglottis
T2 Tumor extends to the vocal cord(s) with normal or impaired mobility.
T3 Tumor is limited to the larynx with vocal cord fixation.
T4 Tumor invades through the cricoid or thyroid cartilage and/or extends to other tissues beyond the larynx (e.g., trachea, soft tissues of neck, including thyroid, esophagus).

MAXILLARY SINUS

T1 Tumor is limited to the antral mucosa with no erosion or destruction of bone.
T2 Tumor causes bone erosion or destruction, except for the posterior antral wall, including extension into the hard palate and/or the middle nasal meatus.
T3 Tumor invades any of the following: bone of the posterior wall of maxillary sinus, subcutaneous tissues, skin of cheek, floor or medial wall of orbit, infratemporal fossa, pterygoid plates, ethmoid sinuses.
T4 Tumor invades orbital contents beyond the floor or medial wall including any of the following: the orbital apex, cribriform plate, base of skull, nasopharynx, sphenoid, frontal sinuses.

(continued)

TABLE 17.2. TNM Classification (5th Edition) for Head and Neck Cancers (continued)

T Category—Primary Tumor
ETHMOID SINUS
T1 Tumor is confined to the ethmoid with or without bone erosion.
T2 Tumor extends into the nasal cavity.
T3 Tumor extends to the anterior orbit and/or maxillary sinus.
T4 Tumor with intracranial extension, orbital extension including apex, involving sphenoid, and/or frontal sinus and/or skin of external nose

SALIVARY GLANDS—PAROTID, SUBMANDIBULAR, AND SUBLINGUAL
T1 Tumor 2 cm or less in greatest dimension without extraparenchymal extension
T2 Tumor more than 2 cm but not more than 4 cm in greatest dimension without extra-parenchymal extension
T3 Tumor having extraparenchymal extension without seventh nerve involvement and/or more than 4 cm but not more than 6 cm
T4 Tumor invades base of skull, seventh nerve, and/or exceeds 6 cm in greatest dimension.

N Category—Regional Lymph Nodes
ALL SITES EXCEPT NASOPHARYNX
NX Regional lymph nodes cannot be assessed.
N0 No regional lymph node metastasis
N1 Metastasis in a single ipsilateral lymph node, 3 cm or less in greatest dimension
N2 Metastasis in a single ipsilateral lymph node, more than 3 cm but not more than 6 cm in greatest dimension; or in multiple ipsilateral lymph nodes, none more than 6 cm in greatest dimension; or in bilateral or contralateral lymph nodes, none more than 6 cm in greatest dimension
  N2a Metastasis in a single ipsilateral lymph node more than 3 cm but not more than 6 cm in greatest dimension
  N2b Metastasis in multiple ipsilateral lymph nodes, none more than 6 cm in greatest dimension
  N2c Metastasis in bilateral or contralateral lymph nodes, none more than 6 cm in greatest dimension
N3 Metastasis in a lymph node more than 6 cm in greatest dimension

NASOPHARYNX
NX Regional lymph nodes cannot be assessed.
N0 No regional lymph node metastasis
N1 Unilateral metastasis in lymph node(s), 6 cm or less in greatest dimension, above the supraclavicular fossa
N2 Bilateral metastasis in lymph node(s), 6 cm or less in greatest dimension, above the supraclavicular fossa
N3 Metastasis in a lymph node(s)
  N3a Greater than 6 cm in dimension
  N3b Extension to the supraclavicular fossa

M Category—Distant Metastasis
ALL SITES
MX Distant metastasis cannot be assessed.
M0 No distant metastasis
M1 Distant metastasis

TABLE 17.3. TNM 5th Edition Stage Groupings: Head and Neck Cancers

Stage—Excluding Nasopharynx				Stage—Nasopharynx			
0	Tis	N0	M0	0	Tis	N0	M0
I	T1	N0	M0	I	T1	N0	M0
II	T2	N0	M0	IIA	T2a	N0	M0
				IIB	T1	N1	M0
					T2a	N1	M0
					T2b	N0, N1	M0
III	T1	N1	M0	III	T1	N2	M0
	T2	N1	M0		T2a, T2b	N2	M0
	T3	N0, N1	M0		T3	N0, N1, N2	M0
IVA	T4	N0, N1	M0	IVA	T4	N0, N1, N2	M0
	Any T	N2	M0				
IVB	Any T	N3	M0	IVB	Any T	N3	M0
IVC	Any T	Any N	M1	IVC	Any T	Any N	M1

Exceptions in stage groupings:
  Salivary gland:
    Both T1/T2 N0 are stage I.
    T3 N1 M0 is stage IV.
    There are no subgroups (A, B, or C) in stage IV.
  Paranasal sinus:
    AnyT N2 M0 is IVB.

In addition to the N categories, an additional component of the description of neck node involvement concerns the localization of lymph nodes to levels in the neck (Fig. 17.1).

Level I: Contains the submental and submandibular triangles bounded by the posterior belly of the digastric muscle, the hyoid bone inferiorly, and the body of the mandible superiorly.

Level II: Extends from the level of the hyoid bone inferiorly to the skull base superiorly.

Level III: Extends from the hyoid bone superiorly to the cricothyroid membrane inferiorly.

Level IV: Extends from the cricothyroid membrane superiorly to the clavicle inferiorly.

Level V: Is the posterior triangle bounded by the anterior border of the trapezius posteriorly, the posterior border of the sternocleidomastoid muscle anteriorly, and the clavicle inferiorly.

Level VI: Contains the anterior neck compartment from the hyoid bone superiorly to the suprasternal notch inferiorly. On each side the lateral border is formed by the medial border of the carotid sheath.

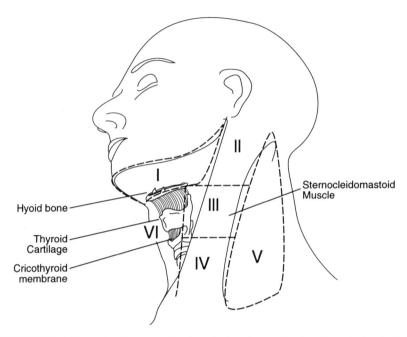

FIGURE 17.1. Schematic diagram indicating the location of the lymph node levels in the neck as described in the text. (Reproduced with permission of the AJCC, 1997.)

Level VII: Contains the lymph nodes inferior to the suprasternal notch in the upper mediastinum.

In NPC, the neck description also requires an appreciation of the triangular supraclavicular fossa or zone described by Ho (Fig. 17.2) which includes caudal portions of levels IV and V. Nodes (whole or part) in the fossa are considered N3b.

MULTIMODALITY TREATMENT

Philosophy of Management

The definitive treatment of head and neck cancer remains controversial because of the existence of two valid curative treatment options for many presentations of these diseases. Indeed evidence exists that much of what is recommended as "best therapy" for laryngeal cancer is determined as much by "accidents of geography and pattern of referral" and not only knowledge of the cancer or an impartial representation of the available treatment options. It is likely that the same situation exists for many of the other head and neck cancers with competing therapeutic options. In general, treatment should be offered with several objectives and with attention to the ability to access medical care, the economics of therapy delivery, and available resources.

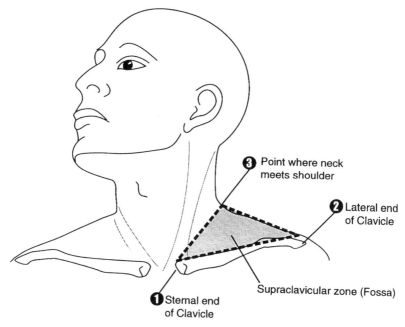

FIGURE 17.2. Shaded triangular area corresponds to the supraclavicular fossa used in the staging of nasopharyngeal carcinoma. (Reproduced with permission of the AJCC, 1997.)

Achievement of cure should be paramount, while also maximizing best functional and cosmetic outcomes. However, patients who are unlikely to attend for regular follow-up are not ideal candidates for approaches requiring vigilant surveillance for early salvage, most usually for radiation treatment failure.

In general, standard therapy consists of surgery or radiotherapy for early disease (T1 and T2 categories), while combined treatment may be used in the more advanced presentations (T3 and T4 categories or when regional lymph nodes are involved). Combined treatment may consist of elective combined radiotherapy as a pre- or postsurgical adjuvant, or in a delayed combined approach with surgery following radiotherapy if planned surveillance does not confirm an adequate response (e.g., histologically proven disease 3 months after radiotherapy). The advantage of the latter is that surgery may not be needed, a major dividend if loss of function is of grave concern. More recent strategies for "organ conservation" promote the use of chemotherapy with response assessment and are discussed later.

Surgery

The main principle in the surgical management of head and neck cancer regardless of site is tumor-free margin resection of the disease. Adjuvant radiotherapy should be considered if there is concern about resection margins on the primary tumor or infiltration beyond the surgery field as may occur with perineural invasion. Surgical

options in the treatment of the primary lesion include the use of formal scalpel resection, electrodesiccation, or laser resection. Regardless of the modality of ablation,
intraoperative pathology consultation to ensure disease-free margins is essential. In
addition to surgical ablation, the head and neck surgical oncologist faces the challenge of reconstruction for acceptable cosmetic result and maintenance of function.

Primary surgical treatment is recognized as a mainstay of therapy for malignancies of the oral cavity. Surgical approaches include transoral for small tumors,
mandibulotomy for larger tumors without bone involvement, and mandibulectomy
for tumors with bone invasion. Reconstruction of the oral cavity is dedicated to reconstitution of the mandibular arch for contour and cosmesis, often using free fibular
flaps. Soft tissue reconstruction necessitates use of low-bulk, pliable tissue with potential for reinnervation as afforded by the radial forearm flap.

Pharyngeal and laryngeal malignancies are treated in many centers with primary
radiation with surgery for residual or recurrent disease. The exception to this general philosophy is in T4 laryngeal and hypopharyngeal cancer, for which combined
modality treatment with surgery as primary therapy may be recommended. Surgery
for pharyngeal cancer adheres to the concept of margin-free resection. Primary closure is employed for partial pharyngectomy and regional myocutaneous flaps are
employed for more extensive ablation. However, where a total circumferential resection is performed free jejunal interposition or gastric pullup is employed depending
on the length of pharyngoesophageal segment that is ablated.

Surgical management of laryngeal cancer can include endoscopic resection, external conservation surgery, and total laryngectomy. Endoscopic resection may be performed with a microdissection technique or can employ the CO_2 laser. Generally endoscopic resection can be used for superficial tumors limited to the midcord with no
involvement of the anterior commissure. External conservation surgery, where indicated, can preserve voice and deglutition and maintain the airway. Although in most
cases patient will regain normal swallowing function after conservative laryngeal
surgery most patients will have significant aspiration in the postoperative period. It
is essential, therefore, to ensure that the patient has acceptable pulmonary reserve
($FEV1 > 60\%$ of predicted) to tolerate aspiration in the recovery period. Conservative laryngeal surgery can include laryngofissure with cordectomy, hemilaryngec-
tomy, extended or frontolateral vertical partial laryngectomy, and near total laryngectomy. For supraglottic cancer a horizontal supraglottic laryngectomy may be employed. However, all forms of conservation laryngeal surgery in early stage disease
remain alternatives to radiotherapy, which continues to provide the highest level of
tumor control and voice quality when case selection is accounted for.

Treatment of the neck is considered if the risk of occult spread is greater than
15% to 25%. The rate of occult regional disease is largely dependent on the site and
T category of the primary disease. More recently, conservative regional disease management has been advocated for the N0 neck. This includes modified radical neck
dissection (e.g., functional neck dissection of levels I to V), and selective neck dissection (e.g., supraomohyoid neck dissection of levels 1 to III, and anterolateral neck
dissection of levels II to IV). The advantages include preservation of the sternocleidomastoid muscle, internal jugular vein and accessory nerve. Radical neck dissection

is employed for advanced regional disease in which the risk of extracapsular extension of nodal metastases is high, necessitating sacrifice of muscle, vein, and nerve. Adjuvant radiotherapy should be considered for large metastatic lymph nodes (> 3 cm), multiple nodes, or when extracapsular disease is present.

Radiation Therapy

Radiation therapy has been a mainstay of curative treatment for head and neck cancer for decades. The modern era is characterized by superior technology permitting higher precision in treatment delivery. Better imaging techniques coupled to superior methods to conform irradiation planning volumes permit a greater volume of normal tissue to be spared. In turn, this has opened the door to dose escalation with radiotherapy alone or combined with concurrent chemotherapy in the investigational setting.

In radiotherapy, a wide range of daily fractionation protocols are used across the world ranging from schemes delivering doses of 50 Gy in as short as 3 weeks at one extreme compared to 70 Gy in 7 weeks at the other. Tumor control rates for these schedules appear similar although the shorter courses are associated with more intense acute radiation reactions. However, clinical and laboratory studies have suggested that protocols associated with more prolonged treatment administration require higher total doses to counteract the effect of accelerated proliferation of tumor cells, believed to commence after a lapse of several weeks of radiotherapy. Strategies to spare normal tissues by exploiting the relatively less damaging long-term normal tissue effect of smaller dose per fraction schedules (hyperfractionation) or by offsetting tumor proliferation using shorter treatment time (accelerated fractionation) schemes are becoming widely tested and provide further opportunity for improvement in outcome compared to traditional radiotherapy regimens. Both strategies generally employ more than once daily fractionation and are intended to deliver a biologically more effective total dose to the tumor. They differ in that the fraction size is smaller in hyperfractionation but is usually unchanged in the accelerated regimens compared to conventional daily regimens. Evidence suggests that these "altered fractionation" approaches may be more effective but have yet to be reliably confirmed, and toxicity must also be assessed.

With the anatomic proximity of critical structures in the head and neck, meticulous treatment planning is important. Maximization of local control with minimal damage demands not only optimal fractionation, but also adequate coverage of target, proper protection of normal tissues, reliable immobilization, and accurate set-up.

With the high incidence of lymphatic involvement in NPC, hypopharyngeal, certain oropharyngeal, and supraglottic tumors, there is little controversy that bilateral neck irradiation is indicated irrespective of the lymph node status. Other sites are at lesser risk but generally relate to the size of the primary tumor. In diseases where the neck is also to be treated, it is almost universal practice to treat the primary lesion and upper neck en bloc with opposing lateral portals during the initial phase of treatment. Additional fields are junctioned to encompass the additional lymph node regions. When the spinal cord dose reaches 40 to 45 Gy at conventional daily fractionation of 1.8 to 2 Gy, different field arrangements are used by different centers to boost the primary and the lymphatics. The standard practice is to treat the gross tumor with a total of 65 to 70 Gy in 6.5 to 7.5 weeks, and the elective sites with 50 Gy. A shrinking field technique should be used, and as far as possible, the dose to critical structures should be limited to 50 to 55 Gy.

In addition to altered fractionation, further improvements by escalation of total dose (using brachytherapy or stereotactic radiotherapy) have been advocated for different sites. Although encouraging results have been reported in comparison with historic controls, data from randomized studies are still awaited.

Chemotherapy

Squamous Cell Cancer in General   The median duration of survival of head and neck cancer patients with recurrent or metastatic disease is about 6 months. Factors that are predictive of a better outcome to chemotherapy include a high performance status of the patient, lack of prior treatment with irradiation or surgery, and absence of fixed nodes. The issue of whether chemotherapy conveys increased therapeutic benefit compared with best supportive care alone has not been tested formally in a large study. Prospective quality of life data and functional assessments to address the palliative value of chemotherapy are lacking in this morbid disease, and are of critical importance because chemotherapy might relieve symptoms, even though current drugs do not improve survival.

For locally advanced head and neck cancer, there have been numerous trials of adjunctive chemotherapy given either before, during, or after local treatment with irradiation and/or surgery. Induction or neoadjuvant chemotherapy delivered prior to local therapy has been associated with a high rate of tumor response but has not improved local control or survival when compared in randomized trials with the same local therapy used alone. Possible limitations of induction chemotherapy include a delay in the onset of definitive therapy, repopulation by the rapid proliferation of surviving, drug-resistant tumor cells, and decrease in tumor radiosensitivity after chemotherapy. The results with adjuvant or maintenance chemotherapy administered after completion of locoregional treatment have also been disappointing. Noncompliance is a major problem, as toxicity is often exacerbated when drugs are given after local therapy. Concurrent chemotherapy and radiotherapy with or without surgery has been the most promising method of combining these treatment modalities. Several randomized trials and literature based overviews have suggested a small advantage in survival, albeit at the expense of increased toxicity. Interaction of radiation with concurrent chemotherapy may augment locoregional control, in addition to the potential reduction in distant failure through eradication of micrometastases. The first individual patient-based meta-analysis has recently been performed, and has also failed to demonstrate a benefit for induction and adjuvant approaches, with any survival advantage being confined to the concurrent chemoradiation approach.

Chemotherapy for NPC   The standard treatment for locoregional NPC is radiotherapy. Even if locoregional control can be improved, however, the need for eradication of micrometastases in high-risk cases remains. This tumor type also exhibits greater chemosensitivity than squamous cell cancers in the other sites, and patients with NPC generally are of a younger age and have a better performance status. For locally advanced NPC, randomized trials evaluating the role of induction chemotherapy given prior to radiotherapy have not demonstrated any improvement in overall survival.

In a recently completed Intergroup (Intergroup 0099) study, stages III and IV NPC were randomized to radiotherapy alone versus concurrent cisplatin and radiotherapy with three subsequent cycles of adjuvant cisplatin and 5-fluorouracil (5-FU). Preliminary results have shown significantly improved survival (80% at 2 years) for the chemoradiation arm compared to radiation therapy alone (55% at 2 years). Locoregional and distant control of disease were also improved significantly by the addition of chemotherapy. Information on the long-term follow-up of patient outcome and toxicity from this trial is still needed to determine the optimal management of nondisseminated NPC. A confirmatory trial using similar combined modality therapy would be desirable.

Organ Preservation

Organ preservation strategies have become widely studied in recent years spurred by the results of two trials that randomized patients to either induction chemotherapy with response assessment (ICT) followed by radiotherapy if the chemoresponse was favorable (nonresponders receive ablative surgery), or to radical surgery. These trials were conducted by the VA Laryngeal Cancer Study Group in advanced laryngeal cancer and the European Organization for Research and Treatment of Cancer (EORTC) in hypopharyngeal cancer. Although an alterative to ablative surgery, the goal of organ preservation can also be achieved with subtotal surgery with or without radiotherapy and by definitive radiotherapy, and not only by the ICT approach. Despite this, the ICT approach has been widely accepted by some practitioners as synonymous with "organ preservation" although the merits of induction chemotherapy are being questioned in an ongoing RTOG study (RTOG 91-11) in T3 larynx cancer, and have already been addressed without apparent benefit by French investigators. As already noted, a benefit for induction chemotherapy has not been upheld in meta-analyses of chemotherapy in head and neck cancer (four have been performed), and the concept is at odds with traditional outcomes of advanced disease, especially in laryngeal cancer where definitive radiotherapy without chemotherapy has been a standard practice in Canadian, European, and Australian centers. In the end the major benefit to ICT will likely be that it opened the log-jam that existed in the discussion of the use of ablative surgery for advanced head and neck cancer where the views were becoming entrenched.

Retreatment

For patients with recurrence following high-dose radiotherapy, the general principle is to salvage with surgery whenever feasible. However, for sites where complete resection is difficult (e.g., nasopharynx) or function preservation is important (e.g., larynx), aggressive reirradiation may be considered in selected cases. Chance of success depends on the extensiveness of recurrence and the reirradiation dose. To avoid excessive complications, treatment volumes should be confined to the recurrent lesion with a small margin, and if possible, brachytherapy should be used for a final boost. For recurrence confined to the nasopharynx treated with combined teletherapy and brachytherapy to 60 Gy or above, a 5-year local salvage rate of 45% can be achieved with a complication rate of 36%. Avoidance of large dose per fraction radiotherapy should also reduce the complication rate. Recently, promising results in resection for selected recurrent NPC lesions are becoming available.

Supportive Treatment

It is essential to select those patients who may develop complications during treatment. The main systemic complications that arise during treatment are often related to airway compromise and nutritional depletion. Compromised airway usually requires a planned tracheotomy at the outset. Similarly gastrostomy tube support is highly recommended early in the management to combat the catabolic and nutritionally depleted state commonly present in advanced cases. Dental care is required, as failure to extract or treat decayed or infected dentition carries an unnecessary risk of postradiation osteoradionecrosis, which can also be minimized by limiting the dose to the mandible and the amount treated. In addition, radiation-induced xerostomia accelerates dental decay in the absence of preventative dental maintenance. Dental cleaning and application of topical fluoride to remaining teeth with fluoride trays should be encouraged.

During treatment the acute side effects to the mucous membranes should be managed with pain relievers, oral hygiene by gargling with bicarbonate of soda, and topical applications of local anesthesia (e.g., 2% viscous xylocaine). Hot and spicy foods and commercial mouthwashes must not be used, as they may exacerbate radiation mucositis. Alcohol and tobacco should be avoided, in particular as there is evidence that compromise in radiotherapy control of the cancer can result.

In the long term, patients should be monitored for laryngeal edema, which can present after radiotherapy, but more commonly represents tumor recurrence. Hypothyroidism and hypopituitarism can result from direct radiation to these structures and is readily managed with hormone replacement.

FOLLOW-UP

With the exception of NPC and salivary gland tumors, the majority of recurrences of head and neck cancer occur during the first 2 to 3 years of follow-up, with the risk declining substantially thereafter. The high prevalence of tobacco and alcohol abuse among this patient population is also associated with a continuing threat of developing a second primary tumor of the upper aerodigestive tract, and with a multitude of comorbid illnesses. A reasonable schedule of follow-up is to assess patients several times per year for the first 2 to 3 years, and less frequently thereafter.

The approximate cure rates in head and neck cancer are related to the site and stage of disease. The presence of lymph node metastases does not mean cure is not achievable but generally halves the survival within a given T category. Patients with T1/T2 lesions should attain 70% to 95% probability of 5-year survival, whereas those with T3/T4 lesions do not do as well (20% to 30% 5-year survival).

PREVENTION

Lifestyle modifications following potentially curative treatment of a primary tumor may lead to a decreasing risk of second tumors with increasing time. In general, cessation of alcohol and tobacco use, or areca nut (betel nut) exposure in India, may halt the multistep carcinogenic process, particularly in individuals who have never developed a malignancy.

Chemoprevention is an attempt to use agents to prevent, arrest, or reverse carcinogenesis before progression to invasive malignancy. A randomized, placebo-controlled trial has demonstrated that adjuvant isotretinoin (13-*cis*-retinoic acid) can reduce the incidence of second primary tumors and confirmatory randomized trials are ongoing. Trials of other agents, such as α-tocopherol (vitamin E), selenium, β-carotene, interferon-α, DL-α-difluoromethylornithine (DFMO), and nonsteroidal antiinflammatory drugs (NSAIDS), are also underway to define chemoprevention activity.

The strong association between nasopharyngeal carcinoma and EBV has led to research on the possibility of prevention using an antiviral vaccine.

FURTHER READING

Al-Sarraf M, LeBlanc M, Giri P, et al. (1998) Chemoradiotherapy versus radiotherapy in patients with advanced nasopharyngeal cancer (NPC): Phase III randomized intergroup study 0099. *J Clin Oncol* 16(4):1310–7.

Byers R, Weber R, Andrews T, et al. (1997) Frequency and therapeutic implications of "skip metastases" in the neck from squamous carcinoma of the oral tongue. *Head and Neck* 19:14–19.

Chia K, Lee H (1997) Epidemiology. In: Chong VFH, Tsao SY (eds) *Nasopharyngeal Carcinoma*. Armour, Singapore, pp. 1–5.

Eicher S, Weber R (1996) Surgical management of cervical lymph node metastases. *Curr Opin Oncol* 8:215–220.

Fleming I, Cooper J, Henson D, et al. (eds) (1997) *AJCC Cancer Staging Manual*. Lippincott-Raven, Philadelphia.

Gluckman J, Zitsch R (1995) Early detection and screening for head and neck cancer. *Cancer Treat Res* 74:141–157.

Harari P, Kinsella T (1995) Advances in radiation therapy for head and neck cancer. *Curr Opin Oncol* 7:248–254.

Ho J (1978) Stage classification of nasopharyngeal carcinoma, etiology, and control. *IARC Sci Publ* 20:99–113.

Lee A, Foo W, Law S, et al. (1997) Re-irradiation for recurrent nasopharyngeal carcinoma: Factors affecting the therapeutic ratio and ways for improvement. *Int J Radiat Oncol Biol Phys* 38:43–52.

Lefebvre J, Bonneterre J (1996) Current status of laryngeal preservation trials. *Curr Opin Oncol* 8:209–214.

O'Sullivan B, Mackillop W, Gilbert R, et al. (1994) Controversies in the management of laryngeal cancer: Results of an international survey of patterns of care. *Radiother Oncol* 31:23–32.

Pathmanathan R (1997) Pathology. In: Chong VFH, Tsao SY (eds) *Nasopharyngeal Carcinoma*. Armour, Singapore, pp. 6–13.

Pathmanathan R, Raab-Traub N (1997) Epstein–Barr virus. In: Chong VFH, Tsao SY, (eds) *Nasopharyngeal Carcinoma*. Armour, Singapore, pp. 14–23.

Peters L, Ang K (1992) The role of altered fractionation in head and neck cancers. *Semin Radiat Oncol* 2:180–194.

Rao D, Ganesh B (1995) Epidemiological observations of head and neck cancers. In: *Head and Neck Cancer: A Multidisciplinary Approach for Its Control and Cure*. Desai, PG, Schweitzer, RJ (eds) UICC, Geneva, pp. 1–28.

Sanguineti G, Geara F, Garden A, et al. (1997) Carcinoma of the nasopharynx treated by radiotherapy alone: Determinants of local and regional control. *Int J Radiat Oncol Biol Phys* 37:985–996.

Sobin L, Wittekind C (ed) (1997) *TNM Classification of Malignant Tumors*. Wiley-Liss, New York.

Strong E, Karsdorf H, Henk J (1995) Squamous cell carcinoma of the head and neck. In: Hermanek P, Sobin L, (eds) *Prognostic Factors in Cancer*, UICC, Geneva. Springer-Verlag, Berlin, pp. 23–27.

The Department of Veterans Affairs Laryngeal Cancer Study Group (1991) Induction chemotherapy plus radiation compared with surgery plus radiation in patients with advanced laryngeal cancer. *N Engl J Med* 324:1685–1690.

Vokes EE, Weichselbaum RR, Lippman SM, et al. (1993) Medical progress: Head and neck cancer. *N Engl J Med* 328:184–194.

CHAPTER 18

ENDOCRINE TUMORS

JEFFREY A. NORTON

University of California, San Francisco
and San Francisco Veterans Affairs Medical Center
San Francisco, CA 94121 USA

MULTIPLE ENDOCRINE NEOPLASIAS

MENI

Genetic Abnormalities and Screening   Multiple endocrine neoplasia type I (MENI) is an inherited endocrine disorder that includes hyperplasia of the parathyroid glands, endocrine tumors of the duodenum and pancreas, and tumors of the pituitary. It is associated with carcinoid tumors of the foregut and midgut, adenomas of the thyroid, and adenomas or carcinomas of the adrenal and lipomas. It is inherited as an autosomal dominant trait.

The gene for MENI has been mapped to the long arm of chromosome 11. It has been sequenced and called menin. Its function is unknown. Identification of the gene will allow more effective screening in at-risk individuals. Screening should begin in the second decade of life, before clinical signs of the disorder appear. Currently, individuals are questioned about the clinical components of the syndrome. Blood levels of calcium, glucose, prolactin, gastrin, and pancreatic polypeptide are measured (Table 18.1).

Hyperparathyroidism   Primary hyperparathyroidism (HPT) is the most common endocrine disorder in patients with MENI. The prevalence increases with age and is nearly 100% after age 50. The age at onset is 25 years, which is younger than in

Manual of Clinical Oncology, 7th edition, Edited by Raphael E. Pollock
ISBN 0-471-23828-7, pages 359–383. Copyright © 1999 Wiley-Liss, Inc.

TABLE 18.1. Multiple Endocrine Neoplasia Syndromes and Familial Medullary Thyroid Cancer

	MENI	MENIIA	MENIIB	FMTC
Familial autosomal dominant	+	+	+	+
Location of genetic defect	11q 12–13	10 Pericentromeric region	10 Pericentromeric region	10 Pericentromeric region
Gene	*Menin*	*RET*	*RET*	*RET*
MTC	−	+	+	+
Pheochromocytoma	−	+	+	−
Parathyroid disease	+	+	−	−
Pancreatic endocrine tumors	+	−	−	−
Phenotype	−	−	+	−

sporadic HPT. Clinical manifestations include asymptomatic hypercalcemia, weakness, fatigue, kidney stones, bone pain, and mental symptoms such as depression, inability to concentrate, and memory loss. Diagnosis is made by measurement of elevated serum levels of calcium and parathyroid hormone (PTH). Urinary levels of calcium are also elevated. Patients always have parathyroid hyperplasia or multiple gland disease. The operation of choice is either subtotal three and one half gland parathyroidectomy or total four gland parathyriodectomy with transplant of tissue into the forearm. In patients with MENI, HPT, and Zollinger–Ellison syndrome (ZES), parathyroidectomy normalizes serum levels of calcium and ameliorates the signs and symptoms of ZES.

Pancreatic Islet Cell Tumors   MENI patients also develop pancreatic or duodenal endocrine tumors. Duodenal tumors are commonly associated with ZES, rarely metastasize to the liver (10%), and often metastasize to lymph nodes (55%). Pancreatic endocrine tumors secrete insulin, gastrin, and pancreatic polypeptide or may be nonfunctional. Pancreatic endocrine tumors often metastasize to the liver (30%). There is a direct correlation between size of pancreatic tumor and development of liver metastases.

The most common syndrome from islet cell tumors in MENI patiuents is ZES. The diagnosis is made by detection of elevated fasting serum levels of gastrin and elevated basal acid output. Patients require omeprazole to control the gastric acid hypersecretion. The second most common functional islet cell tumor is insulinoma, which causes severe hypoglycemia and neuroglycopenic symptoms. The diagnosis is made by detection of fasting hypoglycemia and elevated serum levels of insulin. Any funcitonal islet cell tumor may occur in patients with MENI including gastrinoma, insulinoma, glucagonoma, vasoactive intestinal peptide producing tumor (VIPoma), growth hormone releasing factor (GRFoma), somatostatinoma, PPoma, and carcinoid tumor.

Surgery is indicated to remove potentially malignant islet cell tumors and to provide remission from the hormonal effects. The goal of surgery is to remove endocrine tumors without excessive morbidity and mortality. Surgical resection of tumor generally ameliorates the hypoglycemia in patients with insulinoma, although recurrence or persistence of hypoglycemia is possible because of the multifocal nature. Tumor resection seldom completely resolves the hypergastrinemia in MENI patients with ZES; long-term omeprazole is used to control the acid hypersecretion. MENI patients maintained on omeprazole for years may develop gastric carcinoid tumors so that intermittent gastric endoscopy is recommended. Removal of endocrine tumors in MENI patients appears to control the malignant tumoral process in that fewer patients develop liver metastases after resection of the primary. Generally, pancreatic body and tail islet cell tumors are resected by distal pancreatectomy–splenectomy, whereas tumors within the pancreatic head or duodenum are either enucleated or excised with a small margin of duodenum, respectively.

Pituitary and Other Less Common Tumors   Pituitary tumors are seen in 30% to 50% of patients with MENI. The most common is a prolactinoma. Women with prolactinoma have galactorrhea, and men have impotence. Elevated serum levels of prolactin are diagnostic for prolactinoma and have been used as a screening study. Pituitary tumors may secrete other hormones including corticotropin (ACTH), growth hormone, and thyroid stimulating hormone (TSH), which cause Cushing's disease, acromegaly, and hyperthyroidism, respectively. These syndromes are diagnosed by appropriate biochemical and hormonal testing. Patients require a careful visual field examination to exclude bitemporal hemianopsia which may occur as a result of tumor compression of the optic chiasm. Further, magnetic resonance imaging (MRI) scan of the sella is obtained to determine the size of the pituitary tumor and to assess resectability. Prolactinomas are treated with bromocryptine, which shrinks tumor mass and ameliorates symptoms. However, side effects may limit its acceptance. Pituitary tumors can also be treated with surgery or radiation.

Less common tumors that are associated with MENI include bronchial or thymic carcinoids, intestinal carcinoids, gastric carcinoids, lipomas, benign adenomas of the thyroid gland, benign adrenocortical adenomas, and rarely adrenocortical carcinomas. Carcinoid tumors may cause the carcinoid syndrome secondary to excessive secretion of serotonin. The carcinoid syndrome includes flushing, diarrhea, wheezing, and bronchospasm and right-sided valvular heart disease possibly resulting in congestive heart failure. It is caused by serotonin and other vasoactive amines. The midgut is the most common primary site. Carcinoid syndrome is usually seen with liver metastases, because serotonin that is secreted into the portal circulation is metabolized to nonfunctional 5-hydroxyindolacetic acid (5-HIAA) by the liver. Foregut or ovarian carcinoids can cause the carcinoid syndrome without metastases, because the hormones are secreted directly into the systemic circulation. Further, foregut carcinoids may produce ACTH and cause ectopic ACTH syndrome. Carcinoid tumors are potentially malignant and should be removed surgically when identified. Adenomas of the thyroid and adrenal require no treatment, unless there is evidence of excessive hormonal function. Adrenal cortical carcinomas require resection. The best method to differentiate an adrenal adenoma from carcinoma is size. Adrenal carcinomas are large tumors at least 6 cm in size and are often associated with hypercortisolism. Cushing's syndrome in MENI can be caused by a pituitary tumor producing ACTH, a foregut carcinoid tumor producing ACTH, or an adrenal tumor producing cortisol. Lipomas in MENI patients are usually large and are excised if symptomatic.

MENII

MENII is divided into MENIIA, MENIIB, and familial medullary thyroid cancer (FMTC). MENIIA is an autosomal dominant inherited condition characterized by medullary thyroid carcinoma (MTC), adrenal pheochromocytoma(s), and parathyroid hyperplasia. MENIIB is an autosomal dominant inherited endocrine syndrome that is characterized by MTC, adrenal pheochromocytoma(s), and a characteristic phenotype that includes mucosal neuromas, puffy lips, bony abnormalities, marfanoid habitus, intestinal ganglioneuromas, and corneal nerve hypertrophy. Unlike in MENIIA, parathyroid disease is not assocoiated with MENIIB. FMTC is characterized by an autosomal dominant inheritance of only medullary thyroid carcinoma without any other endocrine abnormalities.

Gene Defect The gene for MENIIA has been mapped to the pericentromeric region of chromosome 10. It is a transmembrane protein kinase receptor called *RET*. Recent studies have detected missense mutations in *RET* in all individuals with MENIIA, MENIIB, and familial MTC. MENIIA and familial MTC mutations have been identified within the extracellular portion of the molecule, while MENIIB is within the intracellular domain.

Medullary Thyroid Carcinoma In patients with MENIIA, MTC generally develops between the ages of 5 and 25 years prior to the other endocrine disorders. It is always bilateral and multifocal. Total thyroidectomy is always necessary to treat the familial forms of MTC. Detection of *RET* mutations in the periperal white blood cells of individuals from kindreds with MENIIA has been used to select patients for total thyroidectomy prior to any signs or symptoms of MTC. In this setting, either premalignant C-cell hyperplasia or in situ MTC was identified in every patient.

Patients with MENIIB have the most aggressive form of MTC. They usually have a palpable large thyroid mass or enlarged cervical lymph nodes at the time of diagnosis. They are seldom cured by thyroidectomy. Conversely, patients with FMTC have the most indolent form of MTC and the best prognosis. MTC develops at an older age and patients seldom die from it. Thus, in the three different familial forms of MTC, the virulence is different. The most virulent form is MENIIB, the intermediate form is MENIIA, and the least virulent is FMTC. Total thyroidectomy is indicated for each of the familial types of MTC, as it is multifocal and bilateral. Neck dissection is necessary when disease is localized to cervical lymph nodes without distant metastases. Prior to neck dissection, laparoscopy is used to exclude liver metastases that may occur despite a normal appearing CT scan. Further prior to any invasive procedure or surgery on an MENII patient, the presence of a pheochromocytoma must be excluded by measurement of urinary catecholamines.

Pheochromocytoma   Individuals with either MENIIA or MENIIB may develop bilateral benign intraadrenal pheochromocytomas. The diagnosis is made by detection of elevated 24-hour urinary levels of catecholamines. Imaging studies are used to identify the adrenal gland with tumor. Computerized tomography (CT), MRI, and labeled metaiodobenzylguanidine (MIBG) scan each have utility. However, CT has the broadest applicability because it is equally sensitive, least expensive, and most available. There is controversy as to the extent of adrenalectomy in patients with MENII. Some recommend bilateral adrenalectomy for all patients with biochemical evidence of pheochromocytoma, because pathology series have demonstrated that 70% are bilateral. However, others recommend adrenalectomy based on the results of CT scan. They contend that bilateral adrenalectomy is associated with episodes of life-threatening Addison's disease and patients may not develop a tumor in the contralateral adrenal. If a unilateral adrenalectomy is performed, careful follow-up is warranted. Because pheochromocytomas in the setting of MENII are usually small and benign, laparoscopic adrenalectomy is used to remove these tumors. It is associated with less pain and shorter hospitalization. Surgery is delayed until the patient is effectively prepared preoperatively with α-adrenergic blocking drugs such as phenoxybenzamine. Alpha blockade restores plasma volume, reverses lactic acidosis, and normalizes blood pressure during the operative procedure.

Parathyroid Disease   Patients with MENIIA may develop symptomatic primary HPT. In this setting, HPT is caused by multiple gland disease or parathyroid hyperplasia. Signs and symptoms of HPT include nephrolithiasis, osteoporosis, weakness, fatigue, altered mental status, and memory loss. The diagnosis is established by concomitant measurement of elevated serum levels of calcium and parathyroid hormone. The proper surgical treatment is either three and one half gland parathyroidectomy or four gland parathyroidectomy with transplant.

Gastrointestinal Manifestations   Some individuals with MENIIA may also have Hirschsprung's disease, which is also associated with a *RET* mutation. Individuals with MENIIB initially have severe constipation that may lead to the development of megacolon or diverticulitis. This is caused by abnormal gut motility secondary to intestinal ganglioneuromatosis. Constipation should be treated as symptoms arise. When the MTC becomes metastatic, patients may develop severe secretory diarrhea secondary to hormones secreted by the tumor. In this setting octreotide may be useful to inhibit diarrhea.

THYROID CANCER

Epidemiology

In 1995, the estimated number of new cases of thyroid cancer in the United States was 14,000 with nearly 10,000 occurring in women. It is the most common endocrine malignancy, and the incidence is increasing. It is responsible for more deaths than any other endocrine tumor; however, the death rate is decreasing. It occurs in both males and females, in any age group including children and the elderly, but it most commonly affects women between the ages of 25 and 65 years. For well-differentiated thyroid cancers, age at diagnosis is an important prognostic variable. Medullary thyroid cancer is inherited in well-documented familial patterns as described previously. Follicular carcinoma of the thyroid occurs more commonly in low-iodine geographic areas in which benign thyroid goiters arise. Thyroid cancer can be among either the most indolent tumors or the most aggressive. Patients with papillary thyroid cancer are usually cured, whereas patients with anaplastic thyroid cancer seldom live longer than 6 months.

Papillary thyroid cancer (PTC) is associated with neck irradiation. A high incidence of papillary thyroid carcinoma was seen following the atomic bombing of Japan and the nuclear accident in Chernobyl. Younger individuals are at the highest risk. The risk increases with increased dose of radiation from 200 to 2000 cGy, and the time interval from radiation exposure. Radiation-induced PTC is usually multifocal and bilateral, and it has the same prognosis as PTC not associated with radiation.

Pathology

Thyroid cancer is divided into four types: papillary, follicular, medullary, and anaplastic. The pathologic classification is based primarily on the cell of origin and the degree of differentiation. Most thyroid cancers arise from the follicular cell (papillary, follicular, Hurthle cell neoplasms, and anaplastic), and most are well differentiated (papillary and follicular). But thyroid cancer can arise from the parafollicular C cell (medullary thyroid cancer) and it can be poorly differentiated (anaplastic). Further, there are some subgroups of papillary with intermediate differentiation (insular, tall cell, clear cell, and sclerosing variant).

Papillary thyroid carcinoma comprises about 80% of thyroid malignancies. It has a variable appearance from cicatrizing white scars to large locally invasive tumors. Most tumors are solid, less than 3 cm in size, firm to palpation, and lie within the capsule of the thyroid. Cystic change, cystic-solid tumors, necrosis, calcification, and ossification may also occur. Microscopically, papillary carcinomas generally have papillary fronds, but some have follicles and are termed the follicular variant of papillary thyroid carcinoma.

Papillary thyroid carcinomas have specific nuclear features. Nuclei are enlarged and ovoid with thick nuclear membranes and intranuclear grooves. They appear clear, the so-called Orphan Annie nuclei. Papillary thyroid carcinoma has a propensity to spread throughout the thyroid gland via lymphatics and to lymph nodes. Occasionally, small primary tumors may present with regional lymph node metastases. Certain types of papillary carcinomas are clearly more aggressive and malignant including the following four variants: tall cell, clear cell, sclerosing, and insular.

Follicular thyroid carcinoma is less common than PTC. It is more common in goitrous areas of the world, but in America it represents only 5% to 10% of thyroid malignancies. Follicular thyroid tumors are generally large (3 to 5 cm), unifocal, and encapsulated. The hallmark of the diagnosis is the presence of capsular or vascular invasion. Tumors are generally follicular, trabecular, or solid, and most cases show combinations of all three. Follicular carcinomas invade veins and not lymphatics. Distant metastases and death are more common with follicular cancers. In the absence of distant metastases, patients do extremely well and the overall long-term survival is between 80% and 85%. Hurthle cell tumors are a subgroup with a similar prognosis.

Medullary thyroid carcinoma arises from the parafollicular C cells. It comprises approximately 3% to 5% of all thyroid cancers depending on different series. It is also inherited in an autosomal dominant fashion in the setting of MENII. Grossly, MTC appears either tan or yellow in color, and is firm and locally infiltrative. Cytologically, the cells are not cohesive and variable with elongated nuclei. Approximately 75% of MTC stain positive for amyloid. Because of considerable variability in the cellular appearance and shape, it is necessary to stain the tumor with antibodies to calcitonin which is diagnostic for medullary thyroid carcinoma. Tumors generally originate as part of a progression from C-cell hyperplasia to invasive cancer. Tumors that occur sporadically and present as thyroid nodules (> 1 cm) often have lymph node metastases at diagnosis.

Anaplastic thyroid cancer represents fewer than 1% of all thyroid malignancies. The median survival is less than 6 months. Anaplastic thyroid cancer is more common in goitrous regions and associated with an iodine-deficient diet. Studies suggest that it may be associated with long-standing untreated PTC. Its incidence is decreasing. Grossly, anaplastic thyroid carcinomas present as large neck masses possibly associated with stridor. Cytologically, the cells are large with pleomorphic nuclei, irregularly distributed chromatin, and evidence of mitoses. Two main patterns have been identified: spindle cell and giant cell. Leukocyte common antigen is used to exclude lymphoma. Anaplastic thyroid carcinoma is commonly unresectable. It generally extends outside the capsule of the thyroid and invades into adjacent structures. Lymph node and distant metastases are common. Death is caused by uncontrolled local disease or widespread dissemination. The median survival is between 6 months and 2 years.

Thyroid Nodule

Thyroid nodules are common. They occur in approximately 4% to 7% of the general population, which results in 250,000 new nodules per year in the United States. The work-up includes the measurement of thyroid function studies and fine-needle aspiration biopsy (FNA). Most patients with thyroid nodules have normal thyroid function studies. If the thyroid function studies suggest hyperthyroidism, a thyroid scan is used to determine if the palpable nodule is functional (hot). In individuals with hypothyroidism, antithyroid antibodies are obtained to exclude Hashimoto's thyroiditis.

The single best, most cost-effective test to select patients for surgery is fine-needle aspiration for cytology. Palpable nodules should simply be aspirated with tactile control. Nonpalpable or difficult to palpate nodules are aspirated with ultrasound guidance. Results of fine-needle aspiration can be divided into benign, atypical, suspicious, or malignant. If a nodule appears benign on FNA, there is only a low probability that it is cancerous (5%), so surgery can be safely avoided. If the FNA result suggests malignancy, there is a high probability of malignancy (90% to 95%), and definitive surgery is planned. FNA is especially useful for diagnosing PTC, MTC, and anaplastic thyroid cancer. However, follicular or Hurthle cell tumors cannot be diagnosed on FNA and require thyroid lobectomy for diagnosis. Definitive surgery should be delayed until a final tissue diagnosis is obtained.

Treatment

For patients with papillary thyroid cancer, a combination of surgery, radioactive iodine treatment, and thyroid suppression therapy is indicated depending on the type, size, and extent of the cancer and age of the patient. Retrospective studies done by Mazaferri have demonstrated that each of these modalities is able to decrease the rate of recurrence. Poor prognosis variables include the tall cell, insular and sclerosing vaiants, large tumor size (> 3 to 4 cm), invasion into muscle, extracapsular extension, distant metastases, male sex, and older age (> 50 years). Patients with these criteria warrant more aggressive treatment. Interestingly, cervical lymph node metastases, multifocal disease, younger patient age (less than 18 years), and history of neck irradiation are not associated with decreased survival, but are associated with a greater propensity of local recurrence (Table 18.2).

Total thyroidectomy or near-total thyroidectomy is recommended for patients with papillary thyroid cancer and poor prognostic variables, and all patients with follicular and medullary thyroid cancer. Only younger patients with small primary papillary thyroid carcinomas may be treated with less than total thyroidectomy. A major concern is safety, and total thyroidectomy should not be performed by individuals with complication rates greater than 1% for recurrent laryngeal nerve injury and hypoparathyroidism. Following thyroidectomy, for patients with well-differentiated thyroid cancer thyroid replacement therapy should be withheld and radioactive iodine is administered when the serum TSH level is greater than 50 UIU/ml. Following radioactive iodine ablation (RAI), L-thyroxine is started at doses designed to keep the serum level of T3 and T4 in the normal range while keeping the serum TSH level suppressed less than 1 UIU/ml. Serum levels of thyroglobulin are used to assess for the presence of recurrent or persistent papillary thyroid cancer. In general, if levels are elevated or if disease is imageable on thyroid scan, more radioactive iodine is administered. Overall, the 10-year survival of patients with papillary thyroid cancer is 90% and for follicular cancer it is 75% to 80%.

MTC may occur in sporadic and familial forms. The familial forms have been described in detail previously. In the sporadic setting, patients present with a thyroid nodule or mass. FNA can reliably ascertain the diagnosis of MTC. The presence of pheochromocytoma should be excluded by urinary catecholamine measurements. Genetic testing for *RET* should be instituted to exclude familial disease. Central compartment lymph node excision and jugular lymph node sampling are indicated to exclude nodal metastases. Additional therapies including RAI, external-beam

TABLE 18.2. Staging of Thyroid Cancer

Definition of TNM

PRIMARY TUMOR (T)
Tx   Primary tumor cannot be assessed
T0   No evidence of primary tumor
T1   Tumor ≤ 1 cm
T2   Tumors > 1 cm and < 4 cm
T3   Tumor > 4 cm
T4   Tumor extending beyond thyroid capsule

LYMPH NODES (N)
Nx   REGIONAL NODES CANNOT BE ASSESSED
N0   NO METASTASIS
N1   REGIONAL NODAL METASTASES

DISTANT METASTASIS (M)
Mx   DISTANT METASTASIS CANNOT BE ASSESSED
M0   NO DISTANT METASTASIS
M1   DISTANT METASTASES

Staging
PAPILLARY OR FOLLICULAR

	PATIENTS < 45 YEARS	PATIENTS > 45 YEARS
STAGE I	ANY T, ANY N, M0	T1, N0, M0
STAGE II	ANY T, ANY N, M1	T2, N0, M0
STAGE III		T4, N0, M0
STAGE IV		ANY T, ANY N, M1

MEDULLARY
STAGE I	T1 N0 M0
STAGE II	T2-4 N0 M0
STAGE III	ANY T N1 M0
STAGE IV	ANY T ANY N M1

UNDIFFERENTIATED
ALL CASES STAGE IV

irradiation, and doxorubicin are ineffective. Surgery is the only potentially curative treatment. L-Thyroxine is prescribed to replace normal thyroid function, but not as an antitumor treatment. Postoperatively, plasma levels of calcitonin are used as a marker to detect recurrence. If elevations of calcitonin are detected following thyroid surgery, persistent or recurrent disease in cervical lymph nodes should be expected and one third of patients can still be rendered disease-free by neck microdissection. Venous sampling of neck veins for calcitonin concentration can be used to indicate which areas of the neck harbor disease and laparoscopy can exclude liver metastases. Survival is dependent on the extent of disease. Patients without lymph node metastases are cured by total thyroidectomy. Patients with lymph node metastases have a 5-year survival of 80%, and with distant metastases, 40%.

The incidence of anaplastic thyroid carcinoma is decreasing. It accounts for only 1% to 3% of thyroid cancers and rarely occurs in individuals younger than age 60. Prognosis is so grave that all patients are termed stage IV. Surgery is generally not indicated unless all tumor can be resected without complications. Debulking is not useful because the tumor regrows rapidly. For most tumors (> 4 cm), trucut needle biopsy or FNA provides the diagnosis and thyroidectomy should not be attempted. RAI is ineffective and hyperfractionated radiotherapy combined with doxorubicin can provide significant local control. Doxorubicin at more conventional doses is then used in an attempt to control tumor at distant sites. Recently, several series have reported long-term survival of a few patients with tumors less than 5 to 6 cm in size. The median survival is 18 months and the 5-year survival is 10%.

PARATHYROID CANCER

Primary HPT is a common clinical condition (Table 18.3). The estimated incidence is 27.7 per 100,000 population. In the majority of patients with HPT, a solitary adenoma or a benign tumor of one of the parathyroid glands (85%) is the cause. The second most common cause is parathyroid hyperplasia (13%). Only approximately 1% to 3% of patients with HPT have parathyroid cancer. This is a rare condition with an estimated incidence in the United States of 1000 new cases per year.

Signs and Symptoms   Patients with parathyroid carcinoma have severe signs and symptoms of HPT. They have serum levels of calcium greater than 13 or 14 mg/dl. They have decreased bone density and bone pain. Nephrolithiasis is common. They experience weakness and easy fatigability. Patients with parathyroid cancer usually have a palpable neck mass. Hoarse voice, shortness of breath, stridor, and signs of aspiration may occur secondary to tumor involvement of the recurrent laryngeal nerve. Families with parathyroid cancer have been reported. In the familial form, the disease may be multifocal. Parathyroid cancer should be considered in patients with severe hypercalcemia, neck mass, hoarse voice, stridor, or aspiration.

Diagnosis

The detection of elevated serum levels of calcium and elevated serum levels of PTH establish the diagnosis of primary hyperparathyroidism. In patients with a clinical suspicion of parathyroid cancer, CT of the neck is obtained to evaluate the extent of disease within the neck and exclude pulmonary metastases.

Pathology

The pathologic distinction between parathyroid carcinoma and adenoma is unclear. It is critical for the surgeon to have a high index of suspicion based on the preoperative findings that have been mentioned previously. Classically, parathyroid carcinoma has five pathologic characteristics that separate it from adenoma. These include trabec-

TABLE 18.3. Etiology of Primary Hyperparathyroidism

Diagnosis	Association	Incidence (%)	Serum Palpable Mass	Calcium (mg/dl)	Serum PTH	Gross Pathology	Surgery	Rate of Recurrence
Hyperplasia	MEN	14	—	11–12	↑	Multiple enlarged glands	Three and one half gland resection or four gland with transplant	Intermediate
Adenoma	Radiation	85	—	11–12	↑	Single enlarged brown gland	Excision of adenoma	Low
Carcinoma of abnormal	Familial?	1	+	>13	↑↑	Single enlarged whitish firm gland	Resection of abnormal gland with ipsilateral thyroid lobe and nodes	High

ular pattern, fibrous bands, mitotic figures, and vascular and capsular invasion. The pathologist also considers the clinical history and the degree of hypercalcemia when determining the diagnosis.

Surgery

At surgery parathyroid carcinoma feels very firm and nodular and is locally invasive. This is markedly different from parathyroid adenoma which is soft, well demarcated, and easily separated from continguous structures. Further, parathyroid adenoma has a reddish-brown color, whereas parathyroid cancer has a white color. Intraoperative recognition is critical, because the surgical procedure is different for cancer. Further, frozen section examination may not precisely determine the diagnosis. If the surgeon ascertains that the patient has parathyroid carcinoma based on the degree of hypercalcemia and characteristics of the abnormal gland (white color, hard feel, and local invasion with indistinct magins), a resection of the abnormal parathyroid should include an ipselateral thyroid lobectomy and dissection of the central lymph node group. For patients with familial cases in whom the pathology may be multifocal, total parathyroidectomy may be indicated.

Distant metastases primarily to the lung may occur and may benefit from resection. Unfortunately, these metastases may be diffuse, involving both lobes, and surgical resection may not normalize serum levels of calcium or prolong survival. This is contrasted to local recurrence which does appear to benefit from reresection. Reresection may normalize serum levels of calcium and prolong survival. However, multiple cervical reoperations for recurrent parathyroid cancer are associated with recurrent laryngeal nerve injury. Unilateral recurrent laryngeal nerve injury may be well tolerated if the contralateral nerve remains intact.

Other Treatments

Radiation therapy has been ineffective in the management of parathyroid cancer. Chemotherapy based on dacarbazine alone or in combination with other drugs may be effective and complete responses have been reported. Drugs to ameliorate hypercalcemia are also indicated and include calcitonin, mithramycin, diphosphonates, gallium nitrate, and etidronate. Five-year survival rates are between 30% and 44%, and 10-year survival is 20%.

ADRENAL CANCER

Pathology

Adrenal cortical carcinoma is a malignant neoplasm of adrenal cortical cells demonstrating partial or complete histologic and functional differentiation. Adrenal cortical carcinomas are rare and comprise between 0.05% and 0.2% of all cancers. This incidence translates to a rate of only 2 per million in the world population. Women develop functional adrenal cortical carcinomas more commonly than men. There is a bimodal occurrence by age with a peak incidence less than 5 years and a second peak in the fourth and fifth decades. Adrenocortical carcinoma has been described as part of a complex hereditary syndrome involving mutations of the *p53* tumor suppressor gene called Li–Fraumeni syndrome. Patients also develop sarcoma and breast and lung cancer.

Carcinomas are greater than 6 cm in size and weigh between 100 and 5000 g (Table 18.4). Areas of necrosis and hemorrhage are common. Invasion and metastases also occur. Microscopically the appearance is variable. Cells with big nuclei, hyperchromatism, and enlarged nucleoli are all consistent with malignancy. Nuclear pleomorphism is more common in tumors larger than 500 g. Vascular invasion and many mitoses are diagnostic of malignancy. Broad desmoplastic bands are associated with metastatic potential of tumors.

Modes of Presentation

Cushing's syndrome is caused by excessive secretion of cortisol by an adrenal tumor. Treatment should aim to cure the hypercortisolism, eliminate the tumor, and minimize the chance of endocrine deficiency or long-term dependence on medications. Signs and symptoms of Cushing's syndrome include type 2 diabetes, obesity, hypertension, infectious complication, truncal obesity with peripheral muscle wasting, osteoporosis, hirsutism, moon facies, buffalo hump, striae, abnormal menstrual periods, and infertility. The diagnosis is established by elevated urinary free cortisol levels, lack of diurnal secretion of cortisol, low levels of ACTH, and failure to suppress urinary cortisol levels following both low-dose and high-dose dexamethasone. Both benign and malignant adrenal cortical tumors may cause hypercortisolism.

TABLE 18.4. Staging of Adrenal Cancer

Stage I	T1, N0, M0, tumor <5 cm without local invasion or nodal or distant metastases
Stage II	T2, N0, M0, tumor >5 cm without local invasion or nodal or distant metastases
Stage III	T1 or T2, N1, M0; T3 N0, M0, tumor >5 cm with local invasion, nodal metastases but no distant metastases
Stage IV	Any T, Any N, M1; T3-4 N1, M0 tumor with local invasion, lymph node metastases, and/or distant metastases
T1	T <5 cm, no invasion
T2	T >5 cm, no invasion
T3	Tumor invasion into fat
T4	Tumor invasion into organs
N0	No nodes
N1	Nodal metastases
M0	No distant metastases
M1	Distant metastases

Primary hyperaldosteronism may be caused by benign and malignant adrenal tumors and idiopathic primary adrenocortical hyperlasia. Although adrenal carcinomas can cause primary hyperaldosteronism, this condition is more commonly caused by small adrenal adenomas or hyperplasia. Patient commonly present with hypertension, weakness, hyokalemia, muscle cramps, polyuria, and polydipsia. Primary hyperaldosteronism is diagnosed by measurement of hypokalemia ($K < 3.5$ mEq/liter), elevated plasma levels of aldosterone, and low or undetectable levels of renin.

Adrenal carcinoma may present with excessive sex hormone secretion. Virilization or feminization may be combined with hypercortisolism, or it results in only increased estrogen or testosterone. The work-up requires measurement of 24-hour urinary 17-ketosteroids, 17-hydroxysteroids, urinary free cortisol, and depending on virilization or feminization, serum determination of testosterone or estrogen. Virilization secondary to an adrenal neoplasm may accompany Cushing's syndrome and if it does occur, it usually indicates adrenal cortical carcinoma. Virilization in the absence of Cushing's syndrome may also occur due to adrenal cortical adenoma or carcinoma. Of course, there are other disorders that cause virilization; however, work-up should include an imaging study of the adrenals to rule out an adrenal neoplasm.

An incidentaloma is an asymptomatic adrenal mass that is detected by CT ordered for another reason. Unexpected adrenal masses are seen in 0.6% of abdominal CT scans. The majority of these adrenal masses are benign adrenal cortical adenomas, which occur in 8.7% of autopsies. Surgery is indicated for these incidentalomas if they are malignant or functional. Functional tumors secrete cortisol, aldosterone, sex hormones, or catecholamines and are diagnosed by appropriate biochemical testing. Adrenal cancer is best determined by the size of the adrenal mass on CT scan. Masses greater than 5 cm in size have a significant probability of being cancerous and should be excised (Fig. 18.1).

Treatment

The mainstay of treatment for adrenal cortical carcinoma is complete resection of all gross tumor. If the carcinoma is intimately associated with adjacent structures, it may be necessary to remove part or all of these structures at the time of surgery. It is important to remember that the best chance for cure is the initial chance. The extent of surgery can be planned by careful assessment of either CT and/or MRI. Images must include the chest to exclude pulmonary metastases. If the inferior vena cava appears compressed, either an inferior vena cavagram or ultrasonography is useful to assess tumor involvement. If resection of one kidney is necessary, function of the other should be evaluated by contrast-enhanced CT or intravenous pyelography (IVP).

Mitotane therapy has been recommended following surgical resection. However, no clear benefit from mitotane has been proven. Patients who undergo definitive resection should undergo monitoring of steroid hormone levels and periodic imaging studies, postoperatively. If a recurrence is detected, it may be possible to remove it surgically. Prolonged remissions have been reported following resection of hepatic,

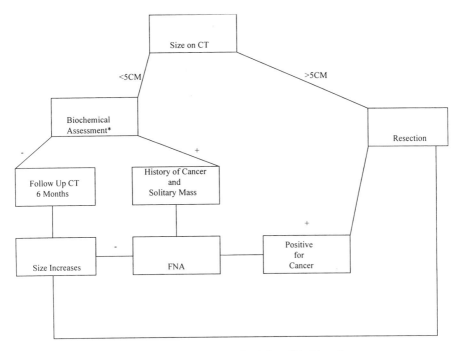

Figure 18.1. Flow Diagram for Adrenal Incidentaloma

pulmonary, and cerebral metastases from adrenal cortical carcinoma. When complete resection of tumor metastases is not possible, near total resection may still be helpful in some hormonally productive, slow growing adrenal cortical cancers. Palliation of bony metastases or local recurrences may be achieved by radiation therapy.

In patients with recurrent and/or metastatic adrenal cortical carcinoma, chemotherapy with o,p-DDD (mitotane) is usually started. Mitotane can decrease serum levels of cortisol and provide amelioration of Cushing's syndrome. Tumor responses usually occur early following the initiation of mitotane treatment. Although most patients subsequently progress on mitotane, there have been a few long-term survivors with metastatic disease. Chemotherapy regimens have been generally ineffective against adrenal cortical carcinoma. Partial responses have been reported with doxorubicin, alkylating agents, cisplatin, and etoposide. For all patients, the 5-year survival rate is between 10% and 35%.

PHEOCHROMOCYTOMA

Pathology

Pheochromocytomas arise from chromaffin cells. Malignant tumors tend to be larger and weigh more, although this is not an unequivocal indicator of malignancy. The only absolute criteria are the presence of secondary tumors in sites where chromaffin cells are not usually located or the presence of visceral metastases. Cellular characteristics, vascular invasion, mitoses, and DNA ploidy have not been useful in the distinguishing between benign and malignant pheochromocytomas.

Clinical Manifestations and Diagnosis

Patients with pheochromocytomas can present with a range of symptoms from mild labile hypertension to sudden death secondary to a hypertensive crisis, myocardial infarction, or cerebral vascular accident. The classic patient describes "spells" of paroxysmal headaches, pallor, palpitations, hypertension, and diaphoresis. The diagnosis is based on measurement of elevated levels of catecholamines and catecholamine metabolites in the urine. Recent studies demonstrate that measurement of metabolites is more sensitive than that of total catecholamines.

Localization Studies and Preoperative Preparation

CT and MRI are the two radiologic (nonnuclear medicine) procedures of choice to localize pheochromocytomas. Both are noninvasive and sensitive, being able to detect tumors approximately 1 cm in diameter. MRI may be more specific because of the increased signal intensity on different image sequences. CT is the study of choice because of lower cost, greater resolution, and greater availability. Another technique for the localization of pheochromocytoma is nuclear scanning following the administration of labeled MIBG. The compound is taken up and concentrated in adrenergic tissue. The sensitivity of MIBG scanning is 78% in sporadic pheochromocytoma, 91% in malignant pheochromocytoma, and 94% in familial pheochromocytoma. The overall sensitivity is 87%. The specificity was nearly 100% in all categories and overall. Metastatic bone involvement by tumor can be imaged by MIBG but bone scan may be more sensitive. In summary, MIBG scanning images catecholamine-producing tumors with a high specificity and sensitivity. Whereas CT and MRI reflect changes in morphology, scintigraphic imaging relies on function.

Once the diagnosis is established and the tumor localized, preoperative preparation includes α-adrenergic blockade. Patients are started on phenoxybenzamine 10 mg PO, bid or tid. If tachycardia develops (heart rate > 100 beats/minute), β-adrenergic blocking agents (propranolol) are added before surgery. Propranolol should never be started prior to α-blockade because unopposed vasoconstriction may worsen hypertension. Phenoxybenzamine increases the total blood and plasma volume in patients with pheochromocytoma.

Malignant Pheochromocytomas

Malignant pheochromocytomas are thought not to occur in MEN syndromes and to be present in approximately 10% of patients with pheochromocytoma. The treatment has been complete surgical resection whenever possible and management of hypertensive symptoms by catecholamine blockade. Bony metastases respond to radiotherapy, if doses of 40 cGy can be administered. Localized or solitary soft tissue masses even when metastatic to the liver or lung may be successfully resected surgically. Chemotherapy regimens based on doxorubicin have not been efficacious in the treatment of malignant pheochromocytomas. Combinations of cyclophosphamide, vincristine, and dacarbazine have produced significant partial responses, but do not appear ro prolong survival. Survival data of patients with malignant pheochromocytoma suggest that the 5-year survival rate is 36%.

PANCREATIC AND INTESTINAL NEUROENDOCRINE TUMORS

Epidemiology

Neuroendocrine tumors of the pancreas and intestine are rare, with an incidence of less than 10 per million population per year. Insulinomas are thought to be the most common islet cell tumor, with a prevalence of approximately one per million population per year, and gastrinomas are the second most common islet cell tumor, with an incidence of 0.1 to 0.4 per million population per year. The remaining pancreatic endocrine tumors occur in less than 0.2 per million population per year. Intestinal carcinoid tumors occur with an incidence of 1 per million population per year (Table 18.5).

Pathology

Neuroendocrine tumors are called apudomas (*A*mine *P*recursor *U*ptake and *D*ecarboxylation). They are composed of monotonous sheets of small round cells with uniform nuclei and cytoplasm. Mitotic figures are unusual. By electron microscopy,

TABLE 18.5. Carcinoid Tumors: Location, Incidence of Metastases, and Carcinoid Syndrome by Primary Location

		Location of Tumors (%)	Incidence of Metastases (%)	Incidence of Carcinoid Syndrome (%)
Foregut				
	Stomach	2	22	10
	Duodenum	3	20	3
	Bronchus	12	20	13
	Thymus	2	25	—
Midgut				
	Jejunum	1	35	9
	Ileum	23	35	9
	Appendix	38	2	< 1
	Colon	2	60	5
	Ovary or testis	< 1	6	50
Hindgut				
	Rectum	13	3	—

these tumors demonstrate dense granules that contain the secretory products. Neuroendocrine tumors appear identical microscopically independent of their site of origin. For example, carcinoid tumors of the ileum look the same as islet cell tumors of the pancreas. In general, microscopic pathologic description of pancreatic endocrine tumors has failed to predict the malignant potential of a specific tumor. In addition, there is no clear correlation between histologic pattern of an islet cell tumor and the type of associated clinical syndrome. At present, the only clear determination of malignancy is detection of metastatic tumor, either in lymph nodes or liver. The benign nature of an individual tumor can be determined only by careful long-term follow-up studies. In general, fewer than 10% of insulinomas are cancerous, fewer than 10% of appendiceal carcinoid tumors are malignant, approximately 60% of gastrinomas are malignant, and 50% to 90% of all neuroendocrine tumors are malignant.

The size of an individual islet cell tumor does not correlate with the severity of the hormonally mediated symptoms. Small tumors such as duodenal gastrinomas may still cause significant symptoms (Table 18.6). There is a correlation between the size of the tumor and the occurrence of malignancy. Appendiceal carcinoid tumors that are less than 2 cm in size are seldom malignant. Insulinomas, such as gastrinomas, are generally small tumors, < 2 cm. Insulinomas are seldom malignant and small (< 2 cm) gastrinomas may metastasize to lymph nodes but seldom spread to the liver. Ileal carcinoid tumors that are approximately 2 cm may still metastasize to the liver. Glucagonomas, somatostatinomas, pancreatic polypeptidomas, and other islet cell tumors are frequently large at the time of detection, > 5 cm. The majority of primary pancreatic endocrine tumors are solitary, encapsulated, and within the pancreas. However, neuroendocrine tumors can also occur in the small intestine, duodenum, and other more unusual locations. When metastatic disease occurs, it initially develops in lymph nodes and subsequently the liver. Late in the course of the disease, neuroendocrine tumors metastasize to other distant sites such as lung, bone, and even the heart.

Pancreatic endocrine tumors occur in either a nonfamilial (sporadic) form or in a familial form associated with MENI (see section on MENI). The exact proportion of patients with pancreatic islet cell tumors who have MENI varies in different series from < 5% to 25%. The recognition that an islet cell tumor occurs in the setting of MENI syndrome is important because these patients may have multiple pancreatic and duodenal tumors. Further, screening of other family members for various features of the syndrome and a menin gene mutation is indicated. Functional islet cell tumors are the second most frequent abnormality in MENI and occur in approximately 80% of individuals. Gastrinomas, insulinomas, glucagonomas, and VIPomas occur in a decreasing incidence in patients with MENI. Finally, MENI patients have a higher probability of developing both foregut and midgut carcinoid tumors.

Almost all insulinomas occur in the pancreas. Insulinomas have a uniform distribution among the head, body, and tail of the pancreas. Glucagonomas generally occur within the pancreas and most commonly in the pancreatic body and tail. In contrast to insulinomas and glucagonomas, gastrinomas occur more commonly within the duodenum, but they may also originate in the pancreas. Approximately 50% to 60% of gastrinomas have recently been identified to be within the duodenal wall. VIPo-

TABLE 18.6. Neuroendocrine Tumors of Pancreas and Duodenum: Incidence Proportion Malignant and MEN-I, Location, Clinical Findings and Diagnosis

Tumor	Incidence	Proportion Malignant	Proportion MENI	Tumor Location	Symptoms	Diagnosis
Insulinoma	4/5,000,000	< 5%	4%	Pancreas	Hypoglycemia Neuroglycopenia	Fasting hypoglycemia and hyperinsulinemia
Gastrinoma	2/5,000,000	60–90%	18–24%	40% Pancreas 60% Duodenum	Peptic ulcer Diarrhea	Elevated gastrin Elevated BAO
Glucagonoma	Rare	> 70%	Occasional	Pancreas	Diabetes mellitus NME Cachexia Hypoaminoacidemia Thrombophlebitis	Elevated glucagon
Somatostatinoma	Very rare	> 90%	—	50% Pancreas	Diabetes mellitus Cholelithiasis Steatorrhea	Elevated somatostatin
VIPoma	Rare	50%	Occasional	90% Pancreas 10% Duodenum	Diarrhea Hypokalemia Achlorhydia	Elevated VIP
Nonfunctional	1/1,000,000	> 60%	20%	Pancreas	Pain Bleeding Obstruction	CT Elevated pancreatic polypeptide

mas are usually in the pancreas. Somatostatinomas, similar to gastrinomas, may be extrapancreatic. In a recent review of 48 primary somatostatinomas, 56% were in the pancreas and 44% were in the duodenum or jejunum. Similar to glucagonomas, somatostatinomas usually are large, > 5 cm at the time of presentation. Only primary insulinomas and gastrinomas are small at the time of presentation, frequently < 2 cm. Nonfunctioning pancreatic islet cell tumors and PPomas are usually > 5 cm in diameter. Other less common functioning islet cell tumors such as those associated with acromegaly, hypercalcemia, or ectopic ACTH production are usually large tumors located within the pancreas.

Cacinoid tumors are divided into foregut, midgut, and hindgut. Foregut tumors usually occur within the thymus or bronchus. Gastric carcinoid tumors are associated with hypergastrinemia, especially in MENI patients. Gastric carcinoid tumors may secrete serotonin, but thymic and bronchial tumors commonly secrete ACTH. Midgut carcinoid tumors most commonly occur in the appendix and ileum. These tumors usually secrete serotonin and other vasoactive amines, but they do not cause the carcinoid syndrome unless they metastasize to the liver. Hindgut carcinoids occur in the rectum, and do not cause the carcinoid syndrome.

Symptoms and Diagnosis

Patients with insulinoma present with neuroglycopenic symptoms secondary to hypoglycemia. These symptoms include seizures, altered mental status, coma, and difficulty arousing after a fast. The diagnosis is established by a standard 72-hour fast during which the patient is observed for neuroglycopenic symptoms. If symptoms occur, blood levels of glucose, insulin, C-peptide, and proinsulin are drawn and the fast is terminated. Patients with insulinoma will develop symptoms and the serum glucose level will be < 45 mg/dl with an insulin level > 5 μU/ml. Patients will also have elevated serum levels of C-peptide and proinsulin. Symptoms may be controlled with increased frequency of feedings and medications such as diazoxide and calcium channel blockers. However, in these patients the medical management of symptoms is poor.

Patients with gastrinoma have severe peptic ulcer disease, diarrhea, and esophageal reflux disease. The diagnosis is made by the detection of elevated fasting gastrin levels and elevated levels of basal acid output. For these studies all gastric antisecretory drugs must be discontinued. Patients with ZES have gastrin levels > 125 pg/ml and basal acid output > 15 mEq/liter. The diagnosis can be further confirmed by the secretin test during which gastrin levels are measured before and after secretin stimulation. Patients with ZES have an increment in serum gastrin level of > 200 pg/ml following 2 U/kg of secretin. Gastric acid hypersecretion is well controlled with omeprazole in doses of 20 to 40 mg/day.

Patients with VIPoma have severe secretory diarrhea (> 5 to 10 liters/day). These patients may also have achlorhydria, hypokalemia, and hypercalcemia. The diagnosis is made by measurement of fasting levels of VIP, which are generally elevated (> 500 pg/ml). The diarrhea can usually be controlled with injections of the long-acting somatostatin analogue octreotide 100 to 150 μg bid or tid.

Patients with glucagonoma have a characteristic skin rash called necrolytic migratory erythema (NME) which involves the groin and ankles. The rash is erythematous and is associated with intense pruritus. Patients are also cachectic with profound muscle wasting, type 2 diabetes, and weight loss. Patients may also have hypercoagulability as seen with repetitive episodes of deep venous thrombosis and pulmonary embolism. The diagnosis is made by measurement of hypoaminoacidemia and elevated fasting serum levels of glucagon (> 1000 pg/ml). Patients require nutritional supplementation; insulin and octreotide often improve the rash.

Patients with somatostatinoma have type 2 diabetes mellitus, gallstones, and steatorrhea. The diagnosis is made by measuring somatostatin levels. Further, most patients have a large tumor within the duodenum or the pancreatic head.

Patients with midgut carcinoid tumors present with no symptoms, carcinoid syndrome, or small bowel obstruction. The most common site for intestinal carcinoid tumor is the appendix and approximately 1 in 300 appendectomy specimens contain an unexpected carcinoid tumor. Size is an important criterion for malignancy in appendiceal carcinoid tumors. Tumors less than 2 cm are seldom malignant and require only simple appendectomy. Tumors greater than 2 cm or tumors present at the base of the appendiceal stump require right hemicolectomy. The second most common intestinal carcinoid tumor occurs within the ileum and these tumors behave in a more malignant fashion than appendiceal carcinoid tumors. Size is not an important dtermination in these tumors, as small tumors can be as malignant as larger ones. In general, involved ileum should be resected with its mesentery. There is an intense local reaction to these tumors with cicatrization and desmoplasia. This reaction can cause obstruction of the small intestine by adhesive bands or narrowing of the lumen. Unfortunately, these tumors commonly metastasize to the liver and patients then develop the carcinoid syndrome which is secondary to the presence of serotonin and other vasoactive amines in the systemic circulation. Carcinoid syndrome includes flushing, diarrhea, bronchospasm, and right-sided heart failure secondary to valvular heart disease. The components of the carcinoid syndrome may be managed with drugs to counteract each of the components, for example, antidiarrhea agents to control the diarrhea and antihistamines to control the flushing. Octreotide, the long-acting somatostatin analogue, can ameliorate each of the components of the carcinoid syndrome except the right-sided heart disease. It is also useful to treat the carcinoid crisis that may occur during induction of anesthesia or surgical procedures to remove liver tumors.

Imaging

Radiologic imaging of pancreatic and intestinal neuroendocrine tumors depends on the size, location, and density of somatostatin receptors. First, large, malignant pancreatic, duodenal, small intestinal, and liver tumors are clearly imaged on CT, but hepatic metastases are best visualized on MRI. Both studies have a resolution of 1 to 2 cm and MRI may have some special sequences that allow detection of smaller tumors. Endoscopic ultrasound has been able to detect small pancreatic endocrine tumors such as insulinoma. These tumors appear sonolucent against an echodense pancreatic backdrop. Conversely, small duodenal gastrinomas are poorly detected by endoscopic ultrasound, possibly because the duodenum lacks the uniform background of the pancreas. Octreoscan has been able to image approximately 80% of neuroendocrine tumors independent of size and location. It images tumors based on density of type 2 somatostatin receptors and predicts response to somatostatin analogue treatment. Imageable tumors will also respond to octreotide therapy. Because most islet cell and intestinal carcinoid tumors are rich in somatostatin receptors, most will appear hot on this scan. However, insulinomas do not have these receptors and therefore are seldom detected.

Treatment

Treatment should be designed to control the signs and symptoms of excessive hormonal secretion and control the tumoral process. The only potentially curative treatment for neuroendocrine tumors is complete surgical resection of all disease. Even localized liver metastases can be removed for apparent amelioration of symptoms and prolongation of survival. Octreoscan should be used to exclude unsuspected metastases outside the liver.

Approximately 30% to 40% of metastatic neuroendocrine tumors respond to Adriamycin, 5-FU, and streptozotocin as single drugs or in combination. Interferon-α has also produced some partial responses. Chemoembolization of liver metastases using interventional radiology techniques and Adriamycin has had a 90% response rate with improvement in symptoms. However, there have been no complete responses and it does not appear to prolong survival. Liver transplantation with postoperative chemotherapy has been used for patients with disease localized to the liver; however, most patients eventually develop extrahepatic recurrence. The tumor may be slowly progressive and indolent. Patients with metastatic disease may survive for long peiods, as patients with liver metastases have a 20% 5-year survival. It is clear that some patients may live for many years with distant disease despite the inadequacies of treatment. Chemotherapy or other potentially morbid treatment is generally not instituted unless there is radiologic evidence of tumor progression.

FURTHER READING

Farndon JR, Leight GS, Dilley WG, et al. (1986) Familial medullary thyroid carcinoma without associated endocrinopathies: A distinct clinical entity. *Br J Surg* 73:278.

Friedman E, Larsson C, Amorosi A, Brandi ML, Bale AE, Metz DC, Jensen RT, Skarulis MC, Eastman RC, Nieman L, Norton JA, Marx SJ (1994) Multiple endocrine neoplasia type 1 pathology, pathophysiology, molecular genetics and differential diagnosis. In: Bilezikian JP, Levine MA, Marcus R (eds) *The Parathyroids*. Raven Press, New York.

Howe JR, Norton JA, Wells SA Jr (1993) Prevalence of pheochromocytoma and hyperparathyroidism in multiple endocrine neoplasia type 2A: Results of long-term follow-up. *Surgery* 114:1070.

Lairmore TC, Ball DW, Baylin SB, Wells SA Jr (1993) Management of pheochromocytomas in patients with multiple endocrine neoplasia type 2 syndromes. *Ann Surg* 217:595.

Lips CJM, Landsvater RM, Hoppener JWM, Geerdink RA, Blijham G, Jansen-Schillhorn van Veen JM, et al. (1994) Clinical screening as compared with DNA analysis in families with multiple endocrine neoplasia type 2A. *N Engl J Med* 331:828.

Metz DC, Jensen RT, Bale AE, Skarulis MC, Eastman RD, Nieman L, Norton JA, Friedman E, Larsson C, Amorosi A, Brandi ML, Marx SJ (1994) Multiple endocrine neoplasia type 1 clinical features and management. In: Bilezikian JP, Levine MA, Marcus R (eds) *The Parathyroids*. Raven Press, New York.

Norton JA, Fromme LC, Farrell RE, Wells SA Jr (1979) Multiple endocrine neoplasia type 2B: The most aggressive form of medullary thyroid carcinoma. *Surg Clin NA* 59:109.

Utiger RD (1994) Medullary thyroid carcinoma, genes and the prevention of cancer. *N Engl J Med* 331:870.

Wells SA Jr, Chi DD, Toshima K, Dehner LP, Coffin CM, Dowton B, Ivanovich JL, DeBenedetti MK, Dilley WG, Moley JF, Norton JA, Donis-Keller H (1994) Predictive DNA testing and prophylactic thyroidectomy in patients at risk for multiple endocrine neoplasia type 2A. *Ann Surg* 220:237.

Wingo PA, Tong T, Bolden S (1995) Cancer Statistics, 1995. *CA Cancer J Clin* 45:8.

Jossart GH, Clark OH (1994) Well-differentiated thyroid cancer. *Curr Prob Surg* 31:937.

Robbins J, Merino MJ, Boice JD, Jr, et al. (1991) Thyroid cancer: A lethal endocrine neoplasm. *Ann Intern Med* 115:133.

Schneider AB, Shore-Freedman E, Ryo JY, et al. (1985). Radiation-induced tumors of the head and neck following childhood irradiation. *Medicine* 64:1.

Mazzaferi EL (1992) Thyroid cancer in thyroid nodules: Finding a needle in a haystack. *Am J Med* 93:359.

Brander A, Viikinoski P, Nickels J, Kivisaari L (1991) Thyroid gland: U.S. screening in an adult population. *Radiology* 181:683.

Gharib H, Goellner JR (1993) Fine needle aspiration biopsy of the thyroid: An appraisal. *Ann Intern Med* 118:282.

Mazzaferri EL (1993) Management of a solitary thyroid nodule. *N Engl J Med* 328:553.

Mazzaferri EL, Young RL, Oertel JE, Kemmerer WT, Page CP (1977) Papillary thyroid carcinoma: The impact of therapy in 576 patients. *Medicine* 56:171.

Cady B, Rossi R, Silverman M, Wool M (1985) Further evidence of the validity of risk group definition in differentiated thyroid carcinoma. *Surgery* 98:1171.

Brennan MD, Bergstralh EJ, van Heerden JA, McConahey WM (1991) Follicular thyroid cancer treated at the Mayo Clinic 1946-1970: Initial manifestations, pathology findings, therapy and outcome. *Mayo Clinic Proc* 66:11.

van Heerden JA, Grant CS, Gharib H, Hay ID, Ilstrup DM (1990) Long term course of patients with persisent hypercalcitoninemia after apparent curative primary surgery for medullary thyroid cancer. *Ann Surg* 212:395.

Mazzaferri EL, Jhiang SM (1994) Long-term impact of initial surgical and medical therapy on papillary and follicular thyroid cancer. *Am J Med* 97:418.

Nikiforov Y, Gnepp DR (1994) Pediatric thyroid cancer after the Chernobyl disaster. *Cancer* 74:748.

Kim JH, Leeper RD (1983) Treatment of anaplastic giant and spindle cell carcinoma of the thyroid gland with combination Adriamycin and radiation therapy: A new approach. *Cancer* 52:954.

Norton JA, Levin B, Jensen RT (1993) Cancer of the endocrine system. In: DeVita VT Jr, Hellman S, Rosenberg SA (eds) *Cancer, Principles and Practice of Oncology*, 4th edition. JB Lippincott, Philadelphia.

Kasperlik-Zaluska AA, Migdalska BM, Zgliczynski S, Makowska AM (1995) Adrenal carcinoma. A clinical study and treatment results of 52 patients. *Cancer* 75:2587.

Luton JP, Cerdas S, Billaud L, Thomas G, Guilhaume B, Bertagna X, Laudat MH, Louvel A, Chapius Y, Blondeau P, Bonnin A, Bricaire H (1990) Clinical features of adrenocortical carcinoma, prognostic factors and the effect of mitotane therapy. *N Engl J Med* 32:1195.

Jensen JC, Pass HI, Sindelar WF, Norton JA (1992) Recurrent or metastatic disease in select patients with adrenocortical carcinoma. *Arch Surg* 126:457.

Decker RA, Elson P, Hogan TF (1991) ECOG mitotane and Adriamycin in patients with ACC. *Surgery* 111:1006.

Haak HR, Van Seters AP, Moolenaar AJ (1990) Mitotane therapy of adrenocortical carcinoma. *N Engl J Med* 322:758.

Pommier R, Brenna MF (1992) An 11 year experience with adrenocortical cancer. *Surgery* 112:1963.

Lairmore TC, Ball DW, Baylin SB, Wells SA Jr (1993) Management of pheochromocytomas in patients with multiple endocrine neoplasia type 2 syndromes. *Ann Surg* 217:595.

Duncan MW, Compton P, Lazarus L, Smythe GA (1988) Measurement of norepinephrine and 3,4-dihydroxyphenylglycol in urine and plasma for the diagnosis of pheochromocytoma. *N Engl J Med* 319:136.

Shapiro B, Copp JE, Sisson JC, Eyre PL, Wallis J, Beierualtes WH (1985) Iodine-131 metaiodobenzylguanidine for the locating of suspected pheochromocytoma: Experience in 400 cases. *J Nucl Med* 26:576.

Krempf M, Lumbroso J, Mornex R, Brendel AJ, Wimeau JL, Delisle MJ, Aubert B, Carpentier P, Fleury-Goyon MC, Gibold C, Guyot M, Lahneche B, Marchandise X, Schlumberger M, Charbonnel B, Chatal JF (1991) Use of [131]IM iodobenzylguanidine in the treatment of malignant pheochromocytoma. *J Clin Endocrinol Metab* 72:455.

Averbuch SD, Steakley CS, Young RC, Gelmann EIP, Goldstein DS, Stull R, Keiser HR (1988) Malignant pheochromocytoma: Effective treatment with a combination of cyclophosphamide, vincristine and decarbazine. *Ann Intern Med* 109:267.

Norton JA (1994) Neuroendocrine tumors of the pancreas and duodenum. *Curr Prob Surg* 31:77.

Doherty GM, Doppman JL, Shawker TH, Miller DL, Eastman RC, Gorden P, Norton JA (1991) Results of a prospective strategy to diagnose, localize and resect insulinomas. *Surgery* 110:989.

Gorden P, Comi RJ, Maton PN, Go VLW (1989) Somatostatin and somatostatin analogue (SMS 201-995) in treatment of hormone-secreting tumors of the pituitary and gastrointestinal tract and non-neoplastic disease of the gut. *Ann Intern Med* 110:35.

Arnold R, Neuhaus C, Benning R, Schwerk WB, Trautmann ME, Joseph K, Bruns C (1993) Somatostatin analog sandostatin and inhibition of tumor growth in patients with metastatic endocrine gastroenteropancreatic tumors. *World J Surg* 17:511.

Lamberts SW, Bakker WH, Reubi JC, Krenning EP (1990) Somatostatin receptor imaging in the localization of endocrine tumors. *N Engl J Med* 323:1246.

Service FJ, McMahon MM, O'Brien PC, Ballard DJ (1991) Functioning insulinoma—incidence, recurrence, and long-term survival of patients: A 60-year study. *Mayo Clin Proc* 66:711.

Norton JA, Doppman JL, Jensen RT (1992) Curative resection in Zollinger–Ellison syndrome: Results of a 10-year prospective study. *Ann Surg* 215:8.

Fraker DL, Norton JA, Alexander HR, Venzon DJ, Jensen RT (1994) Surgery in Zollinger–Ellison syndrome alters the natural history of gastrinoma. *Ann Surg* 220:320.

Norton JA, Sugarbaker PH, Doppman JL, Wesley RA, Maton PN, Gardner JD, Jensen RT (1986) Aggressive resection of metastatic disease in selected patients with malignant gastrinoma. *Ann Surg* 203:352.

Modlin IM, Lewis JJ, Ahlman H, Bilchik AJ, Kumar RR (1993) Management of unresectable malignant endocrine tumors of the pancreas. *Surg Gynecol Obstet* 176:507.

CHAPTER 19

LUNG CANCER

DAVID PAYNE

Department of Radiation Oncology
Princess Margaret Hospital
Toronto, Canada

TSUGUO NARUKE

Division of Thoracic Surgery
National Cancer Center Hospital
Tokyo, Japan

SUMMARY

Lung cancer is the most common cause of cancer death in both sexes. Screening programs are improving but infrequently detect cancer early enough to alter the survival outcome. Prevention programs that effectively decrease the smoking rates in the population would result in a higher number of lives saved than that of people cured by present methods.

The vast majority of malignant tumors are carcinomas arising from bronchial epithelium. Regional spread to mediastinal lymph nodes is frequent, and is predictive of systemic metastases. Clinical staging is based on tumor size, involvement of associated structures, the location of lymph node metastases, and the presence of metastasis in distant organs.

Surgery plays an essential role in diagnosis of all forms of lung cancer, and in the curative treatment of early forms (UICC stages I, II, and some IIIA). Radiotherapy is required in nonsurgical cases of early stage, either as exclusive treatment or as part of combined modality therapy programs for locally advanced disease. Radiotherapy is also highly effective in the palliative treatment of local tumor or distant metastases.

Manual of Clinical Oncology, 7th edition, Edited by Raphael E. Pollock
ISBN 0-471-23828-7, pages 385–405. Copyright © 1999 Wiley-Liss, Inc.

Chemotherapy using current agents produces symptomatic responses and often good systemic palliation, but its impact on overall survival rates is modest, as is that of radiotherapy.

ETIOLOGY

Tobacco smoking is by far the most important risk factor for lung cancer; and is estimated to be the cause of 85% of lung cancer deaths. The extent of exposure to tobacco smoke (carcinogen "dose"), as reflected in numbers of years an individual has smoked, number of cigarettes smoked per day, and tar content of the cigarettes, is correlated with the risk of lung cancer. The carcinogens in tobacco smoke include the polynuclear aromatic hydrocarbons (PAHs), N-nitrosoamines, aromatic amines, other organic and nonorganic compounds, and polonium-210. After smoking cessation, an individual's risk of lung cancer slowly comes to approximate but not equal that of a nonsmoker. It is also suggested that, even among nonsmokers, the "passive" smokers who have been exposed to environmental tobacco smoke have a significantly increased risk of lung cancer.

Other carcinogens that play a role in the development of lung cancer include pollutants in the urban air, such as benzopyrenes, indoor radon, and various occupational respiratory toxic substances. Asbestos exposure is the most widely recognized environmental carcinogen; it acts synergistically with tobacco smoke for lung carcinogenesis, and is also closely associated with the development of mesothelioma. In countries such as China, an excess risk of lung cancer is attributed to indoor air pollution originating from cooking.

Some nutritional elements have long been suggested to act as chemoprotective factors against carcinogenesis. Beta-carotene has been the most widely investigated. However, two large-scale randomized clinical trials have demonstrated no effect of this chemoprevention in reducing the risk of cancer.

Genetic factors appear to be important in lung carcinogenesis in some cases. There are several reports that genetic polymorphisms of carcinogen-metabolizing enzyme systems are associated with the risk of lung cancer. These may determine the different cancer susceptibilities seen in various individuals and families.

None of these "causes" of lung cancer satisfactorily explains the recent increase in incidence of adenocarcinoma. It is clear that human tumors result from a complex sequence of mutational events, and it is likely that still unknown factor(s) play important roles in lung carcinogenesis.

SCREENING AND DIAGNOSIS

The purpose of screening is to accomplish early detection and treatment of as many cancers as possible, especially among smokers, who are at greatest risk. Public awareness of the risk of lung cancer induction by smoking is important. Physicians may screen individuals by means of chest radiograph and sputum cytology for atypical or cancer cells. Suspicious findings should lead to a diagnostic evaluation along the lines of the schema (Fig. 19.1). Note that peripheral lung tumors (surrounded by lung parenchyma) typically produce few symptoms and are best found by chest radiography. The more common central tumors arise from the proximal airways and often attract attention because of cough hemoptysis or dyspnea.

If the screening process proves abnormal, the subsequent diagnostic evaluation depends on the original observation and the method of detection. Thus, while lung cancer screening typically includes chest radiograph and sputum cytology, the workup may differ according to the particular finding and the location of the suspected lesion.

Because lung cancer at the time of presentation is frequently incurable, there is potential for screening of asymptomatic patients to discover cancers at an earlier

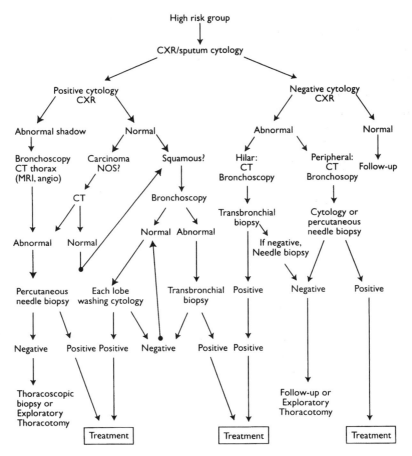

FIGURE 19.1. Diagnosis of lung cancer based on screening by chest radiograph and sputum cytology.

stage, which could result in improved overall survival rates. Large-scale screening programs must utilize simple techniques to be widely applicable. In the case of lung cancer, chest radiography and sputum cytology are the only practical methods currently available to screen large numbers of subjects. However, even these are expensive when applied to a population, and can be justified only if they yield significant numbers of early tumors and better long-term results.

The use of chest radiography and sputum cytology to screen high-risk patients for lung cancer was evaluated in the large-scale, randomized controlled trials sponsored by the National Cancer Institute and conducted at Johns Hopkins Medical Institute, Memorial Sloan-Kettering Cancer Center, and Mayo Clinic. Patients, 45 years old and above who were chronic heavy cigarette smokers, were screened every 4 months using chest radiography with or without sputum cytology. The trial detected more cancers, more resectable cancers, and more early-stage cancers in the sputum-screened group than in the unscreened controls. The 5-year survival rate was higher for the screened groups than the controlled group, explainable by the effect of lead-time bias. However, the cancer-related mortality rates for the screened and control groups were virtually the same. Thus the results did not justify recommending large-scale radiological or cytological screening for lung cancer.

These trials, done over 25 years ago, did not provide sufficient evidence to support large-scale screening by the methods used, even in the high-risk population studied. It should be noted however, that modern technologies now permit greatly improved scrutiny of the airways and parenchyma, and spiral computed tomography (CT) can detect lesions of 3 mm. A large trial of annual chest radiograph screening began in the United States in the early 1990s but will require 16 years and include 148,000 subjects. In addition newer methods of automated sputum cytology collection and immunoanalysis of samples may permit many of molecular and genetic markers to be screened in a single specimen, and provide the capability for early diagnosis. These methods may result in a reappraisal of the need for lung cancer screening.

TECHNIQUES FOR DIAGNOSTIC EVALUATION

The investigation of patients with solitary pulmonary nodules should begin with the search for and examination of previous chest radiographs. Lesions that are new, radiologically suspicious for carcinoma, or increasing in size should be treated as pulmonary malignancies. Calcification is typically a sign of benign lesions, but may be seen in malignant tumors. Radiologic findings are not sufficient for pathologic diagnosis of lung cancer, much less for its subclassification.

The definitive diagnosis of a lung cancer requires histopathologic or cytologic confirmation. Among the four major subtypes of lung cancer (Table 19.1), small cell carcinoma (SCLC) is distinguished from the other, "non-small"-cell lung carcinomas (NSCLC), because of its differences in biologic behavior and clinical course. These tumors exhibit different cellular characteristics, a pronounced tendency for metastasis to distant sites, and typically a marked response to chemotherapy. SCLC and NSCLC often require different treatment strategies. Physicians thus require patho-

TABLE 19.1. Characteristics of Pathologic Cell Types of Lung Cancer

Cancer Type	Major Cell Type	Proportion of All Lung Cancers	Location	Histology	Volume Doubling Time (days)	Cell of Origin
Non-small-cell	Squamous cell	30–35%	Central large or medium bronchi	Intercellular bridges (desmosomes); keratin pearls	100	Multipotential epithelial cells
	Adenocarcinoma; subtype: bronchiolo-alveolar	25–30%	Peripheral	Gland formation; intra-cellular mucous	187	Goblet cells
	Large-cell	10%	Peripheral	Undifferentiated large cells	100	—
Small-cell	Small-cell; subtypes: oat cell, inter-mediate cells	20–25%	Central	neurosecretory granules	33	Kulchitsky's (K; neuro-ectodermal) cell

389

logic information about the disease to perform therapeutic decision-making. In some cases, pathologists may require more tissue to determine whether an adenocarcinoma within the lung represents a primary lung cancer, or a metastatic focus from a metachronous or a synchronous cancer, be it from a source in the breast, colon, or a different part of the lung. An aggressive approach to diagnosis is usually justified, unless specifically contraindicated, to determine prognosis and a basis for management decisions. Multiple diagnostic procedures for a lung cancer are available, each with specific indications.

Sputum Cytology

Sputum cytology is positive in more than 50% of cases. Positive cytology is more likely when the suspected lesion is central in the thorax but has a negative prognostic significance when the cancer is located in the peripheral lung field. However, positive sputum cytology can result from a radiologically occult lesion such as a centrally located bronchogenic carcinoma or an upper airway cancer (e.g., from the larynx). Therefore, bronchoscopic examination is necessary before determining that a radiologically suspicious lesion is the source of the positive sputum cytology.

Bronchoscopy

The vast majority of lung cancer patients are diagnosed by transbronchial biopsy or cytology. Hilar lesions such as centrally located squamous cell carcinomas often present as endobronchial tumors, diagnosed by biopsy, brush cytology, or wash cytology. Submucosal infiltration or an invasive nodal metastasis may be visible by bronchoscopy and the tumor diagnosed by biopsy or aspiration cytology. Even a bronchoscopically negative, peripherally located tumor may be diagnosed by fluoroscopy-guided transbronchial biopsy or cytology (taken by curettage, brush, lavage, or fine-needle aspiration). When a peripherally located tumor is too small or too faint in density to be detected by conventional X-ray fluoroscopy, transbronchial biopsy with CT-fluoroscope guidance may be helpful. Major complications of transbronchial biopsy include hemorrhage, pneumothorax, and exacerbation of infection.

Transthoracic Needle Biopsy

Transthoracic needle biopsy can provide a definite diagnosis of lung cancer more easily than bronchoscopic examination when the suspicious lesion is peripherally located. It is usually performed with X-ray fluoroscopy guidance, but ultrasound guidance may be more appropriate when the lesion contacts the chest wall. CT-guided needle biopsy is helpful when the lesion is difficult to visualize on fluoroscopy or when it is located near vital organs such as major vessels. Pneumothorax is the most frequent complication of transthoracic needle biopsy.

Cytologic examination of other tissues such as pleural fluid, or biopsies of pleura, lymph nodes, liver, or bone marrow are sometimes the most appropriate way to make a diagnosis of lung cancer. A solitary mass in an adrenal gland or in the liver in a patient with otherwise potentially resectable lung cancer should be confirmed with needle biopsy before classifying it as a metastasis.

Mediastinoscopy

Mediastinoscopy is a surgical procedure in which some of the mediastinal lymph nodes, which are often involved with metastases, can be evaluated and biopsied. It is performed under general anesthesia using a rigid scope through a suprasternal incision, providing access to pre- and paratracheal and subcarinal lymph nodes. Access to the aortopulmonary region requires a left parasternal incision. Although it can be diagnostic for a case in which no other lesions are available for biopsy, mediastinoscopy usually is a staging procedure for the evaluation of the N-category (see below for TNM classification). Those with mediastinoscopy-proven nodal disease have a poorer prognosis, compared to cases where the nodal involvement was detected by postoperative pathologic examination only.

Thoracoscopy

Thoracoscopy can be used as a staging procedure for the diagnosis of pleural dissemination or malignant effusion in a patient with lung cancer who otherwise may be suitable for curative resection or definitive radiotherapy. Thoracoscopy is also a useful tool when the diagnosis remains elusive after less invasive measures. Video-assisted procedures allow examination of much of the pleural space, to identify and biopsy nodules or plaques of disease. Although more invasive than bronchoscopy, thoracoscopy is less so than open lung biopsy and can be done under local anesthesia.

Open Lung Biopsy

Open lung biopsy is the most invasive diagnostic procedure but may be required when all other diagnostic procedures have failed. The "wait-and-see" attitude in an otherwise good-risk patient with a solitary pulmonary nodule is seldom justified unless radiologic or clinical evidence strongly suggests that it is benign. Even tumors with a diameter of less than 2 cm can metastasize to regional lymph nodes and spread systemically.

Search for Extrathoracic Metastases

A thorough systemic survey should be done as staging procedures in clinical trial patients (Table 19.2), and in most SCLC patients, as they frequently harbor asymptomatic metastases. In NSCLC patients without clinical findings suggestive of extrathoracic cancer, a chest X-ray film and chest CT scan are recommended to stage locoregional disease, with biopsy of mediastinal lymph nodes found on CT scan to be greater than 1 cm in shortest transverse diameter. Pretreatment bone scan and head CT scan are recommended only when signs or symptoms of disease are present, unless required by a specific research protocol.

TABLE 19.2. Recommended Staging Procedures for Patients with Lung Cancer

Procedure	Standard care	Patients on Clinical Trials
Complete physical examination	Yes	Yes
Hematology with differential, WBC, and platelet count	Yes	Yes
Biochemistry with electrolytes, liver function tests, lactate dehydrogenase	Yes	Yes
Chest radiograph	Yes	Yes
CT scan of thorax	Only for limited disease patients to facilitate radiotherapy planning	Yes
Ultrasound or CT scan of abdomen	Yes[a]	Yes
Radionuclide bone scan	Yes[a]	Yes
Skeletal radiographs	If bone scan is indeterminate	If bone scan is indeterminate
CT or MRI of brain	Yes[a]	Yes[a]
MRI of spine	Only if clinically indicated	Only if clinically indicated
Bone marrow aspiration and biopsies	Only if hematology is abnormal	Only for patients on trials of localized disease
Bronchoscopy	Only if needed for diagnosis	Baseline only necessary unless posttreatment bronchoscopy is required to confirm complete response
Mediastinoscopy	Only if needed for diagnosis	Only if needed for diagnosis
Lumbar puncture	Only if clinically indicated	Only if clinically indicated
Liver biopsy	No	Only necessary if indeterminate results are obtained from CT or ultrasound of abdomen
Monoclonal antibody scans	No	No, unless the trial is specifically evaluating monoclonal antibodies
Biomarkers	No	No, unless the trial is specifically evaluating the role of biomarkers
Pulmonary function tests	Only if there is concern about the ability to deliver thoracic irradiation	Only if there is concern about the ability to deliver thoracic irradiation

[a]If one of these studies is positive, further tests are not necessary because extensive disease will have been confirmed. The decision as to which scan should be done first should be guided by any abnormalities detected on the baseline history, physical examination, and blood work.

PATHOLOGY AND NATURAL HISTORY

Lung cancers may arise from the epithelial or stromal tissues but the vast majority originate in the bronchial epithelium of the large to mid-size airways. This discussion focuses on these tumors, which form the overwhelming number of lung cancers. The major subtypes are listed in Table 19.1, and reflect carcinomas derived from cells with squamous or glandular features or undifferentiated tumors that cannot be so classified. The "small-cell" subtype is distinguished by the presence of neurosecretory granules on electron microscopy and other clinicopathologic features. Its importance derives from its comparatively rapid growth rate, tendency to metastasize, and chemoreponsiveness. Its management is therefore somewhat different from that of the other carcinomas grouped under the designation "non-small-cell." The vast majority of lung malignancies fall into one of these four categories. The bronchioloalveolar subtype of adenocarcinoma is thought to arise from the glandular epithelium of the small peripheral airways and alveoli. Malignant cells of this type have a tendency to spread in a superficial pattern along the epithelium of these structures. The relatively rare primary tumors of the trachea are predominantly squamous although the glandular adenoid cystic carcinoma subtype is almost as frequent.

Lung tumors have been extensively studied by the methods of immunocytochemistry or molecular biology to identify proteins with functional significance or that may serve as tumor markers. These help to classify the tumor but have not so far led to significant treatment applications. Small-cell cancer has been linked to genetic changes in chromosome 3. Other gene abnormalities (K-*ras*, *HER-2/neu*, *p53*, *Rb*) have been identified to occur frequently in lung cancer, and in some cases (K-*ras*) to convey a poor outlook.

Bronchogenic carcinomas have a strong predilection for spread to the regional lymph nodes. Anatomically these have been categorized as intralobar, hilar, and mediastinal (subcarinal, paratracheal, subaortic, and others). A standardized map and numerical nomenclature has been developed to facilitate accurate description of involved or uninvolved nodes (Fig. 19.2). Some, but not all, of these nodes will be accessible at mediastinoscopy staging, whereas these and others may be visualized by CT or MRI staging. The risk that a node is involved with cancer increases dramatically as its diameter exceeds 1.5 cm; in the range of size 1 to 3 cm, however, many false-negatives or false-positives are possible.

Nodal involvement of lung cancer serves as an indicator of relative difficulty of achieving complete surgical removal, or of definite nonresectability. It also identifies disease for radiotherapy planning. More importantly, it serves as a marker of systemic metastatic spread. The risk of systemic metastases, whether clinical or occult, increases dramatically from the lymph node negative status (N0), through the hilar (N1), ipsilateral mediastinal (N2), or contralateral mediastinal (N3) lymph node involvement. Palpable disease in more distal lymph nodes (supraclavicular or cervical) signifies almost certain presence of distant metastases.

Thus the natural history of lung cancer is characterized by local, regional nodal, and systemic spread, with only modest differences attributable to histologic subtype or grade. Relatively few patients (15%) present with operable stage I disease. Most

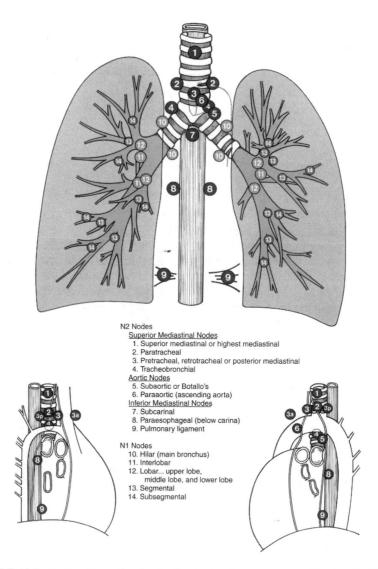

FIGURE 19.2. Regional lymph nodes for the staging for lung cancer. (Reprinted with permission from *TNM Atlas* 4th edit. 1997, Springer-Verlag, New York.)

lung cancer patients will eventually develop distant metastases—typically in liver, brain, and skeleton.

The TNM classification and stage grouping is given in Tables 19.3 and 19.4. The subsequent discussion concentrates on clinical management based on stage. However, lung cancer remains a disease with high overall mortality rates, and series based on selected patients and/or treatment techniques may not be representative

TABLE 19.3. Lung Cancer TNM Staging Classification (5th Edition)

T-Primary Tumor

TX Primary tumor cannot be assessed, or tumor proven by the presence of malignant cells in sputum or bronchial washings but not visualized by imaging or bronchoscopy

T0 No evidence of primary tumor

Tis Carcinoma in situ

T1 Tumor 3 cm or less in greatest dimension, surrounded by lung or visceral pleura, without bronchoscopic evidence of invasion more proximal than the lobar bronchus (i.e., not in the main bronchus (Note 1)

T2 Tumor with any of the following features of size or extent:
   More than 3 cm in greatest dimension;
   Involves main bronchus, 2 cm or more distal to the carina;
   Invades visceral pleura;
   Associated with atelectasis or obstructive pneumonitis that extends to the hilar region but does not involve the entire lung

T3 Tumor of any size that directly invades any of the following: chest wall (including superior sulcus tumors), diaphragm, mediastinal pleura, parietal pericardium; or tumor in the mainbronchus less than 2 cm distal to the carina (Note 1) but without involvement of the carina; or associated atelectasis or obstructive pneumonitis of the entire lung

T4 Tumor of any size that invades any of the following: mediastinum, heart, great vessels, trachea, esophagus, vertebral body, carina; separate tumor nodule(s) in the same lobe; tumor with malignant pleural effusion (Note 2)

N-Regional Lymph Nodes

NX Regional lymph nodes cannot be assessed

N0 No regional lymph node metastasis

N1 Metastasis in ipsilateral peribronchial and/or ipsilateral hilar lymph nodes and intrapulmonary nodes, including involvement by direct extension

N2 Metastasis in ipsilateral mediastinal and/or subcarinal lymph node(s)

N3 Metastasis in contralateral mediastinal, contralateral hilar, ipsilateral or contralateral scalene, or supraclavicular lymph node(s)

M-Distant Metastasis

MX Distant metastasis cannot be assessed

M0 No distant metastasis

M1 Distant metastasis, includes separate tumor nodule(s) in a different lobe (ipsilateral or contralateral)

Notes:

1. The uncommon superficial spreading tumor of any size with its invasive component limited to the bronchial wall, which may extend proximal to the main bronchus, is also classified as T1.

2. Most pleural effusions with lung cancer are due to tumor. In a few patients, however, multiple cytopathological examinations of pleural fluid are negative for tumor, and the fluid is nonbloody and is not an exudate. Where these elements and clinical judgment dictate that the effusion is not related to the tumor, the effusion should be excluded as a staging element and the patient should be classified as T1, T2, or T3

(continued)

TABLE 19.3. Lung Cancer TNM Staging Classification (5th Edition) (continued)

3. Separate tumor nodule(s) in the same lobe is categorized as T4 and synchronous separate tumor nodule(s) in a different lobe (ipsilateral or contralateral) is categorized as M1.

pTNM Pathological Classification

The pT, pN, pM categories correspond to the T, N, and M categories.

pN0: Histological examination of hilar and mediastinal lymphadenectomy specimen(s) will ordinarily include six or more lymph nodes.

of the overall clinical reality. To provide perspective, an overview of treatments and results may be considered (Table 19.5). The survival rates, although approximate, represent the current prognosis by stage when all patients are considered and a reasonably wide range of modern treatments is available. It must be noted that the full spectrum of treatment options may not be available for all patients. In such circumstances single-modality therapy with palliative intent may be all that is possible to offer them.

STAGING SYSTEM FOR LUNG CANCER AND PROGNOSIS

The International Union against Cancer (UICC) staging system is based on anatomic routes of spread, and stage determination depends strongly on the type of diagnostic evaluations that are used. Staging classification does not determine treatment, but rather helps to assign prognosis to patients treated according to the standards and procedures that are current. In addition, staging assists in the comparison of treatment results between different centers. The current UICC and the identical American Joint

TABLE 19.4. Lung Cancer Stage Grouping (5th Edition TNM)

Occult carcinoma	TX	N0	M0
Stage 0	Tis	N0	M0
Stage IA	T1	N0	M0
Stage IB	T2	N0	M0
Stage IIA	T1	N1	M0
Stage IIB	T2	N1	M0
	T3	N0	M0
Stage IIIA	T1	N2	M0
	T2	N2	M0
	T3	N1, N2	M0
Stage IIIB	Any T	N3	M0
	T4	Any N	M0
Stage IV	Any T	Any N	M1

65-70%.
45-55%.
35-50%.

35%.

TABLE 19.5. Management and Survival in Lung Cancer

Stage	Cell Type	Principal Management	5-Year Survival (Approximate)
I	NSCLC	S (some R)	65%
	SCLC	C + R ± S	50%
II	NSCLC	S (some ± R, ± C)	40%
	SCLC	C + R	25%
IIIA	NSCLC	C + R ± S	30%
	SCLC	C + R	20%
IIIB	NSCLC	R ± C	15%
	SCLC	C + R	5%
IV	NSCLC	C or R or C + R	2%
	SCLC	C ± R	2%
Overall	NSCLC		10%
	SCLC		5%

S, Surgery; R, radiotherapy; C, chemotherapy.

Committee on Cancer (AJCC) criteria in lung cancer reflect the use of diagnostic techniques described previously, but their application across regions and nations is highly variable. The 1997 system reflects the importance of local invasion by tumor, and of nodal metastases in the patient's prognosis. Important changes include the recognition of T3 tumors as relatively favorable provided that there is no lymph node invasion. Approximate survival rates anticipated are given by stage of disease in Table 19.5.

PRINCIPLES OF MANAGEMENT BY STAGE OF DISEASE

Non-Small-Cell Lung Cancer

Stage I: Stage IA (T1N0M0) and Stage IB (T2N0M0)   Surgical resection is generally the choice of treatment, taking account of operability and the overall medical risk of the patient. The overall operative mortality is 3% to 4%, more for pneumonectomy and safer for lobectomy. Lesser resections, such as segmentectomy and wedge resection, carry less risk but a higher rate of recurrence. The postresection 5-year survival rate in patients with T1N0M0 lesions is approximately 65% to 70%.

In T2N0M0 cases, lobectomy is generally preferred for lesions within the lung parenchyma or those with invasion of the visceral pleura. Lesions crossing the major fissure generally require pneumonectomy. T2 tumors arising in the lobar bronchus orifice or invading to the main bronchus require sleeve lobectomy or pneumonectomy.

Radiation therapy is appropriate for the minority of patients with localized lung cancer who cannot undergo or will not accept surgery. Five-year survival rates of 15% to 25% reflect the fact that most are unfit for surgery.

Whether initial treatment is by surgery or radiation there is no established role for subsequent treatment such as chemotherapy.

Stage II: Stage IIA (T1N1M0) and Stage IIB (T2N1M0, T3N0M0) In principle a surgical operation is indicated for lesions even in the presence of lymph node metastases, provided a complete resection can be achieved. Curative operation is sometimes possible if lymph node disease is resected by systematic dissection of mediastinal nodes well beyond the involved ones. This may not be possible in the presence of multiple nodes and/or extracapsular invasion. There is no evidence to suggest that "debulking" surgery (incomplete resection) is beneficial. The 5-year survival rate is 45% to 55% in T2N0M0 cases and 35 to 50% in T2N1M0 cases respectively, following histologically confirmed complete resection. Given the frequent local recurrences and organ metastasis observed within these groups, some supplementary treatment may be considered. Postoperative irradiation may reduce the rate of mediastinal or local recurrence, while chemotherapy may reduce systemic relapse; however, neither strategy has been shown to significantly benefit overall survival in randomized trials.

A meta-analysis of eight randomized trials using cisplatin-based chemotherapy after surgery demonstrated a small incremental survival benefit associated with the chemotherapy. Therefore adjuvant treatment has a potential role, although the optimal patient group and drug protocol remains undefined.

The T3N0M0 group, because of its relatively favorable 5-year survival rate following resection, is now classified within stage II, according to the 1997 TNM classification. This group includes the superior sulcus tumor and its prognosis is the poorest of the IIB tumors. This presentation of lung cancer (Pancoast) is due to tumor located at the thoracic inlet. Preoperative radiation has been advocated with the goal of tumor size reduction and an increased resectability rate, but combined modality (chemoradiotherapy) regimens prior to attempted resection are under investigation and may prove more effective. Patients with T3N0M0 due to chest wall invasion are usually treated with tumor and chest wall resection; the 5-year survival rates reported are approximately 35% in these generally fit patients. In cases where the adequacy of surgical margins is suspect, postoperative irradiation should be considered.

A meta-analysis was performed of all nine available randomized trials of postoperative radiotherapy versus surgery alone for completely resected non-small-cell lung cancer. About two-thirds of the patients had stage I or II disease; there were 808 stage III patients analyzed. No patient group or subgroup was seen to benefit from postoperative radiotherapy in terms of overall survival or local recurrence-free survival. Indeed, radiotherapy was actually detrimental, especially in early-stage disease. This effect is almost certainly due to the adverse effect of irradiation on remaining normal lung tissue. Whether there is benefit for incompletely resected patients is not known. If postoperative radiotherapy is given in an effort to reduce the risk of local recurrence, the technique and dose should be chosen so as to avoid irradiating the remaining lung.

Stage III: Stage IIIA and IIIB In general patients are considered for both local and systemic components of therapy in light of their high risk of both types of relapse. The presence of nodal disease is associated with a much increased risk of distant spread and ultimate relapse. On the other hand, many patients have significant comorbid illness and cannot tolerate treatment by multiple modalities. Such patients should be offered treatment by palliative intent, minimizing associated morbidity.

Principles of surgical selection and technique stage III tumors are much discussed but general consensus has not been reached. In T3 disease, pneumonectomy may be required to resect the tumor mass completely but is appropriate only for patients with adequate pulmonary reserve. Bronchial sleeve resection in selected T3 patients is an effective method for pulmonary preservation, with mortality and survival rates comparable to those following pneumonectomy. The prognosis appears to be directly related to the extent of the N category. Surgery can sometimes be considered in T4 cases, but is of doubtful value if mediastinal nodes are involved. Surgery is usually appropriate only for highly selected T4 patients with tumors confined to the carina, or tracheobronchial angle; in such cases, carinal resection with lobectomy or sleeve pneumonectomy may be performed.

The ultimate value of surgical resection is greatly diminished by the fact that nearly half of all patients with non-small-cell lung cancer have mediastinal lymph node involvement. The locations of each lymph node are identified with reference to the lymph node map (Fig. 19.2) to determine the N status. Prognosis can differ depending on the nature of involvement. Generally prognosis is less favorable when nodes are multiple rather than single; extranodal rather than intranodal; and distal rather than proximal to the primary tumor (with respect to lymphatic drainage pathways). Extensive surgical procedures, usually lobectomy or pneumonectomy with complete mediastinal lymph node dissection, may produce 5-year survival rates of 20% to 30% in select series. Some groups advocate preoperative chemotherapy but this experience is based on very small studies.

Radiotherapy as the sole modality is also limited by its inability to control systemic disease and the large population of clonogenic cells in bulky primary and nodal masses. Survival rates at 5 years may range from 5% to 20% but these results also depend on selection of patients, who usually are unfit for surgery. Newer approaches attempt to select smaller tumors, and employ modern three-dimensional shaped planning techniques, to escalate the dose delivered to the tumor without irradiating excessively the nearby normal tissues.

Combined modality regimens adopt one of two strategies for stage III disease. Adjunctive therapies are administered following some form of local therapy. An example would be mediastinal radiotherapy and/or several cycles of chemotherapy administered after complete or incomplete resection. The second associates the systemic therapy with the local one, according to a particular timing schema. The idea is to address multiple, possibly conflicting requirements, including the need to control cells resistant to one modality that might be controlled by multiple non-cross-resistant agents, the tendency for therapy to stimulate repopulation in surviving cells, the presence of occult systemic disease, and the problem of overlapping toxicities. Various timing protocols have been tried including prior chemotherapy (induction or neoadjuvant), concurrent chemoradiotherapy, or schemas in which chemo- and radiotherapy are interdigitated or "alternated."

Most available results from randomized trials concern patients with favorable prognostic factors (good performance status, minimal weight loss) and IIIA disease. The meta-analysis demonstrated a modest (2% at 5 years) increase in survival when cisplatin-based chemotherapy was associated with a high-dose radiotherapy proto-col. The optimal timing of therapies is not known. The encouraging survival results of the influential CALGB trial of using induction chemotherapy prior to thoracic ir-radiation were not supported in a confirmatory trial; testing of the same regimen with concurrent timing is in progress (1998).

Important advances in radiotherapy have established the biologic and clinical im-portance of the dose per fraction (on normal tissue effects), and the overall duration of therapy (on induced tumor repopulation). A British trial treating three times daily over 12 days showed a 2-year survival advantage of 30% vs. 20% and an even larger effect in this squamous cell subgroup. This result is significant compared to survival benefits attributable to chemotherapy, and has influenced practice and encouraged ongoing testing of altered fractionation regimens.

Technical advances in radiotherapy imaging, planning, and delivery now permit more precise targeting of intrathoracic tumors and sparing of critical normal tissues (lung, cord) using computerized three-dimensional shaped (conformational) tech-niques.

The new century is likely to see steady progress in the application of new and established therapies, refined together with newer selection techniques (biomarkers, predictive assays, etc.) to supplement the anatomical TNM system.

Small-Cell Lung Cancer

The mainstay of treatment for small-cell lung cancer (SCLC) is systemic combi-nation chemotherapy, which unquestionably prolongs survival, improves symptoms, and dramatically reduces tumor bulk in the majority of previously untreated cases. Chemotherapy alone, however, is rarely curative, with usual remission duration of less than a year, because of drug resistance. While the staging procedures for small-cell carcinoma do not differ appreciably from those for other forms of lung cancer, for practical purposes the TNM stages are usually collapsed into a simple binary classification. There is no role for exclusive radiation and/or surgery in patients with extensive disease (ED)-SCLC, which has already spread beyond the hemithorax, mediastinum, and supraclavicular nodes. The limited disease (LD)-SCLC patients, whose disease is confined within these limits, are best treated with combination of systemic chemotherapy and thoracic radiotherapy, unless complicated by malignant effusion.

The role of surgery in the treatment of LD-SCLC is not established. Stage I patients (rare) are usually treated by surgical resection of the tumor followed by adjuvant chemotherapy of four to six courses, but its superiority to initial chemo-therapy followed by surgery or chemoradiotherapy remains unproven. In stage II or III patients, surgical resection of tumor after induction chemotherapy has been shown to offer no additional benefit compared to thoracic radiotherapy in a randomized trial.

Surgical salvage of the residual tumor after chemoradiotherapy might be beneficial in selected patients, but it is doubtful whether its merit surpasses its risk.

Thoracic irradiation associated with chemotherapy in limited disease improves both local control and overall survival according to multiple randomized trials and two meta-analyses. The dose of the thoracic radiotherapy should be at least 40 to 45 Gy. The clinical benefit of further dose escalation is not yet proven. Twice-daily radiotherapy of 1.5 Gy b.i.d. to 45 Gy/30 fractions/3 weeks appears to be superior to once-a-day 1.8 Gy to a total of 45 Gy/25 fractions/5 weeks in an American Intergroup randomized trial. However, this accelerated hyperfractionated schedule has never been compared to a standard (once-a-day) regimen with reduced toxicity.

The current chemotherapy standard includes cisplatin/etoposide (PE), carboplatin/etoposide, cyclophosphamide/doxorubicin/etoposide (CAE), alternation of PE with cyclophosphamide/doxorubicin/vincristine (CAV), each for four to six cycles. Schedules containing platinum derivatives seem to be superior, especially combined with thoracic radiotherapy in LD cases.

The optimal timing of combining chemo- and radiotherapy in LD-SCLC remains controversial. Recent controlled trials have suggested that early concurrent combination, in which thoracic radiotherapy is given with the first or the second chemotherapy course, yields the most favorable results. It appears to be superior to other treatment schedules, such as alternating chemoradiotherapy or chemotherapy sequentially followed by radiation, although it also is more toxic to esophagus or bone marrow.

Prophylactic cranial irradiation (PCI) is shown to decrease the frequency of, or at least delay the emergence of, brain metastases. Its contribution to overall survival in SCLC patients is unclear, but is supported by a recent meta-analysis. At present, it is indicated only in LD patients who achieved CR or near CR after induction therapy. The recommended dose is 30 Gy/15 fractions or equivalent, but should be less than 3 Gy per fraction to minimize late toxicity. It is best administered shortly after the induction therapy. Concurrent chemotherapy with PCI should be avoided because of potential toxicity.

PALLIATIVE THERAPY IN LUNG CANCER

For the many lung cancer patients who will relapse eventually, the availability of effective relief of cancer-induced symptoms is essential. Occasionally there are surgical methods (e.g., orthopedic procedures for pathologic fractures or relief of visceral obstruction), but more commonly local palliation is given by radiotherapy. Patients usually respond to simple short courses of radiotherapy delivered in 1 to 10 fractions, usually with very little morbidity. Common symptoms treated are hemoptysis; pain; cough; dyspnea due to airway obstruction and collapse; and visceral metastases in brain, bone, and soft tissue.

Randomized trials have demonstrated the effectiveness of short courses (one to three fractions, using relatively large fraction sizes (3 to 10 Gy). Although these regimens do not usually eradicate the tumors, they provide symptomatic relief in most circumstances (30% to 70% depending on the clinical syndrome). This benefit is usually quite durable in the context of the typical short survival experience of these relapsed patients. Short regimens offer many conveniences to the patient, and in almost all randomized trials have proven to be at least as effective as protracted ones. Current research aims to optimize response and quality of life outcomes.

Severe or emergency complications of lung cancer include superior vena cava obstruction and spinal cord compression. These are relatively common and can be devastating unless treated promptly by radiotherapy.

Systemic chemotherapy can provide useful palliation, especially for patients with systemic symptoms and visceral disease. Modern agents ameliorate greatly the classic adverse effects such as nausea, vomiting, and infection. Therapy for relapse is generally limited to investigational agents with radiotherapy for localized symptomatic disease.

REHABILITATION

The goals of posttreatment rehabilitation are to prevent complications, improve respiratory function, reduce physical and mental pain, and assist the patient's readjustment to the community. The impact of all three treatment modalities must be addressed.

In patients undergoing surgery, control of postoperative pain is essential to maintain thoracic movement and pulmonary expansion. Important techniques besides the use of analgesics include muscle relaxation and psychological support. Measures to improve lung function include early mobilization from bed; deep breathing exercises, preferably in an upright position; and activities to increase expectoration. Bronchoscopic suction may be required to prevent retention of mucous secretions and stasis pneumonia. Major chronic postoperative complications must sometimes be managed, such as bronchopleural fistula, or empyema requiring chronic drainage.

While rehabilitation may not be a major concern after palliative radiotherapy using low to moderate doses, the aftercare of the patient treated with high-dose thoracic irradiation is concerned with maintaining function of the irradiated organs. Skin reactions are rarely troublesome but symptomatic esophagitis must be managed both during and for a few weeks after treatment, particularly if associated with chemotherapy. Lung tissue within the irradiated volume will be subject to an inflammatory reaction and slowly progressive fibrotic changes resulting in loss of some function, in normal as well as in diseased lung. Exercise, mobilization, prompt treatment of infection, and counseling will help the patient adapt to these changes. Uncommonly, patients may develop a symptomatic pneumonitis outside of the limits of the irradiated volume, attributed to an immune response to radiation-induced humoral factors. It requires management with corticosteroids and other measures.

Protracted chemotherapy regimens can be debilitating and may exacerbate the adverse effects of radiation and surgery. However, with careful monitoring of blood and organ function, and the use of supportive agents (modern antiemetics, hematopoietics, etc.) major problems are uncommon. Drug protocols in general use take account of the particular organ sensitivities (hepatic, renal, cardiac, etc.) with dose precautions and criteria for dose adjustment.

Modern approaches seek to optimize the quality of life of patients by finding a balance between the effects of a debilitating and usually lethal disease, and the noxious impact of treatment on normal tissues. Many unresolved questions remain in this field.

FOLLOW-UP FOR LOCAL, REGIONAL, OR DISTANT RECURRENCE

Unfortunately the majority of patients treated for lung cancer will experience a recurrence of their tumor, either locally, in the regional lymph nodes, or in distant organs. Relapses frequently occur at multiple sites. Very few of these clinical events are curable. In essence, the goal will usually be to determine the metastatic nature of the problem, and treat it with palliative intent and minimal treatment related morbidity.

The goals of follow-up may be listed as follows:

1. Early recognition of potentially curable situations (e.g., small localized stump recurrence, early "second primary" lung cancer);
2. Distinguishing genuine metastatic events from other conditions that might simulate them, resulting in either palliative treatment or reassurance to the patient. Examples include skeletal or nerve pain of various causes, and lobar collapse associated with radiation fibrosis or tumor recurrence;
3. Review and reporting of clinical outcomes.

Local recurrences are relatively infrequent when patients are carefully selected and completely resected with generous margins. However, they may arise at the bronchial stump, pleura, drain track, or thoracotomy scar. Mediastinal relapses are more serious and are associated with a high risk of distant metastasis. Both are usually treated with radiotherapy, especially if not previously irradiated.

In nonresected patients local control remains a major problem. Even with modern chemoradiotherapy regimens, long-term control of the primary tumor occurs in only 15% to 20%, taking account of the fact that many patients die of distant disease before the local relapse becomes clinically evident.

Distant organs that are frequently the target of symptomatic metastases are the brain, skeleton, liver, and lungs. There is little variation in the frequency and distribution of metastases among the histological subtypes. However, a degree of organ selectivity has been noted in some series, such as a higher frequency of brain metastases in small-cell and adenocarcinomas. Some controversy exists over the management of the patient with a metastasis determined to be "solitary" after a thorough search for other lesions. Such situations in which the rigors of therapy with curative intent may be justified are quite rare. Autopsy series reveal a pattern of widespread invasion of many other tissues, which may remain clinically silent during life, except insofar as they contribute to the general deterioration of the patient.

Considering that most lung cancer patients will relapse, follow-up should generally be the responsibility of the general physician with specialist support based on the treatment given, the sites of most likely or actual relapse, or anticipated complications. Similarly, frequency of follow-up will depend on the clinical situation, although usually four times per year for the first 2 years following definitive therapy.

PREVENTION

Because interventions are not yet possible at the level of the cellular events involved in lung cancer induction, prevention efforts must focus on the elimination of modifiable risk factors. These include environmental and workplace air pollution, but the overwhelmingly significant and well documented risk factor is the inhalation of tobacco products. Lung cancer is very rare in nonsmokers, and even a modest reduction in rates of tobacco smoking would result in the prevention of a substantial number of cancers.

BIBLIOGRAPHY

Parkin DM, Saxo AJ (1993) Lung cancer: Worldwide variation in occurrence and proportion attributable to tobacco use. *Lung Cancer* 9 (Suppl):1–16.

Schottenfeld M (1996) Epidemiology of lung cancer. In: Pass HI, Mitchell JB, Johnson DH, et al. (Eds.) *Lung Cancer: Principles and Practice*. Lippincott-Raven, Philadelphia/New York, pp. 305–22.

The Alpha-Tocopherol, Beta Carotene Cancer Prevention Study Group (1994) The effect of vitamin E and beta carotene on the incidence of lung cancer and other cancers in male smokers. *N Engl J Med* 330:1029.

National Cancer Institute Cooperative Early Lung Cancer Detection Program (1984) Summary and conclusions. *Am Rev Respir Dis* 130:565–567.

Shaw GL, Mulshine JL (1996) General strategies for early detection: new ideas and future directions. In: Pass HI, Mitchell JB, Johnson DH, et al. (Eds.) *Lung Cancer: Principles and Practice*. Lippincott-Raven, Philadelphia/New York, pp. 329–40.

Stahel RA (1991) Diagnosis, staging and prognostic factors of small cell lung cancer. *Curr Opin Oncol* 3:306.

American Society of Clinical Oncology (1997) Clinical practice guidelines for the treatment of unresectable non-small-cell lung cancer. *J Clin Oncol* 15:2996.

Naruke T, Goya T, Tsuchiya R, et al (1988) Prognosis and survival in resected lung carcinoma based on the new international staging system. *J Thorac Cardiovasc Surg* 96:440–447.

Sibley, GS (1998) Radiotherapy for patients with medically inoperable stage I non small cell lung carcinoma. *Cancer* 82:433–438.

Non-small Cell Lung Cancer Collaborative Group (1995) Chemotherapy in non-small-cell lung cancer: A meta-analysis using updated data on individual patients from 52 randomised clinical trials. *Br Med J* 311:899–909.

PORT Meta-analysis Trialists Group (1998) Postoperative radiotherapy in non-small-cell lung cancer: a systematic review and meta-analysis of individual patient data from nine randomised controlled trials. *Lancet* 352:257–263.

Goss G, Paszat L, Newman TE, Evans WK, Browman G, and the Provincial Lung Cancer Disease Site Group (1998) Use of preoperative chemotherapy with or without postoperative radiotherapy in technically resectable stage IIIA non-small-cell lung cancer. *Cancer Prevent Control* 2:32–39.

Dillman RO, Seagren SL, Propert KJ, Guerra J, Eaton WL, Perry MC, Carey, RW, Frei, EF, Green, MR (1990) A randomized trial of induction chemotherapy plus high-dose radiation versus radiation alone in stage III non-small-cell lung cancer. *N Engl J Med* 323:940–5.

Okawara G, Rusthoven J, Newman T, Findlay B, Evans W, and the Provincial Lung Cancer Disease Site Group (1997) Unresected stage III non-small-cell lung cancer. *Cancer Prevent Control* 1:249–259.

Ihde DC, Ed (1995) Current perspectives in the treatment of small cell lung cancer. *Lung Cancer* 12 (Suppl 3):S1–S95.

Friedland DM, Comis RL (1995) Perioperative therapy of non-small-cell lung cancer: A review of adjuvant and neoadjuvant approaches. *Semin Oncol* 22:571.

Pignon J.P., Arriagada R., Ihde D.C., et al. (1992) A meta-analysis of thoracic radiotherapy for small cell lung carcinoma. *N Engl J Med* 327:1618–1624.

Medical Research Council Lung Cancer Working Party and Macbeth FR, Bolger JJ, Hopwood P, Bleehen NM, Cartmell J, Girling DJ, Machin D, Stephen RJ, Bailey AJ (1996) Randomized trial of palliative two-fraction versus more intensive 13-fraction radiotherapy for patients with inoperable non-small-cell lung cancer and good performance status. *Clin Oncol* 8:167–175.

Medical Research Council Lung Cancer Working Party and Bleehen NM, Girling DJ, Machin D, Stephens RJ (1992) A Medical Research Council (MRC) randomised trial of palliative radiotherapy with two fractions or a single fraction in patients with inoperable non-small-cell lung cancer (NSCLC) and poor performance status. *Br J Cancer* 65:934–941.

Medical Research Council Lung Cancer Working Party. Inoperable non-small-cell lung cancer (NSCLC) (1991) a Medical Research Council randomised trial of palliative radiotherapy with two fractions or ten fractions. *Br J Cancer* 63:265–270.

Saunders M, Dische S, Barrett A, Harvey A, Gibson D, Parmar M, CHART Steering Committee (1997) Continuous hyperfractionated accelerated radiotherapy (CHART) versus conventional radiotherapy in non-small-cell lung cancer: a randomised multicentre trial. *Lancet* 350:161–165.

CHAPTER 20

LIVER CANCER

ZHAO-YOU TANG

Liver Cancer Institute
Zhongshan Hospital
Shanghai Medical University
Shanghai 200032, P.R. China

Hepatocellular carcinoma (HCC) is one of the most frequent malignancies in Southeast Asia and Africa. Owing to the difficulties in early detection and effective treatment, HCC has long been regarded as a hopeless disease. Fortunately, the identification of hepatitis B virus as an important background of HCC, and the detection of subclinical HCC using α-fetoprotein (AFP) and/or ultrasonography screening, have provided important clues to the primary and secondary prevention of HCC. The rapid development of medical imaging procedures, regional cancer therapies, and hepatic surgery have also gradually altered the outcome of HCC. Studies on the molecular biology of HCC have potential clinical implications, particularly in the control of recurrence and metastasis.

EPIDEMIOLOGY AND ETIOLOGY

Parkin et al. (1993) [1] reported that the number of new liver cancer patients globally in 1985 was 315,000; the age-standardized incidence rate was 11.0/100,000 in males and 4.5/100,000 in females, and ranked third in developing countries. However, the global ranking in cancer mortality was seventh in males and ninth in females. HCC was prevalent in Southeast Asia and sub-Saharan Africa. Mozambique, Zimbabwe, Uganda, Malaysia, Indonesia, Singapore, Thailand, Philippines, China, and Japan were among the high-incidence areas. Low-incidence areas included the United States (excluding Alaska), Canada, northern Europe, and Australia. A trend of

Manual of Clinical Oncology, 7th edition, Edited by Raphael E. Pollock
ISBN 0-471-23828-7, pages 407–424. Copyright © 1999 Wiley-Liss, Inc.

increasing incidence was observed in Japan, France, Italy, etc. Of the 315,000 new incidences of liver cancer in 1985, 137,500 (43.7%) occurred in China. In China, HCC has become the second largest cause of mortality from cancer since the 1990s, with a death rate of 20.40/100,000.

The peak age at onset of HCC was around 30 to 39 years in Africa, 45 to 54 in China, 50 to 59 in Japan, and 55 to 64 in the United States. Generally HCC is more predominant in males than in females; however, the male:female ratio is usually greater in high prevalence areas, such as in China, where it was 3:1.

The major etiologic factors of HCC varied in different geographic areas, and included the following: (1) Viral hepatitis infection and cirrhosis. In Southeast Asia, hepatitis B virus (HBV) infection was more common as compared with hepatitis C virus (HCV) infection. In China, around 90% of HCC patients had an HBV infection background, and only 10% to 30% HCV infection, whereas in Japan, France and Italy, HCV-related HCC accounted for around 60% to 80%. The relative risk of HCC in HBV carriers was reported to be 10 to 100 times higher than that of non-HBV carriers. The X gene of HBV was thought important in hepatocarcinogenesis. In high prevalence areas, cirrhosis accounted for around 60% to 80% of the HCC background, of which most are posthepatitic (B or C) cirrhosis, especially the macronodular type. (2) Chemical carcinogens, particularly the intake of aflatoxin B_1 (AFB_1)-containing food, such as peanuts and corn. Epidemiologic data revealed a strong correlation between HCC mortality and intake of AFB_1, and AFB_1 has been proved a strong hepatocarcinogen in experimental animals. (3) Contamination of drinking water. In rural areas of China where HCC is endemic, a strong correlation was found between HCC mortality and contamination of drinking water. People drinking pond-ditch water had a much higher HCC mortality rate than people drinking deep well water. Recently, microcystin was found in the pond-ditch water, and verified to be a strong promoter of hepatocarcinogenesis. (4) Alcohol, smoking, genetics, and other factors. It is estimated that only 15% of HCC cases in North America are attributable to alcohol use, and 12% or less to cigarette smoking. Hemochromatosis and Budd–Chiari syndrome (membranous obstruction of the inferior vena cava) have also been reported as risk factors for HCC. HBV/HCV (particularly the B type), aflatoxin intake, and contamination (such as microcystin) of drinking water in rural areas were the three most common causative factors of HCC in China. A synergistic effect was found among HBV/HCV, AFB_1, and contamination of drinking water epidemiologically and experimentally.

SCREENING

A screening program for early detection of HCC has been in debate for decades. In China, screening a high-risk population using AFP serosurvey and/or ultrasonography (US) has led to detection of resectable subclinical small ($\leq$5S cm) HCC. The 5-year survival associated with small HCC resection was double that with large HCC resection, being 64.9% ($n = 735$) vs. 37.4% ($n = 1050$), and resulted in a large number of long-term HCC survivors. Recently a prospective study of early detection has been conducted in Shanghai urban residents aged 35 to 55 years and with serum evidence of HBV infection or chronic liver disease. The randomized controlled study included a screening group ($n = 8109$) and a control ($n = 9711$). Subjects in the screening group were tested with serum AFP and US every 6 months, and HCC patients detected were treated adequately. Comparison between screening and control groups revealed that the number of HCC patients detected was $n = 50$ vs. 31, subclinical stage HCC being 80.0% vs. 0%, small HCC $n = 22$ vs. 0; resection 80.0% vs. 12.9%; 1-year survival 81.6% vs. 29.6%, 3-year survival 73.7% vs. 0%. The lead time was estimated at 0.45 years. The cost of detecting HCC at the subclinical stage was RMB 12,600 (US \$1500). The detection rate per 100,000 was 616.6 for 3 years, suggesting that screening HBV carriers in China using AFP and US is of value to detect HCC at an early stage, to increase resection rate and to prolong survival with acceptable cost-effectiveness. One of the key points is adequate and effective treatment of patients detected. A similar result was reported in Alaskan Native screening. Instead of AFP and US, only US was used for screening in areas where AFP positivity was low in patients with HCC.

PATHOLOGY AND MOLECULAR BIOLOGY

Gross classifications of HCC have been advocated by several authors: the traditional Eggel's (1901) [2] classification included massive, nodular, and diffuse types; Okuda (1984) [3] divided it into expanding, spreading, multifocal, and indeterminate types; Nakashima and Kojiro (1987) [4] classified it as expansive, infiltrative, mixed infiltrative and expansive, and diffuse types. Gross types differed among geographic areas; the expanding type is common in Oriental patients, whereas the infiltrative type is seen more frequently in the United States.

Histologically, HCC was defined as: "A malignant tumor composed of cells resembling hepatocyte but abnormal in appearance. A platelike organization around sinusoids is common and nearly always present somewhere in the tumor" (Ishak, Anthony and Sobin 1994).[5] For differentiation, Edmondson and Steiner (1954) [6] proposed HCC be graded from I to IV. Cells with different gradings could be found in one HCC nodule. Changes were also found with progress of HCC from early to advanced stages, such as from grade I or II to III or IV, from more diploid to more aneuploid cells, from well encapsulated to poorly encapsulated, from single nodule to multiple nodules. HCC is hypervascular in the majority of cases; arterioportal shunt is frequently found in large tumors. Tumor thrombi are also common in the portal and hepatic veins, which leads to intrahepatic and distant metastases. Fibrolamellar HCC, a variant of HCC more frequent in the West, is abundant with fibrous stroma arranged in parallel lamellae; tumor cells are large and polygonal with granular cytoplasm; and prognosis is better than for classic HCC.

Several methods have been employed for studies on the cellular origin of HCC: (1) Integration of hepatitis B virus DNA was determined. (2) The loss of a heterozygosity (LOH) pattern on chromosome 16 was claimed useful in diagnosis of multifocal HCC. (3) A *p53* loss of heterozygosity or *p53* genotype has also been employed to identify the clonal origin of recurrent HCC. Most of these approaches indicated that both a unicentric and a multicentric origin existed in multiple nodules as well as recurrent HCC.

In most HCC cases associated with cirrhosis, the posthepatitic type accounted for the majority; the macronodular type (with cirrhotic nodule >3 cm) was predominant. Adenomatous hyperplasia has been identified as a precancerous lesion.

Early in 1984, N-*ras* was found overexpressed in HCC; later a spectrum of proto-oncogenes, oncogenes, and growth factors was verified with relation to hepatocar-cinogenesis, such as N-*ras*, c-*myc*, insulin growth factor II (IGF-II), c-*ets*-2, *p53*, etc. In 1994, Tabor summarized molecular events in HBV-related HCC: *p53* mutation was found in 30% to 50%, positivity of Rb was 20% to 25% (in patients with *p53* mutation, the positivity of Rb was 80% to 86%), overexpression was also found in transforming growth factor-α (TGF-α), IGF-II, N-*ras*, c-*myc*, c-*fos*, etc., which might be helpful in explaining hepatocarcinogenesis involved by HBV.

DIAGNOSIS

Clinical Findings

In patients with subclinical HCC detected by screening, usually no symptom or sign exists. In clinical patients, the first complaint is usually pain or palpable mass in the upper abdomen (in the right upper quadrant or epigastric region depending on tumor site). Radiating pain to the right shoulder is common when the tumor is located in the upper part of the right lobe. Acute pain is encountered when rupture of the tumor nodule occurs; subcapsular rupture of HCC nodule in the right lobe is often misdiagnosed as gallbladder disease or appendicitis. Most of the symptoms are nonspecific, originating from HCC or the coexisting hepatitis and cirrhosis, and include hepatomegaly, fullness, decreased appetite, weakness, weight loss, and lower extremity edema. Unexplained fever or diarrhea is often the first complaint of patient with HCC. Jaundice and ascites usually appear in advanced stages. Variceal bleeding is also encountered.

Physical signs include hepatomegaly with or without nodule, splenomegaly, elevated right diaphragm, jaundice, and ascites. Ascites with tension usually indicates thrombus in the portal vein. Reddish liver palm is found in patients with coexisting advanced cirrhosis.

Paraneoplastic syndromes such as erythrocytosis present in 10% of patients, probably as a result of the HCC cell secreting erythropoietin. Hypoglycemia also presents in 10%, especially in patients with large tumors. Coexisting diabetes seems to have been increasing recently.

Metastases in lung, bone, lymph nodes, brain, adrenal gland, or other organs, occur mostly in advanced disease, presenting corresponding symptoms and signs.

Complications include rupture of the HCC nodule, gastrointestinal bleeding, liver dysfunction and liver failure, infection, ascites, right pleural effusion, pulmonary infarct due to tumor thrombus, among others.

Based on the study of subclinical HCC, the concept of natural history of HCC has been renewed. The 1-, 3-, and 5-year survival rates associated with small HCC treated conservatively were reported to be 72.7%, 13.6%, and 0%, respectively. The natural course of HCC was estimated as at least 2 years.

Laboratory Findings

AFP is so far the best tumor marker for HCC. A serum AFP level >20 μg/liter is found in 60% to 70% of HCC patients in the Far East. Although an AFP level >500 μg/liter is acknowledged to be diagnostic, it is recommended that HCC diagnosis be considered and ultrasonography checked when AFP level <500 μg/liter but >20 μg/liter, particularly when the serial change of AFP level is not consistent with serum alanine transaminase (ALT or SGPT) or other liver function tests. An AFP variant is helpful for differential diagnosis between benign and malignant liver diseases. The des-γ-carboxy prothrombin (DCP) test may help in diagnosing AFP-nonproducing HCC.

Liver function tests are needed both for diagnosis and selection of treatment modality. Bilirubin, albumin level and albumin/globulin (A/G) ratio, and prothrombin time are important parameters for surgery. A high γ-glutamyl transpeptidase (GGT) level is usually associated with poor prognosis. Postoperative hepatitic status with high ALT increases risk of recurrence.

Serum HBV and HCV markers are important diagnostic aids for HCC, and are very helpful for differential diagnosis between HCC and other benign/malignant space-occupying lesions in the liver where HBV/HCV are prevalent.

Thrombocytopenia due to hypersplenism is common.

Immunostatus is progressively depressed with advanced disease. However, it is normal in patients with small HCC.

Imaging

The rapid progress of medical imaging procedures has greatly improved HCC diagnosis, localization, as well as effective treatment.

Ultrasonography (US) is the most commonly used noninvasive procedure; a lesion as small as 1 cm can be detected. A hypoechoic space-occupying lesion (SOL) with a halo is the common picture for small HCC. In large HCC, either hyperechoic, isoechoic, or mixed hyper- and hypoechoic lesions are found, and a capsule usually exists. Satellite nodules surrounding the major nodule are often encountered. Tumor thrombus in portal vein, hepatic vein, or inferior vena cava; tumor invasion to the biliary tree; collateral circulation of portal hypertension; and lymph node involvement can also be observed. Color Doppler US can help to identify the vascularity of the lesion. An arterial blood supply is often found in HCC, but usually not in hemangioma. Preoperative US by the surgeon is extremely helpful to select treatment modality as well as to guide surgery. Intraoperative US can help to find deeply seated HCC lesion, as well as to guide the surgical approach, judge the extent of resection, and avoid injury of important vessels and ducts. US can also guide biopsy.

Computed tomography (CT) has been a routine imaging procedure for HCC, providing a more complete picture to the physician. Low-density SOL is a common picture for HCC, and a more clear demarcation found after injection of contrast medium. Spiral CT shows accumulation of contrast medium in the arterial phase, and becomes a low-density area thereafter, which is helpful for differential diagnosis between small HCC and hemangioma. Lipiodol CT can detect HCC as small as 0.5 cm. A strong accumulation of Lipiodol in the SOL is observed after 1 to 2 weeks, which is of both diagnostic and therapeutic value.

Magnetic resonance imaging (MRI) is similar to CT but no-irradiation, three-dimensional imaging can be obtained. The resolution capacity for soft tissue is superior to that of CT, and is good for differential diagnosis between small HCC and hemangioma.

Nuclide imaging is less sensitive. Blood pool scanning remains useful for differentiating between HCC and hemangioma; a strong uptake is usually found in hemangioma. ^{99}Tc-PMT (N-pyridoxyl-5-methyltryptophan) scanning, a hepatobiliary imaging agent, is helpful for diagnosis of hepatic adenoma in the delayed phase. Positive imaging can be found in 60% of well and moderately differentiated HCC, and ^{99}Tc-PMT whole body scanning is of value in detecting a metastatic lesion from HCC. Radioimmunoimaging using radiolabeled specific monoclonal antibody to HCC may be of potential value both for diagnosis and treatment. The value of positron emission tomography (PET) has to be explored. PET using fluorine-18-fluorodeoxyglucose is useful in assessment of the therapeutic effect.

Arteriography remains useful despite its invasive nature. Tumor vessel and tumor stain are two major features for HCC. The combination of CT and arteriography (CTA), is a commonly used procedure; Lipiodol CT is particularly of both diagnostic and therapeutic value.

Laparoscopy and Needle Biopsy

Laparoscopy, an invasive procedure, is less useful because of the rapid progress of medical imaging. US-guided percutaneous fine-needle biopsy is useful when diagnosis is difficult; however, it is not suggested as a routine procedure.

DIFFERENTIAL DIAGNOSIS

When medical imaging shows a solid SOL in the liver, the following diseases should be excluded, and the important points are delineated: (1) Secondary liver cancer—with a history of original cancer, usually no HBV/HCV/cirrhosis background, AFP level ≤20 μg/liter (except for a few instances with liver metastasis from gastric or pancreatic cancer), multiple evenly distributed nodules. (2) Hemangioma—female predominance, usually no HBV/HCV/cirrhosis background, AFP level ≤20 μg/liter, no halo on US, filling of contrast medium beginning from the peripheral zone in CT, strong filling in blood pool scanning. (3) Hepatic adenoma—usually no HBV/HCV/cirrhosis background, with history of oral contraceptive use in some patients, AFP level ≤20 μg/liter, strong imaging in delayed phase of ^{99}mTc-PMT scanning. (4) Inflammatory pseudotumor—usually no HBV/HCV/cirrhosis background, AFP level ≤20 μg/liter, lobular and no halo on US, no arterial blood supply by color Doppler US, not contrasted in CT scan. (5) Focal nodular hyperplasia (FNH) and adenomatous hyperplasia (AH)—difficult to differentiate from small HCC, usually no HBV/HCV/cirrhosis background, AFP level ≤20 μg/liter, no halo on US, but sometimes arterial blood supply can be found, and contrasted in CT scan. (6) Sarcoma—usually no HBV/HCV/cirrhosis background, AFP level ≤20 μg/liter. (7) Liver abscess—usually no HBV/HCV/cirrhosis background, AFP level ≤20 μg/liter, difficult to differentiate when abscess has not yet liquefied.

STAGING

The UICC TNM classification (5th edition, 1997) for liver is summarized as follows. The T, N, and M categories are based on physical examination, imaging, and/or surgical exploration. pTNM pathologic classification corresponds to the T, N, and M categories.

T1   Solitary, ≤2 cm, without vascular invasion
T2   Solitary, ≤2 cm, with vascular invasion
     Multiple, one lobe, ≤2 cm, without vascular invasion
     Solitary, >2 cm, without vascular invasion
T3   Solitary, >2 cm, with vascular invasion
     Multiple, one lobe, ≤2 cm, with vascular invasion
     Multiple, one lobe, >2 cm, with or without vascular invasion
T4   Multiple, more than one lobe
     Invasion of major branch of portal or hepatic veins
     Perforation of visceral peritoneum
N1   Regional lymph node metastasis
M1   Distant metastasis

Stage grouping includes:

Stage I	T1	N0	M0
Stage II	T2	N0	M0
Stage IIIA	T3	N0	M0
Stage IIIB	T1	N1	M0
	T2	N1	M0
	T3	N1	M0
Stage IVA	T4	Any N	M0
Stage IV B	Any T	Any N	M1

Okuda proposed a staging system in 1985,[7] which includes: (1) tumor size: >50% of the liver area measured by CT (+), <50% (−); (2) ascites: (+) and (−);

(c) albumin: <3 g/dl (+) and >3 g/dl (−); and (4) bilirubin: >3 mg/dl (+) and <3 mg/dl (−).

Stage I: all (−)
Stage II: 1 or 2 (+)
Stage III: 3 or 4 (+)

In China, a clinical staging has been used since 1977, particularly for patients who did not receive surgical treatment:

Stage I (subclinical)   Without obvious HCC symptoms and signs
Stage II (moderate)   Between stages I and III
Stage III (late)   With jaundice, ascites, distant metastasis, or cachexia

TREATMENT

Treatment modalities that resulted in prolonging survival include large HCC resection (1950s), small HCC (≤5 cm) resection (1970s), regional cancer therapies (such as transcatheter arterial chemoembolization [TACE], percutaneous ethanol injection [PEI], etc.) (1980s). TACE has surpassed radiotherapy as the first choice of therapy for unresectable HCC. Liver transplantation has been demonstrated effective in treating small HCC. Systematic chemotherapy is less effective. Biotherapy provides hope as a future therapy.

Selection of treatment modality depends on: (1) Tumor status—TNM is the essential classification system, and includes tumor size, number of tumor nodules, involvement, vascular invasion, invasion of major branch of portal or hepatic veins, regional lymph node metastasis, and distant metastasis. Usually T1, T2, and part of T3 are candidates for surgery; part of T3 and T4 are indicated for TACE. (2) Liver function—compensated or noncompensated (high bilirubin, reversed A/G ratio, prolonged prothrombin time, etc.). The Child–Pugh classification is universally accepted. Usually Child A with localized HCC is a good indication for surgery, TACE can be considered with multiple HCC in Child A and part of Child B, and conservative treatment is the choice for Child C. Indocyanine green retention rate at 15 minutes (ICG-R15) is commonly used in Japan to guide indication for surgery as well as extent of resection. (3) General condition—age, cardiac and pulmonary function, coexisting diseases.

For small HCC with compensated liver function or Child A cirrhosis, resection is the first choice. Limited resection is suggested in a cirrhotic liver. For patients with contraindications to resection, regional therapies such as cryosurgery, microwave ablation, and ethanol injection can be chosen. In patients with small HCC and Child B cirrhosis, PEI or superselective TACE can be considered. However, in patients with noncompensated liver function or Child C cirrhosis, only conservative treatment is indicated.

For localized large HCC with compensated liver function or Child A cirrhosis, resection is the best choice. For unresectable localized HCC, cytoreduction and sequential resection is a good approach. Intraoperative hepatic artery cannulation combined with hepatic artery ligation (maintains the patency of the catheter) is effective for cytoreduction. Regional radiotherapy can be added.

For patients with multiple HCC, TACE is the best therapy. TACE can still be tried in individual patients who have tumor thrombus in the main portal vein. A small proportion of unresectable HCC can be converted to resectable if remarkable tumor shrinkage occurs. For HCC with Child C cirrhosis, only symptomatic treatment is indicated.

Surgery

Surgical resection provides the best outcome for patients with HCC. The advances in HCC surgery include: (1) Lobectomy of large HCC. Started in the 1950s, it has benefited 5% to 10% of HCC patients. The operative mortality has decreased from 20% to less than 5%, and 5-year survival increased from 10% to 30%. (2) Small HCC resection. In the 1970s, the application of AFP serosurvey in population screening resulted in early detection of resectable small HCC. The operative mortality was less than 2%, and 5-year survival 50% to 60%. (3) Reresection of subclinical recurrence—in the 1980s, based on periodic follow-up after curative resection using AFP and ultrasonography, subclinical recurrence can be detected, and reresection of subclinical recurrence has resulted in increased 5-year survival, 10% to 15% greater after curative resection of HCC. (3) Cytoreduction and sequential resection of localized unresectable HCC in cirrhotic liver. Advances in multimodality treatment, cytoreduction, and second-stage resection for initially unresectable HCC have provided a curable outcome in a small part of unresectable HCC. The 5-year survival after sequential resection was up to 60%. (4) Liver transplantation for HCC. Liver transplantation was proved superior to resection for small HCC in Western countries; the 5-year survival associated with small HCC (<4 cm) after liver transplantation was 57%. Palliative surgery other than resection, such as hepatic artery ligation/cannulation, cryosurgery, and microwave ablation, has also yielded an acceptable outcome. Recently, basic research in molecular biology has deepened, which is of potential value in further prolonging survival after surgery, particularly in the control of recurrence and metastasis. Based on a nationwide survey in Japan, the 5-year survival was 40.8% after resection, and 8.0% after transcatheter arterial chemoembolization.

Adequate preoperative preparation is extremely important. Preoperative ultrasonography performed by the chief surgeon is very helpful to guide the operative position and incision, estimate the distance between the tumor nodule and major vessels/ducts, and plan the extent of resection. Preoperative treatment is needed in patients with cirrhosis. Right subcostal incision with or without extension to the left subcostal region is commonly used. A strong retractor is very helpful for exposure. In recent years, it has not been necessary to open the chest for any kind of hepatic resection.

The extent of resection is one of the key issues in decreasing operative mortality. In patients without cirrhosis, segmentectomy, lobectomy, hemihepatectomy, or trisegmentectomy can be chosen depending on the extent of tumor. Up to 80% to

85% of the liver can be resected. However, in patients with cirrhosis, particularly of the macronodular type, limited resection, subsegmentectomy, or segmentectomy is the only choice. Intraoperative ultrasonography is extremely helpful during hepatic resection, especially for those with deeply located lesions. Minimizing blood loss is another key issue for hepatic resection. Techniques for this purpose include good exposure, fresh blood transfusion, step-by-step resection and ligation of intrahepatic vessels and ducts, and temporal occlusion of the hepatic hilum. The occlusion time should not exceed 15 minutes for cirrhosis and 10 minutes for severe cirrhosis. Repeated occlusion is needed for complicated operations. The cut end should be approximated by suture or covered by falciform ligament or omentum. Adequate drainage is also important.

With advances in managing patients with cirrhosis, operative mortality (death within 30 days) from HCC resection has decreased from 20% in the 1950s to 1960s to less than 5% in recent years, being less than 2% for small HCC resection. The important elements to a low operative mortality after HCC resection are careful selection of patients, adequate pre- and postoperative care, careful determination of the extent of resection in cirrhotic livers, adequate exposure, limited blood loss, short duration or without occlusion of the hepatic hilum, transfusion with fresh blood, and avoidance of unnecessary surgical procedures in severely cirrhotic livers.

Postoperative complications after HCC resection include the following. (1) Hepatic dysfunction remains the leading issue after major hepatic resection, or resection in a cirrhotic liver, or resection in patients with relatively poor liver function. High pulse rate, rapid increase of serum bilirubin, marked prolongation of prothrombin time, and early appearance of ascites are poor prognostic findings. Early aggressive treatment is important. (2) Postoperative bleeding has been less frequently encountered in recent years. Carefully closing the cut end is a key point. Prolonged prothrombin time and massive bleeding during operation are usually the background. (3) Bile leakage is more often encountered after resection of HCC in the hepatic hilum, and adequate drainage is the treatment of choice. (4) Subdiaphragmatic abscess was less common in recent years because of adequate drainage after resection, and is not difficult to control with ultrasound guided aspiration. (5) Pleural effusion often appeared in the right side after right lobe resection in a cirrhotic liver; aspiration is the treatment. (6) Ascites is common in patients with cirrhosis; albumin and diuretics are needed. (7) Varix or stress ulcer bleeding is also encountered.

In patients with unresectable HCC, hepatic artery ligation (HAL), hepatic artery cannulation with postoperative infusion chemotherapy (HAI), cryosurgery, or microwave ablation can produce significant reduction of tumor nodules. It has been demonstrated that the combination of HAL and HAI was superior to each alone. This combined treatment is performed by inserting a catheter with implanted injection port through the right gastric epiploic artery to the proper right or left hepatic artery according to the location of the tumor. The accuracy of catheterization should be verified by injection of methylene blue. HAL is done to occlude the arterial blood flow to the HCC-affected lobe, and HAL + HAI to occlude the arterial blood supply but maintain the patency of the inserted catheter. Chemotherapeutic agents commonly used are cisplatin, adriamycin (or epirubicin), 5-fluorouracil or flurodeoxyuridine, and mitomycin C. Hepatic artery embolization is done by injecting Lipiodol. Cryosurgery using $-196°C$ liquid nitrogen is performed using a cryoprobe inserted into the tumor for 15 to 20 minutes. If remarkable shrinkage of tumor appears, usually in a small part of localized unresectable HCC, sequential resection is suggested. With advances of regional and multimodality combination therapy, second-stage resection has appeared in recent years as a new approach for treatment of some localized unresectable HCC. Palliative resection with grossly identified residual cancer is not superior to palliative surgery other than resection.

Intrahepatic recurrence is frequently encountered after curative resection. The 5-year recurrence rate is around 60% to 70% after curative HCC resection, being 40% to 50% for curative small HCC resection. Therefore, follow-up using AFP and ultrasonography is suggested at an interval of 2 to 3 months for more than 5 years. This approach has proven effective in detecting subclinical recurrence, and reresection prolongs survival further or even provides another curable outcome. The 5-year survival calculated from the first resection was around 40% to 50%. Limited resection is the only resection type for reresection. Solitary pulmonary metastasis, particularly appearing a few years after the curative resection, is a good candidate for lung lobectomy, and results are very promising.

The results of total hepatectomy and liver transplantation for HCC were disappointing in the past 2 decades because of the high recurrence rate of HCC after the use of immunosuppressors. Until this decade, it was demonstrated that survival is negatively correlated with tumor size. The 5-year survival for single HCC <4 cm was 57%, whereas it was only 11% for HCC >8 cm. Current opinion in Western countries is that only in small HCC is the recurrent rate lower and the 5-year survival is higher in the liver transplantation group than in the resection group. Therefore, liver transplantation is indicated in TNM stage I and part of stage II tumors, confined to one lobe of the liver and without vascular invasion. In the developing countries where HCC is endemic, problems remain to be solved in this regard including the source of donor liver, the expenses, and the recurrence of HBV/HCV infection.

Transcatheter Arterial Chemoembolization

Transcatheter arterial embolization (TAE) or more commonly chemoembolization (TACE) using Seldinger's technique has become the first choice for treatment of unresectable HCC. Most of the HCC nodules are hypervascular, and TACE results in massive necrosis of the HCC nodule. However, most of the blood supply in the peripheral zone of the HCC nodule is from the portal vein; therefore TACE is inadequate as a curative procedure. Combination with percutaneous intrahepatic portal branch chemoembolization was claimed to add weight to TACE. Indications for TACE are patients with unresectable but not far advanced HCC (TNM stage II, IIIA, part of IIIB, and part of IVA), and acceptable liver function (Child A or Child B cirrhosis). Spontaneous rupture of an HCC nodule with internal bleeding is a good candidate for TACE treatment. Complete occlusion of the main portal vein by tumor thrombus is generally a contraindication to TACE. In patients with HCC confined in one side, superselective catheterization to the hepatic artery of the tumor side is suggested. For embolization, Lipiodol (an oily material) and gel-foam are the most commonly used agents. For chemotherapy, a combination of two or three of the following chemotherapeutic agents is routinely used: cisplatin, adriamycin or epirubicin, 5-fluorouracil or fluorodeoxyuridine, and mitomycin C. The procedure can be repeated at intervals of 1 to 3 months depending on the uptake of Lipiodol and recovery of liver function; usually three to six courses are needed to control the tumor. Good accumulation of Lipiodol in the tumor area indicates a good response. The common side effects of TACE include fever and pain. The disadvantages of using TACE include inadequacy of controlling tumor, the downstaging of Child–Pugh classification with increasing TACE courses, and possibly enhanced pulmonary metastasis. The 5-year survival after TACE ranged from 7% to 20%, with superselective TACE yielding better result. Prognostic factors include Lipiodol uptake, number of HCC nodules, and thrombus in the portal vein. The 5-year survival of patients who received sequential resection after marked shrinkage of unresectable tumor was as high as 50%. TACE is generally not indicated in patients with resectable HCC, and increased survival was not found for preoperative TACE in resectable HCC. However, postoperative TACE is helpful to reduce recurrent rate after curative resection. Combination of percutaneous ethanol injection was claimed to improve response. Superselective or segmental/subsegmental TACE is advocated in patients with localized unresectable small HCC.

Other Regional Cancer Therapies

Besides the previously mentioned regional therapies (hepatic artery ligation/cannulation, cryosurgery, microwave ablation) through surgery and TACE through nonsurgical approaches, in recent years, with advances in ultrasonography, ultrasound-guided percutaneous intralesional ethanol injection (PEI) has proved promising in treating small HCC, particularly in patients with contraindications to surgery. The long-term survival was just under that associated with surgical resection. It is important to repeat the procedure for around 10 times over an interval of about 3 to 7 days, and try to cover the entire HCC nodule. The coagulation effect of ethanol prevents further infiltration of ethanol to the peripheral area; therefore, PEI is usually inadequate to cover the entire tumor nodule in one injection. Large HCC is not a good candidate for PEI treatment. Acetic acid (15% to 50%) is an alternative to ethanol. Percutaneous microwave therapy is a new approach as regional cancer therapy for HCC.

Radiotherapy

Radiotherapy has been one of the treatment choices for unresectable HCC. Recently, TACE has surpassed radiotherapy as the first choice of treatment for unresectable HCC. In China, treatment of unresectable HCC using radiotherapy has resulted in acceptable palliation. Factors that favor better response include larger dosages of irradiation, smaller tumor size, and use in combination with Chinese herbs that can strengthen host immunity.

Other internal radiotherapies, such as radioimmunotherapy using ^{131}I-antiferritin, ^{131}I-anti-HCC monoclonal antibody, and ^{131}I-anti-AFP have been tried. Human antimurine antibody (HAMA) remains one of the problems, and humanized or chimeric antibody might be the solution. Intrahepatic–arterial ^{131}I-Lipiodol also yielded acceptable responses, and use of a ^{90}Y-microsphere and ^{32}P-microsphere was also reported.

Chemotherapy and Biotherapy

Chemotherapeutic agents commonly used for treatment of HCC include cisplatin, Adriamycin or epirubicin, 5-fluorouracil or fluorodeoxyuridine, and mitomycin C. Intrahepatic arterial infusion is effective in most of patients. Unfortunately, intravenous administration has been disappointing. The multidrug resistance gene product p-glycoprotein was found in up to 67.4% of HCC patients, which might explain the dismal outcome of systematic chemotherapy. The effect of Tamoxifen in the treatment of advanced HCC has not yet been established.

Biotherapy is considered the fourth therapy for cancer other than surgery and radio- and chemotherapy, and is particularly important in control of residual cancer. Instead of the old BRMs (biological response modifiers, such as Bacillus Calmette-Guerin [BCG], Coley toxin, OK432), interferon-α, interleukin-2 (IL-2), lymphokine activated killer (LAK)/IL-2, and tumor infiltrating lymphocyte (TIL) are commonly used preparations; however, the responses are not yet satisfactory.

Palliative care includes cancer pain control, diuretics, and supportive therapies.

COMPARISON BETWEEN SMALL HCC AND LARGE HCC

As had been reported in a large series, comparison between small HCC ($\leq$5 cm) and large HCC revealed higher limited resection rate (70.1% vs. 40.8%), higher resectability (93.2% vs. 49.9%), lower operative mortality (1.3% vs. 4.0%), and higher 5-year survival (60.0% vs. 22.2%) as well as 10-year survival (42.7% vs. 16.1%). In the pathologic aspect, more solitary tumor (79.1% vs. 54.1%), more well-encapsulated tumor (74.2% vs. 36.4%), lower incidence of tumor thrombus in the portal vein (31.3% vs. 45.2%), and slightly lower percentage of Edmondson Grade III to IV HCC (9.7% vs. 16.7%) were also noted in small HCC patients. It was also found that 66.7% of small HCC was diploid, associated with less incidence of invasion to capsule (16%); whereas aneuploid amounted to 92.3% of large HCC with 84% of capsule invasion. In short, pathologic studies on small HCC revealed well-differentiated, more diploid, single encapsulated tumor in the majority, which became progressively less differentiated, more aneuploid, with more multiple nodules and poor encapsulation during their development to large HCC. These findings strongly support the strategy for early detection and early effective treatment of small HCC.

CONVERSION OF LARGE HCC INTO SMALL HCC

"Cytoreduction and sequential resection of unresectable HCC" is an extension of a small HCC study. Small HCC could be found from screening/monitoring using AFP/ultrasonography in high-risk populations (HBV carrier, chronic viral hepatitis B/C, and cirrhosis), and from follow-up of patients after curative resection. Recently, with the progress in regional cancer therapies and multimodality treatment, it was possible to convert some of the localized unresectable large HCCs to resectable small HCCs. It has been reported that in 72 of 663 patients surgically verified unresectable HCCs were converted to resectable. Successful cytoreduction was mainly a result of the triple or double combination treatment with HAL, HAI, intrahepatic arterial radioimmunotherapy, and fractionated regional radiotherapy. The operative mortality was 1.4% for sequential resection, and 5-year survival was 62.1%, which was comparable to that associated with small HCC resection, because the median tumor size was reduced from 10 cm to 5 cm. Analysis revealed that single-nodule, well-encapsulated tumors, situated at the right lobe or hepatic hilum, associated with micronodular cirrhosis, and treated with triple or double combination modalities had higher sequential resection rates as compared to their counterparts. Solitary tumors confined in one lobe, without tumor thrombus and without residual cancer in specimens from sequential resection, were associated with longer survival. For cytoreduction, a double or triple combination treatment was more effective as compared with single-modality treatment. The recent advance of TACE has provided a non-surgical approach for cytoreduction of unresectable HCC, and the 5-year survival associated with sequential resection after TACE for initially unresectable HCC was around 50%.

RECURRENCE AND METASTASES: CLINICAL AND BASIC ASPECTS

HCC resection has played an important role in improving prognosis of HCC. Unfortunately, the recurrence rate after curative resection remained high, which is mainly a result of intrahepatic "metastasis" and multicentric origin of HCC. As had been reported, the 5-year recurrence rates after curative HCC resection were as high as 61.5%, being 43.5% for small HCC resection. Therefore, recurrence and metastasis are probably important targets for study.

In the clinical aspect, preoperative TACE was not advocated for resectable HCC; however, postoperative intrahepatic arterial chemoembolization seemed acceptable to reduce recurrence rate. As previously mentioned, reresection is effective in prolonging survival further when recurrence is in the subclinical stage. TACE is good for multiple recurrent lesions, and PEI is the choice for small recurrent lesion when surgery is contraindicated. Early detection and reresection of subclinical recurrence are important issues after HCC resection. For early detection of subclinical recurrence, monitoring AFP and ultrasonography every 2 to 3 months for more than 5 years after curative resection are emphasized. Reresection remained the choice of treatment for subclinical recurrence in the liver or solitary lung metastasis. It has been reported that the 5-year survival rate after recurrence was 40.8% in 90 patients who underwent reresection, whereas it was only 2.2% in 95 patients who were treated by other palliative methods.

The molecular aspect of HCC invasiveness is a major target of recent studies. It has been found that *p16* and *p53* mutation, *p21*, c-*erbB*-2, *mdm*-2, TGF-α, EGF-R, MMP-2 (matrix metalloproteinase), uPA (urokinase-type plasminogen activator), uPA-R, PAI-1 (inhibitor of uPA), ICAM-1 (intercellular adhesion molecule), and vascular endothelial growth factor (VEGF) were positively related to invasiveness of HCC, whereas *nm23-H1*, *Kai-1*, TIMP-2 (tissue inhibitor of metalloproteinase), E-cadherin, and integrin-$\alpha5$ were negatively related to invasiveness. Some of these parameters may have potential clinical implications as prognostic indicators. Interestingly, only a slight difference was found between small HCC and large HCC concerning the positivities of these factors, indicating that biologic characteristics remain the leading issue to be studied even in small HCC.

Experimental intervention of metastasis is also an attractive field because of its potential clinical implications. To clarify the mechanism and develop new treatment approach of recurrence and metastasis, a metastatic model of human HCC in nude mice (LCI-D20) has recently been established using orthotopic implantation of histologically intact tissues, the model maintained 100% of intrahepatic metastasis as well as metastasis in lungs and lymph nodes after more than 50 passages, and demonstrated expression of some of the invasiveness related genes and growth factors.

For experimental intervention, antisense H-*ras*, bispecific antibody (anti-CD3/anti-HBx), BB-94 (matrix metalloproteinase inhibitor), TNP470, and Suramin (antiangiogenesis) have been demonstrated to inhibit tumor growth and lung metastasis in this (LCI-D20) model. Gene therapy and novel tumor vaccines are also promising.

PROGNOSIS

In the United States, the relative 5-year survival rates in 1974–76, 1980–82, and 1986–92 were 4%, 4%, and 7% for Whites; and 1%, 2%, and 5% for Blacks, respectively. However, the long-term results in some centers were encouraging.

Factors that influence prognosis can be grouped into four aspects: clinicopathologic features, treatment modalities, biologic characteristics, and coexisting hepatitis and cirrhosis.

1. Clinicopathologic features. Analysis of the factors influencing the prognosis of HCC revealed that patients discovered by screening, with subclinical HCC, normal values of serum γ-glutamyl transpeptidase (GGT), small HCC ($\leq$5 cm), single tumor nodule, well-encapsulated tumor, nonhepatic hilum located tumor, and no cirrhosis or micronodular cirrhosis had better outcomes than patients discovered in the clinic, with symptomatic HCC, abnormal GGT, large HCC, multiple tumor nodules, poorly encapsulated tumor, hepatic hilum located tumor, and macronodular cirrhosis. TNM classification correlates well with prognosis.

2. Treatment modalities. The 5-year survival rates for patients treated with hepatic resection were around 30% to 50%, being 50% to 60% for small HCC resection, and 20% to 30% for large HCC resection. Palliative surgery other than resection such as hepatic artery ligation/cannulation (HAL/HAI), and cryosurgery yielded 10% to 20% of 5-year survival rates. The 5-year survival for large series of TACE was around 7% to 10%, with better results for segmental/subsegmental TACE. Radiotherapy or internal irradiation using ^{90}Y-microsphere or ^{131}I-Lipiodol achieved results comparable to those using TACE. Unfortunately, systemic chemotherapy remained disappointing. Recently, cytoreductive therapies using HAL/HAI or repeated TACE for unresectable HCC have led to remarkable tumor shrinkage in a small number of patients, and sequential resection yielded 50% to 60% of 5-year survival rates.

3. Biologic characteristics. Biologic characteristics remain the major prognosis-influencing factors of HCC. It has been found that patients without intrahepatic venous tumor thrombus, with diploid cancer, low positivity of proliferating cell nucleus antigen (PCNA), with expression of antimetastatic gene *nm23-H1*/tissue inhibitor of metalloproteinase-2 (TIMP-2), and without expression of TGF-α/epidermal growth factor receptor (EGF-R) in HCC had higher 5-year survival rates than did patients with tumor thrombi, aneuploid cancer, high positivity of PCNA, without expression of *nm23-H1*/TIMP-2, and with expression of TGF-α/EGF-R.

4. Coexisting hepatitis and cirrhosis. HCC patients with hepatitic status and Child C cirrhosis often have poor prognosis.

PREVENTION

Primary strategies implemented in China for prevention of HCC involve a combination of hepatitis B vaccination in newborn babies, change of the main food from corn to rice in rural areas to minimize the intake of aflatoxin, and change of drinking water from pond-ditch water to deep-well or tap water. However, the effect of primary prevention comes relatively late as compared to secondary prevention; therefore both primary and secondary prevention is advocated in high-risk areas.

CONCLUSION

HCC remains a common fatal malignancy in many geographic areas. Epidemiologic and etiologic findings suggest a multifactorial and multistep process, with a close relationship to viral hepatitis B and C as well as aflatoxin intake. Primary prevention is feasible using a combination of HBV vaccination in newborn babies and avoidance of food with high aflatoxin and contaminated drinking water. Secondary prevention using AFP/ultrasonography detection in high-risk populations has resulted in detection of resectable small HCC, and small HCC resection remains the major approach to improve series survival. For clinical treatment, aggressive surgery including resection of segment I and VIII tumor, reresection for subclinical recurrence, as well as cytoreduction and sequential resection for unresectable HCC are important. TACE and other regional cancer therapies are new trends in nonsurgical treatment. Invasiveness related recurrence will be the next target of study. With progress in tumor biology, particularly at the molecular level, novel approaches to the prevention and treatment of recurrence and metastasis are predicted.

Problems in the clinical aspect include: (1) The "cost-effectiveness" remains a practical issue for detection of small HCC. (2) The biologic characteristics, particularly the intraportal venous invasion even in very small HCC, remain the leading factors that influence prognosis. (3) Evidence of the multicentric origin of HCC is another obstacle of managing "recurrence" after HCC resection. (4) Liver transplantation will play an important role; however, the problems of obtaining donor organs, the expenses involved, and the recurrence of viral hepatitis are difficult to solve, particularly in developing countries. (5) Coexisting cirrhosis, particularly in Child C stage, remains a great challenge.

FURTHER READING

Aoki K, Kurihara M, Hayakawa N, Suzuki S (eds) (1992) *Death Rates for Malignant Neoplasms for Selected Sites by Sex and Five-Year Age Group in 33 Countries, 1953–57 to 1983–87.* UICC, The University of Nagoya Coop Press, Nagoya, pp. 205–218.

Iwatsuki S, Starzl TE (1993) Role of liver transplantation in the treatment of hepatocellular carcinoma. *Semin Surg Oncol* 9:337–340.

Kawasaki S, Makuuchi M, (eds) (1995) *Novel Regional Therapies for Liver Tumors.* RB Landes, Austin, TX, pp. 1–200.

Livraghi T, Makuuchi M, Buscarini L (eds) (1997) *Diagnosis and Treatment of Hepatocellular Carcinoma.* Greenwich Medical Media, London, pp. 1–454.

Okuda K, Ishak KG (eds) (1987) *Neoplasms of the Liver.* Springer-Verlag, Tokyo, pp. 1–420.

Ravikumar TS (guest ed) (1996) Management options in primary and secondary liver cancer. *Surg Oncol Clin North Am* 5:215–481.

Tabor E, Di bisceglie AM, Purcell RH (eds) (1991) *Etiology, Pathology and Treatment of Hepatocellular Carcinoma in North America.* Portfolio, The Woodlands, TX, pp. 1–365.

Tang ZY (ed) (1985) *Subclinical Hepatocellular Carcinoma.* Springer-Verlag, Berlin, pp. 1–366.

Tang ZY, Wu MC, Xia SS (eds) (1989) *Primary Liver Cancer.* Springer-Verlag, Berlin, pp. 1–495.

Tang ZY, Yang BH (1995) Secondary prevention of hepatocellular carcinoma. *J Gastroenterol Hepatol* 10:683–690.

Tang ZY, Yu YQ, Zhou XD, Ma ZC, Lu JZ, Lin ZY, Liu KD, Ye SL, Yang BH, Wang HW, Sun HC (1995) Cytoreduction and sequential resection for surgically verified unresectable hepatocellular carcinoma—evaluation with analysis of 72 patients. *World J Surg* 19:784–789.

Tang ZY (1996) Studies on small hepatocellular carcinoma—clinical aspects and molecular biology. *Hepatol Rapid Lit Rev* 1:VII–XVI.

Wanebo HJ (ed) (1997) Surgery for gastrointestinal cancer, a multidisciplinary approach—V. Liver, bile duct, and gallbladder. Lippincott-Raven, Philadelphia, pp. 483–606.

Yu SZ (1995) Primary prevention of hepatocellular carcinoma. *J Gastroenterol Hepatol* 10:674–682.

Zhou XD, Yu YQ, Tang ZY, Yang BH, Lu JZ, Lin ZY, Ma ZC, Xu DB, Zhang BH, Zheng YX, Tang CL (1993) Surgical treatment of recurrent hepatocellular carcinoma. *Hepato-Gastroenterol* 40:333–336.

Parkin DM, Pisani P, Ferlay J (1993) Estimates of the worldwide incidence of eighteen major cancers in 1985. *Int J Cancer* 54:1–13.

Eggel H (1901) Ueber das primare Carcinom der Leber. *Beitr Pathol Anat* 30:506–604.

Okuda K, Peters RL, Simson IW (1984) Gross anatomic features of hepatocellular carcinoma from three disparate geographic areas. Proposal of new classification. *Cancer* 54:2165–2173.

Nakashima T, Kojiro M (1987) *Hepatocellular Carcinoma—An Atlas of its Pathology.* Springer–Verlag, Tokyo, pp. ?.

Ishak KG, Anthony PP, Sobin LH (1994) *Histological Typing of Tumours of the Liver*, 2nd ed., WHO international histological claassification of tumours. Springer-Verlag, Berlin, p. 20.

Edmondson HA, Steiner PE (1954) Primary carcinoma of the liver: A study of 100 cases among 48,900 necropsies. *Cancer* 7:462-503.

Okuda K, Ohtsuki T, Obata H, Tomimatsu M, Okasaki N, Hasegawa H, Nakajima Y, et al. (1985) Natural history of hepatocellular carcinoma and prognosis in relation to treatment. Study of 850 patients. *Cancer* 56:918–928.

CHAPTER 21

ESOPHAGEAL CARCINOMA

DOUGLAS E. WOOD, ERIC VALLIÉRES, and CARLOS A. PELLEGRINI

Department of Surgery
University of Washington
Seattle, WA 98195, USA

Cancer of the esophagus is one of the most frequent malignancies world-wide. It is the seventh most common cause of death from cancer after lung, breast, uterine cervical, stomach, colon, and oral pharyngeal cancers. The enormous variability in the incidence of esophageal cancer between countries and regions within countries has created a compelling study of dietary, environmental, and hereditary factors in carcinogenesis. Nearly a 100-fold difference in incidence makes esophageal cancer an unusual neoplasm in some regions and a significant public health problem in others.

More than 90% of patients diagnosed with esophageal cancer will die of their disease. Although surgical therapy has been the mainstay of treatment for esophageal cancer in the past, multimodality therapy, combining various combinations of chemotherapy, radiation, and surgery, shows promising results in North America and Europe. Earlier diagnosis utilizing screening programs in endemic areas and studying genetic risk factors in patients with Barrett's metaplasia provides the potential for improved results.

EPIDEMIOLOGY

Squamous cell carcinoma and adenocarcinoma make up more than 95% of esophageal cancers, with the remaining histologies all extremely uncommon. Squamous cell carcinoma is the most frequent histologic subtype with enormous geographic variability. However, in the past two decades the incidence of adenocarcinoma

Manual of Clinical Oncology, 7th edition, Edited by Raphael E. Pollock
ISBN 0-471-23828-7, pages 425–438. Copyright © 1999 Wiley-Liss, Inc.

has surpassed squamous cell carcinoma in the United States and Europe. The overall incidence of esophageal cancer is approximately 5/100,000 in the United States, although the incidence of squamous carcinoma in black males is as high as 18/100,000. Most of Africa, Central America, Western Asia, and Polynesia have extremely low rates of esophageal cancer, in general less than 1.5/100,000. Areas of Northern Europe, Japan, and South Africa have intermediate rates of approximately 8 to 12/100,000, and Iran and China have a significantly higher rate of approximately 20/100,000.

Regional trends reveal dramatic variability. In the United States, higher incidences occur in the Washington, DC area and southeastern coastal areas. In France, Brittany and Normandy have a higher than usual incidence, whereas southern Thailand, northern Argentina, and mountainous areas of Japan have significantly higher incidences than these countries overall. The highest incidences occur in Iran along the Caspian Sea and in the Linxian and Hebei provinces of China, with incidences as high as 100 to 150/100,000.

The incidence of esophageal cancer increases with advancing age and it is uncommon in individuals under the age of 40. In endemic areas such as China and Iran, the highest mortality rates occur between 60 and 70 years of age although the average age is higher in areas with a lower incidence. Men are more frequently affected than women overall, but again a significant variability exists. In the United States, the male:female ratio for squamous cell carcinoma ranges from 2 to 4:1, although the ratio for adenocarcinoma is as high as 13:1. In general, the ratio is decreased in high incidence areas and is even reversed along the Caspian coast of Iran.

Smoking and heavy alcohol intake have both been implicated as risk factors for esophageal carcinoma. Smoking has been shown to produce a 3- to 8-fold increase in incidence and alcohol a 7- to 50-fold increase in incidence, both in squamous cell carcinoma. Combined heavy smoking and heavy alcohol use result in a 150-fold increase in squamous cell carcinoma of the esophagus. There is no clear relationship, however, between adenocarcinomas and these risk factors. Dietary factors have also been implicated, with a higher incidence associated with diets that are low in vegetable and fruit intake and deficient in vitamins or trace elements. On the other hand, supplementation of the diet with carotinoids, vitamin C, and vitamin E may provide some protection against esophageal carcinoma. Dietary carcinogens may have a role in inducing esophageal cancer. Nitrosamines and their precursors induce esophageal tumors experimentally in laboratory animals and are common in the high-incidence regions of Northern China and Iran. Pickled vegetables, moldy or fermented foods, and cured meats or fish are major sources of nitrosamines.

While the worldwide incidence of squamous cell carcinoma has remained relatively stable, there has been an alarming increase in the incidence of adenocarcinomas of the esophagus in North America and Europe over the past 2 decades. In these regions, adenocarcinoma has increased at a rate of almost 10% a year, far exceeding increases in any other cancer. This increase is predominantly seen in the white male population. The reasons for this increase in incidence are unclear, although some have suggested a relationship to the increased use of histamine blockers in this population.

Patients with certain benign esophageal conditions may be at increased risk for the development of esophageal carcinoma. Plummer–Vinson syndrome, lye-induced esophageal stricture, and achalasia are associated with an increased incidence of squamous cell carcinoma of the esophagus. Most importantly, the columnar epithelium lined (Barrett's) esophagus is a common problem and intimately linked with the increased incidence of adenocarcinoma of the esophagus in the West. It is estimated that the prevalence of Barrett's esophagus is approximately 10% in those patients with symptoms of gastroesophageal reflux and 1% in asymptomatic patients. This is important because Barrett's esophagus is associated with a 30- to 40-fold increase in the incidence of esophageal adenocarcinomas.

Barrett's esophagus has been studied extensively as a model of neoplastic progression. Mutations of the *p53* tumor suppressor gene are detected early in Barrett's dysplasia. It has been shown that patients with Barrett's dysplasia with a high aneuploid or increased G_2/tetraploid population are at increased risk of developing an invasive adenocarcinoma. Further study of these genetic factors may provide information regarding patients at risk for developing adenocarcinoma, as well as therapeutic interventions to prevent or reverse neoplastic progression.

SCREENING

In endemic areas, cytologic screening may be useful in providing an early diagnosis of esophageal cancer in the asymptomatic patient. Cytologic samples are obtained from a swallowed inflatable balloon and, if an intramucosal cancer is detected, cure rates as high as 80% to 90% may be expected. Precise correlation has not been defined between the cytologic and histologic diagnosis, however. Currently cytology should be considered for screening only and does not provide the definitive tissue diagnosis of primary esophageal neoplasm necessary to initiate therapy.

No widely accepted or cost-effective protocols for surveillance of patients with achalasia or lye stricture have been established. However, protocols have been defined for surveillance in patients with Barrett's epithelium and moderate to severe dysplasia. These routinely involve endoscopy with multiple biopsies at variable time intervals, and are expensive and labor intensive. However, these protocols are also productive, not only in the successful diagnosis of early curable esophageal cancers, but also in producing genetic material for prognosticating the risk of developing an invasive adenocarcinoma in the future.

Diagnosis and Staging

Unfortunately the best chance for cure in esophageal carcinoma is if it is detected at an early asymptomatic stage. This has been possible in endemic areas through screening cytology. In other parts of the world, small incidental tumors discovered at endoscopy for unrelated reasons or surveillance endoscopy in patients with Barrett's metaplasia provide the only opportunity for detecting esophageal carcinomas in the absence of symptoms. The majority of patients present with a characteristic pattern of progressive dysphagia, initially for solid foods and later for liquids as esophageal obstruction becomes more severe. Dysphagia is present in nearly 95% of symptomatic patients, with regurgitation and weight loss occurring in 40% to 50% of patients and pain or cough in 20% to 25% of patients.

A careful history provides clues to the local effects of the primary tumor, possible metastatic sites, and the general physiologic status of the patient. Physical examination provides information on the general nutritional status, pulmonary complications due to aspiration or the development of tracheal esophageal fistula, and signs of metastasis including lymphadenopathy or hepatomegaly.

Symptoms or signs suggestive of esophageal carcinoma should be followed by an esophagogram and esophagoscopy. Contrast studies usually show mucosal irregularity and stricture that may be nearly diagnostic of tumor. However, patients with very early lesions may have a normal esophagogram. Esophagoscopy is important to detect radiologically occult carcinomas, obtain a histologic diagnosis, and for estimation of the endoluminal extent of tumor.

Computed tomography (CT) has become an essential part of esophageal cancer staging during the last 20 years. It is the most frequent noninvasive investigation that provides information about the primary esophageal tumor (T), regional lymph nodes (N), and distant visceral metastases (M). Intravenous and oral contrast improves definition of the posterior mediastinal structures, vascular tissue planes, differentiation of adenopathy from normal surrounding structures, and detection of liver metastases. Scanning should include the chest and upper abdomen with extension into the neck or lower abdomen dependent on tumor location or signs of more extensive disease. The primary tumor site can be seen either as a focal area of wall thickening or more commonly as an area of circumferential involvement. Malignant neoplasms are typically irregular and asymmetric soft tissue masses. Longitudinal measurements frequently underestimate the pathologic extent of tumor owing to the frequency of radiologically occult submucosal infiltration.

Tumor stage and prognosis are determined by (1) depth of tumor infiltration into or through the esophageal wall, (2) presence or absence of regional lymph node metastases, and (3) presence or absence of distant metastatic disease (Table 21.1). CT scanning cannot reliably delineate the layers of the esophagus and is thus not useful in differentiating between T1, T2, or T3 tumors. Tumor invasion of adjacent structures (T4) is critical for patient management decisions, as invasion of the aorta or tracheobronchial tree precludes surgical resection.

Multiple radiologic criteria have been investigated regarding their predictive value in identifying tracheobronchial or aortic invasion. Specific findings of tracheobronchial invasion include the demonstration of a tracheobronchial fistula or extension of tumor into the airway lumen. Indentation of the airway, thickening of the wall of the trachea or bronchus, and absence of the fat plane between the esophagus and tracheobronchial tree are all potential but nonspecific indicators of airway invasion. CT findings suggesting aortic invasion include loss of the fat plane between the aorta and esophagus, and interface of $> 90°$ of the aortic circumference by esophageal tumor. Invasion of the pericardium is suggested by pericardial thickening or pericardial effusion and distal esophageal tumors may invade the diaphragm

TABLE 21.1. Staging of Esophageal Carcinoma

Primary Tumor (T)

T1	Invades lamina propria or submucosa.
T2	Invades muscularis propria.
T3	Invades adventitia.
T4	Invades adjacent structures.

Regional Lymph Nodes (N)

N0	No metastasis
N1	Metastasis present

Distant Metastasis (M)

M0	No distant metastasis
M1	Distant metastasis present

Stage Grouping

Stage I	T1N0M0
Stage IIA	T2–3N0M0
Stage IIB	T1–2N1M0
Stage III	T3N1M0
	T4N0–1M0
Stage IV	T1–4N0–1M1

with the CT appearance of a soft tissue density obliterating fat planes that normally surround the crura.

Several prospective comparisons of CT scan and surgical staging have established that the accuracy of CT is poor, with a sensitivity of 0% to 67% and a specificity of 71% to 100%. Preoperative underestimation of tumor stage is common and is due to the poor sensitivity in detecting mediastinal and abdominal lymph node involvement. Radiologically normal nodes may have microscopic metastatic disease. More importantly, overestimation of stage may produce incorrect decisions regarding therapy. Loss of periesophageal fat planes and even circumferential growth around mediastinal structures such as the aorta do not correlate well with invasion of these organs and cannot be taken as signs of unresectability. Enlarged mediastinal or celiac axis lymph nodes detected by CT are nonspecific, as lymph nodes may be enlarged for reasons other than tumor metastases. Owing to the significant incidence of both false-positive and false-negative interpretations of regional lymph nodes, the accuracy of CT scans alone for nodal staging (N) is only about 55%.

In contrast to the limitations of CT for determining primary tumor (T) stage and regional lymph node (N) stage, CT scanning is highly sensitive and specific for detecting metastatic disease of the lung, liver, or adrenal glands. CT or radionuclide scanning of other sites for metastatic disease is usually performed selectively based on suggestive symptoms, signs, or laboratory investigations. Experience with magnetic resonance imaging (MRI) has shown similar limitations in sensitivity and specificity as CT and currently has no routine role in the preoperative staging of esophageal carcinoma.

Endoscopic ultrasound (EUS) combined with CT scanning has been shown to significantly improve the accuracy of staging. EUS provides detail consisting of five ultrasonic layers of alternating echogenicities. The superficial mucosa are hyperechoic, the deep mucosa and musclaris mucosa is hypoechoic, the submucosa is hyperechoic, the muscularis propria is hypoechoic, and the adventitia is hyperechoic. Local structures such as the left atrium, aorta, vena cava, and azygous vein may be identified. Lymph nodes appear as discrete round or elliptical structures. Esophageal cancer appears as an irregular, hypoechoic disruption of the normal esophageal layers. Staging of the primary tumor (T1 to T4) with EUS has an accuracy of 80% to 90%. Overstaging can occur as a result of local inflammation and understaging can occur if there is microscopic invasion below the spatial resolution of EUS. Lymph node metastases are usually irregular, hypoechoic, and round, whereas inflammatory lymph nodes are usually more homogeneous, echogenic, and less well defined. EUS is also reported to be 80% to 90% accurate in detecting mediastinal lymph node metastases. Esophageal ultrasound is limited to evaluation of the esophagus and periesophageal structures and so there is virtually no utility in the detection of visceral metastases. Therefore, EUS and CT are complementary studies in the staging of esophageal cancer, with EUS highly accurate for primary tumor (T) and regional nodal (N) staging, whereas CT is useful and accurate in detecting metastatic disease (M).

A major limitation of EUS is tumor stenosis that prevents passage of the endoscope or ultrasound probe past the tumor. The proximal portion of the tumor may still be staged and this limitation may be solved by development of smaller caliber ultrasound probes. The other major limitation of EUS is dependence on experienced endoscopists in interpretation of ultrasound images. Although experience and criteria for CT staging are widely disseminated, operators with extensive experience in endoscopic ultrasound are less common and institutionally variable. This limits the utility of EUS to regions or centers with significant experience in this modality.

Bronchoscopy should be performed for all tumors in proximity to the airway including all cervical and upper thoracic tumors abutting the trachea, carina, or mainstem bronchi. Indentation of the membranous wall by an underlying esophageal cancer in the absence of mucosal involvement does not preclude resection. However, evidence of transluminal invasion or tracheoesophageal fistula is considered a contraindication to surgical resection.

Preoperative lymph node biopsies have been investigated by a number of techniques including mediastinoscopy, scalene lymph node biopsy, video-assisted thoracoscopic and laparoscopic biopsy, and transesophageal needle biopsy under esophageal ultrasound. Experience in each of these areas is limited to date and currently does not have proven utility in improving esophageal cancer staging and subsequent therapeutic decisions. The role of invasive staging requires prospective clinical trials to determine its efficacy.

TREATMENT AND PROGNOSIS

Surgery

Esophagectomy continues to be the primary therapy for local and locoregional disease in esophageal cancer. The primary goal of treatment is cure, although palliation of dysphagia is an important secondary objective. Although many improvements have been made in chemotherapy, radiation, and multimodality therapy, the best chance for cure includes an operation that encompasses the entire tumor and draining lymph nodes with adequate proximal and distal margins (Fig. 21.1). The optimal surgical approach for the management of esophageal cancer has been vigorously de-

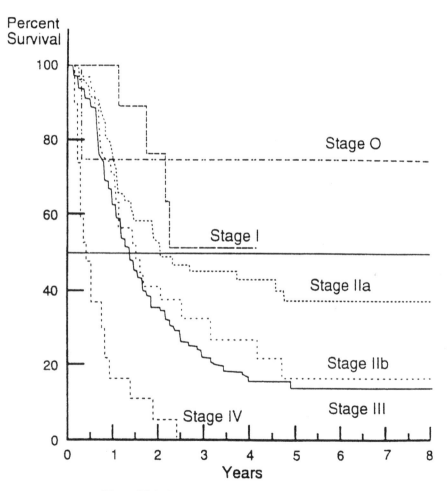

Figure 21.1. Esophageal cancer survival by stage.

bated and is not well established. Esophageal resection is a major procedure with significant mortality and morbidity. Nearly all specialized centers report mortality rates of <10% and even as low as 3%, but operative mortality of nearly 20% has been reported. Major morbidity affects 20% to 40% of patients after esophagectomy and primarily consists of cardiorespiratory complications and anastomotic complications. Careful preoperative staging, good patient selection, and experience in esophageal resection are the most important factors in minimizing operative morbidity and mortality.

Nearly all patients undergoing esophagectomy are reconstructed with the stomach, with a primary esophagogastric anastomosis performed in the neck or chest. Therefore, mobilization of the stomach as a pedicled conduit based upon the right gastroeploic and right gastric arteries is an integral part of nearly every esophagectomy. This is normally performed through a laparotomy but can be performed through an abdominal extension of a left thoracoabdominal approach. The most common approaches for esophageal resection are: (1) an Ivor–Lewis approach utilizing a laparotomy for gastric mobilization and right thoracotomy for esophageal resection and mobilization with an anastomosis in the upper thorax, (2) a transhiatal esophagectomy utilizing a cervical and abdominal incision without thoracotomy with a cervical anastomosis, and (3) a left thoracoabdominal approach for one-field mobilization of the stomach and distal esophagus with an anastomosis below the aortic arch.

An Ivor–Lewis esophagectomy has the advantages of direct mediastinal exposure for intrathoracic esophageal dissection and mobilization. This is especially useful for tumors in the middle third of the esophagus or abutting the tracheobronchial tree. It has the disadvantage of requiring two incisions and an intrathoracic anastomosis with more severe implications of anastomotic leakage. A transhiatal esophagectomy is a good approach for gastroesophageal junction tumors, cervical esophageal tumors, or early stage Barrett's adenocarcinoma. The benefits include the avoidance of thoracotomy and a cervical anastomosis, but the procedure is limited by poor exposure to most of the intrathoracic esophagus, requiring a "blind" dissection and an inability to obtain a good radial dissection with inclusion of periesophageal lymph nodes. A left thoracoabdominal esophagogastrectomy provides excellent exposure for tumors of the gastroesophageal junction with the ability to obtain an en bloc dissection of all regional lymph nodes. This approach is not useful for higher esophageal tumors because in general it is limited to dissection and anastomosis below the aortic arch. Major limitations of this approach are the morbidity associated with a thoracoabdominal incision, limited ability to obtain extensive proximal longitudinal margins, an intrathoracic anastomosis, and the potential for more severe problems with postoperative gastroesophageal reflux.

Variations of these three techniques are commonly employed for more challenging tumors. An Ivor–Lewis approach or a left thoracoabdominal approach combined with a cervical incision and anastomosis provide the benefits of direct intrathoracic dissection and mobilization together with the benefits of a cervical anastomosis which include extensive longitudinal margin, lower morbidity from an anastomotic leak, and a decreased incidence of symptomatic reflux. More radical surgical approaches have been advocated involving a total esophagogastrectomy with cervical, mediastinal, and abdominal lymph node dissection. Proponents of this approach contend that improved local control may result in an improvement in survival, but this must be weighed against the increased morbidity and mortality associated with a more extensive procedure.

When the stomach is unavailable as a conduit, alternative conduits include a pedicled left or right colon interposition that may be used for total esophageal replacement, a pedicled jejunal interposition that can effectively replace the lower half of the esophagus, or a free jejunal graft with microvascular anastomosis that can replace up to 15 to 20 cm of esophagus, most commonly in the cervical and upper thoracic esophagus.

In spite of vigorous debate regarding the relative merits of one approach over the other, surgical series have indicated comparable operative morbidity and mortality, as well as oncologic outcomes, in nonrandomized comparisons of these three basic techniques. It is important to recognize the advantages and disadvantages of each approach and select the operation appropriately according to the patient's disease, tumor location, patient comorbidities, and goals of therapy. Unfortunately, regardless of which approach is taken, 85% to 90% of patients will die of recurrent disease.

Radiation

Radiation therapy has been used as an alternative to surgery in primary treatment of esophageal carcinoma. In most series, radiation has been used to treat patients with extensive disease or patients ineligible for surgery, so it is not surprising that these patients with advanced disease would have a 1-year survival of 18% and a 5-year survival of only 6%. Radiation commonly treats the primary tumor site and lymph node drainage with an optimum radiation dose of 55 to 65 Gy. Unfortunately a major cause of death in patients treated with primary radiotherapy is persistent tumor at the primary site. Used alone, radiation may provide a temporary palliation but is rarely curative and in many cases does not provide durable palliation.

Chemotherapy

Multiple chemotherapeutic agents have been examined extensively in both locally advanced and metastatic esophageal cancer. Chemotherapy can result in palliation of symptoms in a small but significant number of patients with advanced disease, although the duration of this response is brief. None of these chemotherapeutic regimens has so far induced complete remission in any substantial percentage of patients. Combination chemotherapy has most commonly been employed owing to the modest single agent activity and the knowledge of improved results in combination therapy in other tumors. Cisplatin-based chemotherapy is the most common regimen utilized and may be combined with vindesine, bleomycin, and 5-fluorouracil. Response rates of 25% to 50% are commonly reported in cisplatin-based combination chemotherapy.

Multimodality Therapy

Unfortunately, results have been poor with any single therapy for esophageal carcinoma. Surgical therapy has produced the best single therapy results, with 5-year survival rates of 10% to 15%, although this may be due to the selection of favorable patients for surgical resection. However, most patients do fail after surgery and this is rarely due to locoregional recurrence, but instead due to metastatic disease. The implications are that the majority of patients with locally advanced squamous cell or adenocarcinoma of the esophagus have systemic disease at the time of presentation and require consideration of systemic therapy. It is this realization that has led to the investigation of multimodality therapy, combining a systemic therapy with a therapy for locoregional control. These regimens typically involve chemotherapy with radiation and/or surgery.

Combination therapy in the past usually utilized adjuvant chemotherapy or radiation after surgical resection, but neither of these have been shown to improve cancer survival. The current emphasis is on neoadjuvant chemoradiation owing to the favorable results seen in other tumors and for several oncologic principles. Preoperative chemotherapy or chemoradiation has the benefits of: (1) decreasing tumor extent and size to improve resectability, (2) early treatment of micrometastatic disease, and (3) assessment of the response to the preoperative therapy. This latter factor provides individual patient information regarding prognosis and the possible efficacy of postoperative therapy, as well as epidemiologic information regarding the effectiveness of presurgical treatment. The only disadvantage of neoadjuvant chemotherapy is the delay in local control of disease. This is rectified by utilizing concomitant chemotherapy and radiation with the advantages of chemosensitization of the tumor to radiation and the combined treatment providing even more locoregional response improving resectability. A typical neoadjuvant regimen utilizes two to three cycles of cisplatin-based combination chemotherapy with concurrent radiation to 45 Gy, followed by restaging and surgical resection 3 to 6 weeks after completion of the induction protocol. Patients undergoing aggressive multimodality therapy obviously suffer the combined morbidity of each treatment alone, but surprisingly there is no evidence that surgical morbidity or mortality is higher in those patients treated with neoadjuvant therapy.

The results of multimodality therapy involving chemotherapy and surgery, or chemoradiation followed by surgery, are encouraging but far from conclusive. Several phase II trials and two single institution phase III trials have shown complete pathologic response rates of 20% to 40% with most 5-year survivals between 30% and 40%. Not surprisingly complete pathologic responders have the most favorable prognosis, with a 2-year survival rate of over 70%.

Given the promising results in neoadjuvant therapy with chemoradiation, several investigators have questioned whether surgery adds to palliation and survival or simply adds to treatment morbidity and mortality. Several phase II and phase III trials of chemoradiotherapy show significant 5-year survival rates of 20% to 30%. Although these are not as good as trimodality therapy results, the appropriate combination of therapy and role of surgery in multimodality therapy remain to be established in multiinstitutional prospective randomized trials.

PALLIATION OF ADVANCED DISEASE

Metastatic esophageal carcinoma is clinically apparent in approximately 50% of patients at diagnosis and is an incurable disease with a median patient survival of 5 to 8 months. Although response rates of 25% to 40% can be seen with cisplatin-based chemotherapy, the benefit to overall survival is minimal, and is not currently an established therapy for the management of metastatic esophageal carcinoma. Palliation of dysphagia or odynophagia is very important for patients with locally advanced and/or metastatic esophageal carcinoma. Traditionally, radiotherapy has been used to palliate the primary site with or without chemotherapy. Although this provides a reasonable expectation for temporary palliation, the response to therapy is not seen immediately and the delivery of treatment takes several weeks.

Endoscopic palliation can provide immediate relief of dysphagia without the morbidity, delayed response, or time investment of systemic therapy or radiation. Endoscopic techniques include dilatation, placement of an endoluminal prosthesis, laser ablation, endoluminal brachytherapy, or photodynamic therapy. Dilatation of obstructing esophageal tumors can often provide temporary relief of severe dysphagia and is most useful when awaiting results of a more definitive therapy, as a preliminary step to placement of an endoluminal stent, or for the preterminal patient who requires short-term palliation. Historical results with solid plastic stents have shown a significant risk of esophageal perforation (5% to 15%) and have usually limited the patient to a liquid or a pureed diet. Expandable stents coated with silicone rubber have markedly improved the ability to provide effective endoluminal palliation. These stents have the advantages of being easier to place, deployed through a flexible delivery device under endoscopic and fluoroscopic control. They require less dilatation before insertion and subsequently are at less risk of perforation. Expandable stents also provide a larger intraluminal diameter and many patients have been able to resume a nearly normal diet subsequent to stent placement. Laser ablation or photodynamic therapy palliate dysphagia by decreasing the bulk of endoluminal tumor. Both provide temporary palliation and may be combined with planned placement of an endoluminal stent, or used repeatedly to maintain an esophageal lumen if stenting is contraindicated or unavailable. Endoluminal brachytherapy provides an additional modality delivering high-dose radiation within the esophageal lumen for improvement in local control and palliation. Although esophageal resection or bypass was considered for palliation of dysphagia in the past, this is rarely considered today owing to the effectiveness of these endoscopic techniques.

POSTOPERATIVE FOLLOW-UP

Despite aggressive surgical techniques and multimodality therapy, 5-year survival rates for patients who have undergone surgical resection remain between 15% to 35%. Exceptions are those patients with early tumors and no lymph node metastases and those with complete pathologic responses after neoadjuvant therapy. Recurrences can be local—in the bed of the resected tumor, regional—in the lymphatic drainage of the esophagus, or distant—from hematogenous metastases to other organs. Isolated local recurrence is the only disease that is potentially treatable for cure. Small series from Japan have shown that isolated esophageal remnant recurrences are uncommon, occurring with an incidence of 3% to 7%, with an average disease-free interval of 18 months. Unfortunately, mean survival after esophageal stump recurrence was < 6 months with only anecdotal reports of long-term survivors.

Regional lymph nodes are the first sign of recurrent disease in 40% to 50% of patients and are more common in those patients with involvement of lymph nodes at the time of surgery or tumors with evidence of lymphatic invasion in the primary tumor. Unfortunately, survival is rare in these instances, even with aggressive therapy.

Metastatic disease is present in 95% of patients dying of esophageal cancer, predominantly affecting the lungs, liver, and bone. The mean disease-free interval in patients developing metastatic disease after esophagectomy is 17 months, but there is a wide range of 4 to 52 months. However, survival after the diagnosis of distant recurrence is uniformly poor, with a mean survival of only 4 months.

The only incidence of recurrence with a reasonable possibility of curative therapy is a local esophageal recurrence in the esophageal remnant or a second primary esophageal carcinoma. These patients will most likely present with a typical history of progressive dysphagia 6 months to 3 years after esophagectomy. Routine follow-up esophagoscopy would be the only modality likely to discover asymptomatic and potentially curable disease. This may be warranted in patients with a close resection margin or remnant of Barrett's esophagus, but is not cost-effective on a routine basis owing to the low incidence of isolated local recurrences. Currently there is no evidence that routine radiologic studies, serum cancer screening panels, carcinoembryonic antigen (CEA) levels, or nuclear scans provide early detection of treatable recurrent disease.

Unfortunately, no effective therapy for regional or metastatic disease has been established and so it seems unlikely that any investigations would significantly change a patient's treatment or natural history. Therefore, a history and physical exam alone remain the most sensitive and cost-effective follow-up for treated esophageal cancer patients. Because most recurrences occur in the first 2 years, history and physical exams should be performed every 4 months within the first 2 years of surgery. Although curable local recurrences and symptomatic metastatic disease can still occur, the exam interval could then increase to every 6 months for years 3 and 4 and then lengthen to 12-month intervals. Surveillance endoscopy can be considered for patients with a high risk of local esophageal recurrence or remnant of Barrett's esophagus but other follow-up modalities are probably not warranted given both the lack of documented success in early detection of recurrence as well as the lack of effective treatment for recurrent esophageal carcinoma.

PREVENTION

There are currently no proven strategies for prevention of esophageal carcinoma except for the avoidance of risk factors such as smoking and heavy alcohol use. The discovery of columnar-lined epithelium (Barrett's esophagus) warrants aggressive medical and surgical therapy for gastroesophageal reflux disease. Unfortunately, however, these therapies do not seem to decrease the risk of developing a subsequent adenocarcinoma in these patients. Surveillance protocols have been well defined for patients with Barrett's esophagus and dysplastic epithelium that allow for the early detection of an adenocarcinoma at a treatable and curable stage. Some authors recommend prophylactic esophagectomy for patients with Barrett's esophagus and severe dysphagia because of a reported high incidence of incidental adenocarcinoma discovered in the resected esophagus in these patients. Others follow aggressive surveillance protocols combined with genetic analysis and assessment of the aneuploid cell population. Further recognition of markers for the development of esophageal carcinoma such as the *p53* mutation may allow better differentiation of patients at risk for esophageal cancer to provide early definitive therapy. These same factors may provide an opportunity for effective topical or systemic gene therapy for the prevention of esophageal cancer.

Patients in endemic areas where esophageal cancer is common provide a special opportunity and problem in cancer prevention. Continued analysis of these populations may provide recognition of changeable environmental factors to decrease the incidence of esophageal cancer in the population overall. Until then, however, aggressive screening provides the only opportunity for improving survival in patients with esophageal cancer by detecting them at an early stage.

FURTHER READING

Akiyama H, Tsurumaru M, Kawamura T, Ono Y (1981) Principles of surgical treatment for carcinoma of the esophagus: Analysis of lymph node involvement. *Ann Surg* 194:438–446.

Blot WJ, Devesa SS, Kneller RW, Fraumeni JF (1991) Rising incidence of adenocarcinoma of the esophagus and gastric cardia. *JAMA* 265:1287–1289.

Coia LR, Sauter ER (1994) Esophageal cancer *Curr Prob Cancer* 18:191–247.

Ellis FH Jr, Watkins E Jr, Krasna MJ, Heatley GJ, Balogh K (1993) Staging of carcinoma of the esophagus and cardia: A comparison of different staging criteria. *J Surg Oncol* 55:231–235.

Forastiere AA, Heitmiller RF, Lee D-J, Zahurak M, Abrams R, Kleinberg L, Watkins S, Yeo CJ, Lillemoe KD, Sitzmann JV, Sharfman W (1997) Intensive chemoradiation followed by esophagectomy for squamous cell and adenocarcinoma of the esophagus. *Cancer J Sci Am* 3:144–152.

Ilson DH, Kelsen DP (1996) Management of esophageal cancer. *Oncology* 10:1385–1401.

Isono K, Onada S, Okuyama K, Sato H (1985) Recurrence of intrathoracic esophageal cancer. *Jpn J Clin Oncol* 15:49–60.

Lee JG, Lieberman D (1997) Endoscopic palliation for esophageal cancer. *Dig Dis* 15:100–112.

Levine DS, Haggitt RC, Blount PL, Rabinovitch PS, Rusch VM, Reid BJ (1993) An endoscopic biopsy protocol can differentiate high-grade dysplasia from early adenocarcinoma in Barrett's esophagus. *Gastroenterology* 105:40–50.

Rosch T (1995) Endosonographic staging of esophageal cancer: A review of literature results. *Gastrointest Endosc Clin NA* 5:537–547.

Urba SG, Orringer MB, Perez-Tamayo G, Bromberg J, Forastiere A (1992) Concurrent preoperative chemotherapy and radiation therapy in localized esophageal adenocarcinoma. *Cancer* 69:285–291.

Walsh TN, Noonan N, Hollywood D, Kelly A, Keeling N, Hennessy TPJ (1996) A comparison of multimodal therapy and surgery for esophageal adenocarcinoma. *N Engl J Med* 335:462–467.

Wolfe WG, Vaughn AL, Seigler HF, Harhorn JW, Leopold KA, Duhaylongsod FG (1993) Survival of patients with carcinoma of the esophagus treated with combined-modality therapy. *J Thorac Cardiovasc Surg* 105:749–755.

Wood DE, Pellegrini CA (1977) Esophageal Carcinoma. In: Johnson FL, Virgo KS (eds) *Cancer Patient Follow-up*. Mosby-Yearbook, St. Louis, pp. 78–81.

CHAPTER 22

CANCER OF THE STOMACH

JIN-POK KIM

Inje University Seoul Paik Medical Center
Korea Gastric Cancer Center
Seoul, Korea

In contrast to Western countries, where the incidence of gastric cancer has notably declined over the last 30 years, gastric cancer is still the second most common cancer worldwide. It represents a good example of recent improvements in cancer therapy; early diagnosis and curative surgery have been the main factors contributing to higher cure rates. However, several differences in pathology and therapy exist between Western and Eastern countries. Modern molecular genetics methodology has provided possible resolutions to these problems.

EPIDEMIOLOGY AND ETIOLOGY

The incidence of gastric cancer has decreased markedly to about one fourth of the 1950 level in most Western countries (Fig. 22.1), but Asian countries such as Korea, China, and Japan continue to have a high rate. In Latin America, Chile and Costa Rica also have high incidences. About twice as many males suffer from stomach cancer as females; however, women less than 30 years old have a higher frequency than men of the same age. The peak age incidence is in the sixth decade.

The incidence of gastric cancer varies from country to country as well as regionally within countries. Studies of immigrants from Japan to the United States indicate only a moderate decrease in risk, even if they emigrated at an early age. Second-generation Japanese in the United States have gastric cancer risk rates much closer to those of the general United States population. This suggests that environmental factors are important early in life.

Manual of Clinical Oncology, 7th edition, Edited by Raphael E. Pollock
ISBN 0-471-23828-7, pages 439–452. Copyright © 1999 Wiley-Liss, Inc.

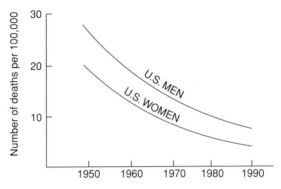

FIGURE 22.1. Decrease in mortality from stomach cancer in the United States since 1950. The reasons are unknown.

Although no specific causal factors have been demonstrated, suggested etiologic factors for gastric cancer include dietary habits such as high-salt diets, consumption of smoked foods containing possible carcinogens or carcinogen precursors (such as nitrates), and diets low in fresh fruits and vegetables. Nitrates and nitrites can clearly be converted to active carcinogens, the N-nitrosamines. Certainly, free-radical-induced injury by nitrosamines and bacterial byproducts of *Helicobacter pylori* are potentially damaging. Both ascorbic acid and β-carotene found in fresh fruits and vegetables act as antioxidants; further, ascorbic acid can prevent the conversion of nitrites to nitrosamines.

Epidemiologic studies have consistently demonstrated an association between *H. pylori* infection and the risk of gastric cancer. Prospective serologic studies have reported that persons with *H. pylori* infection have a three- to sixfold higher risk of gastric cancer than those without infection. This association seems largely restricted to intestinal-type cancers and cancers of the distal stomach. Nevertheless, gastric carcinoma develops in only a small proportion of infected persons, suggesting that genetic or environmental cofactors are required.

An etiologic pathogenetic hypothesis based upon pathologic and epidemiologic studies has been proposed, with sequential stages of chronic gastritis, atrophy, intestinal metaplasia, and dysplasia (Fig. 22.2). The initial stages of gastritis and atrophy have been linked to excessive salt intake and infection with *H. pylori*. The intermediate stages have been associated with the ingestion of ascorbic acid and nitrate, determinants of intragastric nitrosation. The final stages have been linked with the supply of β-carotene and with excessive salt intake. Nitrosating agents are candidate carcinogens and could originate in the gastric cavity or in the inflammatory infiltrate.

Some pathologic conditions have been considered as possible precursors of gastric cancer. Atrophic gastritis, achlorhydria, pernicious anemia, intestinal metaplasia, and hypertrophic gastritis have all been implicated. Patients with achlorhydria are four to five times more likely to develop gastric cancer than people of the same age with normal gastric acid production, and patients with pernicious anemia have a

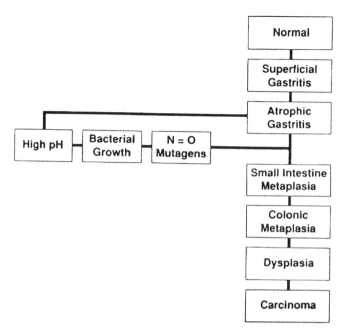

FIGURE 22.2. General hypothesis of gastric carcinogenesis. **(Right)** Postulated successive phenotypic changes in the gastric mucosa. **(Left)** Changes in the gastric cavity. (Adapted from Correa, 1992.)

risk 18 times greater than the average. Peptic ulcer itself is not considered a precursor condition for gastric cancer. However, chronic recurrent gastric ulcer resistant to therapy should be biopsied to rule out gastric cancer. The risk of developing cancer in adenomatous polyps is thought to be between 10% and 20% and is greatest if polyps are 2 cm or greater in diameter. There is considerable evidence that gastric surgery for benign conditions increases the risk of gastric cancer by two- to sixfold. Most cases have occurred after Billroth II anastomosis, 15 to 20 years after the original surgical procedure.

Several cohort and case-control studies have shown a 1.5- to 3.0-fold increase in the risk of gastric cancer among smokers, although most studies have failed to demonstrate a clear dose–response relationship. Studies of the relationship between alcohol consumption and the risk of gastric cancer have been largely inconclusive.

Gastric cancer displays multiple gene alterations involving oncogenes, growth factors or cytokines, cell cycle regulators, tumor suppressor genes, cell adhesion molecules, and genetic instability. However, the scenarios of multiple gene changes in gastric cancer differ depending on the histologic type, as different types may have different genetic pathways.

PATHOLOGY

Gastric adenocarcinoma can arise from gastric mucosal cells anywhere within the stomach. Tumors arose with much greater frequency in the antral and pyloric regions. However, recent series from Western countries indicate a much higher rate of involvement of the cardia and gastroesophageal junction than in the past. But in some series of Eastern countries such as Korea and Japan, the prevalence of proximal cancer was not increased.

Borrmann proposed a gross classification of gastric cancer in 1926. It has been used by many investigators as the standard for the macroscopic classification of advanced gastric cancer. Listed in ascending order of degree of malignancy, they are polypoid (Borrmann type I), ulcerating (Borrmann type II), ulceroinfiltrating (Borrmann type III), and diffuse linitis plastica (Borrmann type IV) lesions.

The concept of early gastric cancer was defined by the Japanese Society for Gastric Cancer Study in 1963. According to the Society, early gastric cancer is a primary carcinoma of the stomach that invades either the mucosa or the submucosal layer, regardless of the presence or absence of lymph node metastasis (now defined as a T1 lesion in the TNM staging system). Early gastric cancer was not included in the Borrmann's classification but has been classified as type 0 in recent years. The macroscopic classification of early gastric cancer includes type I (protruding type), type II (superficial type), and type III (excavated type).

There are numerous systems for histologic typing of gastric carcinoma. In 1977, the WHO introduced a relatively simple and reproducible classification. However, conventional WHO typing does not carry much prognostic or therapeutic significance. Therefore, in the second edition of the *WHO International Histological Classification* two other classifications have been included, that is, that of Lauren, predominantly used in middle and northern Europe, and that of Ming. Stomach cancer is divided into two types, intestinal and diffuse, according to the Lauren classification, which has proven useful for epidemiologic purposes and clinical planning of therapy. Curative resections are more frequently possible in intestinal carcinoma. The diffuse type of carcinoma is generally more advanced in stage, so it carries a worse prognosis. The two types are possibly different in etiology.

NATURAL HISTORY AND SPREAD

Adenocarcinoma of the stomach progresses by continuity, reaching its maximum in linitis plastica, a widespread scirrhous infiltration of the gastric wall, producing a rigid structure.

In more advanced cases the tumor invades adjacent organs, particularly the omentum, liver, pancreas, transverse mesocolon, and colon, and, by transperitoneal spread, the pouch of Douglas (Blumer's rectal shelf). There is an affinity for ovarian metastases, which are often bilateral (Krukenberg's tumor), and with locally advanced disease there is often serous and serosanguinous ascites from extensive peritoneal and omental involvement.

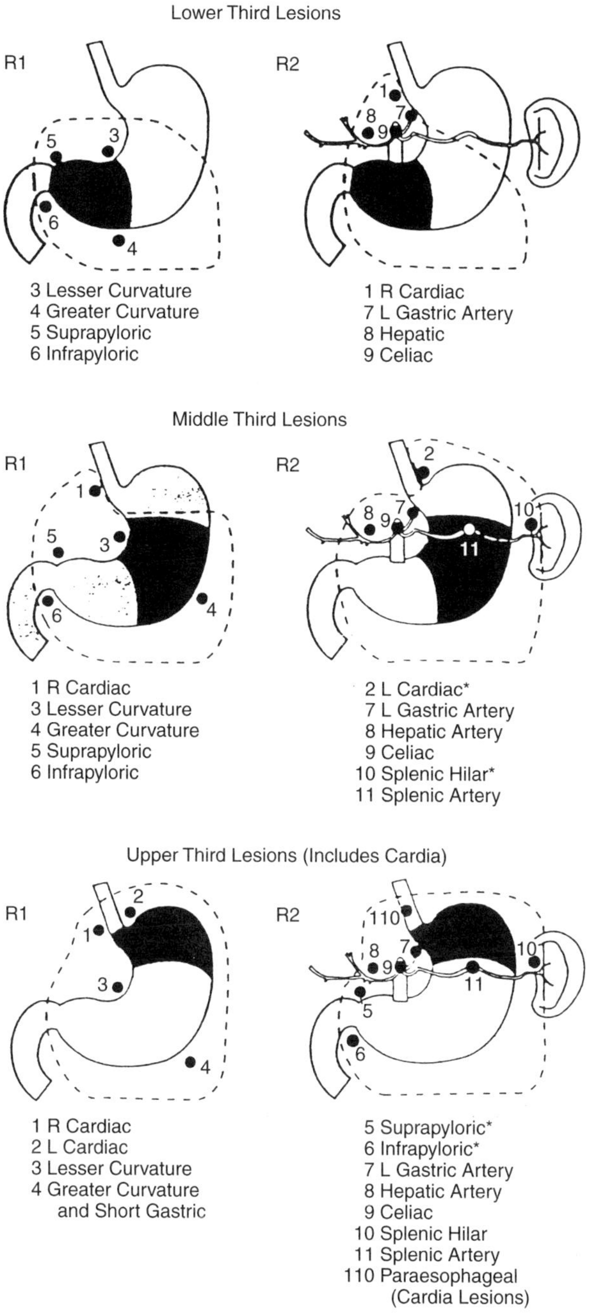

Lower Third Lesions

R1

5 3

6

4

3 Lesser Curvature
4 Greater Curvature
5 Suprapyloric
6 Infrapyloric

R2

1
8 7
9

1 R Cardiac
7 L Gastric Artery
8 Hepatic
9 Celiac

Middle Third Lesions

R1

1

5 3

6

4

1 R Cardiac
3 Lesser Curvature
4 Greater Curvature
5 Suprapyloric
6 Infrapyloric

R2

2

8 7
9   10

11

2 L Cardiac*
7 L Gastric Artery
8 Hepatic Artery
9 Celiac
10 Splenic Hilar*
11 Splenic Artery

Upper Third Lesions (Includes Cardia)

R1

2
1

3

4

1 R Cardiac
2 L Cardiac
3 Lesser Curvature
4 Greater Curvature
  and Short Gastric

R2

110

8 7
9   10

11

5

6

5 Suprapyloric*
6 Infrapyloric*
7 L Gastric Artery
8 Hepatic Artery
9 Celiac
10 Splenic Hilar
11 Splenic Artery
110 Paraesophageal
    (Cardia Lesions)

FIGURE 22.3. Scope of gastric lymphadenectomy as practiced in Japan and as currently being adapted in some United States cancer centers. **(Top)** Lower-third lesions. **(Middle)** Middle-third lesions. **(Bottom)** Upper-third lesions (including cardia). D, Scope of lymphadenectomy (*broken line*). *Asterisks* indicate optional lesions. To qualify as D2, all D1-designated nodes and most D2-designated nodes must be removed. (From Smith et al. 1991. Reprinted with permission from the American Medical Association.)

Lymphatic spread occurs along the gastric vessels to the origin of the celiac axis and through the thoracic duct to the left supraclavicular nodes (Virchow's node). Studies of surgical specimens after total or extended gastrectomies have demonstrated that the nodes of the splenic hilum and those along the body and the tail of the pancreas are also frequently involved. Extensive Japanese studies have shown that there are primary, secondary, and tertiary echelons of nodal metastasis, the exact locations of which vary according to whether the primary tumor lies in the upper, middle, or lower third of the stomach (Fig. 22.3). Distant metastases occur via the portal system primarily to the liver, but also to the lungs, bone marrow, and occasionally skin.

SIGNS AND SYMPTOMS

Symptoms or signs of early gastric cancer are vague and nonspecific. They may mimic symptoms of benign gastric ulcer disease and may either be ignored by the patient or treated medically without further evaluation. The first symptoms are epigastric discomfort, fullness, pain, and unexplained indigestion. Common signs are epigastric mass, weight loss, and an enlarged liver. Dysphagia (in the patient with cancer at the cardia) and vomiting (in the patient with pyloric or prepyloric cancer) may be present at an early stage.

Cancers of the fundus usually have few symptoms and are often missed on radiologic examination (even when the patient is tilted head down to force the barium into the fundus) or on gastroscopy. Following local progression of the disease, obstruction, gastric hemorrhage, and perforation may occur, requiring urgent treatment.

DIAGNOSIS AND STAGING

Double-contrast upper gastrointestinal barium swallow radiography (GI series), fluoroscopy, and endoscopy with multiple biopsies and gastric brushing for cytology are the usual studies that confirm diagnosis. Cytology will pick up some lesions missed by biopsy. In Japan, experienced radiologists using fluoroscopy can be 90% to 95% accurate in diagnosing early gastric carcinoma. If biopsy and cytology studies are nondiagnostic and clinical suspicion for cancer is high, repeat biopsies are necessary.

In Korea, the tumor is considered to be resectable if on a GI series the stomach can be moved more than one vertebral space between the upright and the supine position. If the movability is less than half a vertebral space up and down, then the tumor is considered to be unresectable. Although significant understaging as well as overstaging can occur, ultrasonography and computerized tomography (CT) scans can also be used to help determine the resectability of the tumor, especially when liver metastasis or pancreatic invasion is suspected. Recently endoscopic ultrasound has been used to determine the depth of cancer invasion and enlargement of peri-

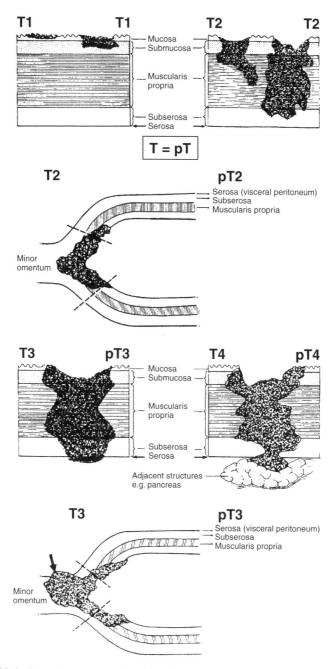

FIGURE 22.4. Stomach cancer staging. N staging was changed in new TNM classification, 1997. (From the *TNM Atlas. Illustrated Guide to the TNM/pTNM Classification of Malignant Tumours*, 3rd edition, 2nd rev., UICC, Springer-Verlag, 1992.)

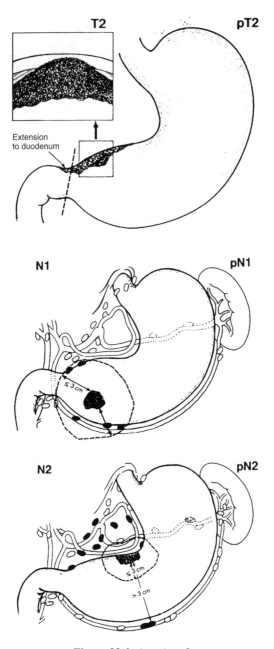

Figure 22.4. (*continued*)

TABLE 22.1. Some Differences in Gastric Cancer in Western and Asian Populations

Features	Western	Asian
Incidence	10/100,000	90–100/100,000
"Curative" resection	20%–30% of all cases	70% of all cases
"Cures"	10%	40%–50% of all cases
		80%–90% of early gastric cancer
Early gastric cancer	4%–7%	30%–60%[a]

[a]With an incidence of 1/1000, the Japanese feel justified in mass screening and therefore find "early gastric cancer" in 30%–60% of all cases. This translates into a much higher rate of "curative" resections and of cures.

gastric nodes. Diagnostic laparoscopy with ultrasound are being attempted to reduce useless laparotomy especially in advanced cancer.

The Japanese have used screening procedures extensively, especially double-contrast radiography, in certain high-risk populations, so that today 30% to 60% of all cases in Japan fall into this category (Table 22.1). Left alone, patients with early gastric cancer (EGC) may develop advanced cancer. Following the Japanese lead, Western investigators are now identifying an increasing fraction of patients with EGC; in the United States about 4% to 7% of gastric cancers are EGC.

The use of molecular biologic techniques may provide a new approach to cancer diagnosis in the next decade.

Since 1982, UICC staging of gastric cancer has been changed several times and showed the progressive worsening of prognosis with lymph node involvement. The 1992 UICC TNM system (Fig. 22.4) combines the important elements in staging. The two elements critically important in prognosis are the depth of penetration of the tumor through the stomach wall and the involvement by the cancer of increasing echelons of lymph nodes (primary drainage nodes, secondary, and tertiary). This is a topographic system and the primary drainage nodes (i.e., with 3 cm) are different for different parts of the stomach. In 1997, however, the TNM system (Table 22.2) adopted a numeric classification in regional lymph nodes metastasis status. This classification is rather simple compared to prior classifications. So, if this new staging system is used universally, better comparisons of results should help clinical researchers in deciding which treatments are most effective for each stage of stomach cancer.

TREATMENT

Surgery

Radical surgery, usually subtotal gastrectomy, is the only curative treatment for stomach cancer. When adjacent organs are involved, extended surgery is appropriate and may be curative if all disease can be removed. To date, adjuvant radiation and/or chemotherapy have minimal, if any, favorable impact on survival. For 25 years,

TABLE 22.2. TNM Clinical Classification for Stomach Cancer, 1997

T—Primary Tumor

TX	Primary tumor cannot be assessed.
T0	No evidence of primary tumor
Tis	Carcinoma in situ: intraepithelial tumor without invasion of the lamina propria
T1	Tumor invades lamina propria or submucosa.
T2	Tumor invades muscularis propria or subserosa.[a]
T3	Tumor penetrates serosa (Visceral peritoneum) without invasion of adjacent structures.[a–c]
T4	Tumor invades adjacent structures.[a–c]

N—Regional Lymph Nodes

NX	Regional lymph nodes cannot be assessed.
N0	No regional lymph node metastasis
N1	Metastasis in 1 to 6 regional lymph nodes
N2	Metastasis in 7 to 15 regional lymph nodes
N3	Metastasis in more than 15 regional lymph nodes

M—Distant Metastasis

MX	Distant metastasis cannot be assessed.
M0	No distant metastasis
M1	Distant metastasis

[a] A tumor may penetrate muscularis propria with extension into the gastrocolic or gastrohepatic ligaments or the greater and lesser omentum without perforation of the visceral peritoneum covering these structures. In this case, the tumor is classified as T2. If there is perforation of the visceral peritoneum covering the gastric ligaments or omenta, the tumor is classified as T3.

[b] The adjacent structures of the stomach are the spleen, transverse colon, liver, diaphragm, pancreas, abdominal wall, adrenal gland, kidney, small intestine, and retroperitoneum.

[c] Intramural extension to the duodenum or esophagus is classified by the depth of greatestb invasion in any of these sites including stomach.

United States surgeons have been reluctant to perform total gastrectomies unless it was absolutely necessary to resect gross disease, and they have had limited enthusiasm for the extensive lymph node dissection advocated by the Japanese. However, recent American reports have shown some improvement in mortality, morbidity, and survival with Japanese approaches, and this is leading to reevaluation of the concepts of optimal surgery along with radical systematic lymph node dissection.

Japanese studies show that the primary lymph node drainage of the stomach is different for each of the three thirds of the stomach and that there are distinct secondary and tertiary levels of lymph node drainage (Fig. 22.3). Node dissections must include at least the secondary level of nodes (in addition to the primary level) and the tertiary levels of nodes if there is evidence of tumor involvement in the secondary level. Japanese and Korean surgeons report a 5-year survival of 60% for patients with perigastric node involvement; only 17% of such patients in the West are reported to have similar survival. The concepts of identifying the likely areas of involvement by tumor and designing appropriate operations to encompass these areas seem valid.

It is uncertain whether it is appropriate to compare Japanese and Korean experience with that in the West. Japanese and Koreans are rather small in stature and thin, which makes the technical aspects of this surgery less complicated. The very large number of patients operated upon using standardized operative protocols give Far Eastern surgeons much more surgical experience.

We have shown that protruding mucosal lesions less than 2 cm in diameter and flat to depressed well-differentiated lesions less than 1 cm in diameter without ulceration have no lymph node metastasis. Thus limited surgeries such as endoscopic mucosal resection and laparoscopic resection can be alternative therapeutic options for these cases. But preoperative confirmation of depth of invasion, lymph node metastasis, and histologic differentiation are required prior to the limited surgery.

For poor-risk patients who have EGC limited to the mucosa, endoscopic laser therapy and careful follow-up can yield good results.

Radiation

The tolerance of the normal stomach and bowel to radiation is so low that external-beam radiation therapy has little or no value as a primary treatment for gastric cancer. Intraoperative radiation therapy (IORT) or IORT combined with postoperative radiation in tolerable doses may increase survival, but definitive results have not yet been shown. The rationale for continued evaluation of IORT is that only 10% of patients with gastric cancer are cured, and locoregional recurrence is a significant factor in the 90% of patients who die of the disease. It makes sense to try IORT to the tumor bed after gastric resection, with uninvolved sensitive tissues—such as bowel—pushed outside the field of radiation.

Chemotherapy

In disseminated or residual disease after resection, a number of drugs may give a temporary "response," that is, some reduction in the size of the tumor for a limited time. A complete response is rare and usually also temporary. Drugs with some activity against gastric cancer include 5-fluorourcil (5-FU), Adriamycin (doxorubicin hydrochloride), mitomycin C, the nitrosoureas, cisplatin, and methotrexate. Commonly used combinations are 5-FU, Adrimycin, and methotrexate or mitomycin C. Because of significant toxicity and little evidence for improved survival, no drug regimen to date has become standard therapy.

The experience with preoperative (neoadjuvant) chemotherapy is still limited to a few trials in patients with either clinically unresectable tumors or with locally advanced disease. The aim of preoperative chemotherapy is to achieve a downstaging of the gastric carcinoma which would allow complete local tumor resection. The aggressive chemotherapy required to achieve this aim, however, is associated with a substantial risk. In one study, sufficient tumor reduction was induced to enable a subsequent radical gastrectomy in one third of patients with initially unresectable gastric cancer, especially those with extensive lymphatic spread. A prospective randomized study is necessary to confirm the clinical benefit of this treatment.

Immunochemosurgery

Postoperative immunotherapy alone is not yet a single treatment modality. Simultaneous immunotherapy and chemotherapy showed marked improvement of 5-year survival rate. Immunochemosurgery, real radical curative surgery followed by early postoperative immunochemotherapy, needs more study. In Korea, a randomized study with 330 cases and a retrospective study of 8544 cases showed that immunotherapy (from the 4th to 5th postoperative day) and chemotherapy (from the 8th to 10th postoperative day) improved 5-year survival rates (24.4% for surgery alone, 29.8% in postoperative chemotherapy vs. 45.3% in the immunochemosurgery group) (Fig. 22.5).

Palliative Therapy

Palliation of stomach cancer falls into three general categories: palliation of distressing symptoms, prevention of symptoms that would develop without treatment, and prolongation of useful, comfortable life.

Relief of obstruction at the esophagogastric junction or pylorus can be accomplished by resection or bypass. Endoscopic intraluminal resection of obstructing lesions with laser therapy offers another approach. Patients with gastric hemorrhage or perforation usually require resection if possible. Pain can also sometimes be helped by resection. Radiation and/or chemotherapy may possibly extend survival in a few

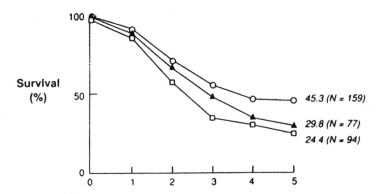

FIGURE 22.5. Survival curves for immunochemosurgery group (○), surgery and postoperative chemotherapy group (▲), and surgery-only group (□) in 330 cases of stage III stomach cancer in a randomized study (1981–1985). The immunochemosurgery treatment included immunotherapy with OK432 (a *Streptococcus pyogenes* preparation) and chemotherapy with mitomycin C and 5-fluorouracil (5-FU) for 2 years after curative surgery. Surgery and chemotherapy treatment was with mitomycin C and 5-FU for 2 years postoperatively. Survival for the 159 patients treated with immunochemosurgery (*top line*) was significantly better than that for the others. (Adapted from Kim et al. 1992.)

cases, but convincing documentation of such is difficult. A response does not necessarily translate into patient benefit when the toxicity of the therapy is taken into account.

PROGNOSIS AND FOLLOW-UP

In Asian countries the operability and resectability of stomach cancer have increased markedly over the past few decades and the morbidity and mortality from surgery have decreased significantly to about 5% to 10% and 1% to 5%, respectively. Patient status-related factors (age, sex, preoperative nutritional status, preoperative immune status); treatment-related factors (R category, type of operation, extent of lymph node dissection, postoperative adjuvant therapy); and pathology-related factors (location, size, Borrmann type, histologic differentiation, Lauren's classification, depth of invasion, number of involved lymph nodes, ratio of involved lymph nodes to resected lymph nodes, distant metastasis, perineural invasion, lymphatic invasion, vascular invasion) have a prognostic significance. Among them, the most important prognostic factors are R category, ratio of involved lymph nodes to resected lymph nodes, and depth of invasion of the tumor. The prognosis of patients may be improved by a complete resection of the primary tumor and its lymphatic drainage, resulting in a UICC-R0 resection. In addition, a detailed preoperative risk analysis and identification of high-risk patients and meticulous attention to the technical details of the surgical procedures to reduce the frequency of postoperative complications may improve the prognosis.

The 5-year survival rate of patients with early gastric cancer can be more than 90%. The survival of patients who have had "curative resection" is about 30%. Overall, the 5-year survival rate of patients with gastric cancer is about 10% in Western countries and 40% in Japan and Korea. There appears to be an increase in recurrences in the gastric remnant after 20 years of follow-up.

Follow-up studies have shown that a significant number of patients with recurrences are found still to be "localized" and potentially treatable. These so-called patterns of failure studies suggest that more extensive operations initially might have prevented some of these recurrences and that further treatment (surgery, radiotherapy, chemotherapy) might be of benefit.

The prevalence of gastric remnant cancer in the literatures varies between 0.8% and 8.9% of patients who undergo gastric operation for gastric cancer, so periodic endoscopic follow-up after gastric resection is very important.

PREVENTION

Based on epidemiologic findings, recommendations for primary prevention of gastric cancer include the avoidance or reduced consumption of foods that are salty, highly spiced, or excessively hot or smoked and cigarette smoking, and the increased consumption of green and yellow vegetables and fruits. Lifestyle in childhood and adolescence is one of the most important determinants for the effective prevention of gastric cancer. So strategy for the prevention of gastric cancer should begin in childhood and in adolescence. Mass screening programs for gastric cancer are now considered to be effective, as they identify a high percentage of early cancers, and there is thus the possibility of a high cure rate. Investigations into the pathogenesis and molecular genetics of the disease are ongoing and may yield clinically applicable strategies in the near future.

FURTHER READING

Blot WJ, Devesa SS, Kneller RW, et al. (1991) Rising incidence of adenocarcinoma of the esophagus and gastric cardia. *JAMA* 265:1287–1292.

Correa P (1992) Human gastric carcinogenesis: A multistep and multifactorial process. First American Cancer Society Award lecture on cancer epidemiology. *Cancer Res* 52:6735–6740.

Greenwald P, Stern HR (1992) Role of biology and prevention in aerodigestive tract cancers. *J Natl Cancer Inst Monogr* 13:3–14.

Japanese Research Society for Gastric Cancer (1981) General rules for the gastric cancer study in surgery and pathology. I. Clinical classification. *Jpn J Surg* 11:127–139.

Kim JP, Kwon OJ, Oh ST, Yang HK (1992) Result of surgery on 6589 gastric cancer patients and immunochemosurgery as the best treatment of advanced gastric cancer. *Ann Surg* 216:269–279.

Kim JP, Lee JH, Kim SJ, Yu HJ, Yang HK (1998) Clinicopathologic characteristics and prognostic factors in 10,783 patients with gastric cancer. *Gastric Cancer* 1:125–133.

Korenaga D, Tsujitani S, Haraguchyi M, et al. (1988) Long-term survival in Japanese patients with far advanced carcinoma of the stomach. *World J Surg* 12:236–239.

Maruyama K, Gunven P, Okabayashi K, et al. (1989) Lymph node metastases of gastric cancer: General pattern in 1931 patients. *Ann Surg* 210:596–602.

Nishi M, Ichikawa H, Nakajima T, Maruyama K, Tahara E (1993) *Gastric Cancer*. Springer-Verlag, Tokyo.

Smith J, Shiu MH, Kelsey L, et al. (1991) Morbidity of radical lymphadenectomy in the curative resection of gastric carcinoma. *Arch Surg* 126:1469–1473.

Wanebo HJ, Kennedy BJ, Osteen R, et al. (1993) Cancer of the stomach—a patient case study by the American College of Surgeons. *Ann Surg* 218:583–592.

CHAPTER 23

CANCER OF THE PANCREAS

DOUGLAS B. EVANS, ROBERT A. WOLFF, and JAMES L. ABBRUZZESE

The University of Texas M.D. Anderson Cancer Center
Houston, TX 77030, USA

Cancer of the exocrine pancreas continues to be a major unsolved health problem, causing approximately 27,000 deaths per year in the United States and 50,000 deaths per year in Europe (excluding the former USSR). Because of difficulties in diagnosis, the aggressiveness of pancreatic cancers, and the lack of effective systemic therapies, only 1% to 4% of patients with adenocarcinoma of the pancreas will be alive 5 years after diagnosis. Thus, incidence rates are virtually identical to mortality rates. In the United States in 1997, pancreatic cancer was the fifth leading cause of adult deaths from cancer (after lung, colorectal, breast, and prostate cancers) and was responsible for close to 5% of all cancer-related deaths.

ETIOLOGIC FACTORS

Recent investigations have identified a number of factors that may contribute to the pathogenesis of pancreatic cancer. A number of important environmental risk factors have been investigated for their role in the etiology of pancreatic cancer. Cigarette smoking is the most firmly established risk factor associated with pancreatic cancer. Pancreatic malignancies can be induced in animals through long-term administration of tobacco-specific N-nitrosamines or by parenteral administration of other N-nitroso compounds. These carcinogens are metabolized to electrophiles that readily react with DNA, leading to miscoding and activation of specific oncogenes such as K-ras. Numerous case-control and cohort studies have reported an increased risk of pancreatic cancer for smokers in both the United States and Europe, and current estimates suggest that approximately 30% of pancreatic cancer cases are due to

Manual of Clinical Oncology, 7th edition, Edited by Raphael E. Pollock
ISBN 0-471-23828-7, pages 453–475. Copyright © 1999 Wiley-Liss, Inc.

cigarette smoking. Recent studies that have explored the dose–response relationship have shown that the risk of pancreatic cancer increases as the amount and duration of smoking increase and that long-term smoking cessation (>10 years) reduces risk by approximately 30% relative to the risk of current smokers. Application of molecular epidemiologic techniques that are being developed for lung cancer may provide greater specificity in linking tobacco exposure with the development of pancreatic cancer and may facilitate the study of chemopreventive strategies.

Over the past 10 years, numerous dietary factors have been implicated in pancreatic cancer development. Generally, high intakes of fat or meat increase risk, and diets high in fruits and vegetables reduce risk. These clinical observations are supported by laboratory studies in animal models in which high-fat and high-cholesterol diets have been shown to promote pancreatic carcinogenesis. Decreased rates for pancreatic cancer have been associated with high consumption of vegetables, citrus fruits, fiber, and vitamin C. The association of diets high in citrus with a reduced risk of pancreatic cancer is particularly interesting given the recent observation that limonene, a natural product found in citrus fruits, is a potent inhibitor of the K-*ras* oncoprotein.

Data regarding the effect of coffee consumption and excessive alcohol consumption appear conflicting. For each of these factors, a few studies have suggested an increased risk of pancreatic cancer, but the majority of studies conducted over the past 10 years have failed to consistently demonstrate such a risk. In some cases, significant methodologic problems may have confounded interpretation of the data, leading to erroneous conclusions.

An association between pancreatitis and an increased risk of pancreatic cancer has long been suspected, although the magnitude of the risk remains uncertain. Clinical studies have suggested that chronic forms of pancreatitis, particularly those accompanied by pancreatic calcifications, were most closely associated with the subsequent development of pancreatic cancer. Calculation of a general estimate of population-attributable risk has suggested that chronic pancreatitis may explain as many as 5% of pancreatic cancer cases. Pathologic examination of lesions along the pancreatic duct have revealed the spectrum of mucous cell hyperplasias (papillary and nonpapillary hyperplastic lesions and atypical hyperplastic lesions) in patients with chronic pancreatitis and patients with pancreatic cancer. The recent report of the identification of mutations in the K-*ras* oncogene, a mutation found almost universally in established pancreatic cancers, in regions of mucous cell hyperplasia in patients with chronic pancreatitis provides the first molecular link between chronic inflammation and the initiation of multistep pancreatic carcinogenesis.

The recent emergence of the importance of inherited genetic abnormalities in gastrointestinal tract neoplasia has led to closer investigation of the potential role for heritable factors in pancreatic cancer. Case reports and formal epidemiologic studies have suggested the possibility of familial aggregations of pancreatic cancer outside the context of these rare familial syndromes. One case-control study estimated that 3% of pancreatic cancers had a hereditary origin. Evaluation of approximately 30 extended families with presumed familial pancreatic cancer has suggested that transmission is consistent with an autosomal dominant pattern. The age at onset, tumor histopathology, male preponderance, and overall survival of persons affected by pancreatic cancer in these families are reported to be similar to those of persons with pancreatic cancer in the general population. Continued study of these patients and their families may provide insight into the critical molecular genetic abnormalities leading to familial pancreatic cancer. Familial genetic abnormalities may then provide insight into the process of pancreatic carcinogenesis for patients with sporadic pancreatic cancer and provide opportunities for early detection and chemoprevention.

MOLECULAR PATHOGENESIS

Attempts to identify premalignant ductal lesions of the pancreas in humans have been limited to autopsy studies, which have produced intriguing but inconclusive results indicating a possible stepwise progression of ductal dysplasia to malignancy. A spectrum of histopathologic changes in proliferating ductal epithelium can be identified, from nonpapillary ductal hyperplasia to papillary hyperplasia, atypical papillary hyperplasia, and carcinoma in situ. The identification of mutated K-*ras* DNA in the majority of patients with invasive pancreatic cancer has provided a possible tool with which these hyperproliferative states can be assessed for their malignant potential based on the frequency of K-*ras* mutations. It may be possible to capitalize on the evolving understanding of the early molecular events that characterize exocrine pancreatic carcinogenesis to develop an effective means of detecting the disease at an early, potentially curable point in its natural history. For example, detection of mutated K-*ras* in bile or pancreatic ductal secretions could suggest the presence of an underlying pancreatic carcinoma. Use of the polymerase chain reaction would allow amplification and detection of extremely small amounts of mutated K-*ras* DNA and, with application of appropriate screening strategies, might identify small, minimally invasive carcinomas, thereby increasing the number of patients able to undergo curative surgical resection or other interventions.

Studies using archival human pancreatic tumor tissue and human pancreatic cancer cell lines have identified an increasing number of characteristic genetic abnormalities. These studies have revealed specific point mutations at codon 12 of the K-*ras* oncogene in 75% to 90% of pancreatic adenocarcinoma specimens. The ras protein is an important signal-transduction mediator for receptor protein tyrosine kinases. Signaling is initiated by the recruitment of guanine nucleotide exchange proteins promoting hydrolysis of GTP to GDP. The *ras* gene bound to GTP is maintained in an active configuration that triggers other enzymatic second messengers leading to nuclear signals resulting in cellular division and proliferation. The mutated *ras* oncogene is not able to convert GTP to inactive GDP, resulting in a constitutively active ras protein product, unregulated cellular proliferation signals, and susceptability to transformation. The K-*ras* mutation in pancreatic carcinogenesis is proposed to be an early event in pancreatic tumor progression.

Additional genetic alterations have been described in human pancreatic cancer, appropriately termed Deleted in Pancreatic Cancer (DPC). These candidate tumor suppressor genes include *DPC-1/2* on chromosome 13q12 (the region of the *BRCA-2* gene), *DPC-3 (p16/MTS-1)* on chromosome 9q21, and *DPC-4* on chromosome 18q21.1. The p16 protein belongs to a class of cyclin-dependent kinase (CDK)-inhibitory proteins (including *p21/WAF1/Cip1*). The p16 protein inhibits the cyclin D/CdK-4 complex which normally acts to phosphorylate the RB protein. Phosphorylation of RB results in the transcription of genes that promote cell cycle progression. Inactivation of *p16* could therefore lead to unregulated cell growth. Allelic deletions involving *p16* were found in 85% of human pancreatic xenographs. *DPC-4* may function as a transcription factor in the transforming growth factor-β (TGF-β) receptor-mediated signal transduction pathway. A functional role for *DPC-4* was suggested by its peptide sequence, which is similar to those of the *Drosophila melanogaster* Mad protein and the *Caenorhabditis elegans* Mad homologues sma-2, sma-3, and sma-4. Mad proteins have been linked to the TGF-β superfamily of cytokines that regulate cell differentiation and are potent inhibitors of cellular proliferation for most normal cells. Based on the frequency with which mutations in K-*ras*, *p53*, *p16*, and *DPC-4* are found, a model of pancreatic carcinogenesis has been suggested whereby the malignant clone evolves from cells driven by a dominant oncogene (K-*ras*) with subsequent deregulation of cell growth precipitated by abnormal cell-cycle control resulting from mutations in *p53*, *p16*, and/or *DPC-4*.

Exactly how the molecular alterations described thus far in human pancreatic cancer interact during pancreatic carcinogenesis is still unclear. However, in vitro studies designed to correct these alterations may lead to novel treatment strategies as well as improve our understanding of the relative roles of these changes in pancreatic cancer.

CLINICAL SIGNS AND SYMPTOMS

The lack of obvious clinical signs and symptoms delays diagnosis in most patients. Jaundice, due to extrahepatic biliary obstruction, is present in approximately 50% of patients at diagnosis and is often associated with a less advanced stage of disease than are other signs or symptoms. Small tumors of the pancreatic head may obstruct the intrapancreatic portion of the bile duct and cause the patient to seek medical attention when the tumor is nonmetastatic and potentially resectable. In the absence of extrahepatic biliary obstruction, few patients present with localized, potentially resectable disease. The pain typical of locally advanced pancreatic cancer is a dull, fairly constant pain of visceral origin localized to the region of the middle and upper back. The pain is due to tumor invasion of the celiac and mesenteric plexus. Vague, intermittent epigastric pain occurs in some patients; its etiology is less clear. Fatigue, weight loss, and anorexia are common even in the absence of mechanical gastric outlet obstruction. Pancreatic exocrine insufficiency due to obstruction of the pancreatic duct may result in malabsorption and steatorrhea. Although malabsorption and mild changes in stool frequency are common, diarrhea occurs infrequently. Glucose intolerance is present in the majority of patients with pancreatic cancer. Although the exact mechanism of hyperglycemia remains unclear, both altered β-cell function and impaired tissue insulin sensitivity are present.

PATTERNS OF TUMOR PROGRESSION

Pancreatic cancer spreads early to regional lymph nodes, and subclinical liver metastases are present in the majority of patients at the time of diagnosis, even when findings from imaging studies are normal. Patient survival depends on the extent of disease and performance status at diagnosis. Extent of disease is best categorized as resectable, locally advanced, or metastatic. Patients who undergo surgical resection for localized nonmetastatic adenocarcinoma of the pancreatic head have a long-term survival rate of approximately 15% to 20% and a median survival of 15 to 24 months. However, disease recurrence following a potentially curative pancreaticoduodenectomy remains common. Local recurrence occurs in up to 85% of patients who undergo surgery alone owing to inaccurate preoperative staging, poor operative technique, and failure to deliver all components of multimodality therapy. With improved local-regional disease control, liver metastases become the dominant form of tumor recurrence and occur in 50% to 70% of patients following potentially curative combined-modality treatment.

Patients with locally advanced, nonmetastatic disease have a median survival of 6 to 10 months. A survival advantage has been demonstrated for patients with locally advanced disease treated with 5-fluorouracil (5-FU)-based chemoradiation compared to no treatment or radiation therapy alone. Patients with metastatic disease have a short survival (3 to 6 months), the length of which depends on the extent of disease and performance status.

STAGING

A standardized system for the clinical and pathologic staging of pancreatic cancer does not currently exist in the United States. The system modified from the American Joint Committee on Cancer (AJCC) and the TNM Committee of the International Union Against Cancer appears in Table 23.1. However, this staging system is most applicable to the pathologic evaluation of resected specimens as accurate measurement of tumor size is difficult to obtain radiographically, and lymph node status cannot be determined without surgical treatment. Pathologic staging can be applied only to patients who undergo pancreatectomy; in all other patients, only clinical staging, based on radiographic examinations, can be done. Treatment and prognosis are based on whether the tumor is potentially resectable, locally advanced, or metastatic, definitions that do not directly correlate with TNM status. For example, both potentially resectable and locally advanced tumors may be stage T4 based on the extent of vascular involvement. As discussed later, isolated involvement of the superior mesenteric vein (SMV) or portal vein in the absence of tumor extension to the superior mesenteric artery (SMA) or celiac axis is amenable to en bloc resection at the time of pancreaticoduodenectomy. In contrast, patients with tumor extension to the SMA or celiac axis are not considered to have potentially resectable disease.

Accurate clinical staging requires high-quality, contrast-enhanced computed tomography (CT) to accurately define the relationship of the tumor to the celiac axis

TABLE 23.1. TNM Staging System

Primary Tumor (T)

TX	Primary tumor cannot be assessed.
T0	No evidence of primary tumor
T1	Tumor limited to the pancreas 2 cm or less in greatest dimension
T2	Tumor limited to the pancreas more than 2 cm in greatest dimension
T3	Tumor extends directly to any of the following: duodenum, bile duct, or peripancreatic tissues.
T4	Tumor extends directly to any of the following: stomach, spleen, colon, or adjacent large vessels.

Regional Lymph Nodes (N)

NX	Regional lymph nodes cannot be assessed.
N0	No regional lymph node metastasis
N1	Regional lymph node metastasis
1a	Single regional lymph node
1b	Multiple regional lymph nodes

Distant Metastasis (M)

MX	Presence of distant metastasis cannot be assessed.
M0	No distant metastasis
M1	Distant metastasis

Stage Grouping

Stage I	T1	N0	M0
	T2	N0	M0
Stage II	T3	N0	M0
Stage III	T1–3	N1	M0
Stage IVA	T4	Any N	M0
Stage IVB	Any T	Any N	M1

From Exocrine pancreas. In: Beahrs OH, Henson DE, Hutter RVP, Kennedy BJ (eds) (1997) *American Joint Committee on Cancer Manual for Staging of Cancer*, 5th edition. JB Lippincott, Philadelphia, pp. 122–123.

and superior mesenteric vessels. The development of objective radiographic criteria for preoperative tumor staging allows physicians to develop detailed treatment plans for their patients, avoid unnecessary laparotomy in patients with locally advanced or metastatic disease, and improve resectability rates. Therefore, a system for clinical staging such as the one illustrated in Table 23.2 is useful to practicing medical oncologists, surgeons, and radiation oncologists.

Similar standardized criteria are needed for the pathologic analysis of pancreaticoduodenectomy specimens to allow accurate interpretation of survival statistics. At The University of Texas M.D. Anderson Cancer Center (MDACC), the surgeon and pathologist evaluate each specimen first by frozen-section examination of the common bile duct transection margin and the pancreatic transection margin. A positive bile duct or pancreatic transection margin is treated with reresection. The retroperitoneal margin is defined as the soft-tissue margin directly adjacent to the proximal

TABLE 23.2. Clinical (Radiographic) Staging of Pancreatic Cancer

Stage: Clinical/Radiologic Criteria

I   Resectable (T1–3, selected T4^a, NX, M0)
       No evidence of tumor extension to the celiac axis or SMA
       Patent SMPV confluence
       No extrapancreatic disease

II   Locally advanced (T4, NX–1, M0)
       Arterial encasement (celiac axis or SMA) or venous occlusion (SMPV)
       No extrapancreatic disease

III Metastatic (T1–4, NX–1, M1)
       Metastatic disease (typically to liver, and peritoneum and occasionally to lung)

SMA, superior mesenteric artery, SMPV, superior mesenteric–portal vein.
^{a}Resectable T4 tumors include those with isolated involvement of the superior mesenteric vein, portal vein, or hepatic artery without tumor extension to the celiac axis or SMA.

3 to 4 cm of the superior mesenteric artery (SMA) (Fig. 23.1), and is evaluated by permanent-section examination of a 2- to 3-mm full-face (en face) section of the margin. The retroperitoneal margin must be taken at the time of tumor resection by the pathologist and the surgeon. Identification of this margin of resection is not possible once the gross examination of the specimen has been completed. The retroperitoneal margin is the most frequent site of margin positivity following pancreaticoduodenectomy and accurate analysis of this margin is critical when performing outcome studies using survival duration or local tumor control as primary study endpoints. Samples of multiple areas of each tumor, including the interface between tumor and adjacent uninvolved tissue, are submitted for paraffin-embedded histologic examination (5 to 10 blocks). Four-microns-thick sections are cut and stained with hematoxylin and eosin. Final pathologic evaluation of permanent sections includes a description of tumor histology and differentiation; gross and microscopic evaluation of the tissue of origin (pancreas, bile duct, ampulla of Vater, or duodenum); and assessments of maximal transverse tumor diameter, lymph node status, and the presence or absence of perineural, lymphatic, and vascular invasion (Table 23.3). When segmental resection of the SMV is required, the area of presumed tumor invasion of the vein wall is serially sectioned and examined in an attempt to discriminate benign fibrous attachment from direct tumor invasion.

The method for classifying subsets of regional lymph nodes in pancreaticoduodenectomy specimens is based on the work of Cubilla. The soft fibrofatty tissue containing regional lymph nodes is divided into six regions as outlined on the anatomic pathology dissection board (Fig. 23.2). If lymph nodes are not identified, fat or other potentially neoplastic tissue is submitted for microscopic examination. Staley and colleagues have demonstrated that the number of lymph nodes identified in the surgical specimen is increased by the use of a standardized system of specimen analysis. The dissection board illustrated in Figure 23.2 provides a simple means of improving lymph node identification and documenting the location of histologically confirmed lymph node metastases. As the use of multimodality treatment strategies for pan-

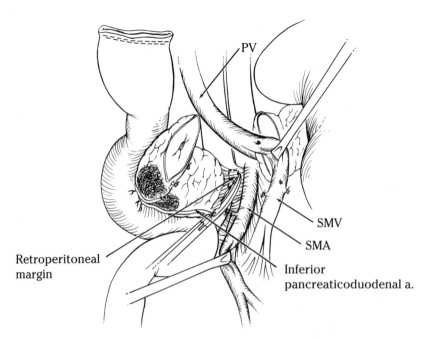

FIGURE 23.1. Illustration of the retroperitonel margin as defined at the time of tumor resection. Medial retraction of the superior mesenteric–portal vein confluence facilitates dissection of the soft tissues adjacent to the lateral wall of the proximal superior mesenteric artery (SMA); this site represents the retroperitoneal margin. PV, portal vein; SMV, superior mesenteric vein. (From Fuhrman GM, Charnsangavej C, Abbruzzese JL, et al. [1994] Thin-section contrast enhanced computed tomography accurately predicts resectability of malignant pancreatic neoplasms. *Am J Surg* 167:106. Used by permission.)

TABLE 23.3. Pathologic Evaluation of the Pancreaticoduodenectomy Specimen

A. Frozen-Section Analysis

   1. Bile duct transection margin

   2. Pancreatic transection margin

B. Permanent-Section Analysis

   1. Retroperitoneal margin

   2. Tumor histopathologic type

   3. Degree of differentiation (tumor histopathologic grade)

   4. Tissue of origin (pancreas, distal bile duct, ampulla of Vater, duodenum)

   5. Maximal transverse tumor diameter

   6. Histologic evidence of invasion:

      Vascular

      Lymphatic

      Perineural

      Superior mesenteric or portal vein (when removed en bloc with the pancreatic head)

   7. Standard pathologic evaluation of lymph node status (anatomic dissection board)

   8. Grade of chemoradiation effect (when applicable)

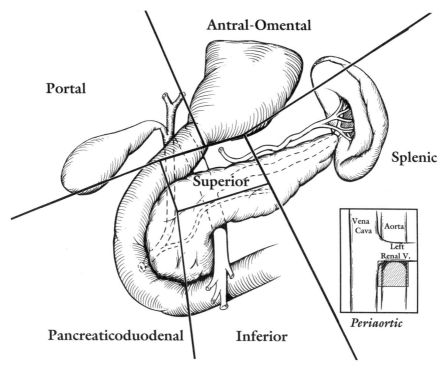

FIGURE 23.2. Illustration of the dissection board used to divide the surgical specimen into regions for lymph node analysis. The periaortic lymph nodes are removed as a separate specimen following completion of the pancreaticoduodenectomy. (From Staley CA, Cleary KA, Abbruzzese JA, et al. [1996] Need for standardized pathologic staging of pancreaticoduodenectomy specimens. *Pancreas* 12:373–380. Used by permission.)

creatic cancer becomes more common, it will be critical to standardize pathologic assessment of tumor specimens.

THE IMPORTANCE OF PRETREATMENT DIAGNOSTIC STUDIES

If the primary tumor cannot be resected completely, surgery (pancreaticoduodenectomy) for pancreatic cancer offers no survival advantage. Therein lies the rationale for accurate preoperative radiographic imaging. Using conventional CT, less than 50% of patients who undergo operation for planned pancreaticoduodenectomy are tumors successfully removed; the remaining patients are found to have unsuspected liver or peritoneal metastases or local tumor extension to the mesenteric vessels. Patients found to have unresectable disease at laparotomy receive no survival benefit from surgery; yet the laparotomy results in a perioperative morbidity rate of 20% to 30%, a mean hospital stay of 14 to 20 days, and a median survival after surgery of only 6 months. Further, in patients whose tumors are resected with positive margins, the survival duration is less than 1 year and no different from the survival duration achieved with palliative chemotherapy and irradiation in patients who have locally advanced, unresectable disease. Therefore, in contrast to the case for selected patients with colorectal or gastric cancer, there are no data in support of palliative (positive-margin) resection for adenocarcinoma of the pancreas.

Our recommended diagnostic schema, based on contrast-enhanced, helical CT, appears in Figure 23.3. A patient is deemed to have locally advanced, unresectable

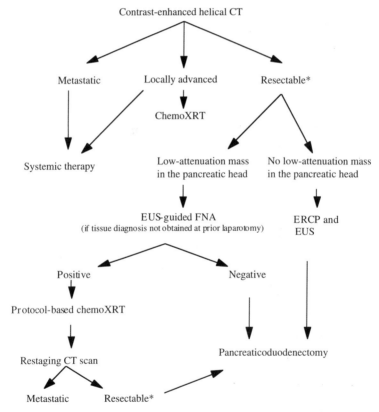

FIGURE 23.3. Management algorithm employed at MDACC for patients with suspected or biopsy proven (from previous laparotomy prior to referral) adenocarcinoma of the pancreatic head. Angiography is performed in patients who have undergone a previous biliary bypass involving the common bile duct to define hepatic arterial anatomy prior to reoperative pancreaticoduodenectomy. Laparoscopy is performed selectively based upon clinical and CT findings. ERCP, endoscopic retrograde cholangiopancreatography; EUS, endoscopic ultrasound; FNA, fine-needle aspiration.

disease when there is clear evidence on CT scans of tumor extension to the SMA or celiac axis or occlusion of the superior mesenteric–portal vein (SMPV) confluence. The accuracy of CT in predicting unresectability is well established; current technology has eliminated the use of laparotomy to assess local tumor resectability. If a low-density mass is not seen on CT scans, patients undergo diagnostic and therapeutic endoscopic retrograde cholangiopancreatography (ERCP) and endoscopic ultrasound (EUS). A malignant obstruction of the intrapancreatic portion of the common bile duct is characterized by the double-duct sign (proximal obstruction of the common bile and pancreatic ducts), which can often be accurately differentiated from choledocholithiasis and the long, smooth tapering seen with chronic pancreatitis. To prevent cholangitis in patients who undergo diagnostic cholangiography in the setting of extrahepatic biliary obstruction, endoscopic stents are routinely placed.

Accurate preoperative assessment of resectability will increase resectability rates and minimize positive-margin resections. A common misconception in pancreatic tumor surgery is that resectability is determined best at laparotomy. In fact, however, resectability is most accurately determined preoperatively by imaging studies, not at the time of "exploratory" laparotomy. Surgeons declare a tumor to be unresectable at the time of laparotomy when unsuspected liver metastases, peritoneal implants, or, most commonly, locally advanced disease is found. The term locally advanced is often poorly defined, leaving the patient, the medical oncologist, and the radiation oncologist without a clear understanding of why the primary tumor was not resected. Improved rates of resectability are achieved when high-quality, contrast-enhanced, helical CT is combined with objective preoperative criteria for resectability. CT criteria for resectability include (1) the absence of extrapancreatic disease, (2) a patent SMPV confluence, and (3) no direct tumor extension to the celiac axis or SMA. Patients whose tumors are deemed unresectable by these radiographic criteria are not considered candidates for a potentially curative resection.

In patients with locally advanced or metastatic disease, operation for palliation is rarely needed. Multiple studies have attempted to compare operative biliary decompression and endoscopic stent placement in patients with jaundice due to obstruction of the intrapancreatic portion of the common bile duct. The higher initial morbidity and mortality rates and longer hospital stay associated with operative biliary bypass are countered by the higher frequency of hospital readmission for recurrent stent occlusion and cholangitis with endoscopic stent placement. Patients with liver metastases or ascites have a median survival of less than 6 months, making endoscopic stent placement an obvious choice. Patients with locally advanced disease treated with chemoradiation have a median survival of 10 to 12 months, with 20% surviving 2 years. Patients with a superior performance status at diagnosis often survive longer, yet it is difficult in most patients to predict, at diagnosis, the tempo of disease progression. Clearly, one would like to avoid operation (with its morbidity and often lengthy recovery period) in patients with rapidly progressive disease. Similarly, one would like to have a durable means of biliary decompression in patients who are expected to survive longer than 6 to 9 months. Therefore, in patients with locally advanced, nonmetastatic disease, it is reasonable to proceed with endoscopic stent placement and reserve operative (open or laparoscopic) biliary bypass for patients who survive long enough to experience recurrent stent occlusion. Innovations in stent construction and the development of the expandable 10-mm metal stent have improved patency rates and are the cause for more widespread application of this technology.

Laparoscopy and angiography have limited value in the diagnostic evaluation of patients with periampullary carcinoma managed according to our suggested diagnostic schema. Laparoscopy has been used in patients with radiographic evidence of localized disease to detect extrapancreatic tumor not seen on CT scans. If extrapancreatic disease is found, laparotomy is avoided, thereby increasing resectability rates. As expected, the more advanced the stage of disease, the greater the yield of positive findings at laparoscopy. If laparoscopy is performed early in the diagnostic sequence, or following poor-quality CT, it will have a higher yield of positive findings. In contrast, if it is used only after high-quality (contrast-enhanced) CT in patients with localized, potentially resectable disease (as defined by objective radiographic criteria), it will have a much lower rate of positive findings. Contrast-enhanced, helical CT can accurately assess vital tumor–vessel relationships, is less invasive and therefore less costly than laparoscopy (which still requires general anesthesia in most centers), and remains the initial study of choice for determining whether a patient has potentially resectable, locally advanced, or metastatic disease. Laparoscopy prevents unnecessary laparotomy in approximately 10% to 15% of patients with presumed localized, potentially resectable pancreatic cancer following state-of-the-art CT. It should be used prior to laparotomy in any patient whose radiographic images or clinical presentation suggests extrapancreatic disease; its routine use prior to laparotomy in all patients with potentially resectable disease remains controversial. Importantly, laparoscopy, angiography, or EUS should not be used in an attempt to compensate for poor-quality CT.

Contrast-enhanced, helical CT has also reduced the role of preoperative angiography. Angiography does not provide the detail that is needed to determine the anatomic relationship between the tumor and the SMA that is provided by high-quality contrast-enhanced CT. Angiography allows contrast enhancement of only the vessel lumen; the surrounding tumor and soft tissue cannot be evaluated. We limit the use of angiography to reoperative cases, in which identification of aberrant hepatic arterial anatomy may prevent iatrogenic injury during portal dissection when there is extensive scarring from a previous biliary procedure.

MULTIMODALITY THERAPY FOR POTENTIALLY RESECTABLE DISEASE

External-beam radiation therapy (EBRT) and concomitant 5-FU chemotherapy (chemoradiation) were shown to prolong survival in patients with locally advanced adenocarcinoma of the pancreas. Those data were the foundation for a prospective randomized study of adjuvant chemoradiation (500 mg/m^2/day of 5-FU for 6 days and 40 Gy of radiation) following pancreaticoduodenectomy conducted by the Gastrointestinal Tumor Study Group (GITSG); that trial also demonstrated a survival advantage from multimodality therapy compared with resection alone. However, owing to a prolonged recovery, 5 (24%) of the 21 patients in the adjuvant chemoradiation arm could not begin chemoradiation until more than 10 weeks after pancreaticoduodenectomy. Further, published studies advocating postoperative adjuvant chemoradiation are prone to selection bias; the patients likely to be considered for protocol entry are those who recover rapidly from surgery and have a good performance status. A similar selection bias is likely in effect when attempts are made to retrospectively compare patients who received postoperative adjuvant chemoradiation with patients who were treated only with pancreaticoduodenectomy. However, recently reported data from Yeo and colleagues at Johns Hopkins University add further support to the use of multimodality therapy. Those investigators reviewed all patients who underwent pancreaticoduodenectomy for adenocarcinoma of the pancreatic head during a 4-year period. One hundred and twenty patients received adjuvant chemoradiation, and 53 underwent pancreaticoduodenectomy alone. Median survival for those receiving adjuvant therapy was 19.5 months compared with 13.5 months for the group who received surgery alone.

Additional data regarding the potential benefit of postoperative adjuvant therapy will come from the European Organization for Research and Treatment of Cancer (EORTC) and the European Study Group for Pancreatic Cancer (ESPCA). The EORTC initiated a study in 1987 comparing adjuvant 5-FU–based chemoradiation following pancreatectomy with surgery alone. Between 1987 and 1995, 218 patients were randomized to receive either chemoradiation or no further treatment following pancreaticoduodenectomy for adenocarcinoma of the pancreas (55%) or periampullary region (45%). Median survival duration, reported in abstract form, was 23.5 months for those receiving adjuvant therapy and 19.1 months for those receiving surgery alone; subset analysis for patients with adenocarcinoma of pancreatic origin has not been reported. Importantly, 22% of those randomized to receive chemoradiation did not receive intended therapy owing to postoperative complications or patient refusal. In 1994, a study was initiated by the ESPCA randomizing patients following pancreatectomy to one of four treatment groups: (1) no adjuvant therapy; (2) 5-FU-based chemoradiation; (3) 5-FU-based chemoradiation followed by systemic 5-FU and leucovorin; and (4) 5-FU and leucovorin without EBRT. Results of the ESPCA study have not been reported.

The risk of delaying adjuvant therapy, combined with small published experiences of successful pancreatic resection following EBRT, prompted many institutions to initiate studies in which chemoradiation was given before pancreaticoduodenectomy for patients with potentially resectable (or locally advanced) adenocarcinoma of the pancreas. The preoperative use of chemoradiation is supported by the following considerations: (1) Radiation therapy is more effective on well-oxygenated cells that have not been devascularized by surgery. (2) Peritoneal tumor cell implantation due to the manipulation of surgery may be prevented by preoperative chemoradiation. (3) The high frequency of positive-margin resections recently reported supports the concern that the retroperitoneal margin of excision, even when negative, may be only a few millimeters; surgery alone may therefore be an inadequate strategy for local tumor control. (4) Patients with disseminated disease evident on restaging studies after chemoradiation will not be subjected to laparotomy. (5) Because radiation therapy and chemotherapy will be given first, delayed postoperative recovery will have no effect on the delivery of multimodality therapy, a frequent problem in adjuvant therapy studies.

In patients who receive chemoradiation prior to surgery, a repeat staging CT scan after chemoradiation reveals liver metastases in 25%. If these patients had undergone pancreaticoduodenectomy at the time of diagnosis, it is probable that the liver metastases would have been subclinical; these patients would therefore have undergone a major surgical procedure only to have liver metastases found soon after surgery. In the MDACC trial, patients who were found to have disease progression at the time of restaging had a median survival of only 6.7 months. The avoidance of a lengthy recovery period and the potential morbidity of pancreaticoduodenectomy in patients with such a short expected survival duration represent a distinct advantage of preoperative over postoperative chemoradiation. When delivering multimodality therapy for any disease, it is beneficial, when possible, to deliver the most toxic therapy last, thereby avoiding morbidity in patients who experience rapid disease progression not amenable to currently available therapies.

The survival advantage for the combination of chemoradiation and surgery compared with surgery alone (Table 23.4) likely results from improved local-regional tumor control. Because of the poor rates of response to 5-FU-based systemic therapy in patients with measurable metastatic disease, it is unlikely that current chemoradiation regimens significantly impact the development of distant metastatic disease.

The first report of standard-fractionation chemoradiation (50.4 Gy over 5.5 weeks with concomitant 5-FU) from MDACC documented gastrointestinal toxic effects (nausea, vomiting, and dehydration) that required hospital admission in one third of patients. A similar experience was recently reported from the multicenter Eastern

TABLE 23.4. Recent Chemoradiation Studies in Patients with Resectable Pancreatic Cancer

First Author (Year)	No. of Patients[a]	EBRT Dose (Gy)	Chemotherapy Agent	Median Survival (mo)
Postop (Adjuvant)				
Kalser (1985)	21	40	5-FU	20
Surgery alone	22	—	—	11
GITSG (1987)	30	40	5-FU	18
Whittington (1991)	28	45–63	5-FU	16
Foo (1993)	29	35–60	5-FU	23
Yeo (1997)	120	>45	5-FU	20
Surgery alone	53	—	—	14
Preop (Neoadjuvant)				
Hoffman (1998)	24	50.4	5-FU,Mito-C	16
Staley (1996)	39	30–50.4	5-FU	19

[a] All patients underwent a pancreatectomy with curative intent.
EBRT, external-beam radiation therapy; 5-FU, 5-fluorouracil; Mito-C, mitomycin C.

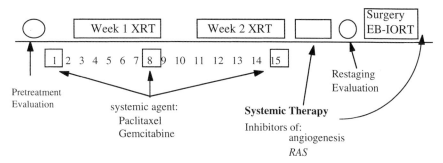

FIGURE 23.4. The evolution of multimodality therapy for patients with potentially resectable adenocarcinoma of the pancreatic head. The future of multimodality therapy for patients with potentially resectable adenocarcinoma of the pancreatic head. Treatment schemas emphasize the importance of minimizing toxicity, and treatment duration, while attempting to improve therapeutic efficacy. Cytotoxicity is enhanced by combining radiation therapy with more potent radiation-sensitizing agents. Systemic therapy is continued after both chemoradiation and surgery with systemic agents of low toxicity directed at specific molecular events involved in pancreatic tumorigenesis (i.e., inhibition of angiogenesis, the use of protease inhibitors [matrix metalloproteinase inhibitors], or inhibition of ras-dependent signal transduction). Abbreviations: EB-IORT, electron-beam intraoperative radiation therapy.

Cooperative Oncology Group (ECOG) trial. The gastrointestinal toxicity of standard-fractionation (1.8 Gy/day; 5.5 weeks) preoperative chemoradiation prompted a change in the treatment program at MDACC to a rapid-fractionation schedule (3.0 Gy/day; 2 weeks) of chemoradiation in an effort to decrease length of treatment and thereby reduce cost, toxicity, and patient inconvenience while attempting to maintain therapeutic efficacy. The evolution of multimodality therapy at MDACC for patients with potentially resectable pancreatic cancer appears in Figure 23.4. Future therapies will capitalize on our expanding understanding of the molecular basis of metastasis, allowing conventional chemoradiation and surgery to be combined with systemic or regional delivery of novel agents that inhibit essential steps in tumor cell growth.

Pancreaticoduodenectomy

Current surgical treatment is based on the procedure of pancreaticoduodenectomy as described in 1935 by Whipple et al. In 1946, Waugh and Clagett from the Mayo Clinic described their modification of the one-stage procedure to its current form. The goals of surgical therapy outlined by Waugh and Clagett have not changed in the past 50 years: (1) there should be reasonable opportunity for cure, (2) the risk of death should not outweigh the prospects for cure, and (3) the patient should be left in as normal a condition as possible.

Recent advances in operative technique, anesthesia, and critical care have resulted in a 30-day in-hospital mortality rate of less than 2% for pancreaticoduodenectomy when performed at major referral centers by experienced surgeons. At such centers, mortality rates remain less than 2% despite the use of multimodality therapy, the frequent need for complex vascular resection and reconstruction, and the referral of many patients following an initial unsuccessful attempt at tumor resection. Recently reported mortality rates from other institutions, including university centers and the Department of Veterans Affairs hospitals, range from 7.8% to more than 10%. Data from New York State have demonstrated that hospitals performing fewer than nine pancreatic resections per year have an unacceptably high perioperative mortality rate (12%). Patient outcome will be optimized and costs minimized by the referral of patients requiring major pancreatic resections for malignant disease to centers with active multidisciplinary treatment programs. Surgical resection, however, benefits only patients who undergo a negative-margin resection. Therefore, it is essential that surgery be done only on patients with localized, potentially resectable pancreatic cancer. In the absence of significant innovations in systemic therapy, the only potential for major improvements in the quality of life of patients with pancreatic cancer lies in our ability to limit surgery-related morbidity to those patients most likely to benefit from surgical intervention (i.e., to avoid laparotomy in patients with unresectable disease).

Pancreaticodudenectomy is performed using a six-step technique that emphasizes complete removal of all tissue to the right of the SMA and celiac axis (Fig. 23.5). Medial retraction of the SMPV confluence facilitates exposure of the SMA, which is then dissected to its origin at the aorta. Total exposure of the SMA avoids iatrogenic injury and ensures direct ligation of the inferior pancreaticoduodenal artery. The soft tissue adjacent to the proximal 3 to 4 cm of the SMA represents the retroperitoneal margin. Margin positivity can result from tumor spread along perineural sheaths and does not always result from direct extension of the primary tumor.

Segmental resection of the SMV or portal vein is performed when the tumor is inseparable from the lateral wall of the vein (Fig. 23.6). Investigators at MDACC

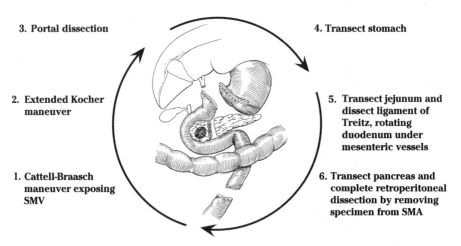

3. Portal dissection

4. Transect stomach

2. Extended Kocher maneuver

5. Transect jejunum and dissect ligament of Treitz, rotating duodenum under mesenteric vessels

1. Cattell-Braasch maneuver exposing SMV

6. Transect pancreas and complete retroperitoneal dissection by removing specimen from SMA

FIGURE 23.5. Six surgical steps of pancreaticoduodenectomy. (From Tyler DS, Evans DB [1994] Reoperative pancreaticoduodenectomy. *Ann Surg* 219:214. Used by permission.)

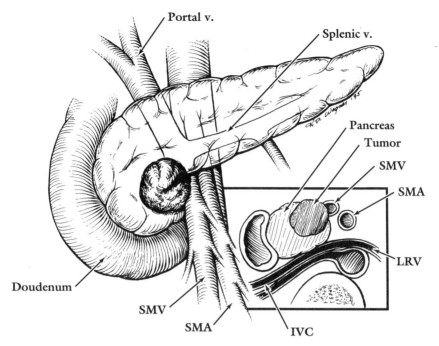

FIGURE 23.6. Illustration of the three-dimensional relationship between a pancreatic head tumor and the superior mesenteric vein (SMV) and artery (SMA). The intimate relationship between the pancreatic head and the lateral and posterior walls of the SMV can result in venous invasion by a pancreatic head carcinoma in the absence of tumor involvement of the SMA (*inset*). IVC, inferior vena cava; LRV, left renal vein. (From Fuhrman GM, Leach SD, Staley CA, et al. [1996] Rationale for en bloc vein resection in the treatment of pancreatic adenocarcinoma adherent to the superior mesenteric–portal vein confluence. *Ann Surg* 223:154–162. Used by permission.)

have demonstrated that invasion of the SMV or portal vein was not associated with histopathologic variables (margin and lymph node positivity), suggesting a poor prognosis. Subsequent data have confirmed that appropriately selected patients who require venous resection at the time of pancreaticoduodenectomy have a survival duration no different than that of patients who undergo pancreaticoduodenectomy without venous resection. Critical to a favorable outcome is the selection of patients (for pancreaticoduodenectomy) who do not have tumor extension to the SMA or celiac axis. Venous involvement in the absence of retroperitoneal tumor extension is a function of tumor location rather than an indicator of aggressive tumor biology. In contrast to previous reports on venous resection, the preferred technique for reconstruction of the SMPV confluence at MDACC involves preservation of the splenic vein–portal vein junction and use of an internal jugular vein interposition graft placed between the SMV and portal vein (Fig. 23.7).

After pancreaticoduodenectomy, gastrointestinal reconstruction is performed in a counterclockwise direction (Fig. 23.8). The transected jejunum is brought through

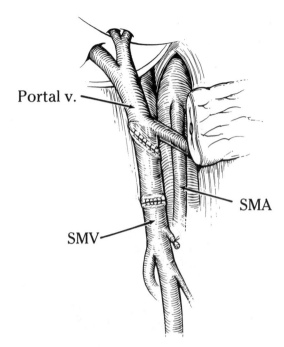

FIGURE 23.7. Illustration of our preferred method of reconstruction of the superior mesenteric vein (SMV) using an internal jugular vein (IJ) interposition graft. The splenic vein–portal vein junction is preserved by tangential excision of the SMV to include a longer segment of the lateral wall of the portal vein. (From Cusack JC, Fuhrman GM, Lee JE, et al. [1994] Management of unsuspected tumor invasion of the superior mesenteric–portal venous confluence at the time of pancreaticoduodenectomy. *Am J Surg* 168:354. Used by permission.)

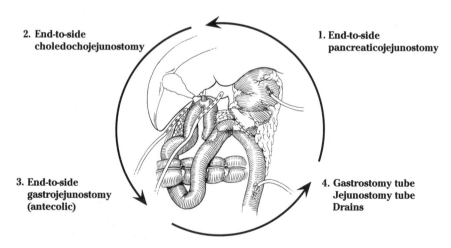

FIGURE 23.8. Four surgical steps of reconstruction following standard pancreaticoduodenectomy. (From Tyler DS, Evans DB [1994] Reoperative pancreaticoduodenectomy. *Ann Surg* 219:214. Used by permission.)

a small incision in the transverse mesocolon to the right or left of the middle colic vessels and a two-layer, end-to-side, duct-to-mucosa pancreaticojejunostomy is performed over a small Silastic stent. A two-layer anastomosis that invaginates the cut end of the pancreas into the jejunum is performed when the pancreatic duct is too small for a primary duct-to-mucosa anastomosis. A single layer biliary anastomosis is then completed, followed by an anticolic, end-to-side gastrojejunostomy constructed in two layers. Gastrostomy and feeding jejunostomy tubes are placed using the Witzel technique, and two closed-suction drains are placed. Delayed gastric emptying is common after standard pancreaticoduodenectomy and may be more frequent with pylorus preservation. The cause is multifactorial but largely due to deinnervation of the upper gastrointestinal tract during resection of the pancreatic head and attached soft tissues and nerves to the right of the SMA. Symptoms of nausea, vomiting, and postprandial fullness resolve in 4 to 12 weeks in virtually all patients. The routine placement of gastrostomy and jejunostomy tubes at the time of surgery avoids needless patient morbidity due to temporary gastric emptying dysfunction. Patients can be discharged while receiving enteral feeding (via jejunostomy tube) and allowed to advance their oral diet as tolerated. In addition, such tube placement prevents the expense and potential complications associated with intravenous hyperalimentation in patients who require prolonged hospitalization because of perioperative or postoperative complications. Poor gastric emptying in the absence of other concomitant intraabdominal pathology should not be the cause of prolonged hospitalization.

TREATMENT OF LOCALLY ADVANCED DISEASE

Patients with clear evidence of encasement of the celiac axis or SMA or occlusion of the SMPV confluence on contrast-enhanced, helical CT do not require laparotomy to confirm that the tumor is unresectable; cytologic confirmation of malignancy can be achieved with fine-needle aspiration performed under the guidance of either EUS or CT. This fundamental advance in pretreatment diagnosis for patients with pancreatic cancer will improve the quality of patient survival and reduce health care costs by avoiding the morbidity and prolonged recovery associated with palliative pancreatic cancer surgery.

A pilot trial of 5-FU and supervoltage radiation therapy in patients with locally advanced adenocarcinoma of the pancreas served as the foundation for a subsequent study of 5-FU-based chemoradiation by the GITSG. All patients were surgically staged; only patients with disease confined to the pancreas and peripancreatic organs, regional lymph nodes, and regional peritoneum were eligible for treatment. The entire area of malignant disease had to be encompassed within a 400-cm^2 area. Radiation therapy was delivered as a split course with 20 Gy given over 2 weeks followed by a 2-week rest. Patients received a total of either 40 or 60 Gy. 5-FU was delivered intravenously at a bolus dose of 500 mg/m^2/day for the first 3 days of each 20 Gy cycle and given weekly (500 mg/m^2) following the completion of chemoradiation. Patients were randomized to receive 40 Gy plus 5-FU, 60 Gy plus 5-FU, or 60

Gy without chemotherapy. Median survival was 10 months in each of the chemoradiation groups and 6 months for patients who received 60 Gy without 5-FU. Additional chemotherapy beyond 5-FU-based chemoradiation increased toxicity without apparent therapeutic benefit.

All patients were entered in the GITSG studies following laparotomy, at which time the disease was deemed unresectable by the operating surgeon. Chemoradiation was reasonably well tolerated following major surgery. Approximately 80% of patients completed chemoradiation, and the two fatal septic events were believed not to be treatment related. The most frequent toxic effects were nausea and vomiting, which were seldom severe. The significant morbidity reported with palliative pancreatic surgery suggests that only patients with a high performance status could have recovered rapidly enough to be eligible for these studies. Thus, although surgical staging made for a more uniform study population, it also introduced significant selection bias: only rapidly recovering patients were considered for treatment. Comparison of future studies to these data must account for this selection bias.

At MDACC, 5-FU–based chemoradiation using prolonged, low-dose, continuous-infusion 5-FU during EBRT has been used for the treatment of advanced pancreatic cancer. Continuous-infusion 5-FU in dosages of 250 to 300 mg/m^2/day for 5 or 7 days/week was given during EBRT employing total doses of 50 to 55 Gy in 5.5 weeks (1.8 Gy/fraction). Treatment was administered in the outpatient setting, and 5-FU was given through a portable pump attached to a percutaneous central venous catheter. Acute side effects included nausea, diarrhea, vomiting, weight loss, fatigue, and hand/foot syndrome, but rarely was leukopenia encountered. The degree of acute toxicity was not related to treatment site, EBRT dose, or 5-FU dose but was associated with the number of days per week of 5-FU infusion. Acute toxicity during 5-FU chemoradiation was decreased by administering 5-FU for 5 days/week rather than 7 days/week. With the 5-day treatment schedule, acute toxicity can be further reduced with the use of enteral nutrition (via jejunostomy tube). The late effects of combined-modality therapy do not appear to be increased compared to those seen with EBRT alone. Paclitaxel and gemcitabine represent two new radiation enhancers that are currently under clinical evaluation.

The increased length of survival for patients treated with chemoradiation is limited largely to patients with higher performance status. Therefore, a program of 5-FU–based chemoradiation is justified in fully ambulatory patients with locally advanced disease who have minimal symptoms. Systemic therapy with gemcitabine also represents a reasonable alternative in these patients. For patients with poor performance status, chemoradiation is probably not indicated. Current pharmacologic and interventional techniques for pain control, including percutaneous injection of alcohol into the celiac plexus, have proven highly successful in patients with pancreatic cancer. Further, adequate pain control improves performance status and quality of life which may translate into increased length of life. The limited therapeutic options available for patients with locally advanced disease and the modest impact of current treatments on survival rates provide the rationale for the entry of patients into trials examining novel systemic agents.

TREATMENT OF METASTATIC AND RECURRENT DISEASE

Most studies of single-agent or combination chemotherapy in patients with advanced adenocarcinoma of the pancreas have documented low response rates and little reproducible impact on patient survival or quality of life. Response rates as high as 15% to 30% occasionally seen in pilot studies of novel agents or combinations have not been reproduced, suggesting that patient selection often accounts for apparent differences between study results. The inherent difficulty in accurately applying bidimensional measurements to pancreatic masses and the problem of interobserver variations in the measurement of metastatic disease may contribute to the poor reproducibility of clinical trials in patients with locally advanced or metastatic pancreatic cancer.

Novel analogues of the topoisomerase I inhibitor camptothecin have undergone limited evaluation in patients with advanced pancreatic cancer. Topotecan administered once daily for 5 days was found ineffective. Irinotecan (CPT-11) was recently evaluated in 34 patients by the EORTC Early Clinical Trials group. Irinotecan was administered intravenously over 30 minutes at a dose of 350 mg/m^2 every 3 weeks; objective partial responses were documented in only three patients, with a median survival for the entire group of 5 months. Despite these discouraging results, the recognized schedule-dependence of these drugs supports further study of topoisomerase I agents using protracted intravenous schedules or daily oral administration.

Gemcitabine (2′,2′-difluorodeoxycytidine, Gemzar) is a deoxycytidine analogue with structural and metabolic similarities to cytarabine. As a prodrug, gemcitabine must be phosphorylated to its active metabolites, gemcitabine diphosphate and gemcitabine triphosphate. In both preclinical and clinical testing, gemcitabine demonstrated activity in solid tumors greater than that of cytarabine. These observations can be potentially explained by the following properties of gemcitabine: (1) it is three to four times more lipophilic than cytarabine, resulting in greater membrane permeability and cellular uptake; (2) it has higher affinity for deoxycytidine kinase; and (3) the intracellular retention of gemcitabine triphosphate is long. Following phase I study, gemcitabine was evaluated in a multicenter trial of 44 patients with advanced pancreatic cancer. Although only five objective responses were documented, the investigators noted frequent subjective symptomatic benefit, often in the absence of an objective tumor response. Based on these observations, two subsequent trials of gemcitabine in patients with advanced pancreatic cancer have been completed. In one randomized trial, gemcitabine was compared to 5-FU in previously untreated patients. Patients treated with gemcitabine achieved modest but statistically significant improvements in response rate and median survival compared to those treated with 5-FU. In addition, more clinically meaningful effects on disease-related symptoms (pain control, performance status, weight gain) were seen with gemcitabine than with 5-FU. Similar effects were documented in patients who were treated with gemcitabine after experiencing disease progression while receiving 5-FU. These results suggest that gemcitabine will become the accepted first-line therapy for patients with advanced pancreatic adenocarcinoma.

Despite the recent encouraging results with gemcitabine, however, median survival for patients with metastatic disease continues to be less than 6 months, with very few patients achieving long-term disease stabilization. Some of the effects attributed to chemotherapy may not be substantially different from what can be achieved with aggressive supportive care alone. Study of novel chemotherapeutic agents based on our improved understanding of the pathobiology of pancreatic cancer represent exciting areas of research. A number of general areas of clinical investigation may yield favorable results including interruption or modulation of growth factors and signal transduction pathways, blockade of the epidermal growth factor (EGF) receptor, inhibition of tyrosine kinase, and chemical inhibition of ras protein function through interruption of posttranslational processing necessary to localize ras proteins to the plasma cell membrane (farnesyl transferase inhibitors). The monoterpene limonene and its more potent metabolite perillyl alcohol decrease farnesylated ras levels, probably through a different mechanism than does lovastatin (which acts via HMG-CoA reductase inhibition). Orally administered perillyl alcohol demonstrated significant in vivo chemotherapeutic activity against pancreatic cancer in a Syrian golden hamster model; this agent is currently in phase I testing in the United States. A second general approach utilizes genetic strategies to inhibit dominant oncogene function. The high frequency with which K-*ras* is altered in exocrine pancreatic cancer and its central function in signal transduction suggest that inhibiting production of this protein could lead to significant growth inhibitory effects. This strategy has been successfully employed in lung adenocarcinoma cells using retroviral constructs coding for K-*ras* antisense RNA. In addition, the evolving ribozyme technologies offer the possibility of improved inhibition compared with traditional antisense approaches.

For patients with metastatic pancreatic cancer who present with a good performance status, treatment with systemic chemotherapy is appropriate. In view of the limited impact of the currently available agents on survival, continued enrollment of patients in phase II trials of new agents or combinations is essential. In the absence of access to a phase II trial, treatment with gemcitabine appears to be the evolving standard. However, it must be recognized that the primary impact of gemcitabine is on quality of life; therefore, continued evaluation of novel agents, especially those targeted against specific molecular events important in the pathogenesis of pancreatic cancer, is crucial. As our understanding of the molecular and biochemical basis of pancreatic cancer expands, we will enter a new era in which treatments are tailored to interact with the specific molecular and biochemical targets thought to be important in the development or maintenance of neoplasia.

FURTHER READING

Burris HA, Moore MJ, Andersen J, et al. (1997) Improvements in survival and clinical benefit with gemcitabine as first-line therapy for patients with advanced pancreas cancer: A randomized trial. *J Clin Oncol* 15:2403–2413.

Evans DB, Abbruzzese JL, Rich TA (1997) Cancer of the pancreas. In: DeVita VT, Hellman S, Rosenberg SA (eds). *Cancer, Principles and Practice of Oncology*, 5th edition. JB Lippincott, Philadelphia, pp. 1054–1087.

Evans DB, Lee JE, Pisters PWT (1997) Pancreaticoduodenectomy (Whipple Operation) and total pancreatectomy for cancer. In: Nyhus LM, Baker RJ, Fischer JF (eds). *Mastery of Surgery*, 3rd edition. Little, Brown, Boston, pp. 1233–1249.

Foo M, Gunderson L, Nagorney D, McLlrath D, van Heerden J, Robinow J, et al. (1993) Patterns of failure in grossly resected pancreatic ductal adenocarcinoma treated with adjuvant irradiation $+/-$ 5 fluorouracil. *Int J Radiat Oncol Biol Phys* 26:483.

Fuhrman GM, Leach SD, Staley CA, et al. (1996) Rationale for en-bloc vein resection in the treatment of pancreatic adenocarcinoma adherent to the superior mesenteric-portal vein confluence. *Ann Surg* 223:154–162.

Gastrointestinal Tumor Study Group (1987) Further evidence of effective adjuvant combined radiation and chemotherapy following curative resection of pancreatic cancer. *Cancer* 59:2006.

Hoffman J, Lipsitz S, Pisansky T, Weese J, Solin L, Benson AB (1998) Phase II trial of preoperative radiation therapy and chemotherapy for patients with localized, resectable adenocarcinoma of the pancreas: An Eastern Cooperative Oncology Group study. *J Clin Oncol* 16:317–323.

Kalser M, Ellenberg S (1985) Pancreatic cancer. Adjuvant combined radiation and chemotherapy following curative resection. *Arch Surg* 120:899.

Leach SD, Lee JE, Charnsangavej C, Cleary KR, Lowy AM, Fenoglio CJ, Pisters PWT, Evans DB (1998) Survival following pancreaticoduodenectomy with resection of the superior mesenteric–portal vein confluence for adenocarcinoma of the pancreatic head. *Brit J Surg* 85:611–617.

Pisters PWT, Abbruzzese JL, Cleary KR, et al. (1997) Pilot study of rapid-fractionation preoperative chemoradiation pancreaticoduodenectomy (PD) and intraoperative radiation therapy (IORT) for resectable pancreatic adenocarcinoma [abstract 16]. In: *Proceedings of the American Society of Clinical Oncology*, p. 1076.

Robinson E, Lee J, Pisters P, Evans D (1996) Reoperative pancreaticoduodenectomy for periampullary carcinoma. *Am J Surg* 172:432–437.

Safran H, King T, Choy H, et al. (1997) Paclitaxel and concurrent radiation for locally advanced pancreatic and gastric cancer: A phase I study. *J Clin Oncol* 15:901.

Spitz FR, Abbruzzese JL, Lee JE, et al. (1997) Preoperative and postoperative chemoradiation strategies in patients treated with pancreaticoduodenectomy for adenocarcinoma of the pancreas. *J Clin Oncol* 15:928–937.

Staley CA, Cleary KA, Abbruzzese JA, et al. (1996) Need for standardized pathologic staging of pancreaticoduodenectomy specimens. *Pancreas* 12:373–380.

Staley C, Lee J, Cleary K, Abbruzzese J, Fenoglio C, Rich T, et al. (1996) Preoperative chemoradiation, pancreaticoduodenectomy, and intraoperative radiation therapy for adenocarcinoma of the pancreatic head. *Am J Surg* 171:118–124.

Yeo CJ, Abrams RA, Grochow LB, et al. (1997) Pancreaticoduodenectomy for pancreatic adenocarcinoma: Postoperative adjuvant chemoradiation improves survival. *Ann Surg* 225:621–636.

CHAPTER 24

CANCER OF THE COLON AND RECTUM

HERMANN KESSLER and JEFFREY W. MILSOM

The Cleveland Clinic Foundation
Department of Colorectal Surgery
9500 Euclid Avenue
Cleveland, OH 44195, USA

EPIDEMIOLOGY

Rates of colorectal cancer vary considerably with geography. This disease is common in the United States, Western Europe, Scandinavia, Australia, and New Zealand and is relatively uncommon in Asia, Africa, and South America. The experience of immigrants suggests an important environmental component to colorectal cancer risk.[1] There were an estimated 138,200 cases of colorectal carcinoma in the United States in 1995, with 55,300 deaths. The lifetime risk of being diagnosed with colorectal cancer in the United States is 6.14% in men and 5.92% in women, and the lifetime risk of dying from this disease is 2.60% in men and 2.65% in women. Colorectal cancer incidence rates increase with age. There has been a progressive improvement in survival from colorectal cancer over the past 20 years. In 1973, the relative survival rate was 45.6%, whereas the rate in 1986 was 61.5%, probably due to improvements in surgical technique, adjuvant chemotherapy, radiotherapy, and early detection. The distribution of cancers has shifted toward the right side of the colon over the past two decades.[1]

Manual of Clinical Oncology, 7th edition, Edited by Raphael E. Pollock
ISBN 0-471-23828-7, pages 477–490. Copyright © 1999 Wiley-Liss, Inc.

ETIOLOGY

There has been more interest in the etiology of colorectal cancer recently, because this disease may provide a particularly good model for the study of interactions of genes and the environment in the etiology of cancer.[2]

Diet

Although the etiology and pathogenesis of colorectal cancer must be perceived as a complex interaction between the genetic make-up of the individual and the environment, experimental evidence suggests a role for dietary factors in the promotion of this disease. Its incidence is greatest in industrialized countries where the per capita consumption of meats, fat, and refined carbohydrates is high.[3]

Inflammatory Bowel Diseases

There is no question that ulcerative colitis predisposes patients to adenocarcinoma, especially when the inflammatory process involves the entire large intestine (pancolitis). Duration of disease greater than 7 to 10 years and onset of colitis at a young age are additional risk factors for development of carcinoma in a patient with ulcerative colitis.[4] The risk for colorectal carcinoma in patients with Crohn's colitis is less pronounced but still significant (4 to 20 times that in the normal population).

Adenomas

Most colorectal carcinomas appear to arise from adenomatous polyps. The best evidence to support the adenoma–carcinoma sequence hypothesis would come from following adenomas over the time until they become malignant. Adenomas are frequently found in association with large carcinomas, although more invasive cancers contain fewer remnants of benign adenomatous tissue. Nowhere has the multistep theory of genetic alterations leading to cancer been more evident than in the molecular biologic work of colorectal adenoma and carcinoma studies. Both share some genetic traits having *ras* gene mutations (adenomas 63%, carcinomas 47%) and allelic loss of chromosome 5 (29%, 36%) and chromosome 18 (47%, 73%).[3]

Genetics

The development of colorectal neoplasia occurs in a series of genetic steps that correspond with the histologic progression from normal colonic epithelium to adenoma to carcinoma. The genetic steps of allelic mutation or loss leading to carcinoma were originally hypothesized by Vogelstein after systematic identification of allelic loss in colorectal cancers and polyps.[5,6] Since the development of this model, the specific genes that reside in the areas of allelic loss have been identified, and their predicted place in the proposed scheme during colorectal carcinogenesis now appears well established.[7] For an adenoma to develop, mutation of one adenomatous polyposis coli (APC) allele on the long arm of chromosome (5q) with subsequent loss of the second APC allele appears to be required. If a K-*ras* mutation on the short arm of chromosome 12 (12p) occurs first, the clonal population develops into a nonneoplastic lesion. If the normal APC proteins are not present, normal growth inhibitory signaling does not occur, permitting the cell to expand clonally into an early adenoma. If one cell in the adenoma acquires another mutation, this time in its K-*ras* proto-oncogene, this mutation allows that cell to expand clonally. This in turn can lead to overgrowth of the original polyp, permitting the adenoma to grow larger. Accumulations of other mutations occur as subclones develop within the mutant APC/K-*ras* clones. These accumulated defects include mutations in the *DCC* (Deleted in Colon Cancer) (chromosome 18q) and *p53* (chromosome 17p) genes. Subsequently loss of heterogeneity (LOH) may occur at the *DCC* locus; when this happens at the *p53* locus, the transition from the benign phenotype to malignancy occurs. These LOH events uncover latent heterozygous mutations at tumor-suppressor gene loci, further abetting neoplastic progression. The consequences are the development of malignancy, invasion, and metastases.[7]

APC Syndromes

*[handwritten: * Analyse mRNA in peripheral blood → find a truncated protein.]*

The APC syndromes include familial adenomatous polyposis (FAP) and Gardner syndrome (autosomal dominant, additional mesenchymal tumors), which account for approximately 1% of all cases of colorectal carcinoma. The APC gene responsible for FAP has been located on the long arm of chromosome 5 (5q), which is a negative regulator of colonic epithelial proliferation. With this autosomal dominant condition patients may develop thousands of adenomatous polyps in the colon. The disease commonly occurs in the second decade of life. The incidence of malignant transformation approaches 100% if left untreated. The mean age at carcinoma diagnosis is approximately 40. However, it may be diagnosed as early as the first decade of life. A blood test for the genetic mutation is now available. The association of familial polyposis and tumors of the central nervous system characterize Turcot's syndrome. Although it is a phenotypic variant of familial polyposis and Gardner's syndrome it is transmitted by an autosomal recessive gene.[8]

HNPCC

[handwritten: Amsterdam Criteria 'Oncology...' pge 109.]

Hereditary nonpolyposis colorectal cancer (HNPCC) is the most frequently occurring hereditary form of colorectal cancer (estimations of up to 10% of all colorectal cancers). It is characterized by an autosomal dominant inherited predisposition to early age at onset (below 45 years) and proximal predominance of colorectal cancer (70% proximal to the splenic flexure). Hemicolectomy or segmental resection, as opposed to subtotal colectomy, is adequate treatment for this syndrome as synchronous and metachronous colorectal carcinomas are very common in the residual large intestine (Lynch syndrome I). The Lynch syndrome II variant additionally shows marked

*DNA mismatch- repair genes ie code for enzymes involved in the correction of errors in replication of DNA.

480 CANCER OF THE COLON AND RECTUM

excess of carcinoma of the endometrium, ovary, small bowel, stomach, pancreas, and transitional cell carcinoma of the ureter and renal pelvis, Meanwhile advances in molecular genetics have implicated the *hMSH-2* gene at chromosome 2p, the *hMLH-* * *1* gene at chromosome 3p, the *PMS-1* gene at chromosome 2p, and the *PMS-2* gene at chromosome 7q in the etiology of HNPCC. Presymptomatic DNA testing for delivering information about the patient's germline status, along with genetic counseling, are mandatory. Prophylactic subtotal colectomy should be discussed as an alternative to continued colonoscopy for patients bearing germline mutations. The cancer family history of such patients has to be taken carefully to detect the disorder and to make the necessary surveillance and treatment options available.[9]

Family History

In addition to the described genetic disorders, a positive family history for colorectal cancer remains an important risk factor for colorectal carcinoma. Individuals with a single first-degree relative with colorectal cancer have about a twofold risk of themselves developing this cancer. When more relatives are affected, the risk is even higher.[1]

SCREENING, EARLY DETECTION, AND PREVENTION

The lives of individuals with colorectal cancers are shortened an average of 13.3 years.[10] Although an effective method of prevention is not available at present for asymptomatic persons at risk, periodic screening may lead to complete removal of precancerous polyps and to the detection of colon cancer at an early stage. In patients with longstanding ulcerative colitis of the entire colon and in FAP either proctocolectomy or colectomy with close follow-up of the rectum prevent colonic cancer formation when carried out regularly. Regarding proposed screening tests, the fecal occult blood test (FOT) has been widely used and seems to be reasonably effective. The incidence of positive results in large screening series is reported to be between 1% and 4%. Approximately 10% to 20% of the positive findings are due to adenomatous polyps, and 5% to 10% result from colorectal cancer.[8] Screening by flexible sigmoidoscopy is associated with a 59% to 80% reduction in the risk of death from cancer located in the part of the colon examined. Double-contrast barium enema and colonoscopy are proven methods of identifying polyps and colorectal cancer but have not been studied as screening tools. The American Gastroenterology Association published an algorithm for colorectal carcinoma screening and surveillance programs according to average and increased risk populations.[11] The efficacy of dietary changes in preventing colorectal cancer by reducing fat and meat consumption and increasing fiber, fruit, and vegetable intake remains to be proved. Aspirin and other nonsteroidal antiinflammatory drugs inhibit carcinogenesis in animal experiments, but a conclusive epidemiologic evidence of their effect is still lacking.[22]

PATHOLOGY/LOCATION

Ninety percent to 95% of all large bowel cancers are adenocarcinomas, the remaining histologic types being squamous cell carcinomas, adenosquamous carcinomas, lymphomas, sarcomas, and carcinoid tumors. Most colonic adenocarcinomas are moderately or well-differentiated tumors. About 20% of adenocarcinomas are poorly differentiated or undifferentiated and are associated with a poorer prognosis. Other factors associated with a poor prognosis include blood vessel infiltration, lymphatic vessel invasion, and absence of a lymphocytic response to the tumor. Using flow cytometry, tumors can be categorized as aneuploid (abnormal DNA content) or diploid (normal DNA content). Patients with aneuploid tumors have been shown to have higher recurrence rates and decreased survival relative to patients with diploid tumors. Forty-five percent of colorectal carcinomas are localized in the rectum, about 30% in the sigmoid colon, 15% in the right or transverse colon, and about 10% in the descending colon.

Spread

The natural progression of colorectal cancer can be determined by three components—local invasion, lymphatic spread, and hematogenous spread. Local growth of an adenocarcinoma is initially characterized by intramural expansion of the tumor into the bowel wall. Lateral invasion into the bowel wall occurs next, usually progressing in a transverse direction rather than longitudinally, thus leading to circumferential involvement of the bowel. There are subgroups of patients with tumors that do *not* invade through the bowel wall who have lymphatic metastases or develop distant disease. In this regard, even patients who are curatively resected for apparently localized colorectal tumors should be viewed as harboring bloodborne metastases. The depth of tumor invasion into the bowel wall (T stage) and involvement of draining lymph nodes (N stage) can predict the risk of developing disseminated disease. The most frequent site of hematogenous spread of colorectal carcinoma is the liver, probably because this is the first capillary network exposed to tumor emboli arriving through the portal system, representing the main venous drainage of the colon and upper rectum. The lower rectum, however, has a bidirectional drainage system—the portal vein by way of the superior rectal vein and the vena cava by way of the middle and inferior rectal veins, respectively. Isolated lung metastases can develop from tumor emboli of lower rectal tumors. Generally the lungs are the second most common sites of metastases from colorectal tumors.[12]

Staging

Dukes described the first practical staging system in 1937 to incorporate the depth of invasion of the primary tumor into the bowel wall and the presence or absence of lymph node metastases. Imperfections of this system, which was strictly confined to rectal tumors lying beneath the peritoneal reflection, resulted in various modifications although this system was fundamentally excellent with regard to depth of bowel wall invasion and presence or absence of nodal metastases being the most important factors determining prognosis of a colorectal cancer. Using the current TNM classification system (which is merely an elaboration of the Dukes system), *numbers* of involved lymph nodes are recorded as stratification criteria for poorer prognosis. There has been strong agreement in the field of oncology regarding adapting the TNM method as the universal colorectal carcinoma staging system (Tables 24.1 and 24.2).

TABLE 24.1. TNM Clinical Classification in Colorectal Carcinoma (1997)[23]

	T—Primary Tumor
TX	Primary tumor cannot be assessed.
T0	No evidence of primary tumor.
Tis	Carcinoma in situ: intraepithelial or invasion of lamina propria[a]
T1	Tumor invades submucosa.
T2	Tumor invades muscularis propria.
T3	Tumor invades through muscularis propria into subserosa or into nonperitonealized pericolic or perirectal tissues.
T4	Tumor directly invades other organs or structures and/or perforates visceral peritoneum.[b]

	N–Regional Lymph Nodes[c]
NX	Regional lymph nodes cannot be assessed
N0	No regional lymph node metastasis
N1	Metastasis in 1 to 3 regional lymph nodes
N2	Metastasis in 4 or more regional lymph nodes

	M—Distant Metastasis
MX	Distant metastasis cannot be assessed.
M0	No distant metastasis
M1	Distant metastasis

pTNM Pathological Classification

The pT, pN, and pM categories correspond to the T, N, and M categories.

pN0   Histologic examination of a regional lymphadenectomy specimen will ordinarily include 12 or more lymph nodes.

From Ref.6.

[a]Tis includes cancer cells confined within the glandular basement membrane (intraepithelial) or lamina propria (intramucosal) with no extension through muscularis mucosae into submucosa.

[b] Direct invasion in T4 includes invasion of other segments of the colorectum by way of the serosa, for example, invasion of sigmoid colon by a carcinoma of the cecum.

[c]A tumor nodule greater than 3 mm in diameter in perirectal or pericolic adipose tissue without histologic evidence of a residual lymph node in the nodule is classified as regional lymph node metastasis. However, a tumor nodule up to 3 mm in diameter is classified in the T category as discontinuous extension, that is, T3.

TABLE 24.2. UICC Stage Grouping in Colorectal Carcinoma[23]

TNM		Stage Grouping		Dukes
Stage 0	Tis	N0	M0	
Stage I	T1	7N0	M0	A
	T2	N0	M0	
Stage II	T3	N0	M0	B*
	T4	N0	M0	
Stage III	Any T	N1	M0	C*
	Any T	N2	M0	
Stage IV	Any T	Any N	M1	

Source: From Ref. 6.

[a] Dukes B is a composite of better (T3N0M0) and worse (T4N0M0) prognostic groups, as is Dukes C (any TN1M0 and any TN2M0)

SIGNS AND SYMPTOMS

The symptoms of colorectal cancer may be nonspecific, such as intermittent pain, bleeding, nausea, and vomiting. Most tumors in their earliest stages produce no symptoms. This is especially true of right-sided lesions. Gross red blood loss is commonly associated with left colon and rectal cancers, and melena may occur with right colon tumors. Lesser amounts of bleeding may be detected with an FOT. Patients with chronic blood loss may develop iron deficiency anemia associated with fatigue. Abdominal pain, nausea, and vomiting may be caused by malignant intestinal obstruction. In the presence of obstruction, there may be a perforation either at the site of the tumor or through the proximal uninvolved bowel. In rectal tumors a change in bowel habits is usual, leading to constipation, straining, or a decreased stool caliber. Further symptoms such as tenesmus, urgency, and perineal pain are characteristic for locally advanced rectal cancers.[12]

DIAGNOSIS

Not all colorectal cancers or adenomas are associated with bleeding, and even when they are, bleeding is often intermittent in nature.

Diagnostic Measures

Stool can be obtained for the evaluation of bleeding by a positive FOT. Several factors affect the utility of this test. Patients need to be instructed to remain on low-peroxidase diets before testing to avoid false-positive results. Certain medications, such as iron, cimetidine, antacids, and ascorbic acid, may interfere with the peroxidase reaction and may lead to a false-negative result. The least expensive and potentially most informative study for rectal tumors is the digital examination. This permits the localization of distal rectal and anal neoplasms. Rigid rectosigmoidoscopy is limited by the length of bowel that can be inspected (15 to 20 cm). An adequate biopsy must be taken, the degree of fixation to surrounding tissue is evaluated, degree of obstruction is reported, size and ulceration of lesions are determined, and the distance from the distal edge of the tumor to the dentate line is measured carefully.

By flexible fiberoptic sigmoidoscopy an examination of the rectum and sigmoid colon up to 60 cm can usually be performed after cleansing enemas. Colonoscopy with a 130 to 180-cm fiberoptic instrument is the most widely used diagnostic study to evaluate the colon. A valuable aspect of this procedure is the ability to obtain mucosal biopsy specimens and perform polypectomies. The incidence of severe complications, such as hemorrhage and perforation, which requires surgical intervention, is 0.1% to 0.3%.

The barium enema is a traditional study for the diagnosis of colonic polyps and cancers. The double-contrast technique using air insufflation is superior to the standard single-contrast barium enema to detect early adenomas or cancers. Proctosigmoidoscopy should also be performed to exclude rectal lesions because visualization of this area is inadequate on barium enema.[12]

A major factor early in the evaluation of a patient with rectal cancer involves determination of the possibility and extent of resectability. After a cancer grows through the wall of the rectum, it can invade any of the surrounding structures. This is usually determined by evaluation of the fixation or tethering of the tumor to these structures. This makes complete examination of these structures necessary. A woman should have a complete pelvic examination with care to determine if the tumor is suspected of invading the vagina or has spread to the ovaries. In a man, evaluation of extension into the prostate or bladder is important. Thorough evaluation may require transanal ultrasound, computerized tomography (CT), magnetic resonance imaging (MRI), or even cystoscopy and biopsy. The depth of tumor invasion can be accurately determined by use of transanal ultrasound. Each layer of the rectal wall can be identified and its penetration by cancer visualized with great accuracy. Although perirectal lymph nodes can be imaged by ultrasound, the presence of cancer within these nodes cannot be exactly predicted. CT scanning of the rectum has been extremely helpful for the evaluation of the cancer itself, but nuclear magnetic imaging, especially with the use of newly available transrectally positioned coils, should be very useful in predicting depth of invasion and involvement of lymph nodes and other pararectal structures by the primary cancer. The advantages of these accurate descriptions of the cancer become evident when the treatment is chosen and decisions must be made regarding extent of operation and use of adjuvant modalities such as chemotherapy or radiation therapy prior to surgery.[8]

Preoperative Evaluation

Taking the family history, physical examination, and hematologic and serologic screening tests are indicated primarily. The determination of distant spread of colorectal cancer is important, because these patients may be considered to be incurable and decisions regarding operative therapy may be altered accordingly. The knowledge of metastases to the liver or to the lungs may significantly modify the surgical management of the primary cancer. Routine evaluation for distant metastatic disease consists of a chest X-ray film, determination of carcinoembryonic antigen (CEA) level, and a CT scan, with contrast, of the abdomen and pelvis. The latter also allows evaluation of the urinary tract. Suspicious lesions in the liver may need further evaluation by MRI or angio-CT. CT will also help in determining metastases to the ovaries or dissemination within the peritoneal cavity. Colorectal cancer rarely metastasizes to the bones or to the brain, and without symptoms, these two areas are not included in routine surveillance.[8]

SURGICAL THERAPY

The surgical goals in the resection of a primary colorectal cancer are to achieve an en bloc removal comprising an adequate length of normal colon proximal and distal to the tumor. If the tumor is adherent to adjacent structures, adequate lateral margins have to be obtained by excising all or a portion of adjacent structures. The regional lymph nodes need to be removed primarily to allow for adequate staging for the presence of nodal metastases. In colonic carcinomas the actual margin of bowel removed is often dependent on the extent of lymph node dissection that is demanded. The paracolic and intermediate lymph nodes along the neighboring two named mesenteric arteries should be removed as part of a curative resection up to the root of the vessel. This is especially important in carcinomas localized in the transverse colon (between the hepatic and splenic flexures), as the lymphatic spread is multidirectional in this region. Resection plus primary anastomosis is the surgical procedure of choice for cancers of the colon and for cancers of the upper and middle third of the rectum, if there is no emergency situation. Whenever possible, a mechanical bowel preparation, along with intravenous antibiotics, should be instituted preoperatively to reduce infectious complications. It depends on the surgeon's preference if the anastomotic technique is hand-sewn or stapled. A left hemicolectomy with removal of bowel from the middle transverse to the distal sigmoid colon can be used for descending colon tumors. A proximal ligation of the inferior mesenteric artery (above the take-off of the left colic artery) is routinely performed. Rectosigmoid cancers and tumors of the rectum can be removed by anterior resection if a distal clearance of 1 cm is achievable in well or moderately differentiated carcinomas and if the carcinoma lies above the puborectalis muscle. In poorly differentiated tumors, the distal clearance should be at least 3 cm. Besides the division of the mesenteric artery at the origin of the vessel close to the aorta and the inferior mesenteric vein below the pancreas, the complete mobilization of the splenic flexure is required to obtain a tension-free anastomosis deep in the pelvis. The introduction of the end-to-end anastomosis (EEA) stapler has increased the possibility of performing a sphincter-saving procedure. An intersphincteric resection with colo–anal anastomosis can be carried out to maintain bowel continuity even in carcinomas located in the lower rectum if their category is not higher than pT3a and the tumor does not extend to the puborectalis muscle (distal clearance of 1 cm achievable). In these cases the colon is brought to the level of the anus and dentate line. If the tumor invades the pelvic floor or if an adequate soft tissue margin around the tumor requires excision of the pelvic floor or anal sphincters, an abdomino–perineal resection must be performed. The procedure involves wide excision of the rectum to include the lateral attachments and pelvic mesocolon and the establishment of a permanent colostomy. In all cancers of the rectum, a complete mesorectal excision is compulsory to minimize the risk of local recurrence.[12] New surgical therapies aimed at minimizing damage to pelvic nerves governing sexual and bladder function are now being developed as well, with evidence that such nerve preservation can be accomplished without compromising chances for cure.

Local treatment options for rectal cancers were initially described for patients with advanced disease or medical contraindications to radical surgery. In addition, selected patients with small (less than 3 cm), well-differentiated tumors histologically without lymph vessel invasion (L0) and in endorectal ultrasonography uT1 and uN0 may be treated locally by transanal excision without elevated risk of recurrence.[13,14] Even in emergency situations of colorectal carcinoma, for example, bowel perforation or acute tumor bleeding, the restoration of intestinal continuity can eventually be achieved, but the surgeon may judge the risk of an anastomotic breakdown in peritonitis to be high and apt to perform a bowel resection in discontinuity according to Hartmann with a temporary stoma. In general, such a stoma can be reversed in 3 to 6 months laparoscopically depending on the medical condition of the patient.

In the past 5 years, there has been a great interest in the use of laparoscopic techniques to resect colorectal cancers. This has permitted avoidance of large incisions and a faster recovery. Long-term results have not been reported, but it does appear that this is a promising new method of colorectal cancer therapy.[15]

ADJUVANT RADIOTHERAPY

The use of radiation therapy has been confined to rectal tumors in which the incidence of local recurrence is significant, that is, for tumors extending through the bowel wall or with lymph node involvement, close proximity to the anal verge and high tumor grade. In these cases the incidence of local recurrence is as high as 30% to 35% but can be reduced with adjuvant radiotherapy. The timing of such therapy can be preoperative, postoperative, or combined. So far, however, no studies clearly indicate that one approach is superior to another; surgeons generally prefer preoperative therapy because irradiated tissue is resected and the neorectum with which the patient must live is nonirradiated.[16]

Combinations of radiation and chemotherapy are being studied because of the recognition that improvement in survival rates will require reduction of the rates of recurrences both at the primary tumor site *and* outside the pelvis, and because so far, radiation and chemotherapy have each been shown to produce relatively limited benefits when used alone. Ongoing trials using combinations of irradiation and chemotherapy have shown a fairly good compatibility, and the risks of serious late morbidity such as enteritis and of treatment-related death were generally similar to those of patients treated with radiation alone.[15]

ADJUVANT CHEMOTHERAPY

Patients who die from colorectal cancer do so from disseminated disease, although tumor control may be locally sufficient. Several randomized prospective studies applying 5-fluorouracil (5-FU) in combination with folinic acid and levamisole have demonstrated that postoperative adjuvant systemic chemotherapy benefits certain subgroups of patients. From these studies it is apparent that patients with stage III *Dukes C* colorectal cancer should be offered adjuvant chemotherapy as standard therapy to improve their survival. The efficacy of adjuvant chemotherapy for patients in lower stages of colorectal cancer (without lymph node involvement) has not been clearly demonstrated in all the reported studies.[12,17]

FOLLOW-UP FOR LOCAL AND DISTANT RECURRENCES

Follow-up programs in patients after curative resection of their primary tumor are often recommended as a subset of patients with recurrent colorectal carcinoma can be cured. It is controversial whether rigorous follow-up programs actually do affect long-term survival. Fifty percent of carcinomas that recur do so within 18 months of surgery, and 90% of recurrences are evident by 3 years. By careful endoscopic follow-up also the 5% of patients who develop a metachronous primary tumor of the large bowels will be identified. Some recurrent tumors are amenable to potential surgical or multimodal cure including anastomotic recurrences and mobile extraluminal pelvic recurrences. Follow-up examinations have been designed according to a careful scheme (Table 24.3).

Hepatic Metastases

Overall, curative surgical resection of hepatic metastases is associated with 25% to 30% 5-year survival rates.[18] Patients eligible for hepatic resection of metastatic disease are those who have no evidence of extrahepatic tumor, no medical contraindications for surgery, and fewer than four lesions amenable to curative resection. Palliative regional chemotherapy of liver metastases by the hepatic artery demonstrated improved tumor response but did not influence survival rates.[12]

Palliative Treatment

More commonly colorectal cancer recurs in multiple sites. No studies have clearly *stage IV* documented that systemic therapies improve survival when metastases are present. Nevertheless chemotherapy is widely used in the patient with advanced disease. The

TABLE 24.3. A Follow-Up Typical Scheme After Resection of a Colon or Rectal Carcinoma[24]

Follow-Up in Colon Cancer

Year After Operation or Adjuant Therapy Resp.	First Year		Second Year		Third Year	Fourth Year	Fifth Year
Months	6	12	18	24	36	48	60
History and clinical examination	X	X	X	X	X	X	X
CEA or CA 19-9	X	X	X	X	X	X	X
Liver sonography	X	X	X	X	X	X	X
Chest X-ray film	X	X	X	X	X	X	X
Rectosocpy		X	X		X	X	
Colonoscopy	X			X			X

Follow-Up in Cancer of the Rectum or Sigmoid

Year After Operation or Adjuant Therapy Resp.	First Year		Second Year		Third Year	Fourth Year	Fifth Year
Months	3 12	6	18	24	36	48	60
History and clinical examination	X	XX	X	X	X	X	X
CEA or CA 19-9	X	XX	X	X	X	X	X
Liver sonography	X	XX	X	X	X	X	X
Chest X-ray film	X	XX	X	X	X	X	X
Colonoscopy		X		X			X
after Operation with Anal Preservation							
Rectoscopy	X	X	X		X		
Transanal ultrasound	X	XX	X	X	X		
CT scan of the pelvis	X						
with Rectal Excision							
Transvaginal Ultrasound	X	XX	X	X	X		
CT scan of the pelvis	X	X	X	X	X		

Source: From Ref. 24.

most frequently employed agent is 5-FU. Promising studies have demonstrated that the antitumor activity of 5-FU can be enhanced by folinic acid, increasing tumor response rates (shrinkage of tumor) to a range of 30% to 40%.[12] Chemotherapy for the treatment of recurrent disease should be considered within clinical trials. In symptomatic patients, maximal palliation may also be achieved by surgical treatments such as resection of the tumor recurrence, fecal diversion, or a bypass procedure. Local palliation for rectal cancer may be accomplished by transmural laser surgery or fulguration in patients with disseminated disease or in poor medical condition. More extensive operations such as sacral resection or pelvic exenterations are reserved for patients with isolated recurrent disease who are in excellent medical condition. Supportive care and pain control using oral or parenteral analgesics are mandatory.[19]

PROGNOSIS

1995

A recent prospective multicenter trial, using uni- and multivariate analyses, was carried out to evaluate the prognostic factors after curative resection of rectal carcinoma for the endpoints of locoregional recurrence and survival.[20,21] Following curative resection survival rates varied according to tumor-related factors such as pT (24% to 74%) and pN (33% to 68%). Stage-dependent survival rates show a range from 9% (stage IV) to 74% (stage I). In stage III prognosis was significantly better for SgCRC pN1 cases (47%) than for pN2 cases (34%) ($p < 0.01$). Treatment-related factors (local spillage of tumor cells, treating institution, and individual surgeon) strongly determined the occurrence of locoregional recurrences. A highly significant correlation exists between locoregional recurrences and observed 5-year survival rate. This study therefore suggests, in analyses of adjuvant treatment results, that stratification according to the treating department and surgeon is needed.

REHABILITATION

As tumor and operative therapy may impair the patient's sexual functions and generally cause psychological problems, comprehensive help may be needed. On the other hand advice in techniques of stoma handling may become necessary. Many of these tasks can be managed adequately by specially trained nurses, and enterostomal therapists.

FURTHER READING

1. Sandler RS (1996) Epidemiology and risk factors for colorectal cancer. *Gastroenterol Clin NA* 25:717–734.
2. Wilmink ABM (1997) Overview of the epidemiology of colorectal cancer. *Dis Colon Rectum* 40:483–493.
3. Milsom JW (1993) Pathogenesis of colorectal cancer. *Surg Clin NA* 73:1–11.
4. Devroede GJ, Taylor WF, Sau WG, et al. (1971) Cancer risks and life expectancy of children with ulcerative colitis. *N Eng J Med* 285:17–21.
5. Fearon ER, Vogelstein B (1990) A genetic model for colorectal tumorigenesis. *Cell* 61:759–767.
6. Vogelstein B, Fearon ER, Hamilton SR, et al. (1988) Genetic alterations during colorectal tumor development. *N Eng J Med* 319:525–532.
7. Carethers JM (1996) The cellular and molecular pathogenesis of colorectal cancer. *Gastroenterol Clin NA* 25:737–754.

8. Chang HR, Kirby IB (1977) Tumors of the colon. In: Zinner MJ, Schwartz SI, Ellis (eds) *Maingot's Abdominal Operations* 10th edition, Vol. II. Appleton & Lange, East Norwalk, CT, pp. 1281–1308.

9. Lynch HT, Lynch JF (1995) Clinical implications of advances in the molecular genetics of colorectal cancer. *Tumori* 81 (Suppl):19–29.

10. Stat Bite (1995): Average years of life lost from cancer. *J N Cancer Inst* 87:956.

11. Winawer SJ, et al. (1997) Colorectal cancer screening: Clinical guidelines and rationale. *Gastroenterol* 112:594–642.

12. Chang AE (1993) Colorectal cancer. In: Greenfield LJ, Mulholland MW, Oldham KT, Zelenock GB (eds) *Surgery—Scientific Principles and Practice*. Lippincott, Philadelphia, pp. 1014–1030.

13. Eckhauser FE, Knol JA (1997) Surgery for primary and metastatic colorectal cancer. *Gastroenterol Clin* NA 26:103–128.

14. Murray JJ, Stahl TJ (1993) Sphincter-saving alternatives for treatment of adenocarcinoma involving distal rectum. *Surg Clin NA* 73:131–144.

15. Milsom JW, Böhm B, Hammerhofer K, Fazio VW, Steiger E, Elson P (1997) A prospective, randomized comparison of laparoscopic vs. conventional resection for colorectal cancer. Presented at the American College of Surgeons Meeting, October 16, 1997.

16. Casillas S, Milsom JW (1997) Adjuvant therapy for colorectal cancer: Present and future perspectives. *Dis Colon Rectum* 40:977–992.

17. Levitan N (1993) Chemotherapy in colorectal carcinoma. *Surg Clin NA* 73:183–198.

18. Registry of Hepatic Metastases (1988). Resection of the liver for colorectal carcinoma metastases: A multi-institutional study of indications for resection. *Surgery* 103:278–288.

19. Asbun HJ, Hughes KS (1993) Management of recurrent and metastatic colorectal carcinoma. *Surg Clin NA* 73:145–166.

20. Hermanek P, Wiebelt H, Staimmer D, Riedl S, German Study Group Colo-rectal Carcinoma (SGCRC) (1995) Prognostic factors of rectum carcinoma—experience of the German multicentre study SGCRC. *Tumori* 81 (Suppl):60–64.

21. Kessler H, Hermonek P, for the Study Group Colo-Rectal Carcinoma: Outcomes in Rectal Cancer Surger Are Directly Related to Technical Factors. *Semin Colon Rectal Surg* (1998) (in press).

22. Kessler H. Mansmann V, Hermanek Pjun, Riedl St, Staimmer D, Hermanek P, for the Study Group Colo-Rectal Carcinoma (SGCRC): Does the Surgeon Affect Outcome in Colon Carcinoma? *Semin Colon Rectal Surg* (1989) (in press).

23. Sobin L, Wittekind Ch (eds) (1997) *TNM Classification of Malignant Tumors* 5th edition. John Wiley & Sons, New York, Chichester, Weinheim, Brisbane, Singapore, Toronto.

24. Hohenberger W, Kessler H, Schenk J (19xx) Recommendations for follow-up in colorectal carcinoma. Edited by the Study Group Colorectal Carcinoma of the University of Erlangen-Nuernberg, Germany (in press).

■■■■■■ CHAPTER 25

BREAST CANCER

UMBERTO VERONESI, VIRGILIO SACCHINI, MARCO COLLEONI,
and ARON GOLDHIRSCH

European Institute of Oncology
Milano, Italy

EPIDEMIOLOGY

Breast cancer represents 20% of all malignancies among European women. It is the most common cancer among women in North America, Europe, Australia, and many Latin American countries. The incidence of breast carcinoma is increasing in many countries at a mean rate of 1% to 2% annually and it is estimated that during the first decade of the third millennium nearly 1 million women will develop this disease yearly throughout the world. Recent reports indicate decreasing breast cancer incidence and mortality in younger cohorts.[1]

Geographic variation of incidence and mortality are well known and extensively described.[2] The incidence rates in Europe decrease from the north to the south and from west to east. Within each country, breast cancer incidence correlates strongly with the per capita income of the population in the various regions.

Of interest are data from migrating populations, which adjust the incidence rates to that of the host countries within a couple of generations, indicating the importance of external factors related to environment and lifestyle.

Breast cancer is very rare before the age of 20 and seldom occurs in individuals under 30 years of age. The incidence rate rises very steadily up to the age of 50 years. Among postmenopausal women the rate of increase declines, although

Manual of Clinical Oncology, 7th edition, Edited by Raphael E. Pollock
ISBN 0-471-23828-7, pages 491–513. Copyright © 1999 Wiley-Liss, Inc.

the incidence continues to rise. Mortality rates for breast cancer in western Europe and North America are of the order of 15 to 25 per 100,000 women, being slightly more than a third of the incidence rate, which is approximately 50 to 60 per 100,000 women.

PATHOLOGY OF BREAST CANCER

Lobular Ca accounts for only 8 % of all can.

Ductal Carcinoma In Situ (DCIS) and Lobular Carcinoma In Situ (LCIS)

DCIS is a peculiar variant of breast cancer, becoming more and more a clinical entity than a variant.[3]

The definition of DCIS has evolved with our enhanced ability to detect earlier forms of breast cancer. Currently, DCIS is defined as a malignancy of the epithelial cells lining the lactiferous ducts, without penetration by these cells of the ductal basement membrane; there is by definition no invasion into the periductal stromal tissue. Pure DCIS thus carries with it no risk of metastasis.

DCIS must be clearly distinguished from LCIS, which arises from the epithelial cells lining the breast lobules. It occurs mainly in premenopausal women, and is multicentric in 50% to 70% of cases. The diagnosis is often made incidentally on removal of breast tissue. The risk of developing homolateral invasive carcinoma after the diagnosis of a lobular carcinoma in situ, not treated with mastectomy, is estimated to be 10% to 15% at 10 years. It is now generally accepted that LCIS should be viewed as a "marker" of increased risk for the subsequent development of invasive breast cancer; in itself, LCIS is now thought to require no intervention besides long-term follow-up. This is in contradistinction to DCIS, which requires good local treatment. Many pathologists refused to use the term "carcinoma" for a noninvasive lesion of this cellular type and coined various definitions, such as "epitheliosis," "small-cell neoplasia," and "lobular neoplasia."

In the past, DCIS was infrequently diagnosed, about 1% to 5% of all breast cancers; was usually detected as either a palpable lesion, Paget's disease, or as bloody nipple discharge; and the treatment was standard—a mastectomy. DCIS now accounts for at least 20% of the mammographically detected carcinomas, and 12% of newly diagnosed breast cancers. Studies on comparison of risk factors for ductal carcinoma in situ and invasive cancer have shown that the risk factors for DCIS are similar to those for invasive breast cancer (family history, nulliparity, age at birth of first child, previous breast biopsies).

There is the perception that many DCIS never progress to invasion and may remain localized in the breast without infiltrating the basal membrane. For this reason few prognostic factors and indicators of invasion have been studied in the last 5 years. Nuclear morphology, increasing nuclear grade, intraductal growth pattern, and extensive comedo necrosis are the most important morphologic prognostic factors, whereas biologic characterization such as extensive apoptosis, genetic changes (gain:1q, 6q, 8q, loss: 17q), angiogenesis (vascular density), and *her-2/neu* and *p53* expression seems to be related to the tendency of invasion.

Four major subtypes of DCIS have been described:

[handwritten margin note: High grade - 30 %. invasion e 5 yrs Low grade - >% e 5yrs]

1. **Papillary/Micropapillary**

   The cuboidal epithelial cells lining the lactiferous ducts proliferate sufficiently to form papillary projections into the ductal lumen. No mitoses or atypia are apparent, and the cells remain well differentiated.

2. **Cribriform**

   The cells proliferate further, become more atypical and occupy more of the lumen of the ducts, forming a bridging network of cells. Open spaces remain apparent within this cellular network, as suggested by the term "cribriform." There may be associated cellular necrosis.

3. **Solid**

   The open spaces of the cribriform pattern become filled in with increasingly anaplastic cells, distending the duct with solid sheets of tumor. Frequent mitotic figures are appreciated.

4. **Comedo**

   The comedo variant is characterized by cellular necrosis extending from the center of the filled ductal lumen toward an outer rim of viable malignant cells. This necrosis is associated with the deposition of calcium, producing the characteristic appearance of microcalcification on mammographic examination.

For several decades, mastectomy was considered the appropriate treatment for DCIS. The theoretical rationale supporting the use of mastectomy includes the incidence of multifocality and multicentricity and the possibility of an occult invasive carcinoma in association with the DCIS. The concept of multicentricity has been reviewed and DCIS seems to be more multifocal (tumoral foci only in the same quadrant of the primary tumor) than multicentric. For this reason conservative surgery had a progressive role in the treatment of this very early stage of the disease. Comedo necrosis and inadequate free margins (carefully evaluated on the removed specimen) are the most important prognostic factors related to local breast recurrences.

Radiotherapy after conservative surgery has been proved to be effective in reducing the risk of local relapses for both intraductal and invasive types (50% of local relapses after conservative surgery for DCIS are invasive).[4] Studies in progress are identifying subgroups of patients in whom radiotherapy may be avoided on the basis of histotype, morphologic and biologic prognostic indicators, and adequate free margins of resection.[5]

[handwritten margin note: No DXT 10 %. local recurrence ½ of which are invasive with DXT risk ↓ 2 %. invasive can. (ie 5 %. vs 2 %. invasive recurrence)]

Invasive Breast Carcinoma

Invasive ductal carcinoma is the most common type of breast cancer, comprising about 70% of all cases. It may contain a more or less extensive component of intraductal carcinoma.

Invasive lobular carcinoma represents 10% to 20% of all breast cancers.

✱ Invasive ductal carcinoma not otherwise specified

Other types of invasive cancers accounting for the remaining 10% of cases include:

> Medullar carcinoma, with sharp tumor borders and lymphoid infiltration
>
> Mucoid carcinoma, with large amounts of extracellular mucus
>
> Papillary carcinoma, with a well-differentiated papillary structure
>
> Inflammatory carcinoma (1% to 2% of all cases), usually an invasive ductal carcinoma with extensive invasion of lymphatic vessels of the dermis.

1 %.

Another distinct pathologic entity is represented by Paget's disease of the nipple, a variant of ductal carcinoma in situ, in which tumor cells invade the ducts without infiltrating the basal membrane and extend into the major ducts of the nipple and the epidermis of the areola. An invasive carcinoma is an associated feature in about 90% of these cases. (lump median survival 42/12 no lump 126/12's)

Other rare types of invasive cancers include adenoid cystic carcinoma, apocrine carcinoma, and carcinoma with squamous metaplasia.

Other Nonmalignant and Malignant Breast Diseases

Several pathologic noncancerous conditions present with a single or multiple breast lumps or with symptoms and signs that simulate breast cancer.

Fibrocystic Mastopathy This is a condition considered in the past to confer an increased risk for breast cancer. Reevaluation of the outcome of this disorder has concluded that the overall increased risk of 1.86 of developing breast cancer, estimated by pooling together many published series, was more likely due to the selection of patients than to the real malignant potential of the disease. The presence of proliferation with cell atypia on pathologic assessment, however, is associated with an increased risk for breast cancer, especially if the patient has a positive family history. Fibrocystic disease occurs more often among individuals 30 to 55 years of age, and is frequently identified by women as multiple, round lumps in one or both breasts. The mammographic patterns of multiple areas of fibrosis and cysts are typical, but represent a difficult background for evaluation of an underlying neoplasia. Another associated pathologic entity is sclerosing adenosis that can even appear in younger ages.

Fibroadenoma This presents as one or more mobile, indolent lumps, commonly in women between 20 and 25 years of age. Occasionally a fibrocystic mastopathy is associated.

Intraductal Papilloma This usually presents in larger ducts as a mobile lump, often associated with bloody or stained nipple discharge requiring surgical removal. Galactography might be necessary for localization of the node. Cell atypia is found in about one quarter of papillomas. Usually, multiple intraductal papillomas carry a higher risk of breast cancer, while the risk is much lower for solitary central papillomas.

Other malignant diseases of the breast that might simulate breast cancer include the following:

Cystosarcoma Phylloides This can appear as early as in adolescence. It presents as a mass in a breast, and the pathologic examination leads to recognition of epithelial and mesenchymal components and to definition of the grade of malignancy. Treatment requires a wide surgical removal that often results in a total mastectomy.[6] High-grade or recurrent disease might require radiation therapy and systemic treatments.

Sarcoma This presents usually as a large fast-growing painless mass. Histopathologic features and clinical behavior are similar to those of sarcomas of other organs.

Malignant Lymphoma This is a very rare presentation, usually of B-cell type. Its evaluation and treatment follow guidelines for this type of disorder.

PROGNOSTIC FACTORS

The histologic type of the disease has at best a very limited prognostic value. On the other hand, other features related to histopathologic and biologic aspects of the disease provide significant information in the determination of prognosis and prediction of response to a given antineoplastic treatment. An increasing number of these factors is currently being investigated.[7] A list of established prognostic and predictive variables is shown in Table 25.1.

In general, prognostic factors are useful for the definition of a baseline prognosis, which helps in the estimation of costs and benefits for a given treatment program. Predictive factors are useful in case where there is a quantitative or even a qualitative difference in response to a given treatment, allowing better use of available approaches. Thus, the evaluation of patients with newly diagnosed breast cancer is composed of several facets, some of which have a specific role in defining the best available therapy. These factors, related to patient and disease at presentation, should be available for making treatment choices.

HEREDITARY BREAST CANCER

Hereditary breast cancer represents 8% of all breast cancers. Mutations of *BRCA-1* and *BRCA-2* genes have been associated with familial breast cancer. The major risks for developing breast cancer are associated with *BRCA-1* mutations. The relative risk for breast cancer in *BRCA-1*-linked families compared to the general popula-

handwritten note (top margin): * Size, stage, grade, nodal involvement, receptor status — major prognostic factors

TABLE 25.1. Prognostic Factors in Patients with Breast Cancer

Factor	Remarks
Tumor size	• Best information if pathologically determined. • Direct relationship between the increase of tumor size and the worsening of the prognosis
Axillary lymph node status	• The most important prognostic variable. At least 10 lymph nodes must be examined to correctly estimate prognosis. The current tendency in several centers to avoid axillary dissection in N0 presentations is still investigational. • Micrometastases identification was also prognostically relevant.
(Internal mammary lymph node status)	• Internal mammary node involvement is an important prognostic factor, but their dissection did not improve prognosis.
Vascular invasion	• Presence indicated worse prognosis, especially in node-negative disease.
Histologic grade	• Histologic grade (composed of several features indicating more or less resemblance to nonmalignant breast tissue) is prognostically relevant. Nuclear grade was considered by many to be the most important component. The mitotic count might be the best predictor of prognosis.
Receptor status: estrogen or progesterone level	• Estrogen receptor expression is associated with increased responsiveness to adjuvant and palliative endocrine therapies, improving disease free interval (DFI) and survival in treated patients. Presence of progesterone receptors also carried a similar prognostic value, especially in premenopausal women.

Cell proliferation indexes
  Thymidine labeling
  Flow cytometry (S phase)
  Ki-67
	• Measured on unfixed tumor material. Higher values indicated a worse prognosis.
	• Measured on fixed material. Determination of proportion of cells in S phase. Higher values indicated a worse prognosis.
	• Measured on fixed material. Higher percentage of stained cells with a anti-Ki67 antibody indicated a worse prognosis.

Receptors (growth factors or growth regulators, including oncogenes)	
Epidermal growth factor receptor (*c-erbB-1*)	• Measured mainly on unfixed material. Higher percentage might predict a worse prognosis.
her-2/neu (*c-erbB-2*)	• Measured on fixed material. Expression might predict a worse prognosis. Good candidate as predictor for response to anthracycline combination chemotherapy, and for resistance to tamoxifen or CMF combination chemotherapy
IGF-IR (insulin-like growth factor receptor)	• Measured in the serum. Lowering of its serum levels was seen during treatment with tamoxifen.
Somatostatin receptor	• Presence in the tumor indicated better prognosis.
Tumor suppressor genes	
p53	• Demonstration of mutants of this gene has no relevant prognostic value. Presence of the mutant protein in serum of patients with breast cancer might be associated with worse prognosis, or resistance to cytoxan methotrexale 5-fluorouracil (CMF) combination chemotherapy. *p53* mutations in DCIS seem prognostically important.
nm23	• Reduced expression of *nm23* in the tumor was associated with high metastatic potential, thus with a worse prognosis.
Miscellaneous	
Cathepsin D	• Lysosomal protease. Increased concentrations in tumor tissue correlated with worse prognosis
• Proteases. Concentrations determined on frozen tissue. Increased levels were associated with a significant worse prognosis in node-negative and node-positive disease.
Angiogenesis	• Neoplastic microvessel density is estimated by staining using platelet endothelial cell adhesion molecule CD31. Increased density was associated with a worse prognosis

tion ranged from 8 to 42 times depending on age. This increased risk is maximal in premenopausal women. A woman with *BRCA-1* mutation has at least a 65% risk of developing breast cancer by age 70. This mutation, mapped to the long arm of 17 chromosome (q21), also increases the risk of ovarian cancer, but to a lesser extent. The risk for ovarian cancer was 23% by age 50 and 63% by age 70, whereas the cumulative probability of ovarian cancer in the general population is 1% to 2%.

[handwritten margin notes: vs. ~ 7 %. life time risk normally]

The other germline mutation increasing the risk of breast cancer is related to the *BRCA-2* gene on chromosome 13q12–13. The lifetime risk of developing breast cancer in *BRCA-2* mutation carriers is lower than in the *BRCA-1* carriers: the cumulative risk of breast cancer in female gene carriers was estimated to be 45% by age 50 and 60% by age 70 years. Families linked to *BRCA-2* are distinguished by a high incidence of male breast cancer (approximately 15% of all male breast cancers). The cumulative risk of breast cancer in male carriers was estimated to be 6.3% by age 70 years. Ovarian cancer appears less prevalent in *BRCA-2* carriers: the risk was estimated to be less than 10 by age 70. The proportion of a high positive family history with these mutations was calculated in linkage studies: 40% of breast cancer kindred were linked to *BRCA-1*, 35% to *BRCA-2*, and probably 5% to other *BRCA* genes.

The diagnosis of *BRCA* mutation is quite complex owing to their extremely large size (22 coding exons in the *BRCA-1* gene and 27 in *BRCA-2*). More than 100 mutations have been documented in the *BRCA-1* gene, but three (185delAG, 5382insC, and 4184delTCAA in codon 1355) seem to be more common.

Indications for individuals requiring genetic testing include people with breast or ovarian cancer with family history for breast and ovarian cancer (two or more first- or second-degree blood relatives); people with breast or ovarian cancer with one blood relative in whom either breast and ovarian cancer developed before 45 years; people with breast and ovarian cancer in premenopausal status; people with breast or ovarian cancer with multiple primary cancers or bilateral disease; and relatives with *BRCA* mutations. People under 18 years of age or cognitively impaired people are not suitable subjects for testing. The American Society of Clinical Oncology[8] recommends that genetic testing be performed in the setting of long-term outcome studies and endorses continued support of patient-oriented research to analyze the psychosocial impact of genetic testing of at-risk populations.

MANAGEMENT OF HIGH-RISK SUBJECTS

BRCA mutations are the major new risk factors for breast cancer. The second important factor with major impact in sporadic breast cancer in the population is age. Other risk factors, previous breast biopsies, number of pregnancies, age at first childbirth, breast feeding, and mammographic density are less important in the definition of the breast cancer risk. Benign breast diseases, discovered with biopsy, confer an increased risk of developing breast cancer (Table 25.2).

Multivariate analysis combining several risk factor was implemented in the definition of individual risk for primary or secondary prevention of breast cancer,[9] but have not still been utilized for a different approach in screening programs or diagnos-

TABLE 25.2. Relative Risk of Subsequent Breast Cancer After Benign Breast Biopsy

Benign Finding	Relative Risk	Study Population	Reference
Any biopsy	1.5	CASH	McDivitt et al. (1992)
Cyst	1.5	Nashville	Dupont and Page (1985)
Fibroadenoma	1.7	BCDDP	Carter et al. (1988)
	1.7	CASH	McDivitt et al. (1992)
	1.42–1.89	Nashville	Dupont et al. (1994)
Fibroadenoma with	3.7	CASH	McDivitt et al. (1992)
hyperplasia, no atypia	2.16–3.47	Nashville	Dupont et al. (1994)
Fibroadenoma with	6.9	CASH	McDivitt et al. (1992))
atypical hyperplasia	4.77–7.29	Nashville	Dupont et al. (1994)
Hyperplasia without	1.9	BCDDP	Carter et al. (1988)
atypia	1.6	NHS	London et al. (1992)
	1.8	CASH	McDivitt et al. (1992)
Atypical hyperplasia	4.4	Nashville	Dupont and Page (1985)
	3.0	BCDDP	Carter et al. (1988)
	3.7	NHS	London et al. (1992)
	2.6	CASH	McDivitt et al. (1992)
Atypical hyperplasia	5.9	NHS	London et al. (1992)
Premenopausal	12.0	BCDDP	Dupont et al. (1993)
Atypical hyperplasia	2.3	NHS	London et al. (1992)
Postmenopausal	3.3	BCDDP	Dupont et al. (1993)

From Kimberly J. Van Zee, Memorial Sloan-Kettering Cancer Center, New York, with permission.

tic management. At present there are no firm data to allow a statement regarding the management of high-risk women, and the advice given is more based on common sense rather than supported by hard facts. In cases where there is a positive family history for breast cancer, physical examination is recommended once a year starting at 20 years, first mammogram at the age of 35 years, and then every 2 years. It is suggested that *BRCA* mutation carriers be screened at 20 years of age followed by physical examination every 3 to 6 months and with mammography beginning at age 25 on an annual basis. Other examinations include pelvic evaluation and transvaginal ultrasound with color Doppler, and CA 125 semiannually beginning between age 25 to 35 years.[10] The lower specificity of mammography in younger women is the major limiting factor in this intensive follow-up program. The roles of ultrasound and magnetic resonance imaging (MRI) are under evaluation in prospective trials.

Prophylactic simple mastectomy, usually with reconstruction, is an option open to the patient that reduces the risk of breast cancer in up to 96% of cases. The failure rate is due to residual breast tissue left behind after the mastectomy (especially subclavicular and parasternal glandular foci). On average, 30-year-old women who carry *BRCA-1* or *BRCA-2* mutations gain from 2.9 to 5.3 years of life expectancy from prophylactic mastectomy and from 0.3 to 1.7 years of life expectancy from prophylactic oophorectomy, depending on their cumulative risk of cancer.[11]

No absolute criteria to determine which patients should undergo prophylactic mastectomy exist. Each patient should be treated on an individual basis with a psychological assessment, preferably in a clinical trial setting. Chemoprevention is another interventional procedure for this high-risk group. Drugs interfering with the initiation and promotion of breast cancer have recently allowed for the development of a new strategy in the reduction of the incidence of this disease. Experimental studies on the possibility of chemically induced tumor prevention with tamoxifen, and the clinical results relating to adjuvant tamoxifen in breast cancer patients over the past years, have emphasized that tamoxifen is the drug that best meets the requirements of effectiveness and tolerability in potentially preventing breast cancer.[12] Myocardial infarction and bone fractures are less frequent in women treated with this drug, which also seems to have a beneficial effect on bone density, and in the prevention of cardiovascular illnesses.

Such observations have led to tamoxifen being considered as a possible agent to prevent or delay the development of breast cancer together with increased control of cardiovascular diseases and osteoporosis in postmenopausal women.

In this framework, chemoprevention of breast cancer with tamoxifen represents a major effort involving the participation of thousands of women in long-term randomized trials, involving taking either tamoxifen or placebo over a 5-year period. Three of such studies (one in the UK, one in the USA, and a third one in Italy) have been concluded and first trends should be available in a couple of years.

Other chemoprevention agents, retinoic acid derivatives and the antiestrogen raloxifen, are under evaluation in clinical trials.[13]

SCREENING

Several randomized studies have demonstrated an important benefit in women more than 50 years old having physical exam and one double view mammogram per year. The advantage in terms of survival ranged from 28% to 38% in different studies. The role of breast self-examination in the early diagnosis of interval cancers is not clear. In March 1997 the American Cancer Society held a consensus meeting to develop guidelines in the early detection of cancer.[14] Although data presented at this meeting were in favor of beginning annual mammographic screening at 40, different opinions were expressed, especially regarding the cost-effectiveness this procedure would entail. Nevertheless the American Cancer Society recommended annual mammography for women beginning at age 40. Age at which screening should be stopped is related to concomitant diseases and performance status of each individual. No studies have proved the effectiveness of ultrasound in breast cancer screening. This method may have a role in the dense breasts of younger women, but cost-effectiveness should be carefully evaluated, especially regarding the issues of false positive cases.

Quality assurance programs, professional training, and self-assessment are fundamental in achieving standard results in mammographic screening.

DIAGNOSTIC WORK-UP IN PATIENTS SUSPECTED TO HAVE BREAST CANCER

The first sign of breast cancer is still a palpable lump. Only 20% of all cancers are nonpalpable and visible only at mammography or ultrasound. Unfortunately physical examination has a low specificity and sensitivity and further examinations are required to decrease the risk of missing cancers.

The first choice examination is mammography. The specificity of modern mammography ranges from 60% to 75% and the sensitivity from 85% to 95%. These variations mainly depend on age, with younger patients with dense breasts having lower specificity and sensitivity. Breast sonography is an invaluable adjunct to mammography in the diagnosis and management of breast diseases, especially in dense breasts.[15] The primary role of sonography in breast imaging is to determine if a focal mass is cystic or solid. If the mass is solid sonography may differentiate benign from malignant lesions with a sensitivity of 90 to 98% and specificity of 50 to 65%.

Fine-needle aspiration for cytologic diagnosis or core biopsy for histology provides the highest overall predictive value for malignancy. The diagnostic accuracy of these examinations together with clinical examination, mammography, ultrasonography, fine-needle aspiration (FNA) cytology, or core biopsy histology in discriminating between benign and malignant breast lesions has been shown to be near 99%.

Other promising techniques are under evaluation. These include breast MRI with gadolinium contrast which may be able to improve the sensitivity and specificity of mammography. The majority of breast cancers demonstrate enhancement after contrast administration whereas benign breast lesions either do not enhance at all or demonstrate slow uptake of contrast. Studies have demonstrated effectiveness of MRI in differentiating breast recurrences from posttreatment changes. In occult breast cancer, in which the first manifestation is axillary metastases with no abnormalities at mammography, MRI is able to identify the primary tumor in 80% of cases. Other indications for MRI include women with silicone augmentation and suspected implant rupture or breast abnormalities.[16,17]

MANAGEMENT OF NONPALPABLE BREAST LESIONS

The widespread use of mammography and ultrasound has resulted in the detection of increasing numbers of suspicious nonpalpable lesions of the breast. A diagnostic balance should be struck between the task to find as many small tumors as possible, minimizing the number of false-negatives, while avoiding unnecessary examinations and biopsies resulting in high anxiety and cost for women and health services involved. The rate of benign biopsies varies depending on the centers and countries. A ratio of benign to malignant of no more than 1:1 is recommended.[18] More refined mammographic projections, ultrasound, FNA cytology, and core-biopsy histology can reduce this ratio.

Core needle biopsy has been shown to have a higher predictive value with an improved probability of definitive diagnosis histologically compared to FNA cytology, owing to the amount of actual tissue removed. This allows the possibility of diagnosing atypical hyperplasia from noninvasive carcinomas, as well as better differentiation of intraductal versus invasive cancer.[19] *False - 5%. false + 1%.*

Preoperative localization must be performed to guide the surgeon to an accurate biopsy, and radiography of the specimen is mandatory to confirm the removal of the lesion.

SURGICAL TREATMENT OF INVASIVE BREAST CANCER

For the most part, surgery for patients with breast cancer is the first treatment. For years Halsted's mastectomy was the treatment of choice for all stages of breast cancer. This operation, which consists of the removal of a large portion of the breast skin, all the breast parenchyma, and the major and minor pectoral muscles en bloc with the axillary lymph nodes, is now the exception and is limited to locally advanced tumors (T3, T4b) in which primary chemotherapy is contraindicated. Less aggressive surgery, with sparing of the pectoral major muscle, was described by Patey in 1948 and was proved to be effective in the local control of most tumors. Many prospective randomized trials carried out in the last 20 years have definitively shown that in many instances it is possible to spare the breast if radiotherapy is administered on the residual breast tissue.[20,21] Conservative surgery was shown to be effective for good local control of the disease given the proper indications. T1–2, N0–1 breast cancer, for example, can be treated with conservative surgery whereas larger tumors (2.5 to 3.5 cm) require larger resection to achieve free margins and this is sometimes incompatible with a good cosmetic result. Neo-adjuvant chemotherapy may reduce the size of the lump, allowing conservative surgery.[22] Many risk factors for local recurrences after conservative surgery have been taken into consideration.[23] The absence of radiotherapy increases the risk of recurrence to 25% to 45%. The presence of an associated extensive intraductal component with the infiltrating cancer is another important determinant of risk. Age of the patient, inadequate tumor-free margins in the resected specimen, grading, and peritumoral vascular invasion also impact on the risk of local failure. Muticentricity (two or more tumors in different breast quadrants) is considered a contraindication to sparing the breast.

At 10 yrs ~8%. to 30%. if no DXT pat- of.

Axillary lymph nodes as well as internal mammary nodes are the most frequent filters of the breast lymphatic drainage. Removal of internal mammary nodes has failed to demonstrate a benefit in survival and it is for this reason that the lymphatic clearance in breast cancer is now limited to the axilla.[24] For this reason the axillary dissection is being considered more and more as a staging rather than a therapeutic procedure. In terms of the prognostic significance of the axillary nodal status, number of involved nodes is still considered the most important determinant for modulating adjuvant systemic treatment. In this framework attempts have been made to determine axillary status noninvasively, but to date no measure has been shown to be successful.

sentinel node

TABLE 25.3. Surgical Options for Operable Breast Cancer

Type of Surgery	Description	Indications
Radical mastectomy (Halsted mastectomy)	Removal of a large portion of skin, nipple–areola complex, breast tissue en bloc with minor and major pectoral muscles and the lymphatics of the I, II, and III levels	T4b tumors. (If the invasion is limited removal of the portion of the major pectoral muscle above the tumor may be enough.)
Modified radical mastectomy (Patey mastectomy)	Removal of loose skin including nipple–areola complex, breast tissue, minor pectoral muscle en bloc with the lymphatics of the I, II, and III level	T2 tumors, T1 tumors in which there is a contra-indication for conservative surgery (multicentricity, psychological attitude toward mastectomy, positive margins at subsequent excisions)
Total mastectomy	Removal of loose skin including nipple–areola complex and all breast tissue	Diffuse DCIS, prophylactic surgery in BRCA1-2 patients, prophylactic surgery for LCI S
Subcutaneous mastectomy	Removal of all glandular tissue, sparing the skin and the nipple–areola complex	No longer used. Risk of left behind mammary tissue and retroareolar ducts.
Skin-sparing mastectomy	Removal of all glandular tissue en bloc with the nipple–areola complex through the areolar incision	Prophylactic surgery for LCIS, *BRCA* mutations, DCIS. Better cosmetic result. Risk of leaving behind breast tissue and flap necrosis.
Quadrantectomy, segmental mastectomy (Veronesi quadrantectomy) plus axillary dissection	Removal of loose skin with the breast parenchyma harboring the tumor. The resection is performed at least 2 cm from the tumor borders.	T1–T2 (< 2.5 to 3 cm) tumors. When an extensive intraductal component is present this conservative surgery may decrease the risk of leaving behind peritumoral foci
Lumpectomy, tumorectomy, wide excision plus axillary dissection	Removal of the breast parenchyma harboring the tumor. The resection is performed at 1 cm from the tumor borders.	T1 tumors
Lumpectomy, tumorectomy, wide excision, quadrantectomy without axillary dissection	No axillary dissection	DCIS, LCI, benign breast disease
Axillary sampling	Removal of five to eight axillary nodes of the first level	Considered sufficient for staging purpose
Sentinel node biopsy	Small axillary incision and removal of the sentinel node	Small infiltrating tumor in which the sentinel node may be predictive of axillary status

The standard axillary dissection consists of the removal of the three axillary levels. The first level conventionally extends from the lateral border of the latissimus dorsi–dorsal muscle to the lateral margin of the minor pectoral muscle; the second is above the minor pectoral and the third between the medial border of the minor to the subclavicular muscle. Removal of the first level or a "sampling" of some lymph nodes of the first level (four to eight) may be representative of the status of the axilla.[25] If metastases are present in these lymph nodes there is the probability of involvement of other nodes in levels I and II. Further surgery or radiotherapy may be advised in this case.

Recently studies have focused on the "sentinel node." Their objectives are to identify the first node that receives lymph from the tumor area. The status of this node may be predictive of axillary involvement.[26] By injecting methylene blue or ^{99m}Tc-labeled human colloid albumin into the skin overlying the tumor it is possible to recognize this node (with probe in the case of a radioactive tracer) and remove it for histologic assessment. The pathologic status of the sentinel node is indicative of the status of the remaining nodes. Thus a negative sentinel node can be used as an indicator that further axillary dissection is not necessary.

Plastic surgery is an option in cases where mastectomy is required. Immediate or delayed reconstruction depends on the local condition of tissue after the mastectomy and on the resources available. Different methods are now used for reconstructing the breast: these include prosthesis implant, latissimus dorsi or rectus abdomus pedunculated flaps, and microvascularized free flaps.

SYSTEMIC TREATMENT

Many breast cancer patients who remain disease free after local and regional treatment eventually relapse and die of, or with, overt metastasis. The current hypothesis ascribes the failure to obtain freedom from disease to occult micrometastatic disease already present at the time of diagnosis and first surgery. This hypothesis has acquired indirect support from the results of clinical trials that have shown no additional advantage in terms of disease-free or overall survival following more radical local therapy.

Despite a large volume of experimental and empirical data, almost all knowledge related to the benefits of adjuvant systemic treatment has derived from randomized trials. Trials were designed to define treatment benefit in terms of disease-free survival (DFS) or overall survival (OS) and focused upon the type of therapies found to produce a significant improvement.

Three main types of treatments, later found to be effective in prolonging disease-free and overall survival, were investigated in the past decades. These include endocrine therapies, cytotoxics administered as single- or multiple-agent regimens, and combined chemoendocrine therapies. These treatments were initially compared with locoregional treatment only. More recently trials have investigated new therapeutic concepts based on the initial results, thus attempting to further improve treatment outcome.

Adjuvant systemic therapy does not provide cure for most of the treated patients. It is estimated that adjuvant therapy averts relapse in one third of the patients who would have relapsed without its use. Such reduction in relapse rate eventually results in lowering the death rate by about one fifth. Cumulative estimates after 5 to 15 years of follow-up indicate that the benefit in terms of reduction of the risk of death is approximately 7% to 12% (e.g., overall survival percentage increases at 10 years from 40% to 50%) in a population of patients with node-positive disease and 2% to 5% in a population with node-negative breast cancer (e.g., overall survival percentage increases at 10 years from 79% to 84%). Newer trials that compare an adjuvant systemic therapy, thought to be better in terms of cost-effectiveness with the best available treatment, are likely to yield smaller differences that might be significant. A larger sample size is required for such studies.

Owing to these sample size considerations the summing up of the results in an overview or meta-analysis from individual trials that compared one therapy to another has become the most powerful tool for identifying treatment outcome differences.[27,28]

The latest update of this international collaborative effort was performed in the autumn of 1995 and a previous overview included trials that started before 1985, with the following comparisons:

- Tamoxifen with no adjuvant therapy, or tamoxifen plus another treatment versus the other therapy alone (e.g., tamoxifen plus radiation therapy versus radiation therapy alone) carried out in 40 trials with 29,892 participants
- Chemotherapy with no adjuvant therapy or with chemotherapy plus another therapy versus the other therapy alone (e.g., chemotherapy and tamoxifen versus tamoxifen alone) carried out in 44 trials with 18,403 participants
- Ovarian ablation with no adjuvant systemic therapy or ovarian ablation plus chemotherapy versus chemotherapy alone in 10 trials with 3072 participants, of whom 1817 patients were < 50 years of age before trial entry
- Trials evaluating immunotherapy with 6300 participants.

Trials of adjuvant systemic therapy have provided information on several other features related to details of treatments and selection of prognostic factors to better tailor the approach to the individual patient. Decision-making for choosing a suitable therapy for a patient is thus based upon a large amount of information, much of which continues to be the subject of clinical investigations. The specific items studied in clinical trials and comments about the results or the current status of research can be summarized in the following sections.

Ovarian Ablation

Overview results showed an estimated relative reduction in the likelihood of relapse or death of 26% and a reduction in the likelihood of death of 25%. The reduction in relapses associated with the use of ovarian ablation appeared late during follow-up.

Chemotherapy-induced amenorrhea was also found to be associated with improved disease-free survival in trials of adjuvant cytotoxic therapies, but it is unlikely that the main therapeutic effect of adjuvant chemotherapy in premenopausal patients is due to ovarian suppression.[29]

Current trials investigate ovarian supresion with gonadotropin releasing hormone (GnRH) analogs and its combination with chemotherapy.

goserelin.

Perioperative and Preoperative Chemotherapy

Overview data on five trials with 6093 participants showed a slight reduction in relapses (reduction of 31% in local recurrences) with perioperative chemotherapy.[30]

Preoperative chemotherapy has been shown to yield a high rate of response in the primary tumors (60% to 95% overall of which 3% to 28% were complete pathologic responses). Results of large trials (e.g., NSABP Trial B-18) failed to provide an advantage in disease-free survival although tumor downstaging was observed. Therefore this modality, commonly used in locally advanced disease, remains investigational. Several regimens were tested as preoperative chemotherapy in early breast cancer, including some new agents and approaches. The advantage of evaluating primary tumor responses to preoperative chemotherapy was used for the definition of new administration modalities (e.g., continuous infusion of 5-fluorouracil given with intermittent 4-epirubicin and cisplatin with an estimated response rate of 98%).[31]

Good prognostic features
1. good ECOG
2. 1 or 2 sites mets esp soft tissue
3. prior hormonal tx

Adjuvant Prolonged Chemotherapy

|Poor|
prior ext / RRT ↓
mets in bone or visera ↑
esp liver
large # ?
mets ?

Overview results showed an estimated relative reduction in the likelihood of relapse or death of 28% and a reduction in the likelihood of death of 16%. Most investigated regimens in surgery-controlled trials were CMF-type. Multidrug regimens were found to be superior to single drug (alkylating agents) and six courses of CMF have an effect similar to that of four courses of an anthracycline combination.[32]

An alternating regimen with doxorubicin followed by CMF compared with the same drugs given in a sequence starting with CMF resulted in an advantage for the doxorubicin-first regimen.[33]

A trial that investigated a dose reduction showed a significant decreased treatment effect for patients treated with the lower dose.[34]

who?
rapid progressive disease
short disease-free interval
refractory to hormone receptor ⊖
pred: visceral mets

Adjuvant Tamoxifen

No effect Age / menopausal status / hormone receptors.

Overview data showed that tamoxifen reduced the annual likelihood of recurrence or death by 25% and the likelihood of death by 17%. Tamoxifen was more effective in patients with tumors classified as estrogen-receptor-positive. Contralateral breast cancer risk was reduced by approximately 35%. Different doses of tamoxifen have not been compared. The recommended dose is 20 mg/day. Treatment duration trials are ongoing. Existing evidence indicates treatment duration to be between 2 and 5 years. Other endocrine therapies using different antiestrogens (Toremifene),

Median duration of response 1-2 years

Factors ass. ÷ greater response:
1. +ER +/- PR ⊕
2. long disease-free interval
3. soft tissue / bone mets
4. prev. response in endocrine tx

5. older age for additive hormonal tx.

specific aromatase inhibitors — formestane, letrozole, anastrozole, vorozole. (pentagron) (arimidex)

500 mgs od

progestins (e.g., medroxyprogesterone acetate), and aromatase inhibitors* (aminoglutethimide) were insufficiently investigated and are the subject of ongoing trials.

Adjuvant Chemoendocrine Therapies

The Overview showed that for patients above 50, chemoendocrine therapy (with tamoxifen) compared with chemotherapy alone reduced the annual likelihood of recurrence by 28% and the likelihood of death by 20%. Similarly, when compared to tamoxifen alone, the reductions in likelihood were 26% and 10%, respectively. For premenopausal women, chemoendocrine therapy with either ovarian ablation or tamoxifen is still being investigated against each of the modalities. The combination doxorubicin and cyclophosphamide with tamoxifen improved treatment outcome when compared with tamoxifen alone. The trial was conducted in patients with tumors classified as endocrine therapy-sensitive (e.g., ER-positive).[35]

The best way to combine chemotherapy and tamoxifen is unknown, especially if the cytotoxic regimen does not include anthracyclines (e.g.,CMF). Laboratory studies have demonstrated that chemotherapy cell kill was inhibited in the presence of tamoxifen.[36]

Clinical data also suggested a negative interaction between cytotoxics (alkylating agents and 5-fluorouracil) and tamoxifen,[37] and this issue is still under study.

High-Dose Chemotherapy

A dose-intense regimen using several drugs on a weekly schedule for 16 weeks was found to significantly improve disease-free and overall survival when compared to six courses of cytoxan adriamyin 5 F-U (CAF).[38]

High-dose chemotherapy with peripheral blood progenitor cell or bone marrow support is a promising treatment modality, and several randomized trials are currently being conducted to investigate this issue. Indirect evidence exists that this approach might be advantageous in terms of treatment results. Although these approaches are promising, they are very costly and toxic, and should be used only in the context of randomized clinical trials.

Adjuvant Immunotherapy

Overview data showed no significant therapeutic effect of immunotherapy (mainly Bacillus Calmette-Guerin (BCG) or its methanol extract, levamisole, and *Corynebacterium parvum*).

The choice of treatment is thus based upon results from clinical trials and evaluation of risk factors derived from disease- and patient-related features. For patients with node-negative breast cancer, factors that have been defined as useful for the determination of prognosis include pathologic tumor size, grade of the tumor, and estrogen receptor status. The latter, together with age and menopausal status, also have been defined as useful for treatment decisions. For node-negative breast cancer patients three risk categories have been defined to select a subpopulation with

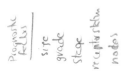

508   BREAST CANCER

TABLE 25.4. Definition of Risk Categories for Patients with Node-Negative Breast Cancer

Factors	Minimal/Low-Risk (All of the Features)	"Good" Risk	"High" Risk (One of the Features)
T-size^a	<1 cm	1-2 cm	>2 cm
ER Status^b	Positive	Positive	Negative
Grade^b	Grade 1 (uncertain relevance for tumors < 1 cm)	Grade 1–2	Grade 2–3
Age^c	>35 Years	—	

^{a}Pathologic tumor size (of invasive component) was the most important prognostic factor for defining additional risk of relapse.
^{b}ER-status and grade are expressions of the malignant transformation of the tumor cell, and it is difficult to precisely dichotomize these features to indicate a good versus bad prognosis.
^{c}Patients who develop breast cancer at a young age are considered to be at high risk of relapse, although an exact age threshold for this increased risk has not been defined. Although acknowledging this fact, the panel did not accept age as a factor to influence treatment choice.

chances of systemic relapse lower than 10% at 10 years. Table 25.4 summarizes the factors useful for allocation of node-negative disease into these three prognostic categories.

For node-positive disease, the number of nodes involved seemed the best indicator of prognosis. Age, estrogen receptor (ER) status, and menopausal status were defined as useful for an appropriate treatment choice. For patients with small screening-detected tumors the only identified useful prognostic factor was nodal status. These prognostic factors were formulated at a consensus conference held in St. Gallen, Switzerland in March 1995.[39]

Treatment choice recommendations for each subpopulation defined by these factors were made. Table 25.5 describes available types of systemic adjuvant therapies based upon baseline prognosis and features influencing treatment outcome.

Treatment of Metastatic Disease

Overt metastases indicate a chronic, incurable disease. Treatments are defined by their efficacy to provide palliation. An important feature influencing treatment choice relates to the heterogeneous course of the disease, with survival times that might vary from a few weeks to several decades. Overall, the median duration of survival is 2 years. Thus, the choice of the treatment should take into account the extent of the disease, its related symptoms, and the estimation of survival. It should aim to increase the total duration of the time with no or few disease-related symptoms, with the lowest costs in terms of side effects of treatment. Systemic therapies, radiation, or surgery should be discussed for this purpose in a multidisciplinary setting.

The choice of primary treatment should take into consideration also certain biological features that define the aggressiveness of the disease and its chance

TABLE 25.5. Adjuvant Treatment for Patients by Nodal Status (Node-Negative, A; Node-Positive, B), Menopausal Status, and Estrogen Receptor Status. For node-negative patients risk categories are displayed in Table 25.4

(A) Node-negative

Patient Group	Minimal/Low Risk	"Good" Risk	"High" Risk
Premenopausal ER positive	Nil versus tamoxifen[a]	**Tamoxifen** Ovarian ablation[a] Chemotherapy GnRH analog[a]	**Chemotherapy** ± Tamoxifen[a] GnRH analog[a]
Premenopausal ER negative	(Not applicable)	(Not applicable)	**Chemotherapy**
Postmenopausal ER positive	Nil versus tamoxifen[a]	**Tamoxifen**	**Tamoxifen** ± Chemotherapy[a]
Postmenopausal ER negative	(Not applicable)	(Not applicable)	**Chemotherapy** ± tamoxifen[a]
Elderly	Nil versus tamoxifen[a]	**Tamoxifen**	**Tamoxifen**; If ER negative: **Chemotherapy** ± tamoxifen[a]

(B) Node-Positive

Patient Group	Treatments
Premenopausal ER positive	**Chemotherapy** ± tamoxifen[a] **Ovarian ablation** ± tamoxifen[a] GnRH analog[a] **Chemotherapy** ± GnRH analog[a] tamoxifen[a]
Premenopausal ER negative	**Chemotheapy**
Postmenopausal ER positive	**Tamoxifen** ± chemotherapy[a]
Postmenopausal ER negative	**Chemotherapy** ± tamoxifen[a]
Elderly	**Tamoxifen**; If ER negative: **Chemotherapy** ± tamoxifen[a]

Bold: Treatments accepted for routine use or baseline in clinical trials.
[a] Indicates treatments still under testing in randomized clinical trials.

for response. Shorter disease-free interval (from diagnosis to appearance of overt metastases), low or no estrogen receptor content in tumor cells, and multiple organ involvement are indicators of aggressive disease and short survival. Host-related factors, best objectively quantified by the performance status, also influence the prognosis because they are associated with lower response rates and shorter duration of response.[40] A short time interval since completion of previous adjuvant therapy to the development of metastatic disease is also associated with a poor prognosis.

The subjective attitude of the patient and the physician toward systemic treatment such as chemotherapy (and its subjective side effects) is one of the major factors that influence the choice and acceptance of a therapeutic program. Time to expected response after treatment is also a feature that may influence the choice of therapy: endocrine manipulations require an average of 6 to 12 weeks, whereas chemotherapy might influence disease symptoms within a shorter time.

The question whether asymptomatic patients with overt metastatic disease should receive immediate systemic therapy upon the detection of metastatic spread is a matter of controversy. It is generally accepted that treatment should be offered immediately after diagnosis of metastases in an attempt to defer the appearance of symptoms.

Endocrine treatments are usually well tolerated, enhancing their acceptability as a therapeutic option.[41] In general, endocrine therapies are offered to a patient with metastatic disease knowing that:

- About one third of an unselected patient population is likely to respond to endocrine therapy. Median duration of response is 8 to 14 months. Chances of response are higher when the tumor is rich in estrogen receptors, leading to 50% to 60% response rates. Responses are more likely to occur in patients with prolonged disease-free interval, with soft tissue or patients whose disease is confined to bone.

- Response to one endocrine therapy predicts a higher chance of effectiveness with subsequent hormonal manipulations.

- Discontinuation of an endocrine therapy such as estrogens, progestins, and tamoxifen at the time of disease progression (usually after a response) might induce a subsequent response. The mechanism of this "withdrawal response" phenomenon is not clearly understood.

- Starting of some hormonal manipulations may be accompanied by an exacerbation of cancer related symptoms ("flare"). This might appear within hours or days, and last for several days or weeks. Flare might be associated with an increase of serum tumor markers, alkaline phosphatase, and hypercalcemia. The incidence of this phenomenon is between 3% and 9%, and is likely to be followed by an objective response to therapy. Flare has been observed after the start of therapy with estrogens, tamoxifen, androgens, and progestins but not after aromatase inhibitors.

Cytotoxic agents are usually used for all patients whose aggressive disease requires a fast objective tumor regression. Overall response rates to chemotherapy are reported to range between 40% and 90%, with complete responses in 5% to 10%. The median time to maximal response varies between 7 and 14 weeks, with a maximum reported to be 16 months. The median duration of response to chemotherapy ranges between 6 months and 12 months. Some patients are described as having been in response for more than a decade. Whether the use of chemotherapy also prolongs survival is a matter of controversy. It is postulated that some improvement in overall survival is limited to patients with aggressive tumors, as opposed to those with less rapidly progressive disease. The most significant factor related to improvement of survival, as well as of quality of life, is response to treatment.[42]

FURTHER READING

1. Hermon C, Beral V (1996) Breast cancer rates are levelling off or beginning to decline in many Western countries: Analysis of time trends, age-cohort and age-period models of breast cancer mortality in 20 countries. *Br J Cancer* 73:955–601.

2. Sturgeon SR, Schairer C, Gail M, McAdams M, Brinton LA, Hoover RN (1995) Geographic variation in mortality from breast cancer among white women in the United States. *J Natl Cancer Inst* 87:1846–1853.

3. Swallow CJ, Van Zee KJ, Sacchini V, Borgen PI (1996) Ductal carcinoma in situ of the breast: Progress and controversy. *Curr Prob Surg* 33:553–600.

4. Fisher ER, Costantino J, Fisher B, Palekar AS, Redmond C, Mamounas E (1995) Pathologic findings from the National Surgical Adjuvant Breast Project NSABP Protocol B-17. Intraductal carcinoma (ductal carcinoma in situ). The National Surgical Adjuvant Breast and Bowel Project Collaborating Investigators. *Cancer* 75:1310–1319.

5. Silverstein MJ, Lagios MD (1997) Use of predictors of recurrence to plan therapy for DCIS of the breast. *Oncol Huntingt* 11:393–406, 409–410, discussion 413–415.

6. Reinfuss M, Mitus J, Duda K, Stelmach A, Rys J, Smolak K (1996) The treatment and prognosis of patients with phylloides tumor of the breast: An analysis of 170 cases. *Cancer* 77:910–916.

7. Weidner N, Cady B, Goodson WH III (1997) Pathologic prognostic factors for patients with breast carcinoma. Which factors are important. *Surg Oncol Clin N Am* 6:415–462.

8. American Society of Clinical Oncology Subcommittee (1996) Statement of the American Society of Clinical Oncology: Genetic testing for cancer susceptibility. *J Clin Oncol* 14:1730–1736.

9. Gail MH, Brinton LA, Byar DP, Corle DK, Green SB, Schairer C, Mulvihill JJ (1989) projecting individualized probabilities of developing breast cancer for white females who are being examined annually. *J Natl Cancer Inst* 81:1879–1886.

10. Burke W, Daly M, et al. (1997) Recommendation for follow-up care of individuals with an inherited predisposition to cancer II. BRCA1 and BRCA2. *JAMA* 277:997–1003.

11. Schrag D, Kuntz KM, Garber JE, Weeks JC (1997) Decision analysis—effects of prophylactic mastectomy and oophorectomy on life expectancy among women with BRCA1 or BRCA2 mutations. *N Engl J Med* 336:1448–1449.

12. Gallo MA, Kaufman D (1997) Antagonistic and agonistic effects of tamoxifen: Significance in human cancer. *Semin Oncol* 24 (Supp 1):S1–71–S1–80.

13. Kelloff GJ, Hawk ET, Crowell JA, Boone CW, Steele VE, Lubet RA, Sigman CC (1996) Perspectives on chemoprevention agent selection and short-term clinical prevention trials. *Eur J Cancer Prev* 5(Suppl 2):79–85.

14. Leitch AM, Dodd GD, Costanza M, Linver M, Pressman P, McGinnis L, Smith RA (1997) American Cancer Society guidelines for the early detection of breast cancer: update 1997. *CA Cancer J Clin* 47:150–153.

15. Stavros AT, Thickman D, Rapp CL, Dennis MA, Parker SH, Sisney GA (1995) Solid breast nodules: Use of sonography to distinguish between benign and malignant lesions. *Radiology* 196:123–134.

16. Harms SE (1996) *Curr Prob Diagn Radiol* 25:193–215.

17. Hall FM (1997) Technologic advances in breast imaging. Current and future strategies, controversies, and opportunities. *Surg Oncol Clin NA* 6:403–409.

18. Tubiana M, Holland R, Kopans DB, Kurtz JM, Petit JY, Rilke F, Sacchini V, Tornberg S (1994) Commission of the European Communities "Europe Against Cancer" Programme. European School of Oncology Advisory Report. Management of non-palpable and small lesions found in mass breast screening. *Eur J Cancer* 30A:538–547.

19. Devia A, Murray KA, Nelson EW (1997) Stereotactic core needle biopsy and the workup of mammographic breast lesions. *Arch Surg* 132:512–515; discussion 515–517.

20. Veronesi U, Luini A, Del Vecchio M, Greco M, Galimberti V, Merson M, Rilke F, Sacchini V, Saccozzi R, Savio T, et al. (1993) Radiotherapy after breast-preserving surgery in women with localized cancer of the breast. *N Engl J Med* 328:1587–1591.

21. Fisher B, Anderson S (1994) Conservative surgery for the management of invasive and noninvasive carcinoma of the breast: NSABP trials. National Surgical Adjuvant Breast and Bowel Project. *World J Surg* 18:63–69.

22. Veronesi U, Bonadonna G, Zurrida S, Galimberti V, Greco M, Brambilla C, Luini A, Andreola S, Rilke F, Raselli R, et al. (1995) Conservation surgery after primary chemotherapy in large carcinomas of the breast. *Ann Surg* 222:612–618.

23. Veronesi U, Marubini E, Del Vecchio M, Manzari A, Andreola S, Greco M, Luini A, Merson M, Saccozzi R, Rilke F, et al. (1995) Local recurrences and distant metastases after conservative breast cancer treatments: Partly independent events. *J Natl Cancer Inst* 87:19–27.

24. Fisher B, Redmont C, Fisher ER, et al. (1985) Ten year results of a randomized clinical trial comparing radical mastectomy and total mastectomy with or without radiation. *N Engl J Med* 312:674–681.

25. Greenall MJ (1995) How should the axilla be treated in breast cancer? Why I favour axillary node sampling in the management of breast cancer. *Eur J Surg Oncol* 21:2–5.

26. Veronesi U, Paganelli G, Galimberti V, Viale G, Zurrida S, Bedoni M, Costa A, de Cicco C, Geraghty JG, Luini A, Sacchini V, Veronesi P (1997) Sentinel-node biopsy to avoid axillary dissection in breast cancer with clinically negative lymph nodes. *Lancet* 349:1864–1867.

27. Early Breast Cancer Trialists' Collaborative Group (1992) Systemic treatment of early breast cancer by hormonal, cytotoxic, or immune therapy. *Lancet* 339:1–15 & 71–85.

28. Gelber RD, Goldhirsch A, Coates AS (1993) Adjuvant therapy for breast cancer: Understanding the Overview. *J Clin Oncol* 11:580–585.

29. Goldhirsch A, Gelber RD, Castiglione M (1990) The magnitude of endocrine effects of adjuvant chemotherapy for premenopausal breast cancer patients. *Ann Oncol* 1:183–188.

30. Clahsen P, van de Velde C, Goldhirsch A, et al. (1995) An overview of randomized perioperative polychemotherapy trials in early breast cancer. *Proc Am Soc Clin Oncol* 14:214.

31. Smith IE, Walsh G, Jones A, et al. (1995) High complete remission rates with primary neoadjuvant infusional chemotherapy for large early breast cancer. *J Clin Oncol* 13:424–429.

32. Fisher B, Brown AM, Dimitrov NV, et al. (1990) Two months of doxorubicin cyclophosphamide with and without interval reinduction therapy compared with six months of cyclophosphamide, methotrexate, and flourouracil in positive-node breast cancer patients with tamoxifen-nonresponsive tumors: Results from the National Surgical Adjuvant Breast and Bowel Project B 15. *J Clin Oncol* 8:1483–1496.

33. Bonadonna G, Zambetti M, Valagussa P (1995) Sequential or alternating doxorubicin and CMF regimens in breast cancer with more than three positive nodes: Ten-year results. *JAMA* 273:542–547.

34. Wood WC, Budman DR, Korzun AH, et al. (1994) Dose and dose intensity of adjuvant chemotherapy for stage II, node-positive breast carcinoma. *N Engl J Med* 330:1253–1259.

35. Fisher B, Redmond C, Legault-Poisson S, et al. (1990) Postoperative chemotherapy and tamoxifen compared with tamoxifen alone in the treatment of positive-node breast cancer patients aged 50 years and older with tumors responsive to tamoxifen: Results from the National Surgical Adjuvant Breast & Bowel Project B-16. *J Clin Oncol* 8:1005–1018.

36. Osborne CK (1994) Interactions of tamoxifen with cytotoxic chemotherapy for breast cancer. In: Jordan VC (ed) *Long-Term Tamoxifen for Breast Cancer*. The University of Wisconsin Press, pp. 181–198.

37. Fisher B, Redmond C, Brown A, et al. (1986) Adjuvant chemotherapy with and without tamoxifen: Five-year results from the National Surgical Adjuvant Breast and Bowel Project Trial. *J Clin Oncol* 4:459–471.

38. Fetting J, Gray R, Abeloff M, et al. (1995) CAF vs a 16 week multudrug regimen as adjuvant therapy for receptor negative, node-positive breast cancer. *Proc Am Soc Clin Oncol* 14:83.

39. Goldhirsch A, Wood WC, Senn HJ, Glick JH, Gelber RD (1995) Meeting Highlights: International Consensus Panel on the Treatment of Primary Breast Cancer. *J Natl Cancer Inst* 87:1441–1445.

40. Fey MF, Brunner KW, Sonntag RW (1981) Prognostic factors in metastatic breast cancer. *Cancer Clin Trials* 4:237–247.

41. Henderson IC (1991) Endocrine therapy of metastatic breast cancer. In: Harris JR, Hellman S, Henderson IC, Kinne DW (eds) *Breast Diseases*. JB Lippincott, Philadelphia, pp. 559–603.

42. Coates AS, Glasziou PP, McNeil D (1990) On the receiving end. III: Measurement of quality of life during cancer chemotherapy. *Ann Oncol* 1:213–217.

CHAPTER 26

CANCER AND PRECURSOR LESIONS OF THE UTERINE CERVIX

MICHELE FOLLEN MITCHELL, GUILLERMO TORTOLERO-LUNA, DIANE C. BODURKA, and MITCHELL MORRIS

The University of Texas M.D. Anderson Cancer Center
Houston, TX 77030, USA

The etiology of cervical cancer is multifactorial. Human papillomavirus (HPV) appears necessary, but not sufficient, as a causal agent. Screening in a systematic fashion has lowered the morbidity and mortality from cervical cancer in every country in which an organized screening program has been established. The diagnosis may begin with an abnormal Papanicolaou (Pap) smear; lesions visible by the naked eye are biopsied. The International Federation of Gynecology and Obstetrics (FIGO) staging system is used. The treatment for stage I and small stage II cancers is radical surgery; for stage II to stage IVA cancers, radiotherapy; and for stage IVB cancers, chemotherapy or palliation. Follow-up strategies concentrate on intense follow-up in the first 2 to 5 years after treatment. Rehabilitation after surgical and radiotherapeutic treatment is symptom based. Prevention currently consists of efforts to increase the number of women who are screened. Chemoprevention and an HPV vaccine may be preventive measures in the future.

ETIOLOGY

Cervical cancer, comprising 12% of all cancers in women, is the second most common cancer among women worldwide, exceeded only by breast cancer. It is estimated that about 500,000 women are diagnosed annually with cervical cancer and that almost half as many die of the disease. Up to 80% of cases are reported in developing countries, but economically disadvantaged women in both developing and developed countries are particularly affected. In the United States, cervical cancer

Manual of Clinical Oncology, 7th edition, Edited by Raphael E. Pollock
ISBN 0-471-23828-7, pages 515–535. Copyright © 1999 Wiley-Liss, Inc.

is the third most common neoplasm of the female genital tract, with an estimated 14,500 new cases (6% of all cancers in women) and 4800 deaths expected in 1997.

A continuous decline in incidence of and mortality from cervical cancer has been observed in most developed countries during the last 50 years. This decline is mainly attributed to early detection using the Pap smear. Despite this decline, cervical neoplasia continues to be an important health problem in women worldwide, particularly in underserved populations. Further, a shift in the declining trend of incidence and mortality has been observed in the United States and other developed countries since the mid-1980s. Since 1986, the incidence rate of cervical cancer in white American women under age 50 years has been increasing by about 3% annually, while rates have continued to decline in African-American women. In England and Wales, Canada, Italy, New Zealand, and Australia, similar trends have been reported. The reasons for this trend among young women are poorly understood, and should be interpreted with caution. Although the increase might be due to changes in the prevalence of risk factors, such as an increase in the prevalence of HPV infection or changes in sexual practices, childbearing patterns, and oral contraceptive use, other factors, such as changes in coding and registration procedures, screening coverage, hysterectomy rates, and the proportion of cases classified as "uterus not otherwise specified (NOS)," must be considered.

The overall 5-year relative survival rate has remained constant. In the United States, for the periods 1970–1973 and 1983–1989, the 5-year relative survival rates were both about 67%. Survival rates are higher for white women and women under 50 years of age. Survival rates are high (~90%) when the disease is diagnosed at early stages and poor (~13% to 14%) when diagnosed at advanced stages.

Epidemiologic evidence has long suggested that cervical neoplasia behaves like a sexually transmitted disease. In support of this hypothesis, several measures of sexual behavior are consistently associated with an increased risk of cervical neoplasia. Risk is higher among women with multiple partners, women whose sexual partners are more promiscuous, and women who first had sexual intercourse at an early age. In addition to sexual behavior, low socioeconomic status, reproductive history, smoking habits, oral and barrier contraceptive use, dietary factors, immunosuppression, frequency of obtaining Pap smears, and the characteristics of the male sexual partners have been implicated in the risk of cervical neoplasia.

Previous studies focused on the etiologic role of several sexually transmitted infections, including herpes simplex virus type 2, *Chlamydia trachomatis, Trichomonas vaginalis*, cytomegalovirus, *Neisseria gonorrhoeae, and Treponema pallidum*. Epidemiologic data obtained during the last 15 years support a strong role of HPV infection in the etiology of cervical neoplasia. This association seems to satisfy the criteria for causality in epidemiologic research: the association is strong, consistent, and specific; there are dose–response and temporal relationships, and the causal relationship is biologically plausible.

In a recent international collaborative study, HPV DNA was detected in 93% (range 75% to 100%) of cervical cancer specimens collected in 22 countries and analyzed by the polymerase chain reaction. The percentages of cases of cervical cancer attributed to HPV infection have been estimated to be about 82% in developed countries and 91% in developing countries. Similarly, HPV has been reported in up to 94% of women with preinvasive cervical lesions and in up to 46% of women who are cytologically normal.

The association between HPV infection and cervical neoplasia is particularly strong with specific HPV types (16, 18, 31, 33, and 35), increasing viral load, and infection with multiple HPV types. This association is consistent and independent of HPV assay method used and epidemiologic study design and appears to explain many of the previously established risk factors for cervical neoplasia, including sexual behavior and cigarette smoking which are now thought to be confounding risks.

The difference between the high prevalence of HPV infection and the low incidence of cervical neoplasia in young healthy women, as well as the low rate of progression of untreated CIN lesions, suggests that HPV may be a necessary but not sufficient risk factor for cervical neoplasia. Although HPV is the most important risk factor, other cofactors seem to be necessary for the development of disease. The availability of more accurate and effective methods for detection of HPV infection will provide the opportunity to conduct epidemiologic studies to assess the role of previously established risk factors as independent factors or cofactors for the development of cervical neoplasia and to assess the effect of interaction between HPV and these factors, particularly smoking habits and hormonal and dietary factors. The role of HPV persistence in the progression of cervical neoplasia and the determinants of HPV persistence need further evaluation. Moreover, the impact of recent trends in risk factors on the occurrence of cervical neoplasia deserves future attention.

SCREENING FOR CERVICAL NEOPLASIAS

Cervical cancer meets the criteria for a disease to be considered for screening: (1) it is a frequent disease and an important health problem; (2) it has a long detectable precancerous stage; (3) there is a screening test, the Pap smear, that is quick, noninvasive, inexpensive, and widely accepted; and (4) there is treatment available, and the treatment of early-stage disease is more effective than the treatment of symptomatic disease.

The main purpose of the Pap smear, which was introduced in the mid-1940s in the United States, is the earliest possible detection of cervical cancer and its precursor lesions. Since the test's introduction, it has been shown to be an effective measure for the prevention of cervical cancer, and it has been credited with the decline in incidence and mortality in cervical cancer observed in most developed countries over the last 50 years. Mass screening with the Pap smear has been considered one of the most successful public health measures in the prevention of cancer and the best available method for the early detection of cancer.

Although the effectiveness of the Pap smear has never been evaluated in a randomized clinical trial, there is substantial evidence from many observational epidemiologic studies, including ecologic, case-comparison, and cohort studies, that the use of the screening is associated with a lower incidence of and mortality from cervical cancer. Cohort data from British Columbia and case-comparison studies from Geneva, Milan, and Toronto demonstrate the protective effect of the Pap smear. Ecologic studies from areas with screening programs, such as Scotland; British Columbia; Iceland; Manitoba; Maribo County, Denmark; Ostfold County, Norway; Sweden; and the United States, show sharp reductions in incidence and mortality after screening was introduced.

However, it is important to remember that the Pap smear is a screening, not a diagnostic, test and as such is not a perfect tool; in recent years, its accuracy has been questioned. Although there are not precise data on the accuracy of the Pap smear, primarily because of methodological problems (study design, study population, gold standard for comparison, etc.), most studies report a sensitivity between 60% and 85% and a specificity greater than 90%. In a recent meta-analysis of the accuracy of the test, Fahey et al. (1995) observed that in 59 studies published between 1984 and 1992 comparing results of Pap smears and histologic analysis, estimates of the sensitivity and specificity of the test ranged from 11% to 99% (median 66%) and 14% to 97% (median 67%), respectively. The large variation in the estimates of the sensitivity and specificity was mainly attributed to differences in the methodology and quality of the studies.

Several sources of error have been identified in the screening for cervical cancer, including sampling error, smearing technique, processing of the sample, visual screening of the smear, laboratory quality control, interpretation of the smear, and reporting errors. Of these sources of error, the two major contributors to the false-negative rate are poor specimen collection (sampling error), accounting for up to 60% of false-negatives, and interpretation error, accounting for approximately 40% of the false-negatives. Because of the potential significance of the adverse effects of both high false-negative and high false-positive rates, several methods, used alone or in conjunction with cytologic analysis, have been assessed to reduce the error rate, particularly the false-negative rate. Among these methods are targeted rescreening, colposcopy, cervicography, speculoscopy, HPV testing, monolayer cell preparations, and automated screening. All of these methods have been shown to increase the sensitivity of the Pap smear to 90% or more; however, most of these methods have the limitations of increasing screening cost and time and requiring highly trained personnel.

In addition to the accuracy of the test, there are several other unsolved issues regarding the Pap test: the ages at which screening should begin and end and the screening interval that will increase the cost-effectiveness of a screening program. In 1988, a consensus panel representing the American Cancer Society, the National Cancer Institute, the American College of Obstetricians and Gynecologists (ACOG), the American Medical Association, the American Nurses Association, the American Academy of Family Physicians, and the American Medical Women's Association agreed on recommendations for Pap smear screening. They recommended annual Pap smears for all women who are or have been sexually active or have reached the age of 18 years. Low-risk women may be screened at 3- to 5-year intervals once two negative smears are obtained, while high-risk women (those with multiple sexual partners and those who commenced sexual activity at a young age) may be screened annually. The consensus panel did not recommend an age at which to discontinue the Pap smear.

Despite this recommendation, the most cost-effective screening interval is unknown. Data from case-comparison studies and mathematical modeling have shown a significant increase (from 64.2% to 83.9%) in the reduction in the risk of invasive cervical cancer by reducing the screening interval from 10 to 5 years, but less impact with shorter screening intervals. With screening at 3-year intervals, the risk of invasive cervical cancer is reduced by 91.4%; at 2-year intervals, 92.5%; and yearly, 93.3%. Therefore, based on these data, it is estimated that annual screening versus a 2- to 3-year screening interval has a very small impact on effectiveness at a two to three times higher cost. The preference for annual screening in the United States is based on the following rationale: (1) more frequent screening compensates for the high false-negative rate; (2) there is concern that long screening intervals may stretch longer, increasing the risk of losing contact with patients and forfeiting the opportunity to conduct screening during routine annual gynecologic examinations; (3) longer screening intervals may deemphasize the importance of screening among high-risk women; and (4) longer screening intervals decrease the number of opportunities to detect rapidly progressing lesions early.

In developing countries, where most cases of cervical cancer occur but where cytologic screening services and medical services for further evaluation and treatment of cervical preinvasive lesions are unavailable or scarce, resources must be allocated in a cost-effective manner. Some of the recommended strategies for screening programs in developing countries include longer screening intervals (5 to 10 years); later age at first screening (>35 years old); "once in a lifetime" screening among women aged 35 to 40 years; screening of all women at least once before any woman is screened twice; downstaging; and the use of colposcopy, HPV testing, cervicography, and automated cytologic analysis.

Despite the long-term presence and recognition of the benefits of Pap smear screening for detecting cervical cancer, the need for further research remains. Some of the areas that deserve future research are: (1) identifying strategies to increase screening rates among socially disadvantaged and elderly women in both developed and developing countries; (2) determining the most cost-effective screening interval; (3) increasing the accuracy of the Pap smear by reducing sampling error; (4) assessing the role of monolayer smear techniques, automated screening devices, and HPV testing in the screening of cervical abnormalities; and (5) determining the most appropriate strategies for the evaluation and management of patients with abnormal cytologic results (considering cost, the emotional impact on women, criteria for referral, and the role of HPV testing in triage and follow-up).

DIAGNOSTIC MEASURES

Preinvasive Lesions

Abnormal Pap smears are classified according to the Bethesda system (Table 26.1). Once abnormal epithelial cell abnormalities are detected by Pap smear, the standard

TABLE 26.1. The Bethesda System for the Classification of Abnormal Papanicolaou Smears[a]

Adequacy of specimen
  Satisfactory for evaluation
  Satisfactory for evaluation but limited by _____ (specify reason)
  Unsatisfactory for evaluation (specify reason)
General categorization (optional)
  Within normal limits
  Benign cellular changes: see descriptive diagnosis
  Epithelial cell abnormalities: see descriptive diagnosis
Descriptive diagnosis
  Benign cellular changes
    Infection
      Trichomonas vaginalis
      Fungal organisms morphologically consistent with *Candida* species
      Predominance of coccobacilli consistent with *Actinomyces* species
      Cellular changes associated with herpes simplex virus
      Other[b]
    Reactive changes
      Reactive cellular changes associated with inflammation (atypical repair)
      Atrophy with inflammation (atrophic vaginitis)
      Changes due to radiation
      Changes due to intrauterine contraceptive device
      Other
  Epithelial cell abnormalities
    Squamous cell abnormalities
      Atypical squamous cells of undetermined significance (qualify[c])
      Low-grade squamous intraepithelial lesion (encompassing HPV positivity, mild dysplasia, CIN 1)
      High-grade squamous intraepithelial lesion (encompassing moderate and severe dysplasia, CIS, CIN 2, and CIN 3)
      Squamous cell carcinoma
    Glandular cell abnormalities
      Endometrial cells, cytologically benign, in a postmenopausal woman
      Atypical glandular cells of undetermined significance (qualify[c])
      Endocervical adenocarcinoma
      Endometrial adenocarcinoma
      Adenocarcinoma, not otherwise specified
    Other malignant neoplasms (specify)
  Hormonal evaluation (applies to vaginal smears only)
    Hormonal pattern compatible with age and history
    Hormonal pattern incompatible with age and history (specify)
    Hormonal pattern not evaluable due to _____ (specify)

[a]HPV indicates human papillomavirus; CIN, cervical intraepithelial neoplasia; CIS, carcinoma in situ.
[b]Cellular changes of HPV, previously termed koilocytosis, koilocytotic atypia, or condylomatous atypia, are included in the category of low-grade squamous intraepithelial lesions.
[c]Atypical squamous or glandular cells of undetermined significance should be further qualified, if possible, as to whether a reactive or a premalignant/malignant process is favored.

of care, where resources permit, is referral for a repeat Pap smear and colposcopically directed biopsies. This group usually includes patients with atypical cells of uncertain significance (ASCUS) and low-grade squamous intraepithelial lesions (LGSILs, those that show HPV and cervical intraepithelial neoplasia grade 1 [CIN 1]) although few cancers are found in these patients and most of these lesions regress. A triage strategy for lesions more likely to progress to higher grades and thus more likely to develop into invasive cancers is needed. Colposcopy, cervicography, and HPV DNA testing are being evaluated for identifying high-risk ASCUS and LGSIL patients, but these tools are expensive. Triage strategies for ASCUS/LGSIL may be a lower priority in developing countries.

At the first colposcopic visit, a complete history should be taken and a physical examination, pelvic examination, repeat Pap smear, and pan-colposcopic examination (including vulva, perineum, vagina, and cervix) should be performed. The colposcopic examination involves the application of 3% to 6% acetic acid, followed by a careful 3- to 6-minute examination of the cervix, identifying the endocervical canal, squamocolumnar junction, transformation zone, and lesions, which typically turn white in acetic acid; lesions may or may not exhibit angiogenesis, for which a descriptive classification has been developed, including fine punctation, coarse punctation, mosaiform atypia, mosaic atypia, and atypical vessels. Atypical vessels are thought to be diagnostic of cancer. Mosaic and coarse punctation are thought to be worse findings than fine punctation and mosaiform atypia. Abnormal areas of the ectocervix are biopsied, and an endocervical curettage is performed. Additional abnormal areas in the vagina, vulva, and perianal area are inspected and biopsied.

Several new approaches to diagnosis of preneoplastic lesions are being developed. They include targeted rescreening, colposcopic screening, cervicography, HPV DNA testing (differentiating low-risk and high-risk viral types), speculoscopy (viewing the cervix under chemiluminescent illumination), digital-imaging colposcopy using computer assistance, fluorescent spectroscopy, and computer-assisted automated image analysis of Pap smear readings. It is hoped that all of these will improve the performance of screening cytologic analysis or better diagnose high-grade lesions at the time of the initial visit. Currently, all of these modalities are expensive and the value they add must be carefully evaluated.

Cervical Cancer

In its early stages, cervical carcinoma tends to be asymptomatic. Early symptoms include vaginal discharge, vaginal odor, and abnormal vaginal bleeding. If the patient is sexually active, there may be postcoital bleeding.

When a gross cervical lesion is visible, a biopsy is indicated. Cervical cancers may be characterized by gross appearance as exophytic or endophytic. Exophytic lesions protrude from the cervical surface and can be easily visualized and measured. Endophytic lesions are more difficult to detect, often not visible on speculum examination. They may considerably expand the endocervix before being detected.

Cervical carcinoma has two predominant spread patterns: direct extension and lymphatic dissemination. Hematogenous spread occurs late in the natural history of the disease. In the first pattern, the cancer spreads from the cervix to adjacent tissues, especially to the upper vagina and the parametrial tissues (cardinal and uterosacral ligaments). These areas are best assessed by a careful pelvic examination. Following speculum examination with good visualization of the entire vagina, vaginal and rectovaginal palpation should be performed to evaluate vaginal or parametrial extension. In many countries, this examination is performed under general anesthesia for patient comfort. If a cytoscopy and proctosigmoidoscopy are planned, they can be performed at the same time.

The tumor may also involve the pelvic sidewall. Sidewall disease can be a result of direct lateral extension of the cervical tumor or medial growth of metastatic lymph node deposits. Direct extension is most common. Sidewall disease can result in pelvic pain, sometimes with associated radiculopathy in the lower extremity. Unilateral leg edema may be the result of lymphatic and venous outflow obstruction. Larger cervical cancers may cause an asymptomatic hydroureter, which may be diagnosed by intravenous pyelography (IVP) or computed tomography (CT) imaging. Uremia may be the presenting sign in a patient with bilateral ureteral obstruction. When the bladder or rectum is involved by direct extension, there may be hematuria, rectal bleeding, or rectal obstruction.

The lymphatic spread pattern of cervical cancer is thought to proceed in a stepwise fashion. It begins with cells spreading into paracervical lymphatic channels, then into the pelvic node chains associated with the obturator, internal iliac, and external iliac vessels. From there, the cells spread cephalad to the common iliac chain and the para-aortic lymph nodes. Finally, extension to the mediastinal and supraclavicular nodes may also be seen.

Hematogenous dissemination is most often seen in women who have been previously treated for cervical cancer and have had a recurrence. When it is seen at primary presentation, it is in patients with very advanced cancer or with early cancer of an aggressive histologic subtype, such as small cell carcinoma. Metastatic disease may involve the lungs, liver, bone, or peritoneal cavity.

STAGING

Preinvasive Lesions

Biopsies showing preinvasive lesions are being read in the United States in similar fashion as are Pap smears: as LGSILs and high-grade squamous intraepithelial lesions (HGSILs). Often the pathologist will further clarify whether the LGSIL is more consistent with HPV or CIN 1 and whether the HGSIL is more consistent with CIN 2, CIN 3, or CIS. Europeans have not yet embraced the Bethesda system and continue to use the classification Richart developed in the 1960s, in which Pap smears and biopsies are classified as atypias, HPV, CIN 1, CIN 2, CIN 3 (which includes CIS), or invasive cancer.

Cervical Cancer

Cervical cancer is staged by clinical evaluation, which enables comparison of treatment results around the world. The rules for staging cervical cancer have been established by the International Federation of Gynecology and Obstetrics (FIGO) and were revised in 1995 (Table 26.2). While the FIGO staging correlates well with survival, treatment planning often includes several other important prognostic variables, such as tumor volume and surgical or radiographic evidence of lymph node metastasis. Poor prognostic factors are advanced FIGO stage, large tumor volume, positive pelvic nodes, certain high-risk histologic types (adenosquamous, small cell), poorly differentiated squamous carcinoma or adenocarcinoma, and the presence of lymphatic or vascular space involvement.

All patients should undergo a thorough evaluation of medical history and a physical examination with attention to the supraclavicular, axillary, and inguinal lymph node chains. Pelvic examination, particularly inspection and palpation at the time of bimanual and rectovaginal examination, is important in determining the size of the lesion and the presence of vaginal or parametrial spread. The risk of complications

TABLE 26.2. FIGO Staging of Cervical Carcinoma

	Preinvasive Carcinoma	
Stage 0		Carcinoma in situ; intraepithelial carcinoma
	Invasive Carcinoma	
Stage I		Carcinoma confined to the cervix (extension to the corpus should be disregarded)
	IA	Preclinical invasive carcinoma, diagnosed by microscopy only
	IA1	Invasion up to 3 mm deep and 7 mm wide
	IA2	Invasion between 3 and 5 mm deep and 7 mm wide
	IB	Clinically apparent lesions confined to the cervix
	IB1	Lesions no greater than 4 cm in diameter
	IB2	Lesions greater than 4 cm in diameter
Stage II		Carcinoma extends beyond the cervix onto either the vagina or parametrium but not to the lower third of the vagina and not to the pelvic wall
	IIA	No obvious parametrial involvement
	IIB	Obvious parametrial involvement
Stage III		Carcinoma extends to either the lower third of the vagina or to the pelvic wall. Hydronephrosis or a nonfunctioning kidney, unless known to be due to another cause, necessitates classification as stage IIIB.
	IIIA	Involvement of lower third of vagina. No extension to the pelvic wall
	IIIB	Extension to the pelvic wall or hydronephrosis or a nonfunctioning kidney
Stage IV		Carcinoma extends beyond the true pelvis or involves the mucosa of the bladder or rectum. Bullous edema does not permit assignment to stage IV.
	IVA	Spread to bladder or rectum
	IVB	Spread to distant organs

from radiotherapy is increased if there is a history of prior abdominal surgery, pelvic inflammatory disease, hypertension, heart disease, or diabetes.

Chest radiography and IVP are mandatory. It is not unusual to find a unilateral or bilateral hydroureter that changes the stage and prognosis. The position of the kidneys prior to pelvic radiation is confirmed by the IVP.

Cystoscopy and sigmoidoscopy are used by FIGO for the evaluation of the bladder and rectum. Invasion must be ruled out before the initiation of therapy because of the proximity of these organs to the cervix. A biopsy specimen, not visual impression, is used to change the stage. Almost all patients, except those with the earliest and smallest lesions, should undergo these procedures.

The barium enema can be a useful procedure for patients who are older or who have glandular lesions. Asymptomatic polyps or diverticular disease may influence the choice of treatment. Most often, younger patients with smaller squamous lesions probably do not require a barium enema. Plain radiographs are permitted in the staging evaluation but have a low yield and are seldom performed.

Often, other radiologic tests are used to aid in the development of a management plan, but results of these tests do not alter the stage. Lymphangiography is extremely useful in determining the presence of pelvic or para-aortic node metastasis; because it can reveal the architecture of nodes, not the just the size, it can detect early lymph node metastasis. The CT scan is often used to evaluate nodal status but is not nearly as accurate as lymphangiography. Confirmation of a metastatic deposit should be obtained by fine-needle aspiration or surgical exploration. The use of magnetic resonance imaging (MRI) has been reported as helpful in determining the extent of cervical cancer. MRI can distinguish tissue density well, hence it may be useful in looking at the nodes, as well as in evaluating pelvic involvement.

Surgical staging of cervical cancer is widely performed around the world, despite the fact that it does not alter the FIGO stage. Surgical staging is used to gain additional prognostic information regarding the extent of disease and to tailor therapy. Transperitoneal approaches to the pelvic and para-aortic lymph nodes led to a significant increase in complications from radiotherapy, predominantly radiation bowel injury, so many surgeons have turned to extraperitoneal lymph node dissection. Surgical staging has the disadvantage of causing a 2- to 4-week delay in the initiation of radiotherapy. There is no evidence that patients who undergo pretreatment surgical staging have better survival rates than patients who have lymphangiography or MRI with fine-needle aspiration of positive nodes.

MULTIMODALITY TREATMENT

Preinvasive Lesions

High-grade intraepithelial lesions, once identified, are usually treated with ablative methods or cone biopsy; chemopreventives are being used experimentally. Cone biopsy, rather than ablation, is mandatory for HGSILs if there is suspicion of invasion on Pap smear, biopsy, or colposcopy; a positive endocervical curettage; a discrepancy between the Pap smear and biopsy (Pap smear suggesting a higher grade lesion than biopsy); an unsatisfactory colposcopy (entire lesion or squamocolumnar junction not entirely visualized); an adenomatous lesion (adenocarinoma in situ or adenocarcinoma); or if the patient is not compliant with follow-up. Low-grade intraepithelial lesions are treated similarly or simply followed every 6 months with repeat Pap smear and colposcopy. Biopsy-proven atypia, the histopathologic correlate of ASCUS, is usually followed without treatment.

The most popular techniques of ablation in the United States are cryotherapy, laser ablation, and the loop electrosurgical excision procedure (LEEP). Although the LEEP is excisional in nature, it removes as much tissue as is destroyed with cryotherapy and laser ablation and is therefore an equivalent therapy. All three techniques destroy a portion of the cervix for which the superior and deep margin is estimated at 6 to 8 mm in height around the endocervical canal and the inferior and ectocervical margin includes the transformation zone of the ectocervix. In nonrandomized series, the failure rates of all three therapies are 10% to 20% over 2 years. Randomized studies of laser ablation and cryotherapy show similar long-term cure rates and complications. A recent randomized trial of the three modalities with 31 months of follow-up showed failure rates of 15% to 20% for all three treatments and no significant differences in complications, either short or long term.

Cone biopsies remove the endocervical canal; specimens include a superior and deep margin 2 to 3 cm in height around the canal and an inferior and ectocervical margin including the transformation zone of the ectocervix. Because the endocervical canal is included, cone biopsies are diagnostic as well as therapeutic treatment. Cone biopsies in the United States are performed using the scalpel ("cold-knife" cone), electrocautery ("hot-knife" cone), laser, and LEEP. A LEEP cone removes the cervix in two to three specimens, whereas the other techniques remove the specimen in one piece. (The additional two specimens are portions of the endocervical canal removed with an endocervical loop that reaches up higher in the canal, giving a tissue specimen 3 cm in height like a cold knife cone.) The advantage of a LEEP cone is that it can be performed in the clinic under local anesthesia in less than 5 minutes, whereas the other techniques are typically performed under general anesthesia in the operating room. One randomized study showed many uninterpretable specimens using LEEP, but other studies showed success rates and specimens for LEEP comparable with those for other types of cones.

Future treatment options may include chemoprevention, the use of micronutrients or pharmaceuticals to prevent or delay the development of cancer. Chemopreventives have the advantage of affecting the patient systemically and may be particularly advantageous in the patient who has multifocal vulvar, vaginal, and cervical disease or who is immunodepressed. Several chemoprevention trials have been carried out in the cervix with both micronutrients and pharmaceuticals. None of the micronutrient studies have demonstrated statistically significant regression of CIN lesions in randomized trials. Topical *trans*-retinoic acid caused significant regression of CIN 2, but not CIN 3, in a trial by Meyskens et al. Chemoprevention may become a treatment in the future but at present should be considered experimental.

Many interesting immunobiologic studies of HPV and patients' humoral and cell-mediated immunity have been published. All these studies suggest that patients who are able to mount an immune response to the virus are less likely to develop lesions or less likely to have a recurrence once a lesion has been treated. These results suggest that eventually initial cervical infections might be prevented by a humoral vaccine aimed at the capsid proteins L1 and L2, possibly administered before the onset of sexual activity in population-based vaccination programs. Once persistent infection has occurred or a lesion is present, efforts might eventually better be aimed at cell-mediated immunity using HPV type-specific peptides with the intention of causing regression of disease. This vaccine would be therapeutic and would be used in a well-defined group of women with disease.

Cervical Cancer

Careful choice of a primary therapy for cervical carcinoma is critical because recurrent disease is seldom curable. The primary approaches are surgery, radiotherapy, and multimodality therapy.

Microinvasive Cervical Carcinoma   The classification of microinvasive carcinoma of the uterine cervix is limited to squamous lesions. The distinction between adenocarcinoma in situ and microinvasive adenocarcinoma is not yet well defined. Invasive adenocarcinoma of the cervix should be treated by either radical surgery or radiotherapy. The diagnosis of microinvasion is made by cone biopsy.

For treatment planning, most clinicians in the United States use the functional definition of microinvasion described by the Society of Gynecologic Oncologists (SGO); this definition limits the depth of invasion to 3 mm and excludes patients with lymphatic or vascular space involvement. For patients with lesions with depths of invasion between 3 and 5 mm, options such as radiotherapy or radical surgery with either a type II (modified radical) or type III (radical) hysterectomy should be considered. Note that the FIGO definition of stage IA1 carcinoma, as modified in 1995, closely resembles the SGO definition of microinvasion.

For patients who have a depth of invasion of less than 3 mm and no lymphatic or vascular space involvement, hysterectomy by either the vaginal or abdominal route is appropriate. With this approach, the cure rate approaches 100%. Women of childbearing age who have a strong desire to maintain fertility and are compliant with follow-up can be treated with conization alone. Conization is acceptable only when the margins of the specimen are negative for invasive or preinvasive disease. Continued surveillance with colposcopy, cervical cytologic analysis, and endocervical curettage is indicated.

Invasive Cervical Carcinoma

Radical Hysterectomy   Radical hysterectomy has long been the standard therapy for stage IB1 and small stage IIA cancers. Simple hysterectomy had been attempted with poor results; the spread pattern of cervical carcinoma showed that the uterine ligaments and pelvic lymphatics were at risk. When described in 1900 by Wertheim, the radical hysterectomy was successfully being used as a treatment for invasive cervical cancer; nodes were removed only if involvement was suspected. However, there was a high mortality rate for the procedure. During the same period, radiotherapy was being successfully used as well. Meigs modified the radical hysterectomy procedure in the late 1940s, taking a wider margin on the parametrial tissues and routinely dissecting the pelvic lymph nodes. With Meigs' approach and the use of blood transfusions and antibiotics, results of the surgical treatment of early cervical cancer soon equaled those of radiotherapy.

The radical hysterectomy begins with abdominal exploration, including careful inspection of the peritoneal surfaces, liver, bowel, ovaries, and other pelvic organs. Pelvic and para-aortic lymph nodes should be carefully palpated for clinically evident metastatic disease. The paravesical and pararectal spaces are then opened with careful palpation of the cardinal and uterosacral ligaments. Most surgeons will discontinue the surgery and treat the patient with radiation or multimodality therapy when extrauterine disease or parametrial extension is present.

Younger patients who are in good health and preferably not obese are the ideal candidates for radical hysterectomy. Cancer should be confined to the cervix, although some patients with upper vaginal involvement may be adequately treated with radical hysterectomy. The most important criterion is that the cervical lesions should not, in most cases, exceed 4 cm in size. Larger lesions are best treated by radiotherapy or multimodality therapy. Because ovarian metastases from early cervical cancer are exceedingly rare, the ovaries may remain in premenopausal patients.

Further prognostic and treatment planning information can be obtained by analysis of the surgical specimen. Most patients are treated with postoperative pelvic radiotherapy when lymph node metastases, close or positive surgical margins, or parametrial spread is detected. Results of radiotherapy after radical hysterectomy have been mixed. While pelvic radiation following a radical dissection certainly adds morbidity, most gynecologic oncologists feel that the potential benefits outweigh the risks in these patients. Several prospective randomized trials evaluating the role of postoperative radiotherapy are underway.

The results for patients treated with radical hysterectomy are excellent, with 5-year survival rates ranging from 77% to 93%. A variety of authors have reported their experiences with laparoscopic lymphadenectomy, laparoscopic modified radical hysterectomy, and laparoscopy-assisted radical vaginal hysterectomy. To date, no large prospective randomized trials have compared abdominal radical hysterectomy with laparoscopic radical hysterectomy; these will be important to establish the value added by the laparoscopic approach.

Radiotherapy Ionizing radiation is the most commonly used therapy for patients with stage II to IVA disease, the majority of women who present with cervical carcinoma. Treatment involves delivery of radiotherapy in two separate phases, using an external beam and internal implants. Initially, external-beam radiotherapy (EBRT) is given to the pelvic area. The purpose of EBRT is twofold: it sterilizes microscopic disease that may exist in the pelvic lymph nodes, and it shrinks the central tumor in the cervix and paracervical tissues to provide better geometry for placement of the radiation implant. External therapy is given in a series of small fractions, most commonly 1.8 to 2.0 Gy daily for 4 to 5 weeks, for a total of 40 to 50 Gy. Delivery in multiple small fractions allows for maximal tumor cell kill with preservation of normal tissues.

Standard treatment areas measure 15×15 cm, and treatment fields may be divided between two separate fields (anterior and posterior) or four separate fields (anterior, posterior, and lateral fields). The lower border of the field is generally placed at the mid pubis or 4 cm below the lowest level of vaginal disease, which can be marked by placing silver pellets in the tumor that can be seen on X-ray examination. The upper border is placed at L4–L5 or L5–S1 unless the para-aortic nodes are believed to be at risk. The lateral borders are placed at least 1 cm lateral to the pelvic margins. The borders of the radiation field are tailored to the distribution of the tumor and the patient's anatomy.

The EBRT field is extended above the pelvis for patients who have known or suspected disease in the para-aortic nodes. When used for patients with surgically documented *microscopic* disease, extended-field EBRT has the potential to cure nearly 50% of patients. The results for patients with *gross* para-aortic metastases are very poor. Extended-field radiation exposes a greater volume of normal tissue to ionizing radiation, hence the risk of complications is significantly increased. More patients experience myelosuppression with extended-field therapy, and complications involving the small intestine are also more common.

Following external radiation, patients usually receive two intracavitary radiation implants, also referred to as brachytherapy. A variety of applicator devices have been designed to give an intense dose of radiation to the central pelvis while sparing surrounding tissues. The most widely used applicator is the Fletcher–Suit–Delclos afterloading tandem and ovoid. This system is inserted about 1 week after the conclusion of EBRT and left in place for 48 hours; the sequence is repeated 2 weeks later. The system consists of a curved tandem that is placed within the uterine cavity and two ovoids that lie in the upper vaginal fornices. It produces a distribution of high-intensity radiation that treats the upper vagina, cervix, and uterine cavity. Shielding in the ovoids limits the dosage of radiation delivered to the bladder and rectum. The placement of the device by an experienced practitioner is of vital importance to ensure dose distribution that will improve local control of the cancer without increasing serious complications. In many places, hollow "afterloading" devices are used, which allow the radioactive source to be inserted in the patient's room following verification of proper placement by pelvic radiograph and transfer from the recovery room. This type of system minimizes the dose of radiation to hospital staff, a major improvement over the older "hot" systems.

The tandem and ovoids are loaded with radium or, more commonly, cesium. The major portion of the dose delivered by the implant is to the immediate surrounding tissues, as the energy from the radiation source decreases over distance. Treatment results with radiotherapy for stage IB disease are excellent and comparable to those achieved with radical surgery.

Intracavitary brachytherapy has traditionally been delivered at a low dose rate (LDR) of 0.4 to 0.8 Gy per hour. There has recently been a dramatic increase in interest, however, in high-dose-rate (HDR) brachytherapy. Although HDR is defined as a dose rate greater than 0.2 Gy per minute, 2 to 3 Gy per minute is usually administered, a rate similar to that of EBRT. Potential advantages of HDR include the outpatient nature of the procedure (each application lasts only 10 to 15 minutes), decreased cost, decreased anesthetic requirement, and minimization of applicator movement. Randomized trials will be needed to establish how the cure and morbidity rates with HDR compare with those of LDR.

Alternative Therapies for Large Lesions   The effectiveness of EBRT is directly related to the size and oxygenation of the tumor. Whereas large hypoxic tumors tend to be radioresistant, those with a rich blood supply are more radiosensitive. Several strategies have tried to improve the radiosensitivity of large lesions, including hyperbaric oxygen therapy, radiotherapy with particles such as neutrons, and the addition of radiosensitizers, such as chemotherapy. None of these therapies has shown a significant advantage over standard therapy to date, but all remain under active investigation.

Radiosensitizers potentiate the effect of radiation on tumors. The mechanism of this action is not completely understood. The most commonly used radiosensitizer for cervical cancer has been hydroxyurea. Initially, several nonrandomized studies have shown superior treatment results with the combination of hydroxyurea and radiotherapy compared with radiation alone. Randomized studies are currently ongoing. The other widely used group of radiosensitizing agents are the chemotherapeutic agents 5-fluorouracil and cisplatin. The risk–benefit ratio of radiosensitizers in the treatment of cervical cancer is being investigated; only randomized studies will reveal the most beneficial strategy.

An alternative to the use of radiosensitizing agents is neoadjuvant chemotherapy, in which patients are treated before radiation with two to four cycles of chemotherapy. Initial studies indicated a good response to chemotherapy, as measured by tumor shrinkage. Randomized studies have failed to demonstrate a significant survival advantage, however.

Intra-arterial chemotherapy has also been used before radiation with the purpose of shrinking the tumor. In the 1960s, researchers at The University of Texas M.D. Anderson Cancer Center found that intraarterial chemotherapy before or during radiotherapy might improve response. Because of the morbidity, expense, and complexity of the procedure, however, little further work was done in this regard until the early 1980s, when Kavanagh and co-workers reported that patients receiving intraarterial cisplatin, mitomycin C, bleomycin, and floxuridine had good results. Advances in catheter and pump technology have allowed innovative constant intraarterial infusions during the course of radiotherapy, as reported by Morris and associates. These procedures are expensive and labor intensive. The role of intraarterial therapy in the treatment of cervical cancer remains under investigation.

Recurrent Cervical Cancer   The great majority of patients with recurrent disease are unfortunately incurable. Recurrent or metastatic cervical cancer may occur in one of four sites: the pelvic sidewall, para-aortic or other distal lymph nodes, lung, or bone (most commonly the vertebral bodies). A few patients will have a central pelvic recurrence. One reason for careful follow-up after treatment is to identify this last group of patients because they are candidates for curative therapy through a radical surgical procedure, exenteration.

The treatment of recurrent disease is based on the type of primary therapy delivered. Pelvic recurrence after radical hysterectomy can be treated with radiotherapy. For the patient who has already received pelvic radiation, additional radiotherapy is usually not possible. For disease outside the pelvis, radiation plays a palliative role in controlling the size and spread of metastatic deposits.

If a patient has a very small cervical recurrence after primary therapy with radiation, radical hysterectomy has been used as a less radical alternative to pelvic exenteration. Patients must be carefully selected for this approach, as the potential for complications is high. Most patients with a central pelvic recurrence of cervical cancer following radiotherapy should be considered for pelvic exenteration.

Pelvic Exenteration   Pelvic exenteration involves removal of the pelvic reproductive organs, including the uterus, tubes, ovaries, and vagina; the bladder and distal ureters; the rectum and anus; the pelvic floor, including the pelvic peritoneum and levator muscles; and usually the pelvic lymph nodes. Occasionally, a more limited procedure may be performed, such as an anterior exenteration (preserving the rectum and anus) or a posterior exenteration (preserving the bladder and ureters). The initial experience with pelvic exenteration carried a very high mortality rate. In recent years, several technical advances (the continent conduit, vaginal reconstruction with muscle flap grafts, and distal rectal anastomosis) and refined patient selection have made pelvic exenteration a curative and well tolerated operation for women with recurrent pelvic carcinomas. Other factors that have influenced the drop in mortality rate (from 13% to 4%) may include the liberal use of total parenteral nutrition in the postoperative setting, use of modern antibiotics prophylactically as well as for treatment of the frequent infectious complications that occur, and intensive care unit monitoring in most patients in the postoperative setting.

The operative procedure itself can be broken down into three phases: the operative evaluation, surgical extirpation, and reconstruction. During the operative evaluation, a vertical midline incision is made with a thorough exploration of the abdominopelvic cavity. Washings are taken and sent for immediate evaluation to rule out the presence of peritoneal metastases. The liver, spleen, and other abdominal organs are carefully palpated and inspected and any suspicious areas are biopsied. If gross peritoneal disease is discovered or washings are positive for malignant cells, the procedure is abandoned. The para-aortic lymph nodes are selectively sampled and pelvic lymph nodes, if not previously removed, are excised. The paravesical and pararectal spaces are opened, and the surgeon ensures that there is adequate clearance of the tumor from the pelvic sidewall. It is estimated that about 20% to 30% of exploratory laparotomies performed in expectation of exenteration are abandoned because of adverse factors not detected preoperatively. If no adverse factors are found, surgical extirpation is then carried out with en bloc removal of the aforementioned organs. Anesthesia and blood bank support should be available; significant blood loss often occurs at this point. Surgery is most commonly performed with two teams, one working through the abdominal incision and the other working to excise the surgical specimen through the perineum. Many advances have been made in the reconstructive phase in recent years. A urinary conduit is constructed and can now be made to allow continence by catheterization. A low rectal anastomosis may be performed, sparing the anus and allowing rectal continence. The vaginal reconstruction can be performed with a variety of muscle flaps, often gracilis muscle flap grafts.

Acute complications of pelvic exenteration are the same as those associated with radical surgery, including cardiac decompensation, pulmonary embolism, deep vein thrombosis, and hemorrhage. Most patients require blood transfusion during and after the surgery. Infections are common, including necrosis of the myocutaneous graft with secondary infection, pyelonephritis, or sepsis. Complications involving the urinary conduit include obstruction at the ureteral conduit junction, fistula formation, and anastomotic leak. Long-term complications often involve the urinary diversion, for example, recurring bouts of pyelonephritis. Psychosocial adjustments must also be considered after this surgery, and the patient's support system should include family and hospital staff. With the appropriate assistance, most women can resume an essentially normal lifestyle following pelvic exenteration. Following pelvic exenteration for a recurrent carcinoma of the cervix, 5-year survival, including death from all causes, is 44%.

Chemotherapy   Chemotherapy for recurrent cervical carcinoma should be regarded as a palliative treatment. The palliation is perhaps realized as decreased pain because of shrinkage of tumor mass. The opportunity for cure is very small and is limited to patients with a single lesion that can be resected. Even the best chemotherapeutic regimens have complete response rates of less than 10%.

The most active agent in the treatment of recurrent cervical cancer appears to be cisplatin. Used as a single agent, the expected response rate is about 30%. Other active agents include 5-fluorouracil, methotrexate, cyclophosphamide, melphalan, doxorubicin, mitomycin C, bleomycin, and carboplatin, with response rates of 10% to 23%.

Combination chemotherapy may provide an additional chance for response when compared with cisplatin alone. The use of cisplatin in combination with other agents has resulted in response rates that range from 30% to 50%. However, responses tend to be short lived, with median survival in the range of 7 to 10 months.

Palliative Therapy   Perhaps one of the most important roles of a physician with a patient with recurrent cervical cancer is delivering proper palliative treatment. The management of pelvic pain, renal failure, and infection are important aspects of the total care of the patient. Advanced cervical cancer often results in severe pelvic pain. A lesion on the pelvic sidewall may involve the sacral nerve roots or directly invade the bone. It is not uncommon for patients to have pain that radiates down the leg. The importance of adequate pain control with narcotics, antiinflammatories, and antidepressants and judicious use of radiation for bone metastases cannot be overemphasized. When local pain is resistant to these measures, patients may be helped by the use of epidural analgesia or ambulatory intravenous patient-controlled analgesia.

Recurrent or progressive cervical cancer may result in bilateral ureteral obstruction. This obstruction can cause infection, which can be treated with non-nephrotoxic antibiotics. In a patient who has not received radiotherapy, urinary diversion by percutaneous nephrostomy or ureteral stenting is indicated, which will allow the patient to proceed to radiation. In the patient with recurrent or progressive cancer after radiation, performing urinary diversion is controversial. Because there is no effective second-line therapy, saving a patient from death by uremia only to have her suffer with progressive pelvic pain may not be wise. The patient and her family must be counseled on the severity of the problem and the natural history of cervical carcinoma so that she can make an informed decision regarding urinary diversion and the use of chemotherapy.

FOLLOW-UP

It is estimated that 75% of cervical cancer recurrences occur within 2 years of therapy. Ninety-five percent of patients who will develop recurrent disease will have relapsed by the end of 5 years. Several studies suggest that for recurrences in early stages, survival is prolonged if recurrences are caught early and managed aggressively. Surveillance programs should focus on more visits (three or four per year) in the first 2 years and fewer (two per year) in the next 3 years. Yearly follow-up should occur thereafter. Each visit should include a thorough review and update of the patient's medical history, a review of systems, and a complete physical exam. Pap smears should be performed yearly. Chest X-ray films should be obtained at least yearly. Other studies can be ordered based on the review of systems.

REHABILITATION

Complications of Radical Hysterectomy

Many of the technical aspects of radical hysterectomy and pelvic lymphadenectomy have been refined in the last few decades, which has led to a reduction in the incidence of serious long-term complications. Great care is now taken in the handling of the ureters and their removal from the cardinal ligament, which leads to fewer ureteral fistulae. The patient who undergoes radical hysterectomy and pelvic lymphadenectomy is at risk for the typical acute postoperative complications from abdominal surgery, such as prolonged ileus and postoperative bowel obstruction. Particular to this procedure, however, is the long-term complication of an increase in constipation, which may be due to transection of the parasympathetic fibers in the uterosacral ligaments. Constipation, when present, may last for many years. The best management approach is to counsel the patient to begin a high-fiber diet, using laxatives only in resistant cases. The most common alteration in the urinary tract following radical hysterectomy involves the bladder, with women reporting an altered sensation of bladder fullness, with or without the urge to void. Urinary retention is a common problem during the postoperative period and sometimes longer.

There are several management approaches, but a common one is using the technique of self-catheterization. Another complication can result from excision of up to half of the vaginal tube during radical hysterectomy; in some cases, the vaginal shortening may cause sexual dysfunction. Finally, as a result of the interruption of lymphatic channels in the pelvis, some patients develop a collection of lymphatic fluid, a lymphocyst. Patients with a lymphocyst may present postoperatively with pain, a pelvic mass, or ureteral obstruction. Some lymphocysts resolve spontaneously, but if patients are symptomatic or have signs of ureteral or intestinal obstruction because of mass effect, lymphocysts can be drained percutaneously.

Complications of Radiotherapy

Portions of the gastrointestinal tract will receive a significant radiation dose during the delivery of pelvic radiotherapy. The sigmoid colon is within the radiation field, and portions of the small intestine often enter the pelvis as well. With the intimate anatomic relationship of the sigmoid to the cervix, it is understandable how a tandem and ovoid system with a relatively posterior placement could result in a high dose of radiation to the sigmoid. The acute effects of radiation on the sigmoid are described as proctosigmoiditis. They include diarrhea, at times with passage of blood and mucus, and occasionally tenesmus. Patients with chronic narrowing of the rectosigmoid usually present with diarrhea alternating with constipation. Bloating, gaseousness, and crampy abdominal pain are not uncommon. As a result, patients will often have anorexia and weight loss. Patients with a high-grade obstruction require surgical intervention. Chronic radiation injury to the sigmoid may also result in progressive ischemia, leading to necrosis and perforation requiring aggressive surgical management.

The acute reaction of the small intestine to radiotherapy is often manifested as diarrhea and abdominal cramping, sometimes associated with nausea and vomiting. Often, this is a short-lived side effect that promptly disappears with the cessation of irradiation. As with rectosigmoid injury, however, chronic injury can take years to become manifest. The section of small bowel most prone to injury is the terminal ileum, although other small bowel segments can be involved, especially in patients who have had prior abdominal surgery. Patients who receive extended-field EBRT are at particular risk for small bowel complications. Patients who have mild to moderate symptoms can often be managed expectantly with a low-residue diet and careful observation. Patients with more severe symptoms, especially repeated episodes of partial obstruction, warrant surgical intervention.

During EBRT to the pelvis, patients will sometimes note urinary frequency, usually a short-lived side effect of treatment. A small percentage of patients, however, may develop chronic problems, such as a contracted fibrotic bladder, leading to frequent urination and, in some cases, incontinence. Hemorrhagic cystitis may also be present in some women. This may be an incidental microscopic finding, although occasional severe exacerbations with gross hematuria may occur. When the bleeding is significant enough to cause clot formation in the bladder, emergency intervention is indicated, with continuous irrigation and possibly even fulguration.

It is expected that patients who undergo a combination of EBRT and brachytherapy will have very high-dose radiation delivery to the superficial vaginal and cervical
tissues. It is not uncommon to see some necrosis of these tissues in the weeks following completion of treatment. Treatment of cervicovaginal necrosis should be conservative, usually using cleansing douches and gentle debridement. The long-term
sequelae are vaginal stenosis, vaginal dryness, and shortening of the vaginal vault.
These defects can be treated with both systemic and local application of estrogen and
the regular use of a vaginal dilator to maintain patency of the canal.

PREVENTION

There are many ways to strengthen efforts for prevention and early detection of cervical cancer. The most promising areas of research include those that focus on understanding and preventing HPV infections and understanding the process of cervical carcinogenesis and how it can be interrupted with chemopreventives. Preventing
HPV infections with a humoral-based vaccine should eventually receive worldwide
interest. Eventually, treating lesions with a cell-mediated-based vaccine would be exciting. Once the role of other cofactors (e.g., smoking, use of oral contraceptives, and
diet) is assessed, specific behavioral interventions will be of interest. In general, the
use of barrier contraception, delaying the onset of sexual activity, and limiting the
number of partners should be encouraged as preventive behaviors. Early detection
could be improved by increasing the use of the Pap smear in unscreened women, decreasing the false-negative rate of the Pap smear, automating the screening process to
lower the cost, and better defining which patients need to be referred for colposcopy,
which is expensive. Prompt evaluation and treatment of cervical cancer precursors
should be encouraged, and technologies that automate or shorten the process should
be vigorously developed.

FURTHER READING

American Cancer Society (1997) *Cancer Facts and Figures—1995.* American Cancer Society,
    Inc., Atlanta.

Carcinoma of cervix (1992) In: Coppleson M (ed) *Gynecologic Oncology: Fundamental Prin-
    ciples and Clinical Practice.* Churchill Livingstone, Edinburgh, pp. 543–728.

Eddy DM (1990) Screening for cervical cancer. *Ann Intern Med* 113:214–226.

Fahey, MT, Irwig L, Macaskill P (1995) Meta-analysis of Pap test accuracy. *Am J Epidemiol*
    141:680–689.

Franco E, Monsonego J (1997) *New Developments in Cervical Cancer Screening and Preven-
    tion.* Blackwell, Malden, MA.

Hakama M, Miller AB, Day NE (1986) Screening for cancer of the uterine cervix. IARC
    Scientific Publication No. 76

International Agency for Research on Cancer Working Group on Evaluation of Cervical Can-
    cer Screening Programs (1985) Screening for squamous cervical cancer: duration of low

risk after negative results of cervical cytology and its implications for screening policies. *Br Med* 293:659–664.

Invasive cervical cancer (1997) In: DiSaia PJ, Creasman WT (eds) *Clinical Gynecologic Oncology*. Mosby-Year Book, St. Louis, pp. 51–106.

Kaufman RM, Henson DE, Herbst AL, et al. (1994) Interim guidelines for management of abnormal cervical cytology. *JAMA* 271:1866–1869.

Meyskens FL, Surwit EA, Moon TE, Childers JM, Paris JR, Dorr RJ, et al. (1994) Enhancement of regression of cervical intraepithelial neoplasia II (moderate dysplasia) with topically applied all trans-retinoic acid: a randomized trial. *J. Natl Cancer Inst* 86:539–543.

Mitchell MF (1990) Diagnosis and treatment of preinvasive disease of the female lower genital tract. *Cancer Bull* 42:71–76.

Mitchell MF (1993) Preinvasive diseases of the female lower genital tract. In: Gershenson DM, DeCherney AH, Stephen L (eds) *Operative Gynecology*, WB Saunders, Philadelphia, pp. 231–256.

Mitchell MF, Hittelman WN, Hong WK, et al. (1994) Review: The natural history of cervical intraepithelial neoplasia: An argument for intermediate endpoint biomarkers. *Cancer Epidemiol Biomark Prev* 3:619–626.

Mitchell MF, Tortolero-Luna G, Wright T, et al. (1995) Cervical human papillomavirus infection and intraepithelial neoplasia: A review. *J Natl Cancer Inst Monogr* 21:17–25.

Morris M, Burke TW (1983) Cervical cancer. In: Copeland LJ, Jarrell JF, McGregor JA (eds) *Textbook of Gynecology*. WB Saunders, Philadelphia, pp. 989–1013.

Morris M, Tortolero-Luna G, Malpica A, et al. (1996) Cervical intraepithelial neoplasia and cervical cancer. *Obstet Gynecol Clin NA* 23:347–410.

Muñoz N, Bosch F, Shah KV, et al. (1992) The epidemiology of human papillomavirus and cervical cancer. IARC Scientific Publication No. 119.

National Institutes of Health Consensus Conference on Cervical Cancer (1996) National Institutes of Health Consensus Conference on Cervical Cancer. Bethesda, Maryland, April 1–3, 1996. *J Natl Cancer Inst Monogr* 21:1–6.

Pisani P, Parkin DM, Muñoz N, et al. (1997) Cancer and infection: estimates of the attributable fraction in 1990. *Cancer Epidemiol Biomark Prev* 6:387–400.

Rubin SC, Hoskins WJ (1996) *Cervical Cancer and Preinvasive Neoplasia*. Lippincott-Raven, Philadelphia.

Shingleton HM, Orr JW (1983) *Cancer of the Cervix: Diagnosis and Treatment* 1st edition. Churchill Livingstone, New York.

Shingleton HM, Orr JW Jr (1987) *Cancer of the Cervix: Diagnosis and Treatment* 2nd edition. Churchill Livingstone, New York.

Tumors of the cervix (1993) In: Morrow CP, Curtin JP, Townsend DE (eds) *Synopsis of Gynecologic Oncology*. Churchill Livingstone, New York, pp. 111–152.

CHAPTER 27

GYNECOLOGIC CANCER

J. L. BENEDET and D. M. MILLER

Division of Gynecologic Oncology
BC Cancer Agency & University of British Columbia
Vancouver, British Columbia, Canada

CANCER OF THE ENDOMETRIUM

Incidence

Endometrial cancer has become the most common gynecologic cancer in many industrialized countries and particularly in North America. In Canada and the United States, endometrial cancer is approximately three times as common as invasive cervical cancer. In part this change is due to a decrease in the incidence and mortality of cervical cancer secondary to widespread screening for this disease and its precursors. In addition, the longer life expectancy of women in these countries is a contributing factor.

Epidemiology and Etiology

Endometrial cancer is predominantly a disease of postmenopausal women, with the peak incidence occurring in women of approximately 60 years of age. The basic mechanism in the development of endometrial cancer seems to be prolonged unopposed estrogen stimulation of the endometrium. A natural history model for this disease has been granulosa–theca cell tumors of the ovary, in which approximately 5% to 10% of cases at the time of diagnosis will have a concomitant endometrial carcinoma. Other states of altered hormone activity, characterized by chronic anovulation such as seen in polycystic ovarian disease, have also been associated with an

Manual of Clinical Oncology, 7th edition, Edited by Raphael E. Pollock
ISBN 0-471-23828-7, pages 537–561. Copyright © 1999 Wiley-Liss, Inc.

TABLE 27.1. Risk Factors for the Development of Endometrial Cancer

Endogenous	Exogenous	Demographic
Obesity	Hormone replacement therapy with unopposed estrogen	Higher social economic status
Infertility		
Chronic anovulation	Diet	Caucasian or Jewish
Nulliparity		Family history of breast, colon, or endometrial cancer
Polycystic ovarian disease		

increased frequency of endometrial cancer. Table 27.1 lists the associated risk factors for this disease. These risk factors fall broadly into three main categories: endogenous, exogenous, and demographic.

Obese women are known to convert androstenedione from adrenal or ovarian sources to estrone in their adipose tissue. Both increased precursor and more efficient conversion have been reported in these women.

In the late 1960s and early 1970s an increased incidence of endometrial cancer was noted in the United States owing to the then common practice of prescribing unopposed estrogens to women mainly for the control of menopausal symptoms. The use of oral contraceptive tablets containing both an estrogen and a progestin is thought to decrease the risk for the subsequent development of this cancer.

Screening

Although endometrial sampling and ultrasonography have been proposed as a screening modality for this cancer, they do not meet the criteria for a good screening test. These methods are not cost effective. Given the low prevalence of this disease in asymptomatic women it is difficult to justify routine screening. However, women who are at high risk because of family history (Lynch syndrome type II), obesity, or estrogen or tamoxifen therapy might benefit from annual endometrial sampling and in specific instances ultrasonographic assessment for endometrial thickness.

Pathology

Approximately 90% of all endometrial cancers have an endometrioid pattern, with the majority being well-differentiated lesions. Clear cell carcinomas and papillary serous cancers as well as adenosquamous cancers make up the remainder and generally are more virulent and aggressive. A clearly identified precursor lesion for endometrial cancer is atypical adenomatous hyperplasia or complex atypical hyperplasia, with estimates that 25% of such patients will progress to endometrial cancer if left untreated. Minor degrees of such hyperplasias generally respond well to hormone therapy with progesterone.

Most endometrial cancers are well-differentiated tumors with superficial invasion only. Tumor grade is also related to depth of invasion, with the more deeply invasive tumor usually being of higher grade. Most endometrial cancers arise in the fundus, and spread by surface extension to the cervix, tube, ovaries, and ultimately to other peritoneal surfaces. These lesions also invade the underlying myometrium, where they can also involve lymphatic or vascular spaces and in turn this can lead to pelvic and peri-aortic lymph node involvement. Peri-aortic node involvement, without pelvic node involvement, does occur but it is uncommon.

Clear cell and papillary serous adenocarcinomas of the endometrium generally are very aggressive tumors with a poor prognosis. To date there have been no identified precursor lesions for these variants and also there is no agreement as to what percentage of an endometrial cancer needs to show clear cell or papillary serous features to be classified into these categories.

Diagnosis

Endometrial cancer has a classic presenting symptom, namely that of postmenopausal bleeding or spotting and this symptom should be regarded as endometrial cancer until proven otherwise. Even though only 35% of such patients will be found to have endometrial cancer or other forms of pelvic malignancy, this disease remains the most important cause. Clear attention to this distinctive symptom by both the patient and the physician is undoubtedly responsible for the majority of cases being diagnosed in a stage I category, resulting in a usually favorable prognosis.

Diagnosis is made by tissue sampling, usually by fractional dilatation and curettage (D&C). Other methods of assessment such as endometrial sampling and biopsy with an accompanying endocervical curettage, hysteroscopy, and biopsy are also commonly employed methods and are accurate alternatives to D&C.

Staging

Staging for endometrial carcinoma is surgical and the existing staging system is presented in Table 27.2. Figure 27.1 diagrammatically illustrates stage I disease. Although the staging system was changed to a surgical system in 1988, clinical staging is still important in terms of preoperative assessment and planning for surgery. Clinical staging correlates well with surgical staging and also prognosis. In the majority of cases, if the uterus is not enlarged and there is no evidence of extrauterine disease or of cervical involvement, further assessment consists of a screening chest X-ray film and the usual preoperative blood work and chemistry. More complex preoperative assessment such as computerized tomography (CT) scan, barium enema, cystoscopy, etc. are indicated for patients whose disease features suggest involvement of other organ systems or spread. CA-125 may also have a role in following patients with advanced disease or as a possible indicator of extrauterine involvement.

Approximately 10% to 15% of patients with clinical stage I disease have evidence of more advanced disease on surgical staging. It is recommended that in patients with what appears to be clinical stage I disease, peritoneal washings should be obtained on

TABLE 27.2. Corpus Uteri. TNM Clinical Classification. Staging for Tumors and FIGO Surgical Staging

TNM Categories			FIGO Stages	
TX				Primary tumor cannot be assessed.
T0				No evidence of primary tumor
Tis			0	Carcinoma in situ
T1			I	Tumor is confined to corpus.
	T1a		IA	Tumor is limited to endometrium.
	T1b		IB	Tumor invades up to or less than one half of myometrium.
	T1c		IC	Tumor invades to more than one half of myometrium.
T2			II	Tumor invades cervix but does not extend beyond uterus.
	T2a		IIA	Endocervical glandular involvement only
	T2b		IIB	Cervical stromal invasion
T3 and/or N1			III	Local and/or regional spread as specified in T3a, b, N1 and FIGO IIIA, B, C below
	T3a		IIIA	Tumor involves serosa and/or adnexa (direct extension or metastasis) and/or cancer cells in ascites or peritoneal washings.
	T3b		IIIB	Vaginal involvement (direct extension or metastasis)
	N1		IIIC	Metastasis to pelvic and/or para-aortic lymph nodes
T4			IVA	Tumor involves bladder *mucosa* and/or bowel *mucosa*.
M1			IVB	Distant metastasis (*excluding* metastasis to vagina, pelvic serosa, or adnexa, *including* metastasis to intraabdominal lymph nodes other than para-aortic and/or inguinal lymph nodes)

entering the abdominal cavity. Careful exploration of the entire abdominal and pelvic cavity should be carried out with biopsy of any suspicious areas followed by transabdominal hysterectomy/bilateral salpingo-oophorectomy (TAH/BSO) in straightforward cases. Examination and exploration of the retroperitoneal areas with biopsy of any enlarged or suspicious lymph nodes is then carried out.

Some individuals have advocated TAH/BSO be performed after washings are taken for clinical stage I patients. The removed uterus should then be carefully examined pathologically with frozen sections to assess adverse features such as high-grade differentiation and/or deep invasion, or unusual histologic types, for example, unsuspected clear cell or papillary serous carcinomas. If these findings are positive then further staging with nodal biopsy and dissection of the pelvic, para-aortic areas are carried out.

Although surgical staging with pelvic and para-aortic node removal clearly offers the most thorough assessment of disease extent it should be remembered that many of those patients are elderly, obese, with complicating disease, such as diabetes and hypertension. In these situations clinical judgment should be used as careful surgical–pathologic assessment of the removed tissues can generally accurately predict likelihood of risk of recurrence and the need for adjunctive therapy.

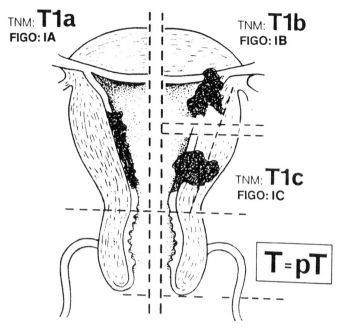

Figure 27.1. Stage I cancer, corpus uteri.

Postsurgical Treatment

Once surgical staging has occurred and a careful histopathologic assessment of the removed tissue has been made, a decision is then made as to whether or not postoperative adjunctive therapy is needed. Cases can be classified as high or low risk for recurrence based on a variety of factors. High-risk patients are generally those with grade 2 or 3 disease, deep myometrial invasion, or where evidence of lymphatic–vascular space involvement is noted. Also extrapelvic or extrauterine disease are high-risk features as are nodal metastases. Individuals with well-differentiated grade 1 tumors confined to the endometrium or minimal superficial myometrial invasion have an excellent prognosis with surgery alone and do not require adjuvant therapy. A variety of hormonal and radiotherapeutic schemes have been used as adjunctive therapy in stage I cases with high-risk features. It is generally agreed that postoperative radiotherapy, either in the form of vault irradiation or pelvic irradiation, can help lower the incidence of local recurrence but does not appear to have any beneficial effect in terms of survival. Fortunately the vast majority of cases are diagnosed with stage I, low-risk disease and are successfully treated with simple hysterectomy.

Primary radiotherapy or preoperative intracavitary radiotherapy followed by hysterectomy is no longer commonly used, as results are no better than with primary surgery.

Effective therapy for advanced stage disease or recurrent disease to date has proven to be elusive. Generally a combination of radiotherapy and/or chemotherapy has been used in these situations. Currently, combinations of platinum and taxol chemotherapy are favored for recurrent or metastatic disease. These agents generally produce a good response but the duration of response, unfortunately, is in most cases not more than 12 months. Other medications with documented response in endometrial cancer have been Adrimycin and 5-fluorouracil (5-FU). Hormonal therapy with progestational agents can lead to gratifying responses in some patients with recurrent or advanced disease; in general the better differentiated tumors are those most likely to respond.

Prognosis

The 5-year survival rate for stage I disease is approximately 90% with survival falling to 75% and 50% for stage II and III disease respectively. Clearly identified prognostic factors for endometrial carcinoma consist of stage, grade, depth of myometrial invasion, lymphatic–vascular space involvement, and histologic subtype.

Summary

Endometrial adenocarcinoma is a common tumor, which fortunately most often presents with a distinctive symptom enabling a diagnosis at a stage I level. Stage I disease generally has a favorable outcome and is usually treated with primary surgery with or without adjunctive radiotherapy depending on subsequent surgical pathologic findings.

CANCER OF THE OVARY

Introduction

Although death from cervical cancer remains the most common cause of death from gynecologic malignancy worldwide, ovarian cancer is the leading cause of death in most industrialized countries. Although our approach and knowledge of epithelial ovarian cancer has changed in the past 25 years, the overall survival has not been affected because approximately 65% to 70% of all cases continue to be diagnosed with stage III or stage IV disease.

Epidemiology/Etiology

It has been estimated that a woman's risk for developing ovarian cancer is 1 in 70, with the disease being most common in women in the fifth to seventh decade. Borderline or low malignant potential tumors are often diagnosed in younger premonopausal women. The etiology of epithelial ovarian cancer remains unknown. In a small percentage of cases (5%), genetic and hereditary factors appear to play a role. For the vast majority the occurrence of the disease is sporadic with no known etiologic agents or factors. Identified risk factors for epithelial ovarian cancer are nulliparity, delayed menopause, and early menarche, while high parity, breast feeding, and prolonged use of oral contraceptive medications seem to confer a degree of protection. These observations have led to the concept of incessant ovulation as being one of the underlying mechanisms in the production of these tumors. It is postulated that repeated rupture of the surface epithelium at the time of ovulation with regeneration and repair may lead to some subsequent change in cell regulatory mechanisms resulting in tumor development.

Patients with a family history of ovarian cancer need a careful pedigree assessment to determine their particular risk profile. Individuals with two or more first-degree relatives with the disease may have risk as high as 40% for site-specific autosomal-dominant inheritance pattern for ovarian cancer. In addition, individuals with breast–ovarian cancer pedigree and also breast–colon–endometrial–prostate $\overline{\text{Lynch II}}$ pedigrees are also at increased risk, although not as high for familial site-specific disease. Mutations of the *BRCA-1* gene have been linked to some 80% to 90% of breast–ovarian cancer families. Somatic *BRCA-1* mutations have also been noted in approximately 10% of sporadic ovarian cancers. The lifetime risks for developing cancer based on *BRCA-1* mutations are 60% ovary, 80% breast, as well as a three- to fourfold increase of colon and prostate cancer. In the future *BRCA-1* testing may be a potentially useful adjunct in the assessment of women at risk for ovarian cancer.

Pathology

Table 27.3 lists a modified WHO classification of ovarian tumors. This system basically divides tumors of this complex organ into three major categories: those arising from surface epithelium, which are the most common tumors by far; tumors arising from ovarian stromal tissues, both specialized ovarian stroma as well as supportive stromal elements such as fibrous tissue, blood vessels, etc.; and tumors arising from germ cells.

The common epithelial ovarian cancers, serious mucinous, endometrioid and clear cell, generally behave in a similar fashion on a stage-for-stage basis. Epithelial ovarian cancer has a propensity for spread along peritoneal surfaces, probably aided by the circulation of peritoneal fluid. The common sites for spread are the opposite ovary, pelvic peritoneum, pelvic organs, peritoneal surface on the abdomen, mesentery, omentum, and diaphragmatic surfaces. Lymphatic spread of this disease is more common and widespread than was once thought.

Pathologic criteria for serous and mucinous tumors of low malignant potential (LMP) have been well defined. Invasiveness of tumor implants and tumor DNA ploidy have been shown to be of prognostic value for this group of lesions. The ovary is a common site of spread for other tumors, particularly those arising from the breast or gastrointestinal (GI) tract.

Germ cell tumors constitute the second most common group of ovarian malignancies, with the majority occurring in women less than 40 years of age. At one time, with the exception of dysgerminomas, these tumors were universally and rapidly fatal. With the advent of effective system chemotherapy, the majority of these women will survive their cancer and many will maintain fertility.

TABLE 27.3. Modified WHO Classification of Ovarian Epithelial Tumors

I. *Common "Epithelial" Tumors*
   A. Serous
   B. Mucinous   (a) Benign
   C. Endometrioid   (b) Of borderline malignancy
   D. Clear cell (mesonephroid)   (c) Malignant
   E. Brenner
   F. Mixed epithelial
   G. Undifferentiated carcinoma
   H. Unclassified
II. *Sex Cord Stromal Tumors*
   A. Granulosa—theca cell   (a) Benign
   B. Androblastoma (Sertoli–Leydig) (b) Malignant
   C. Gynandroblastoma
   D. Unclassified
III. *Lipid Cell Tumors*
IV. *Germ Cell Tumors*
   A. Dysgerminoma
   B. Endodermal sinus tumor
   C. Embryonal carcinoma
   D. Polyembryoma
   E. Choriocarcinoma
   F. Teratomas
      Immature; mature (solid or cystic);
      monodermal (struma ovarii and/or
      carcinoid, others)

Tumors from the sex cord stroma tend to behave in an indolent fashion. These tumors may be hormonally active, producing excess estrogen or androgen.

Screening and Diagnosis

No effective, acceptable screening test is currently available for epithelial ovarian cancer. The most commonly used tumor marker, CA-125, although helpful in monitoring disease states, unfortunately does not have sufficient sensitivity and specificity to be used as an effective screening test. Abdominal and transvaginal ultrasonography has also been evaluated as a potential screening tool, either alone or in combination with CA-125, but to date results have been disappointing. Nonetheless, individuals at risk for familial ovarian cancer may benefit from assessment with these modalities in a regular manner. α-Fetoprotein and β-human chorionic gonadotropin (β-hCG) are tumor markers that are helpful in patients with germ cell tumors.

Because the early stages of this disease tend to be asymptomatic, most women present with advanced stage disease at diagnosis. The most common presenting complaints seem to be of a vague GI nature and consist of bloating and indigestion, resulting ultimately from ascites and tumor deposits on intraabdominal peritoneal and bowel surfaces.

In the past it was hoped that annual Papanicolaou (Pap) smear screening, accompanied by bimanual pelvic examination, might lead to improved diagnosis of early stage asymptomatic lesions. Unfortunately this has not occurred. Compounding the problem are cases of primary peritoneal neoplasia with lesions with widespread involvement of peritoneal surfaces similar to papillary serous ovarian cancer and that appear to have arisen primarily from the peritoneum and not the ovaries.

Any adnexal enlargement greater than 5 cm on routine pelvic examination should raise the suspicion of a possible ovarian cancer and its assessment should be pursued. Cystic ovarian lesions with intracystic excrescences or septae on ultrasound examination are highly suggestive of ovarian malignancy.

Staging

The TNM and FIGO staging systems for ovarian cancer are listed in Table 27.4.

Ovarian cancer is a surgically staged disease and Fig. 27.2 illustrates the features of stage III cancer.

Treatment

Primary treatment of epithelial ovarian cancer is surgical, with the objective being to remove all bulk disease so that if possible zero residual, or tumor deposits less than 1 cm in size, are left at the completion of surgery. TAH/BSO and omentectomy are the main objectives of surgical treatment although some variations of these may occur depending on tumor distribution, age of the patient, stage of disease, and desire for fertility.

There is ample evidence available to suggest that this approach followed by combination chemotherapy produces the best results in terms of disease-free survival, even though overall survival and cure of the disease has been disappointingly low and largely unchanged over the past 25 years.

Current concepts of interval debulking and neoadjuvant therapy are also gaining some popularity. Patients with the findings of advanced stage disease and in whom clinical and radiologic findings suggest that the likelihood of achieving zero residual may be poor with primary surgery are given three cycles of chemotherapy followed by debulking surgery. This approach may relieve symptoms of ascites, distention, and pressure much more quickly than a primary surgical approach and also result in improved nutrition and ultimately, depending on the response to chemotherapy, make subsequent surgery much easier. There has also been evidence to suggest that the likelihood of getting zero residual postoperatively is higher with this approach.

Most epithelial ovarian cancer patients are managed according to risk categories based on the stage, grade of disease, and the amount of residual disease following surgery. Patients with stage Ia grade 1 disease do not need any further adjuvant therapy post-surgery and have a good prognosis. Patients with more advanced disease and with residual positive disease are generally treated with postoperative

TABLE 27.4. Ovary. TNM Clinical Classification and FIGO Staging

TNM Categories		FIGO Stages		
TX				Primary tumor cannot be assessed.
T0				No evidence of primary tumor
T1		I		Tumor is limited to ovaries.
	T1a		IA	Tumor is limited to one ovary; capsule intact; no tumor on ovarian surface; no malignant cells in ascites or peritoneal washings.
	T1b		IB	Tumor is limited to both ovaries; capsules intact, no tumor on ovarian surface; no malignant cells in ascites or peritoneal washings.
	T1c		IC	Tumor is limited to one or both ovaries with any of the following: capsule ruptured, tumor on ovarian surface, malignant cells in ascites or peritoneal washings.
T2		II		Tumor involves one or both ovaries with pelvic extension.
	T2a		IIA	Extension and/or implants on uterus and/or tube(s); no malignant cells in ascites or peritoneal washings
	T2b		IIB	Extension to other pelvic tissues; no malignant cells in ascites or peritoneal washings
	T2c		IIC	Pelvic extension (2a or 2b) with malignant cells in ascites or peritoneal washings
T3 and/or N1		III		Tumor involves one or both ovaries with microscopically confirmed peritoneal metastasis outside the pelvis and/or regional lymph node metastasis.
	T3a		IIIA	Microscopic peritoneal metastasis beyond pelvis
	T3b		IIIB	Macroscopic peritoneal metastasis beyond pelvis 2 cm or less in greatest dimension
	T3c and/or N1		IIIC	Peritoneal metastasis beyond pelvis more than 2 cm in greatest dimension and/or regional lymph node metastasis
M1		IV		Distant metastasis (*excludes peritoneal metastasis*)

Liver capsule metastasis is T3/stage III, liver parenchymal metastasis M1/stage IV. Pleural effusion must have positive cytology for M1/stage IV.

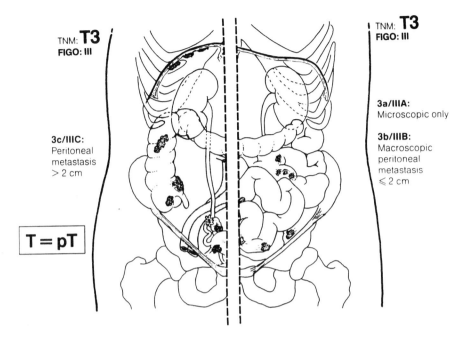

Figure 27.2. Stage III cancer, ovary.

chemotherapy. A large number of agents alone or in combination have been shown to be effective in epithelial ovarian cancer. Currently, combination chemotherapy is generally recommended with agents of different toxicity, profiles, and mechanisms of actions being utilized. Since the mid-1970s platinum-based chemotherapy regimens have been the most commonly used and to date have consistently produced the best results.

Platinum and taxol combinations most recently have become the favored combination. Substitution of carboplatinum for cisplatin has led to less neural and renal toxicity but unfortunately the cost of carboplatinum is substantially higher, which may be a factor in its use where limited resources exist.

Bowel resection surgery is currently thought not to be indicated unless obstruction is imminent or unless resection of a segmental bowel will lead to zero residual.

Although radiotherapy was used extensively to treat ovarian cancer in the past, currently it is used much less frequently. It is still useful in combination therapies in certain cases of low-residual, low-stage disease, where further consolidation may be achieved. Basic limitations to radiotherapy for ovarian cancer have been the large field size needed and the necessary shielding of kidneys and liver which may, to a degree, also shield peritoneal tumor deposits in these areas.

TABLE 27.5. Survival Rates, Epithelial Ovarian Cancer by Stage

Stage	Survival Rate (%)
Stage Ia	90
Ib	65
II	45
III	25
IV	5

Prognosis

Prognosis is largely dependenet on the stage of presentation and the effectiveness of surgical therapy and the response to chemotherapy. Table 27.5 gives the survival of patients by FIGO stage at presentation. In all groups, patients with no residual disease post-surgery have a much better survival rate.

In most patients with ovarian cancer who ultimately die from this disease, the disease is still confined to the abdominal cavity, which usually produces malnutrition, cachexia, and ultimately bowel obstruction and death.

CANCER OF THE VULVA

Introduction

Vulvar cancer is one of the least common of all the major gynecologic tumors and is responsible for approximately 5% of all gynecologic cancers. Invasive carcinoma of the vulva is essentially a disease of older women.

Epidemiology/Etiology

The etiology of this disease is unknown and factors that may be operative for other squamous cancers of the epithelium, such as exposure to sunlight and ultraviolet radiation, do not seem to be likely factors in the production of these lesions. In recent years interest has also focused on the possible role of previous human papillomavirus (HPV) infections, given the role that these agents have in squamous cell carcinoma of the cervix and the not infrequent occurrence of patients with lesions that involve the cervix, vagina, and vulva, either in a synchronous or metachronous fashion. There is also some evidence to suggest different etiologic mechanisms in young patients with invasive disease as compared to older patients.

Pathology

The most common lesions histologically are squamous cell cancers followed by malignant melanoma, Paget's disease of the vulva, and basal cell carcinoma. Adenocarcinoma of Bartholin's gland is another lesion, which fortunately is uncommon and usually arises from the gland itself. Lesions also may arise from Bartholin's duct with some lesions from this structure showing patterns consistent with transitional cell carcinoma.

It seems likely that carcinoma in situ is a precursor lesion for invasive cancer, given the age difference of the two and the positive past history of carcinoma in situ (CIS) in some patients, and the presence of CIS at the margins of invasive lesions.

Diagnosis

Most patients present with some vulvar symptom such as pruritus, irritation, discharge, or lesion noted. The appearance of vulvar cancer can be variable and is based often on the duration, site, and histologic type. Invasive carcinomas of the vulva may be exophytic or ulcerative lesions and most commonly involve the labia and lateral structures on the upper half of the vulva, in contrast to CIS, which often involves the lower half of the vulva. Lesions arising from the clitoris or perineal body are less common but not infrequent primary sites for vulvar cancer. Biopsy usually confirms the diagnosis and histology of the lesions and is recommended in all cases prior to definitive therapy. Vulvar cancer generally spreads by direct extension and also via lymphatics in a rather predictable manner. When the diagnosis is suspected, careful examination of the inguinal areas should be carried out to assess the possibility of clinically suspicious or positive lymph nodes. Following involvement of groin lymph nodes tumors may spread to the pelvic nodes and ultimately to the para-aortic chain.

Lesions involving the perineal body or in the perianal area can follow pararectal lymph node drainage patterns, which may not be addressed with the standard inguinal–femoral lymph node dissections.

Staging

Table 27.6 presents the current FIGO/TNM staging systems for vulvar cancer. Figure 27.3 also illustrates the features of a stage II tumor.

TABLE 27.6. 1995 FIGO Staging for Carcinoma of the Vulva

	Stage 0
TIS	Carcinoma in situ; intraepithelial carcinoma
	Stage I
T1 N0 M0	Tumor is confined to the vulva and/or perineum, 2 cm or less in greatest dimensions; nodes are negative.
Stage IA	Lesions 2 cm or less in size confined to the vulva or perineum with stromal invasion no greater than 1.0 mm. No nodal metastases. The depth of invasion is defined as the measurement of the tumor from the epithelial–stromal junction of the adjacent most superficial dermal papilla to the deepest point of invasion.

TABLE 27.6. 1995 FIGO Staging for Carcinoma of the Vulva *(continued)*

	Stage 0
Stage IB	Lesions 2 cm or less in size confined to the vulva or perineum with stromal invasion greater than 1.0 mm. No nodal metastases.
	Stage II
T2 N0 M0	Tumor is confined to the vulva and/or perineum, more than 2 cm in greatest dimension; nodes are negative.
	Stage III
T3 N0 M0	Tumor of any size with
T3 N1 M0	(1) Adjacent spread to the lower urethra and/or the vagina, or the anus, and/or
T1 N1 M0	(2) Unilateral regional lymph node metastasis
T2 N1 M0	
	Stage IVA
T1 N2 M0	Tumor invades any of the following:
T2 N2 M0	upper urethra, bladder mucosa, rectal mucosa, pelvic bone, and/or bilateral regional node metastasis.
T3 N2 M0	
T4 any N M0	
	Stage IVB
Any T	Any distant metastasis including pelvic lymph nodes
Any N, M1	
	TNM Classification of Carcinoma of the Vulva
T—Primary Tumor	
Tis	Preinvasive carcinoma (carcinoma in situ)
T1	Tumor is confined to the vulva and/or perineum <2 cm in greatest dimension.
T2	Tumor is confined to the vulva and/or perineum >2 cm in greatest dimension.
T3	Tumor of any size with adjacent spread to the urethra and/or vagina and/or the anus
T4	Tumor of any size infiltrating the bladder mucosa and/or the rectal mucosa, including the upper part of the urethral mucosa and/or fixed to the bone
N—Regional Lymph Nodes	
N0	No lymph node metastasis
N1	Unilateral regional lymph node metastasis
N2	Bilateral regional lymph node metastasis
M—Distant Metastasis	
M0	No clinical metastasis
M1	Distant metastasis (including pelvic lymph node metastasis)

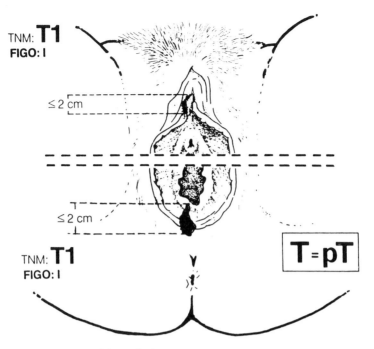

Figure 27.3. Stage II cancer, vulva.

Treatment

Treatment of vulvar cancer is primarily surgical, although combination surgery and radiotherapy is also used in specialized situations. Current recommendations regarding vulvar cancer treatment is for the individualization of therapy based on a variety of clinical–pathologic parameters. In the past, en bloc radical vulvectomy and node dissection was the mainstay of therapy and used routinely for all cases, if the patient's general medical condition permitted. Radical treatment of vulvar cancer can be associated with significant physical and psychological complications. In addition to the usual surgical complications of bleeding, infection, and postoperative deep vein thrombosis, complications related specifically to this type of radical surgery include groin morbidity, for example, lymphocysts, lymph edema, hernia, and delayed wound healing. Complications related to vulvar surgery depend on the extent and whether or not clitoral or other central structures were removed. These complications include decreased sensation, dyspareunia, introital stenosis, and stricture with voiding difficulties. Psychosexual identity and body image problems are also common after radical vulvectomy surgery.

Surgical management should be individualized based on the size, site, depth of invasion, histology, age of the patient, and whether or not lymphatic vascular space invasion is noted. The most important prognostic factor is whether or not disease has spread to regional lymph nodes.

The number of positive nodes and whether or not bilateral versus unilateral nodes are involved, as well as the size of the nodal metastasis itself and whether or not any extranodal disease is present, are important prognostic factors.

Tumor thickness relates well to the incidence of nodal disease, particularly with small sized tumors.

Small, laterally located lesions can be merged with wide local excision with an attempt to obtain a 2-cm margin and unilateral inguinal–femoral node dissection. If the nodes are negative, no further surgery is usually needed and prognosis is good. Central lesions require bilateral node dissection and unfortunately more radical vulvar resection.

Radiotherapy is often used to radiate pelvic node areas in patients found to have positive groin nodes and also may be used in patients with positive margins. In patients with lesions that are close to or encroach on the anal sphincter, radiotherapy as a primary adjuvant therapy may be used in an attempt to shrink lesions and may permit less radical excision with preservation of sphincter and anal continence.

Late central recurrences are not uncommon and many of these can be successfully managed by repeat wide local excision, which seems to indicate that there are variants of this disease that seem to be locally invasive with little propensity for early distant spread. Nonetheless, the seriousness of this disease should never be underestimated, as spread to extravulvar sites does occur with advanced disease and can produce a dismal end for patients suffering from terminal metastatic vulvar cancer.

Chemotherapy has not generally shown to be helpful in these patients and limited experience is available. It has been used, however, as a radiosensitizer similar to its use in certain anal or rectal cancers.

In patients with malignant melanoma of the vulva routine node dissection is no longer thought to be therapeutic but enlarged or suspicious nodes should be resected as a palliative measure.

Prognosis

Prognosis for stage I and stage II tumors or tumors with no nodal metastasis has been extremely good, with disease-free 5-year survival rates approaching 95%. Also, patients with only one positive lymph node without extranodal disease also have an excellent prognosis. Clearly identified prognostic factors for nodal disease are related to: (1) depth of invasion, (2) number of nodes positive, (3) bilateral nodes, (4) extranodal spread or extracapsular disease, and (5) size of deposits in nodes.

GESTATIONAL TROPHOBLASTIC DISEASE

Gestational trophoblastic disease (GTD) is a term that refers to a variety of neoplastic disorders arising from the blastocyst. The trophoblast is a fascinating and important tissue in human biology and is the ectodermal covering of the blastocyst that erodes into the uterine mucosa and through which the developing embryo receives nutrition from the maternal circulation. This tissue has metabolic, hormonal, and immunologic functions, which are all important in terms of the diagnosis of these disorders and their response to therapy. This tissue is classified on the basis of its anatomic location and morphologic features in the three cell types: cytotrophoblast, intermediate trophoblast, and syncytial trophoblast. In recent years specific histologic diagnosis has become less important.

Epidemiology/Etiology

The incidence of GTD varies geographically, ranging from a low of approximately 1/200 pregnancies in North America to a high of 1/120 to 1/200 pregnancies in Asia. One consistent etiologic factor that has been identified has been increasing maternal age. Diets that are low in calories, deficient in protein, and poor in vitamin A have all been implicated as causing an increased risk for this disorder.

Classification of GTD

The classification for GTD is documented in Table 27.7.

Complete Mole

A complete hydatidiform mole is a lesion in which no fetus or embryo is noted. These lesions have a diploid chromosomal pattern, which are paternally derived. Clinically the uterus usually appears larger than gestational age and patients most often present with abnormal bleeding. Hyperemesis gravidarum and pregnancy associated hypertension are also common accompaniments of this disorder. Complete moles are usually characterized by markedly elevated levels of hCG and a classic ultrasound picture often called a "snowstorm pattern." Ten percent to 30% of complete moles persist after evacuation. Both complete and partial moles are essentially chromosomally abnormal pregnancies.

Partial Mole

Partial moles have a triploid chromosomal pattern with two sets derived paternally and one set maternally. They may also have an accompanying fetus or embryo and

TABLE 27.7. Classification of Gestational Trophoblastic Disease

1. Hydatidiform mole
   (a) Complete
   (b) Partial
2. Invasive hydatidiform mole
3. Choriocarcinoma
4. Placental site trophoblastic tumor
5. Other lesions

the degree of partial mole can be minor or major. Often, the uterus will be small-for-dates with hCG levels that are only slightly elevated or not at all. Five percent to 10% of partial moles persist after evacuation.

Invasive Moles

Invasive moles are characterized by the presence of hydropic villi in the myometrium or in vessels and are usually diagnosed from plateauing or persisting hCG titers following evacuation of one of the above lesions. Invasive moles may also regress spontaneously.

Placental Site Trophoblast Tumor

These are uncommon tumors that are characterized by proliferation of intermediate cytotrophoblast tissue. These tumors generally do not produce high titers of hCG and may have elevated levels of human placental lactogen. These tumors also do not respond well to chemotherapy so that hysterectomy is a good treatment for these rather uncommon lesions.

Choriocarcinoma

The only known risk factor for choriocarcinoma is advancing maternal age and this lesion may have a variable presentation. The most common method of presentation is with abnormal uterine bleeding but it may also present with symptoms related to the metastatic lesions in the lung, vagina, brain, or liver. Choriocarcinoma can occur following any type of gestation including hydatidiform mole, spontaneous abortion, or ectopic or term pregnancy.

Staging

The FIGO staging system for GTD is presented in Table 27.8.

Management or Treatment

Lesions are generally divided according to good or poor prognosis based on a variety of assessment schemes. One of the simplest is that derived by the National Institutes of Health, shown in Table 27.9. Metastatic work-up in cases of choriocarcinoma should include CT scan of lung, abdomen and pelvis, and brain. Pelvic ultrasound may also be helpful and routine blood counts and renal and liver function tests are also helpful prior to therapy. Metastatic sites most common in order of frequency are lung, vagina, brain, liver, GI tract, and kidney.

The other prognostic scoring system is that presented by the World Health Organization based on the experience of Bagshawe and co-workers at Charing Cross Hospital in London. Their scoring system is presented in Table 27.10 and based on the sum of the prognostic score cases may be divided into low- and high-risk cases.

TABLE 27.8. FIGO Staging for Gestational Trophoblastic Tumors

Stage I	Disease is confined to the uterus.
Stage Ia	Disease is confined to the uterus with no risk factors.
Stage Ib	Disease is confined to the uterus with one risk factor.
Stage Ic	Disease is confined to the uterus with two risk factors.
Stage II	GTT extends outside of the uterus but is limited to the genital structures (adnexa, vagina, broad ligament).
Stage IIa	GTT involves genital structures without risk factors.
Stage IIb	GTT extends outside of the uterus but limited to genital structures with one risk factor.
Stage IIc	GTT extends outside of the uterus but limited to the genital structures with two risk factors.
Stage III	GTT extends to the lungs with or without known genital tract involvement.
Stage IIIa	GTT extends to the lungs with or without genital tract involvement and with no risk factors.
Stage IIIb	GTT extends to the lungs with or without genital tract involvement and with one risk factor.
Stage IIIc	GTT extends to the lungs with or without genital tract involvement and has two risk factors.
Stage IV	All other metastatic sites
Stage IVa	All other metastatic sites without risk factors
Stage IVb	All other metastatic sites with one risk factor
Stage IVc	All other metastatic sites with two risk factors

TABLE 27.9. NIH Clinical Classification of Malignant GTD

I. Nonmetastatic/persistent GTD
II. Metastatic
  A. Good prognosis, low risk (absence of high risk factors)
    • includes lung metastases
  B. Poor prognosis, high risk (presence of any of following high-risk features):
    • Interval to treatment > 4 months
    • Pretreatment hCG > 40,000 mlU/ml
    • Brain or liver metastases
    • Antecedent term pregnancy
    • Prior failed chemotherapy

TABLE 27.10. World Health Organization Prognostic Index Score for GTD

	Score			
Prognostic Factor	0	1	2	4
Age (yr)	≤ 39	>39	—	—
Antecedent pregnancy	Mole	Abortion	Term	—
Interval (mo)	<4	4–6	7–12	>12
hCG (mIU/ml)	$<10^3$	10^3–10^4	10^4–10^5	$>10^5$
ABO groups	—	O or A	B or AB	—
Largest tumor, including uterine	—	3–5 cm	>5 cm	—
Site of metastases	Lung, pelvis, vagina	Spleen, kidney	GI tract, liver	Brain
Number of metastases	—	1–3	4–8	>8
Prior chemotherapy	—	—	Single	Multiple

Risk category for failing initial therapy given Total score:

Low Risk	0–4
Intermediate Risk	5–7
High Risk	>8

Generally, a score of 7 or less is considered to be low risk. A variety of treatment protocols have been advocated for this tumor.

Choriocarcinoma was the first solid gynecologic tumor and one of the first solid tumors in humans to be cured with chemotherapy. Methotrexate and actinomycin have been the mainstays of treatment since the introduction of methotrexate for this disease in 1956. Figure 27.4 shows an example of a protocol for low risk cases. Figures 27.5 and 27.6 shows protocols that have been used successfully for high-risk cases.

Prophylactic chemotherapy has also been advocated in certain situations. Arguments for the use of such an approach consist of the following. Approximately 20% of cases will have persistent disease after evacuation of a mole. Trophoblast is generally a highly sensitive tumor to chemotherapy and chemotherapy at the time of evacuation should reduce the incidence of both locally invasive and metastatic GTD. Conversely, such an approach would indicate that 80% of patients would receive treatment that they do not need and that serious side effects can accompany the chemotherapy medications used for prophylaxis. There is also some concern that this may lull individuals into a false sense of security and follow-up may be inadequate. Patients who might benefit from such an approach would be individuals with thecal lutein cysts greater than 6 cm in diameter, with presenting hCG at the time of the molar pregnancy of greater than 100,000, and a uterus that is larger than expected for dates, or patients with medical complications such as thyroid storm.

Hysterectomy is also a useful adjunct to therapy in cases where persisting moles are present and where reproductive function is no longer important.

Day 1   Prehydration

Antiemetics

Actinomycin D   0.6 mg/m^2 IV Push

MTX, then   100 mg/m^2 IV Push

MTX   300 mg/m^2 in 500 ml Over 4 Hr

Day 2   Actinomycin D   0.6 mg/m^2 IV Push

And start

Folinic Acid   15 mg P.O. Q6h x 9 doses

Figure 27.4. Gestational trophoblastic disease low-risk protocol.

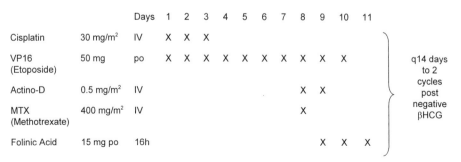

		Days	1	2	3	4	5	6	7	8	9	10	11	
Cisplatin	30 mg/m^2	IV	X	X	X									
VP16 (Etoposide)	50 mg	po	X	X	X	X	X	X	X	X	X	X		q14 days to 2 cycles post negative βHCG
Actino-D	0.5 mg/m^2	IV								X	X			
MTX (Methotrexate)	400 mg/m^2	IV								X				
Folinic Acid	15 mg po	16h									X	X	X	

VP16 = Etoposide

Figure 27.5. Gestational trophoblastic disease high-risk protocol.

Course A EMA

Day 1	Etoposide	100 mg/m^2 IV Over 30 Min.
	MTX	300 mg/m^2 Iv as a 12 Hr. Infusion
	Actinomycin D	0.5 mg/m^2 IV Push
Day 2	Etoposide	100 mg/m^2 IV Over 30 Min.
	Actinomycin D	0.5 mg/m^2 IV Push
	Folinic Acid	15 mg P.O./IM q 12 Hr. x 4 doses Start 24 Hrs. after MTX

Course B CO

| Day 1 | Vincristine | 1.0 mg/m^2 IV Push |
| | Cyclo | 600 mg/m^2 IV Infusion Over 30 Min |

Figure 27.6. Gestational trophoblastic disease EMA/CO protocol.

Rarely patients may present with brain, liver, and lung metastases. Hemorrhage from these metastatic foci in some individuals may be life threatening, and unless controlled to enable chemotherapy to have its desirable effect, can cause death of the patient. Urgent radiotherapy may be necessary to prevent or control an intracranial lesion.

FURTHER READING

Cancer of the Endometrium

Abeler VM, Vergote IB, Kjorstad KE, Trope CG (1996) Clear cell carcinoma of the endometrium. Prognosis and metastatic pattern. *Cancer* 78:1740–1747.

Bokhman JV, Chepick OF, Volkova AT, Vishnevsky AS (1985) Can primary endometrial carcinoma stage I be cured without surgery and radiation therapy? *Gynecol Oncol* 20:139–155.

Boronow RC (1997) Surgical staging of endometrial cancer: Evolution, evaluation, and responsible challenge—a personal perspective. *Gynecol Oncol* 66:179–189.

Boronow RC, Morow CP, Creasman WT, DiSaia PJ, Silverberg SG, Miller A, Blessing JA (1984) Surgical staging in endometrial cancer: Clinical–pathologic findings of a prospective study. *Obstet Gynecol* 63:825–832.

Burke TW, Gershenson DM, Morris M, Stringer CA, Levenback C, Tortolero-Luna G, Baker VV (1994) Postoperative adjuvant cisplatin, doxorubicin, and cyclophosphamide (PAC) chemotherapy in women with high-risk endometrial carcinoma. *Gynecol Oncol* 55:47–50.

Creasman ST, Morrow CP, Bundy BN, Homesley HD, Graham JE, Heller, PB (1987) Surgical pathologic spread patterns of endometrial cancer. *Cancer* 60:2035–2041.

Granberg S, Wikland M, Karlsson B, Norstrom A, Friberg L (1991) Endometrial thickness as measured by endovaginal ultrasonography for identifying endometrial abnormality. *Am J Obstet Gynecol* 164:47–52.

Morrow CP, Bundy BN, Kurman RJ, Creasman WT, Heller P, Homesley HD, Graham JE (1991) Relationship between surgical–pathological risk factors and outcome in clinical stage I and II carcinoma of the endometrium. A Gynecologic Oncology Group Study. *Gynecol Oncol* 40:55–65.

Potish RA, Twiggs LB, Adcock LL, Savage JE, Levitt SH, Prem KA (1985) Paraaortic lymph node radiotherapy in cancer of the uterine corpus. *Obstet Gynecol* 65:251–256.

Randall TC, Kurman RJ (1997) Progestin treatment of atypical hyperplasia and well-differentiated carcinoma of the endometrium in women under age 40. *Obstet Gynecol* 90:434–440.

Cancer of the Ovary

Bristow RE, Lagasse LD, Karlan BY (1996) Secondary surgical cytoreduction for advanced epithelial ovarian cancer. Patient selection and review of literature. *Cancer* 78:2049–2062.

DePriest PD, Gallion HH, Pavlik EJ, Kryscio RJ, van Nagell JR Jr (1997) Transvaginal sonography as a screening method for the detection of early ovarian cancer. *Gynecol Oncol* 65:408–414.

Gayther SA, Warren W, Mazoyer S, Russell PA, Harrington PA, Chiano M, Seal S, Hamoudi R, van Rensburg EJ, Dunning AM, et al. (1995) Germline mutations of the *BRCA-1* gene in breast and ovarian cancer families provide evidence for a genotype–phenotype correlation. *Nat Genet* 11:428–433.

Gershenson DM (1994) Chemotherapy of ovarian germ cell tumors and sex cord stromal tumors. *Semin Surg Oncol* 10:290–298.

Heintz APM, Van Oosterom AT, Baptist J, Trimbos MC, Schaberg A, Van Der Velde EA, Nooy M (1988) The treatment of advanced ovarian carcinoma (I): Clinical variables associated with prognosis. *Gynecol Oncol* 30:347–358.

Hoskins WJ (1993) Surgical staging and cytoreductive surgery of epithelial ovarian cancer. *Cancer* 71:1534–1539.

McGuire WP, Hoskins WJ, Brady MF, Kucera PR, Partridge EE, Look K, Pearson DL, Davidson M (1996) Cyclophosphamide and cisplatin compared with paclitaxel and cisplatin in patients with stage III and stage IV ovarian cancer. *N Engl J Med* 334:1–6.

NIH (1994) NIH Consensus Development Conference on Ovarian Cancer: Screening, treatment and follow-up. *Gynecol Oncol* 55:S1 73.

Surwit E, Childers J, Atlas I, Nour M, Hatch K, Hallum A, Alberts D (1996) Neoadjuvant chemotherapy for advanced ovarian cancer. *Int J Gynecol Cancer* 6:356–361.

Swenerton K, Jeffrey J, Stuart G, Roy M, Krepart G, Carmichael J, Drouin P, Stanimir R, O'Connell G, MacLean G, Kirk ME, Canetta R, Koski B, Shelley W, Zee B, Pater J (1992) Cisplatin–cyclophosphamide versus carboplatin–cyclophosphamide in advanced ovarian cancer: A randomized phase III study of the National Cancer Institute of Canada Clinical Trials Group. *J Clin Oncol* 10:718–726.

van der Burg MEL, van Lent M, Buyse M, Kobierska A, Colombo N, Favalli G, Lacave AJ, Nardi M, Renard J, Pecorelli S for the Gynecological Cancer Cooperative Group of the European Organization for Research and Treatment of Cancer (1995) The effect of debulking surgery after induction chemotherapy on the prognosis in advanced epithelial ovarian cancer. *N Engl J Med* 332:629–634.

Cancer of the Vulva

Cunningham MJ, Goyer RP, Gibbons SK, Kredentser DC, Malfetano JH, Keys H (1997) Primary radiation, cisplatin and 5-fluorouracil for advanced squamous carcinoma of the vulva. *Gynecol Oncol* 66:258–261.

Homesley HD (1995) Management of vulvar cancer. *Cancer* 76:2159–2170.

Homesley HD, Bundy BN, Sedlis A, Adcock L (1986) Radiation therapy versus pelvic node resection for carcinoma of the vulva with positive groin nodes. *Obstet Gynecol* 68:733–740.

Homesley HD, Bundy BN, Sedlis A, Yordan E, Berek JS, Jahshan A, Morrel R (1993) Prognostic factors for groin node metastasis in squamous cell carcinoma of the vulva: A Gynecologic Oncology Group Study. *Gynecol Oncol* 49:279–283.

Iversen T, Aberler V, Aalders J (1981) Individualized treatment of stage I carcinoma of the vulva. *Obstet Gynecol* 57:85–89.

Stehman PB, Bundy BN, Dvoretsky PM, Creasman WT (1992) Early stage I carcinoma of the vulva treated with ipsilateral superficial inguinal lymphadenectomy and modified radical hemivulvectomy: A prospective study of the Gynecologic Oncology Group. *Obstet Gynecol* 79:490–497.

Thomas G, Dembo A, DePetrillo A, Pringle J, Ackerman I, Bryson P. et al. (1989) Concurrent radiation and chemotherapy in vulvar carcinoma. *Gynecol Oncol* 34:263–267.

Gestational Trophoblastic Disease

Bagshawe KD (1969) *Choriocarcinoma: The Clinical Biology of the Trophoblast and Its Tumors.* Williams & Wilkins, Baltimore.

Bagshawe KD (1976) Risk and prognostic factors in trophoblastic neoplasia. *Cancer* 38:1373–1385.

Berkowitz RS, Goldstein DP, Bernstein MR (1990) Methotrexate infusion and folinic acid in the primary therapy of nonmetastatic gestational trophoblastic tumors. *Gynecol Oncol* 36:56–59.

Berkowitz RS, Goldstein DP, Bernstein MR, Sablinska B (1987) Subsequent pregnancy outcome in patients with molar pregnancy and gestational trophoblastic tumors. *J Reprod Med* 32:680–684.

DuBeshter B, Berkowitz RS, Goldstein DP, Cramer DW, Bernstein MR (1987) Metastatic gestational trophoblastic disease: Experience at the New England Trophoblastic Disease Centre, 1965 to 1985. *Obstet Gynecol* 69:390–395.

Finkler NJ, Berkowitz RS, Driscoll SG, Goldstein DP, Bernstein MR (1988) Clinical experience with placental site trophoblastic tumors at the New England Trophoblastic Disease Center. *Obstet Gynecol* 71:854–857.

Goldstein, DP, Berkowitz RS (1995) Prophylactic chemotherapy of complete molar pregnancy. *Semin Oncol* 22:157–160.

Hammond CB, Weed JC Jr, Currie JL (1980) The role of operation in the current therapy of gestational trophoblastic disease. *Am J Obstet Gynecol* 136:844–858.

Newlands ES, Bagshawe KD, Begent RHJ, Rustin GJS, Holden L (1991) Results with EMA/CO (etoposide, methotrexate, actinomycin D, cyclophosphamide, vincristine) regimen in high risk gestational trophoblastic tumours, 1979–1989. *Br J Obstet Gynaecol* 98:550–557.

Redline RW, Abdul-Karim FW (1995) Pathology of gestational trophoblastic disease. *Semin Oncol* 22:96–109.

Soper JT (1995) Identification and management of high-risk gestational trophoblastic disease. *Semin Oncol* 22:172–184.

CHAPTER 28

CANCER OF THE PROSTATE

LOUIS J. DENIS

Algemeen Ziekenhuis Middelheim
Antwerp, Belgium

G.P. MURPHY

Pacific Northwest Cancer Foundation
Seattle, WA 98125, USA

Prostate cancer became a major health problem with significant morbidity, mortality, loss of quality of life, and cost in societies with increased life expectancy. It is a slow but continuous heterogeneous tumor that covers a wide range of disease over a wide age range, however, with a peak incidence and mortality around the seventh decade.

The dramatic division between localized and curable prostate cancer versus advanced incurable disease has created heated controversies regarding diagnosis and treatment schedules. The use of prostate-specific antigen (PSA) and the painless biopty gun have created a shift to the diagnosis of earlier and curable stages of the disease with surgery or radiotherapy as recognized treatment. Patients at the earlier stages of advanced incurable disease receive primary hormonal therapy, sometimes as neo-adjuvant treatment. About 70% of patients with extensive disease profit from endocrine treatment but a median survival of 18 months is not improved.

Hormone-independent cancers are debilitating and sometimes require palliation over available treatment. Clinical research is focused on prevention and control of hormone-independent disease.

Manual of Clinical Oncology, 7th edition, Edited by Raphael E. Pollock
ISBN 0-471-23828-7, pages 563–574. Copyright © 1999 Wiley-Liss, Inc.

EPIDEMIOLOGY AND NATURAL HISTORY

Clinical prostate cancer is a disease of aging men, with a peak incidence and mortality around 70 years of age. Prostate cancer accounts for 10% to 30% of clinical reported tumors in men and 13% of all male cancer deaths. While the incidence rate varies enormously between and within continents, there is evidence that the mortality rate does not correlate with the incidence rate. The incidence of clinical cancer is low in Asia, intermediate in Latin America and southern Europe, and high in northern Europe and North America.

It is estimated that there are approximately 1 million patients alive with prostate cancer throughout the world, and this represents 16% of all 5-year prevalent cancer cases in males. Of these cases approximately 900,000 originate in the developed countries and the rest in developing countries. These figures will increase in the early part of the 21st century as a result of the increasing life expectancy of the involved populations.

It is important to note that latent prostate cancer, that is, prostate cancer clinically unsuspected throughout life, and discovered only at autopsy or incidentally at surgery for other causes, remains evenly distributed throughout the male world population in a range from 12% to 16%. In contrast, clinical cancer, with volumes over 0.5 cc being larger and less well differentiated, show a geographic and national distribution similar to clinical symptomatic cancer directly related to increasing age.

It is accepted that the development of clinical prostate cancer is a multistep process. The initial distribution of early stages of the histologic microscopic forms of the disease are stimulated by external and possibly avoidable factors, which opens the case for lifestyle causes and possibly primary prevention. The natural history concept shows prostate cancer to be a slow growing tumor with variable occurrences of malignant transformation or differentiation. The age at the time of diagnosis and the volume (stage of the tumor) explain an apparent controversy that watchful waiting may be acceptable in elderly patients with small and differentiated tumors whereas active treatment is recommended in elderly patients with less well differentiated tumors and a volume greater than 0.5 cc. Decreasing differentiation and increasing size are existing proof of the biologic activity of the tumor. This concept of relativity does not always apply to the individual patient because we lack understanding of the total biologic potential growth of each diagnosed prostate cancer.

ETIOLOGY AND PREVENTION

There is agreement that androgens mediate normal programmed cell death through the androgen receptors that regulate the genes that determine secretion, proliferation, or programmed cell death of the prostate. In the progression of prostate cancer this process is influenced by secreted growth factors in an autocrine manner, resulting in continuous growth. It has been shown that even prostate cancer cells of the hormone-independent type require some form of growth factor stimulation. There is no evidence of any primary endocrine disturbance that would be a risk factor in the etiology of prostate cancer or that could explain the variability of the incidence of clinical cancer in the different populations. The hypothesis that the inhibition of the intraprostatic 5-α-reductase activity would reduce the incidence of prostate cancer is being challenged in a randomized trial of 18,000 men over 55 years of age, and to be followed for 7 years, who will receive an 5-α-reductase inhibitory drug. Other explanations rest with lifestyle differences in nutritional practices. Prostate cancer risk appears to be associated with the intake of saturated fat, vitamins A and E, as well as carotenes. However, the differences in diet fat intake alone can account for only at most 10% of the variation between reported incidence of race and the community. These factors have to be taken into account for the reported risk of prostate cancer for first-degree relatives of patients with prostate cancer, as familial clustering may have a genetic etiology as well as a cultural feature. Thus the genetic etiology factor appears to account for 13% of reported cancers. The concept that Asian men have a low risk for clinical prostate cancer as a result of a diet containing potential anticarcinogenic agents is seriously considered as a possibility for a study of such agents that could induce effective primary prevention. This concept is based on the observation that sons of Japanese immigrants in the United States show an incidence between that of native Japanese and the native US population. Of direct clinical importance is the observation that transurethral resection of the prostate for benign prostatic hyperplasia (BPH), as well as the diagnosis of BPH and vasectomy, are not related to prostate cancer. Further epidemiologic and etiologic studies related to genetic epidemiology of prostate cancer are a research priority.

PATHOLOGY

The great majority of prostate cancers are adenocarcinomas of a heterogeneous nature. The differentiation or grade of the tumor is recognized dominating prognostic factor to predict the outcome of the disease in localized or metastatic disease independent of the therapy applied. The Gleason grading score system is now widely accepted to assess the histologic differentiation of prostate cancer (Figure 28.1). The primary cancer may be unifocal or in more cases multifocal. The majority of the lesions are at the periphery of the gland in the so-called peripheral zone, where they may be palpated by the examining finger from a palpable size on rectal examination.

About 25% of the cancers also arise in the transition zone. These latter tumors are reported to follow a better prognostic pattern because they must penetrate the surgical capsule. Peripheral cancers are better situated for early capsule invasion and extracapsular extension (ECE).

PIN (prostate intraepithelial neoplasia) has been identified as a precursor of prostate cancer. High-grade PIN is generally regarded as the potential, aggressive lesion. Screening for prostate cancer became an accessible approach with the clinical introduction of the prostate-specific antigen (PSA) serum test and the transrectal ultrasound (TRUS) guided and spring-loaded biopsy device. The latter technique allows to take a number of biopsies of the prostate without excessive burden to the patient.

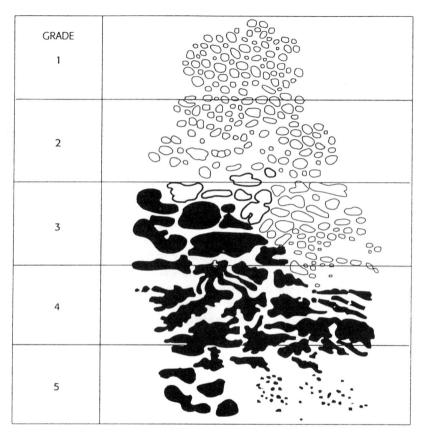

FIGURE 28.1. The Gleason score is based on the glandular and cellular characteristics and adding the grades. In grade 1 the glands look almost normal while in grade 5 sheets of undifferentiated cancer are present. The sum of the two most prominent grades is the score.

Most of our preoperative clinical assessment of the local tumor relies on the histologic sampling of the biopsies to assess the grade and extent of the tumor. The system is not perfect, but a definitive poor prognosis starts with a Gleason score of 7 (4 + 3). Additional predictive markers such as PSA or tumor volume, when available, allow a good treatment selection in individual cases. The development of new markers of progression such as prostate-specific membrane antigen (PSMA) and proliferative and molecular genetic markers are a current clinical research priority.

SCREENING AND DIAGNOSIS

Screening should be designed to find cancer in the early curable stages of the disease in an asymptomatic population, which is totally different from case finding or the early diagnosis in symptomatic patients. Population-based screening is still debated at the moment because specific beneficial effects on mortality or improvement of quality of life (QOL) as a result of prospective randomized trials have not yet been demonstrated by screening technology in selected populations. However, several large demonstration series in different parts of the world have contributed to the recognition that there are available early detection procedures in suspected cases that can result in early diagnosed cancer. A few randomized screening trials are accruing well and may ultimately may provide the missing data. A specific improvement would be to increase the specificity of the biopsy diagnostic test to limit the indications for biopsy and decrease possible overtreatment. Underdiagnosis in locally advanced disease is another fallacy of early diagnosis and treatment of prostate cancer.

Early diagnosis will, however, detect cancers in the localized stage of the disease, which offers the best chance for cure if effective treatment is provided. Advanced prostate cancer means there is an incurable disease but ongoing awareness programs reduced the number of patients diagnosed with locally advanced or metastatic disease. The diagnosis of prostate cancer is mainly based on the suspicion of cancer by three tests. The digital rectal examination (DRE) feels for zones of induration in the prostate or asymmetry of the gland. The PSA is a nonspecific marker for prostate cancer but is representative in the serum for prostatic volume increase or for disease. The TRUS may demonstrate echo-poor lesions in the prostate sonogram. None of the three tests have a high sensitivity to detect early prostate cancer. The combination of DRE and PSA provides a reliable risk combination to indicate the need for a confirming biopsy.

STAGING AND PROGNOSIS

Clinical and pathologic staging tries to determine the anatomic extent and total tumor burden in the primary tumor (T), the original lymph nodes (N), and the metastasis (M) in the TNM system. The 1997 staging system is advocated by the Union Internationale Contre le Cancer (UICC) and the American Joint Committee on Cancer (AJCC). The details of the system are summarized in Table 28.1. The T-classification covers a wide variety of tumors, ranging from category T1a, which is a small, well-differentiated cancer with a median time of progression of 13.5 years, to T1b tumors with higher volumes and less differentiation, where the median time to progression is 4.7 years. The category T1c classifies all tumors that are nonpalpable on the DRE and not visible on TRUS but detected usually by confirming biopsies on the basis of an abnormal serum PSA level. It is now recognized that the T1c classification is mainly composed of several types of clinically significant tumors. The staging is completed by the grading (G) of a positive biopsy. PSA above 10 ng/ml with overlap for benign disease may indicate metastatic disease. The tumor volume that can be estimated through systematic biopsies may improve the staging accuracy which at this moment is characterized for a significant level of clinical understaging (40%) and overstaging (20%).

TABLE 28.1. TNM Classification of Prostate Cancer (ICD-O C61) in Schematic Form

T1		Not palpable or visible
	T1a	≤5%
	T1b	≥5%
	T1c	Needle biopsy
T2		Confined within prostate
	T2a	One lobe
	T2b	Both lobes
T3		Through prostatic capsule
	T3a	Extracapsular
	T3b	Seminal vesicle(s)
T4		Fixed or invades adjacent structures: bladder neck, external sphincter, rectum, levator muscles, pelvic wall
N1		Regional lymph node(s)
M1a		Nonregional lymph node(s)
M1b		Bone(s)
M1c		Other site(s)

There is no pathologic stage equivalent for clinical stage T1c, and these tumors are usually upstaged after pathologic examination to pathologic stages T2 or T3. The prediction of the invasion of the regional lymph nodes (N) correlates to increasing tumor grade, tumor volume, and high PSA levels. Currently this is generally achieved by the lymph node sampling of the obturator region. Clinical metastasis (M) is usually demonstrated on a positive radionuclide bone scan, computerized tomography (CT) scan, or magnetic resonance imaging (MRI) scan of the abdomen. False-positive results are possible with a bone scan owing to either metabolic activity in the bone, for example, post fracture or arthritis, and the accuracy of the imaging decreases for small lesions. Patients with a small tumor burden survive longer than patients with extensive disease.

At the present time, there is no clear foolproof prognostic index that guarantees a specific prognosis for each individual patient but evaluation of a prognostic index based on tumor grade, stage, volume, and PSA provides enough accuracy to enable one to make treatment decisions. More specific prognosis is expected from the introduction of PSMA in the clinic.

TREATMENT

There is a dramatic separation in the ultimate outcome of patients with prostate cancer over the presence of extraprostatic extension (EPE) and patients with disease limited to the prostate in this stage. Even high-grade tumors are curable, either by surgery or by radiotherapy, brachytherapy, or cryosurgery. Surgery involves a total

**TABLE 28.2. Treatment Options for Clinically
Localized Tumor**

Total anatomic prostatectomy (retropubic or perineal)
Radiotherapy (external-beam, brachytherapy, conformal)
Watchful waiting
Cryotherapy (under investigation)

anatomic prostatectomy usually with the elimination of all prostatic tissue, whereas radiation and cryotherapy aim to destroy the tissue without the elimination of all prostatic tissue. There may be a problem of overtreatment in that some insignificant tumors might be better followed or further evaluated by watchful waiting programs and a far greater problem of undertreatment by the demonstration of EPE in the surgical specimen or PSA increase after any treatment. The treatment options are presented in Table 28.2.

Total prostatectomy involves the removal of the entire prostate, the seminal vesicles, and adjacent tissues. It is best employed in patients with localized disease (T1–T2), and with a life expectancy over 10 years, with no comorbidity, and no other contraindications to surgery. Selection is the key to success and many series show survival curves that match the normal survival of a given age group. The comorbidity is urinary incontinence (2% to 5%), erectile dysfunction, or impotence (more than 50%) and urethral strictures (0% to 5%), and a potential mortality of less than 0.3%. The appeal is the radical approach, which provides precise histologic pathologic information and definitive cure with the relief of the patient's anxiety. Of course, it also shows immediate persistent disease requiring secondary treatment if the surgical margins are positive and PSA remains detectable.

External-beam radiotherapy using new technology to focus the radiation more precisely, as well as brachytherapy, in which radioactive seeds are implanted in the prostate, offer valid alternatives to surgery. The morbidities associated with their use include rectal and bladder irritation (5% to 10%), impotence, but rarely incontinence. These treatments provide opportunities for also treating regionally localized disease but are contraindicated if colorectal comorbidity is present. Increased disease-free survival and even increased survival have been reported in randomized trials by adding neo-adjuvant and adjuvant hormonal treatment to the radiation dose. No treatment can be selected as best treatment, as a proper randomized trial the treatment entities of surgery or radiation is unavailable.

Watchful waiting is really deferred treatment, and appropriate in patients over 70 years of age with a minimal tumor volume, well-differentiated disease, and significant comorbidity. In selected instances, this conservative approach provides disease-specific survival rates similar to those for surgical treatment after 10 years of treatment. Two ongoing randomized trials may provide a clarification of these published results. The actual survival after treatment for T2 prostate cancer has been reported by a clinical guidelines panel of the American Urological Association and is presented in Table 28.3. The outcome figures all look positive but direct comparison is excluded by the different characteristics in the reported patients.

TABLE 28.3. Survival Results of Different Treatment Series for Localized Cancer from a Literature Review

	Radical Prostatectomy			External-Beam Radiotherapy			Brachytherapy			Surveillance		
	No.	Min. (%)	Max. (%)	No.	Min. (%)	Max. (%)	No.	Min. (%)	Max. (%)	No.	Min. (%)	Max. (%)
5-Year survival												
Overall	10	68.9	95.0	39	51.4	93.0	8	57.0	93.0	7	67.0	92.0
Progression free	2	81.9	92.0	29	32.0	93.0	14	38.0	90.0	1	68.0	68.0
10-Year survival												
Overall	7	44.4	88.0	11	41.4	70.0	0			5	34.0	70.7
Progression free	1	82.0	82.0	10	40.0	64.0	7	50.0	90.0	1	53.0	53.0

Source: Adapted from Middleton

These outcome results cannot be compared because they concern patients with different prognostic factors.

Cryoablation of the prostate uses frozen temperatures to destroy the prostatic tissue by means of cryogenic probes that are inserted via the perineum under TRUS guidance into the prostate. Excellent early results are also reported but the original goal to sterilize failed radiotherapy-treated cancer does not seem to answer the high expectations.

ADVANCED DISEASE

The term advanced disease emcompasses small extraprostatic disease to widespread metastasis. Both stages, however, have in common that they are incurable. Increased survival due to the lead time is recognized and it is just for these early stages that treatment opinions are very divergent. It is evident that surgery alone, even with wide excision, is not ideal to offer cure for these patients and attempts for downstaging by introducing neo-adjuvant hormonal treatment hoping to improve the results have failed so far in T3 cancers. The first results from combinations of external-beam radiotherapy together with neo-adjuvant and adjuvant hormonal therapy offer more hope but until the endpoints in some of the randomized trials are met, these treatment strategies should be regarded as investigational.

Even the option of watchful waiting can be proposed to patients with significant comorbidity but some form of androgen suppression seems to improve the morbidity and to increase the survival of the patients in randomized trials with M0 patients comparing early versus deferred endocrine treatment. The option of intermittent androgen suppression for locally advanced prostate cancer is under investigation and intends to minimize the side effects of the treatment. Important is the fact that not only are the usual endpoints of time to progression and specific cause of death researched but also the quality of life of the affected patients.

METASTATIC DISEASE

There is consensus that immediate endocrine treatment is indicated for patients with symptoms. The case to provide endocrine treatment in patients without symptoms is still debated but the trend seems to go to immediate treatment. There is a wide choice of endocrine treatment available where the mainstay is designed to lower the circulating levels of plasma androgens or to block the uptake of plasma androgens by the cancer cells. The available array of endocrine treatment is listed in Table 28.4. A choice has to be made between chemical and surgical castration if androgen withdrawal is chosen as a first-line approach. Controversy remains if maximal androgen blockade (MAB) is superior to monotherapy. A series of consensus meetings brought the information of a meta-analysis on all available randomized treatments including MAB. The published results show a marginal advantage for the MAB treatment which looks not very clear in terms of clinical advantage. However, there is agreement that MAB is indicated for a limited time to prevent a surge in plasma testosterone when medical castration by luteinizing hormone releasing hormone agonist

TABLE 28.4. **Array of Current First-Line Endocrine Treatments Utilized in Daily Praxis to Palliate Prostate Cancer**

Androgen Withdrawal	
1. Castration:	Bilateral orchiectomy
	Subcapsular orchiectomy
	Subepididymal orchiectomy
2. Medical castration:	Estrogens
	Depot preparations
	LHRH A
Androgen Blockade	
Antiandrogens:	Cyproterone acetate 300 mg/d
	Flutamide 750 mg/d
	Nilutamide 300 mg/d
	Bicalutamide 150 mg/d
Combination Treatment	
Maximal androgen blockade:	LHRH A antiandrogen castration-anti-androgen

(LHRH A) is preferred. There is also agreement that responses are quicker with the combination treatment.

A number of questions remain open, such as if the MAB treatment should be the control arm in randomized, prospective trials on metastatic prostate cancer, and if monotherapy with nonsteroidal antiandrogens might be appropriate in patients with locally advanced cancer to retain their potency if cohorts of patients with good prognostic factors would profit from the combination treatment.

The use of female sex hormones such as diethylstilbestrol (DES) and the possibility of introducing intermittent endocrine treatment to lessen the effects of long-term androgen withdrawal in elderly men remain intriguing options to close the search for the best endocrine treatment over the last 5 decades.

Classically chemotherapy is given when clinical prostate cancer after response to endocrine treatment eventually relapses into new growth, known as hormone-independent cancer. It is not generally accepted that after the initial start of the endocrine treatment about 20% to 30% of the cancers do not react to the treatment, which is probably due to a tumor composed of androgen-independent cell lines. Here the prognosis is generally poor and a number of second-line treatments remain an option to delay the progression of symptoms.

Second-line treatments for relapsed prostate cancer include cytotoxic chemotherapy, chemohormonal therapy, treatment against growth factors, differentiation treatment, and biologic response modifiers with the inclusion of vaccine therapy.

A multitude of small phase II trials have been introduced, mainly resulting in a number of partial responses, which questions the significance of justifying the high toxicity related to this therapy. The median survival in these patients has been in the order of 6 to 12 months, which is comparable to the survival achieved by standard palliative treatment. Combinations are most widely used such as estramustine phosphate, combinations of estramustine phosphate and vincristine or vinblastine, epirubicin, and paclidaxil. All these treatments have significant side effects in these weakened patients, creating the need to evaluate their quality of life and the cost of treatment in these trials.

PALLIATIVE CARE

Bone pain and a general feelings of tiredness are the most crippling effects of terminal prostate cancer and specific treatment of pain by biphosphonates and radioactive isotopes such as strontium 89 are modern pain treatments and indicated in selected cases.

The correct use of analgesics, steroids, and other supportive treatments are vital in these stages of the disease where palliation and quality of life are most important study endpoints.

Great attention should be paid to the nutritional and psychological state of the patient in specific palliative care programs.

FURTHER READING

Abbas F, Scardino PT (1997) The natural history of clinical prostate carcinoma. *Cancer* 80:827–833.

Bostwick DG (1997) Staging of prostatic cancer. Current methods and limitations. *Eur Urol* 32(Suppl. 3):2–14.

Denis L (1993) Primary hormonal treatment. *Cancer* 71:1050–1058.

Denis LJ, Murphy GP, Schröder FH (1995) Report of the Consensus Workshop on Screening and Global Strategy for Prostate cancer. *Cancer* 75:1187–1207.

Denis LJ (1997) Endocrine therapy of prostate cancer: A view from Europe. *Mo Urol* 1:231–241.

Fair WR, Israeli RS, Heston WDW (1997) Prostate-specific membrane antigen. *The Prostate* 32:140–148.

Gleason DF (1992) Histological grading of prostate cancer: A perspective. *Human Pathol* 23:273–279.

Griffiths K, Adlercreutz H, Boyle P, Denis L, Nicholson RI, Morton MS (1996) *Nutrition and Cancer*. ISIS Medical Media, Oxford, England.

Isaacs JT (1994) Role of androgen in prostate cancer. *Vit Horm* 49:433–502.

Kirby RS, Oesterling JE, Denis LJ (1996) *Fast Facts on Prostate Cancer*. Health Press, Oxford, England.

The Medical Research Council Prostate Cancer Working Party Investigators Group (1997) Immediate versus deferred treatment for advanced prostate cancer: Initial results of the Medical Research Trial. *Bri J Urol* 79:235–246.

Middleton G (1996) The management of clinically localized prostate cancer: Guidelines from the American Urological Association. *CA Cancer J Clin* 46:249–253.

Murphy G, Griffiths K, Denis L, Khoury S, Chatelain C, Cockett AT (1997) *First International Consultation on Prostate Cancer*, Monaco, June 20–21, 1996. SCI, Paris.

Pacelli A, Bostwick DG (1997) Clinical significance of high-grade prostatic intraepithelial neoplasia in transurethral resection specimens. *Urology* 50:355–359.

Parkin DM, Pisani P, Ferley J (1995) Worldwide burden of cancer. In: *Biannual Report 1994–1995*. IARC, Lyon, France, pp. 14–15.

Partin AW, Yoo J, Carter HB, Pearson JD, Clan DW, Epstein J, Walsh PC (1993) The use of PSA, clinical stage and Gleason score to predict pathological stage in men with localized prostate cancer. *J Urol* 150:110–117.

The Prostate Cancer Trialists' Collaborative Group (1995) Maximum androgen blockade in advanced prostate cancer: An overview of 22 randomized trials with 3283 deaths in 5710 patients. *Lancet* 346:265–269.

Sobin LH, Wittekind Ch (1997) *TNM Classification of Malignant Tumors*, 5th edition. Wiley-Liss, New York.

Tannock IF, Osoba D, Stockler MR, et al. (1996) Chemotherapy with mitoxantrone plus prednisone or prednisone alone for symptomatic hormone-resistant prostate cancer: A Canadian randomized trial with palliative end points. *J Clin Oncol* 14:1756–1764.

CHAPTER 29

NON-PROSTATE TUMORS GENITOURINARY CANCER

MARY K. GOSPODAROWICZ

University of Toronto
Princess Margaret Hospital
Toronto, Ontario, Canada

The term *genitourinary cancer* covers a wide variety of cancers arising in the human genital and urinary systems. By convention, cancers arising in the female genital tract are discussed as gynecologic cancers, and those arising in the male genital system and the urinary tract as genitourinary cancers. The etiology, pathology, and management of these tumors are so heterogeneous that they should be discussed as distinct disease entities. The most common cancer, prostate cancer, is discussed in a separate chapter. Of the cancers discussed in this chapter, cancer of the urinary bladder is the most common, with the other urothelial cancers, of the renal pelvis and ureter, being much less common. Kidney cancer is much less common, but an important disease with significant mortality. Testis cancer is an uncommon but very important disease that affects young men, and it is the only nonskin cancer in which appropriate therapy cures the majority of patients. Finally, cancer of the penis, a very rare disease in the Western world, continues to be an important cancer with a significant mortality in underdeveloped countries of Africa and South America.

CANCER OF THE KIDNEY

Cancer of the kidney is relatively uncommon, accounting for approximately 3% of all adult cancers. The incidence has been increasing in recent years, but this is thought to be due to increased detection of small incidental cancers found on abdominal ultrasound or computerized tomography (CT) scan in asymptomatic patients. The histopathologic classification is outlined in Table 29.1. Adenocarcinomas, or renal

Manual of Clinical Oncology, 7th edition, Edited by Raphael E. Pollock
ISBN 0-471-23828-7, pages 575–606. Copyright © 1999 Wiley-Liss, Inc.

TABLE 29.1. Pathologic Classification of Renal Cell
Carcinoma

Benign Neoplasms	Malignant Neoplasms
Papillary adenoma	Conventional (clear cell) renal carcinoma
Renal oncocytoma	Papillary renal carcinoma
	Chromophobe renal carcinoma
	Collecting duct carcinoma
	Renal cell carcinoma, unclassified

cell carcinomas, comprise nearly 85% of these tumors. The tumor occurs mainly in the fifth to seventh decade of life, with men affected twice as often as women.

Etiology

The etiology of renal cell carcinoma is uncertain. Epidemiologic studies have suggested a correlation between smoking and renal cell carcinoma. Urban living, thorotrast exposure, and family history of renal cancer are among reported risk factors. Although uncommon, familial cases of renal cell carcinoma have been reported and specific chromosomal abnormalities (3 to 8 translocation) have been described in members of one family. The autosomal dominant hereditary von Hippel–Lindau disease is frequently associated with renal cell carcinoma associated with the presence of the *VHL* gene on chromosome 3.

Screening

Currently there are no accepted screening programs in the general population to detect kidney cancer. Screening of high-risk populations, such as those with familial cancers or Von Hippel–Lindau syndrome, has been conducted in some centers.

Presentation

The primary renal lesions usually produce few early symptoms, with one fourth of patients presenting with advanced stages of disease. Progression is by direct extension, regional lymphatics, or hematogenously. The most common sites of metastases at presentation include the regional nodes, lungs, bone, and skin. As the disease progresses, the liver, brain, adrenal, and contralateral kidney are often involved. There is a wide variation in clinical presentation of renal cancers. The classic triad of hematuria, flank pain, and palpable mass is found only in 10% of patients; however, at least one of these findings can be found in 40% of patients. An uncommon presentation in patients with adenocarcinoma of the left kidney (2% to 3%) is that of a sudden onset of left-sided varicocele. Approximately 20% of patients have slowly progressive disease and remain relatively asymptomatic for several years even in face of metastatic disease. Approximately 30% of patients present with a paraneoplastic syndrome, occurrence of which is not necessarily indicative of distant metastases. Tumor related overproduction of renin, erythropoietin, prostaglandins, insulin, glucagon, enteroglucagon, β-human chorionic gonadotropin (β-hCG), ferritin, ectopic production of adrenocorticotropic hormone (ACTH) and parathormone have been reported. The finding of abnormal liver functions can be present in the absence of liver metastases (Stauffer's syndrome). Renal cell carcinoma may produce hypertension through a variety of mechanisms including hyperreninemia, renal arteriovenous fistulae, polycythemia, hypercalcemia, ureteral obstruction, and elevated intracranial pressure secondary to intracranial metastases. Paraneoplastic syndromes are not known to have an adverse prognostic impact, and their presence should not preclude curative management.

Pathology

Renal cell carcinomas, referred to as hypernephromas, arise from the epithelium of the proximal convoluted tubule. Local growth is usually well defined and the tumor is encompassed by the renal parenchyma or perinephric fibrous tissue. Invasion of the renal vein is common. There is direct correlation between both size and differentiation of the primary tumor and the propensity for metastatic spread. The sarcomatoid histologic type has been found to be associated with poor survival, whereas clear cell type and papillary growth pattern infers better survival. A large proportion of clear cell tumors, both sporadic and hereditary, share a common cytogenetic abnormality, namely, the loss of a portion of the 3p chromosome. A tumor suppressor gene for renal cell carcinoma lies along chromosome 3p. It appears that papillary renal cell carcinomas arise by a different cytogenetic mechanism, with trisomies and tetrasomies of chromosomes 7 and 17 as the initiating event.

Diagnostic Measures

CT scan is the method of choice for detection and staging of kidney tumors. Magnetic resonance imaging (MRI) is superior to delineate extent of tumor in patients with renal vein or vena cava involvement. Assessment also includes a complete blood count, liver function studies, and a chest X-ray film. Radioisotope bone scan is appropriate in patients with bone pain. The current UICC TNM staging classification is based on the size of the primary tumor, the presence of extrarenal extension, renal vein invasion, and nodal or distant metastases (Table 29.2). The overall 5-year survival for patients with stage I disease is 60% to 85%; for stage II, 45% to 80%; for stage III, 30% to 50%; and for stage IV, 5% to 10%.

Prognostic Factors

The clinical presentation of renal cell carcinoma is often diverse and outcome is notoriously difficult to predict. The only therapy for renal cell carcinoma with curative potential is radical surgery for patients presenting with localized disease. To date there is no evidence that treatment affects the outcome of patients with surgically unresectable or metastatic disease. Therefore stage, which reflects the anatomic extent of

TABLE 29.2. TNM Classification of Renal Cell Carcinoma (1997 5th Edition)

Primary Tumor (T)

TX   Primary tumor cannot be assessed.
T0   No evidence of primary tumor
T1   Tumor 7.0 cm or less in greatest dimension, limited to the kidney
T2   Tumor more than 7.0 cm in greatest dimension, limited to the kidney
T3   Tumor extends into major veins or invades adrenal gland or perinephric tissues
     but not beyond Gerota fascia.
    T3a   Tumor invades adrenal gland or perinephric tissues but not beyond Gerota fascia.
    T3b   Tumor grossly extends into renal vein(s) or vena cava below diaphragm.
    T3c   Tumor grossly extends into vena cava above diaphragm.
T4   Tumor invades beyond Gerota fascia.

Regional Lymph Nodes (N)

NX   Regional lymph nodes cannot be assessed.
N0   No regional lymph node metastasis
N1   Metastasis in a single regional lymph node
N2   Metastasis in more than one regional lymph node

Distant Metastasis (M)

MX   Distant metastasis cannot be assessed.
M0   No distant metastasis
M1   Distant metastasis

Stage Grouping

I	T1	N0	M0
II	T2	N0	M0
III	T1	N1	M0
	T2	N1	M0
	T3	N0, N1	M0
IV	T4	N0, N1	M0
	Any T	N2	M0
	Any T	Any N	M1

disease, is the most important factor predicting survival. Histologic grade and DNA ploidy measurement are also important prognostic factors, with well-differentiated and diploid tumors being associated with better outcome. The presence of anemia and an elevated erythrocyte sedimentation rate herald a poor prognosis in all stages of the disease whereas a poor performance status and weight loss indicate poor prognosis in patients with metastatic disease.

Multimodality Treatment

Philosophy of Management   Surgery is the mainstay of curative management of renal cell carcinoma. The other treatment methods do not result in a cure. Therefore, radical surgery is recommended in the majority of patients including those with locally extensive disease and minimal metastatic disease such as those with limited lymph node involvement and those with solitary distant metastases.

Surgery The principles of surgical management in renal cell carcinoma are well established in patients with confined tumors. Radical nephrectomy involves extrafascial removal of the entire kidney en bloc with the contents of the Gerota's fascia. Gerota's fascia is an excellent barrier to local tumor extension and is only rarely involved. Perinephric fat involvement occurs in approximately 30% of patients. Regional lymphadenectomy should be performed because the status of local nodes cannot be determined otherwise. Complete excision of a localized lesion provides a greater than 70% chance of 5-year survival. Renal cell carcinoma can be large and very vascular at the time of diagnosis, thereby making excision difficult. Preoperative percutaneous angioinfarction has been used to reduce operative complications. Roughly 15% of patients with renal cell carcinoma will have vena cava involvement, and extension to the level of the diaphragm and even into the right atrium is not uncommon. Although many patients with vena cava involvement at or above the hepatic veins have concomitant metastases, about 50% will not at the time of diagnosis. Techniques of cardiopulmonary bypass and circulatory arrest have made removal of large thrombi, even those extending into the right atrium, surgically feasible. Such undertakings are justified only in the absence of hematogenous metastases because, in their presence, death will almost invariably come within 6 to 18 months. In patients with renal vein or vena cava involvement, cure rates of 30% to 60% have been achieved, and hence extensive surgical procedures are clearly indicated. Spontaneous regression of metastatic disease has been reported in rare patients undergoing nephrectomy. However, because the chance of spontaneous regression is very low, and far exceeded by the surgical morbidity and mortality, the hope for spontaneous regression should never be an indication for surgery. Nephrectomy should be considered for palliation in the following situations: reasonably good performance status or low performance status due to local symptoms only, the only symptoms are due to local tumor, and resectable tumor identified by imaging studies. Because of the unpredictable natural history of the renal cell carcinoma, the resection of metastatic lesions may be occasionally undertaken to improve the quality of life and survival. This is usually considered in patients with solitary metastases with good performance status. Resection of solitary lung and brain metastases has been occasionally reported to be associated with prolonged survival.

Radiation Therapy Radiation therapy (RT) has no established role in the curative management of early renal cancer. Postoperative radiation has been used as adjuvant postnephrectomy in patients with extrarenal involvement, but there is no definitive evidence that such treatment improves survival. Palliative RT may be used to control the bleeding from the primary tumor or to palliate symptoms from metastases to the brain, bones, and soft tissues. Palliative RT in patients with bone or soft tissue metastases produces symptomatic relief in 50% of patients.

Chemotherapy and Immunotherapy   The unusual natural history of renal cell carcinoma, including spontaneous regression of the primary tumor, delayed growth of metastatic lesions, and varying tumor doubling times, suggests that host immune factors may be important in this tumor. Spontaneous regression of renal cell carcinoma is reported in fewer than 0.5% of patients. Progestins have been used to treat patients with metastatic disease. Tumor responses have been reported in fewer than 15% of patients. Chemotherapy has produced negligible effects on metastatic renal cell carcinoma and there is no evidence that its use affects survival. The reason for almost universal resistance to all effective chemotherapeutic agents is widespread overexpression of the *MDR-1* gene and its product p-glycoprotein. Agents such as vinblastine, nitrosoureas, and hydroxyurea have been reported to produce occasional responses. Advances in immunology and molecular biology have opened the way for promising new treatment modalities of metastatic renal cell carcinoma. These approaches use the cytokines interferon and interleukin-2 (IL-2), alone and in combination, or cells from the patient's own immune system expanded ex vivo by IL-2. Cytokine therapy with recombinant interferons has been shown to have a 5% to 27% response rate. Interferon-α monotherapy has a response rate of up to 16%. The median duration of response averaged 6 to 10 months with few durable complete remissions being observed. Toxicity of interferon therapy includes flulike symptoms, fatigue, and gastrointestinal upset. IL-2 is a lymphokine produced by T lymphocytes. The intravenous bolus or continuous infusion of IL-2 has produced response rates of 13% to 19%. Some durable responses were observed. The toxicity of IL-2 includes fevers, chills, malaise, nausea, vomiting, diarrhea, and other constitutional symptoms. IL-2 therapy is also associated with a vascular leak syndrome that can progress to hypotension, fluid retention, respiratory failure, prerenal azotemia with oliguria. Combinations of interferon-α and IL-2 have response rates between 12.5% and 31%. Trials of IL-2 and LAK (lymphokine-activated killer) cells currently do not suggest a major contribution by LAK cells to IL-2 therapy. Trials of TIL (tumor-infiltrating lymphocytes) therapy have also been conducted with little effect. The ability to introduce and express foreign genes in cells has raised hopes for application of such technology in clinical oncology. Current studies are underway attempting to incorporate genes coding for tumor necrosis factor into TILs and to use these modified cells in clinical trials. Another approach evolving from this technology uses genetically modified tumor cells as a vaccine.

Organ Preservation

Although radical nephrectomy is the procedure of choice for localized renal cell carcinoma, no randomized studies have shown a survival advantage over less aggressive surgical approaches. A number of studies have shown that partial nephrectomy in selected cases, at least with short-term follow-up, offers equivalent survival to radical nephrectomy, and the local recurrence rates have been minimal. At present parenchyma sparing surgery for renal cell carcinoma is indicated for patients with bilateral tumors, tumors in solitary kidney, and von Hippel–Lindau disease or familial renal cell carcinoma, and in patients whose remaining kidney is compromised by significant medical illness. Once the tumor has metastasized, the role of nephrectomy is less well defined. In patients with severe local symptoms, nephrectomy may offer significant palliative relief.

Follow-Up

The majority of patients with renal cell are treated with surgery. The risk of recurrence is related to the stage of the disease and the completeness of surgical resection. The role of routine follow-up investigations to detect recurrence is controversial because of the paucity of effective treatments for relapse. Regular clinical visits with abdominal ultrasound allow detection of retroperitoneal recurrence that can occasionally be managed with further surgery and also detect contralateral primary tumors. Chest X-ray film is useful to detect solitary pulmonary metastasis that can be resected. Other routine follow-up tests are not considered cost effective in this disease.

CANCER OF THE URINARY BLADDER

Bladder carcinoma is the most common malignant tumor of the urinary tract. It accounts for 4% of all visceral cancers. The disease is 2.5 times more common in men than in women and most often occurs in the sixth and seventh decades of life. The prognosis and management of bladder cancer is related to the depth of bladder wall invasion. Tumors that invade detrusor muscle are associated with high risk of lymph node and distant metastases, whereas those limited to the bladder mucosa and submucosa can be managed with local therapies, as they have very low risk of extravesical spread.

Etiology

According to the current paradigm, bladder cancer results from the genetic alteration of normal bladder mucosa. The mechanisms by which DNA is altered, the nature of these changes, and the genes involved are not known. Some environmental factors that are associated with bladder cancer have been determined. It is estimated that about one half of bladder cancers result from tobacco exposure and one quarter from occupational exposure. The association between the exposure to aromatic amines and the development of bladder cancer is very strong. Aniline dyes used in textile, rubber, and cable industries are among the known industrial factors associated with bladder cancer. The latency period for occupational exposure is often very long, generally in excess of 15 years. The relationship between infection with *Schistosoma hematobium* and squamous cell bladder cancer is well established, but its pathogenesis poorly understood. In Egypt, where the prevalence of schistosomiasis is as high as 45%, almost 70% of bladder cancers are squamous cell carcinomas and tumors occur at a younger age. There appears to be an association between urinary stasis and recurrent urinary tract infections and bladder cancer, with the majority of such cases being squamous cell carcinomas. The pathogenesis of bladder cancer associated with urinary tract infections is uncertain, but may be due to nitrate production by bacteria. Long-term administration of cyclophosphamide appears to be associated with an increased risk of bladder cancer. Most chemically induced cancers are transitional cell carcinomas (TCCs), but some are squamous cell carcinomas. The association between excess phenacetin use and TCC of renal pelvis and ureters is well established, but the association with bladder cancer is less well documented. The association between dietary factors and bladder cancer is controversial. Several reports on the use of artificial sweeteners and coffee consumption provided ambiguous results.

Screening

There are no prospective randomized trials to document that routine screening for bladder cancer improves survival. However, studies suggest that bladder cancer screening in healthy men age 50 and older by repeated home hematuria testing significantly decreases bladder cancer morbidity and mortality and is cost effective. Routine screening with urine cytology may be useful in high-risk populations such as those with known industrial exposure to urinary carcinogens. Early detection of bladder cancer depends on prompt evaluation of patients with hematuria or other irritative urinary symptoms.

Presentation and Natural History

Approximately 70% of patients with newly diagnosed transitional cell carcinoma have tumors that are confined to the epithelium or the underlying lamina propria. It is unusual for such tumors to be associated with concomitant metastases and thus all are theoretically curable by local means. However, once the tumor has invaded into the muscle wall of the bladder or beyond, the likelihood of nodal or distant metastases is much higher. Indeed, only a small proportion of patients with extensive involvement of perivesical tissues survive for more than a couple of years. The majority of patients, almost 75%, present with gross or microscopic hematuria. The degree of hematuria is generally unrelated to the seriousness of its underlying cause. Also, hematuria associated with bladder cancer may be intermittent. Urination frequency, bladder irritability, and dysuria occur in about one third of patients. In the later stages of the disease symptoms of upper tract obstruction also occur. However, bladder cancer is almost never found incidentally at autopsy, indicating that it is likely to cause symptoms at some time during the patient's life. Systemic symptoms are rare, but fever (>39°C) can be present in up to 20% of patients.

Pathology

In Europe and North America, more than 90% of bladder tumors are transitional cell carcinomas derived from the uroepithelium. Approximately 6% to 8% are squamous cell carcinomas and 2% are adenocarcinomas. Adenocarcinomas may be either of urachal origin or nonurachal origin; the latter type is thought to arise from metaplasia of chronically irritated transitional epithelium. The frequency of SCC is very high in Egypt and other areas endemic for *Schistosoma hematobium*. Many tumors show a mixed pattern with transitional cell carcinoma with squamous or adenomatous hyperplasia. Although tumors may arise from any part of the bladder, they most commonly arise from the trigone and the lateral walls. Pathologic grade, which is based on cellular atypia, nuclear abnormalities, and the number of mitotic figures, is of prognostic importance. Carcinoma in situ (CIS), a cytologically malignant epithelium, may coexist with other transitional cell tumors or occur by itself as a separate and distinct entity. It may appear on cystoscopy as a flat, reddish lesion with a granular surface. Configuration of macroscopic tumor may be exophytic (papillary) or flat and solid (nodular). The solid configuration is usually associated with muscle invasive disease, whereas a papillary configuration is common in low-grade noninvasive and superficial tumors.

Diagnosis

The cornerstones of the diagnostic evaluation have traditionally been intravenous pyelography (IVP) and cystoscopy, with the latter being the most common diagnostic test. Once cystoscopic examination has revealed that a bladder tumor is present, the tumor should be endoscopically resected in its entirety. This is therapeutic and also provides important staging and grading information. Cytologic examination of urine should be performed in conjunction with those tests, particularly if the IVP and cystoscopy were not diagnostic. Urine cytology is more sensitive for high-grade urothelial cancers than for the low-grade ones, with between 50% and 80% of high-grade lesions being detected as opposed to only 20% of low-grade tumors. This difference is so pronounced that an abnormal urine cytology in the presence of a low-grade tumor suggests the presence of a coexistent high-grade lesion.

Staging and Prognostic Factors

Although some clinical and pathologic prognostic factors have been defined, the more fundamental and potentially more discriminating molecular and biologic factors remain unknown. The most important prognostic factor in bladder cancer is the depth of bladder wall invasion. Many other clinical and pathologic prognostic factors such as grade, tumor size, multiplicity, tumor configuration, vascular invasion, positive urine cytology, or coexistent carcinoma in situ have been described. There is an increasing body of evidence that tumors with *p53* mutations have more aggressive behavior independent of the other prognostic factors.

The clinical staging of carcinoma of the bladder rests upon determining the depth of invasion of the bladder wall by the tumor. Cystoscopic examination with biopsies, and examination under anesthesia with assessment of the size and mobility of palpable masses, the degree of induration of the bladder wall, and the presence of extravesical extension or invasion of adjacent organs are required for staging. Clinical staging, even when CT and or MRI scans are employed, often underestimates the pathologic extent of tumor. The TNM UICC staging system was modified in 1997

TABLE 29.3. TNM Classification of Urinary Bladder Cancer (1997 5th Edition)

Primary Tumor (T)

TX   Primary tumor cannot be assessed.
T0   No evidence of primary tumor
Ta   Noninvasive papillary carcinoma
Tis   Carcinoma in situ
T1   Tumor invades subepithelial connective tissue.
T2   Tumor invades muscle.
      T2a   Tumor invades superficial muscle (inner half).
      T2b   Tumor invades deep muscle (outer half).
T3   Tumor invades perivesical tissue
      T3a   Microscopically
      T3b   Macroscopically (extravesical mass)
T4   Tumor invades any of the following: prostate, uterus, vagina, pelvic wall, abdominal wall.
      T4a   Tumor invades prostate, uterus, vagina.
      T4b   Tumor invades pelvic wall, abdominal wall.

Regional Lymph Nodes (N)
Regional lymph nodes are those within the true pelvis; all others are distant lymph nodes.

NX   Regional lymph nodes cannot be assessed.
N0   No regional lymph node metastasis
N1   Metastasis in a single lymph node 2 cm or less in greatest dimension
N2   Metastasis in a single lymph node more than 2 cm but not more than 5 cm in greatest dimension or multiple lymph nodes none more than 5 cm in greatest dimension
N3   Metastasis in a lymph node more than 5 cm in greatest dimension

Distant Metastasis (M)
MX   Distant metastasis cannot be assessed.
M0   No distant metastasis
M1   Distant metastasis

Stage Grouping

0a	Ta	N0	M0
0is	Tis	N0	M0
I	T1	N0	M0
II	T2a	N0	M0
	T2b	N0	M0
III	T3a	N0	M0
	T3b	N0	M0
	T4a	N0	M0
IV	T4b	N0	M0
	Any T	N1	M0
	Any T	N2	M0
	Any T	N3	M0
	Any T	Any N	M1

to reflect the prognostic impact of extravesical tumor extension (Table 29.3). Distant metastases are distinctly uncommon in patients with superficial disease, that is, without invasion of muscularis propria. However, in patients with muscle invasive disease, assessment with chest X-ray film, bone scan, and CT of the abdomen and pelvis is indicated to exclude distant metastases.

Multimodality Treatment

Prolonged survival in most patients with superficial cancers can be achieved by transurethral resection and intravesical chemotherapy. Although recurrence is common, progression to muscle invasive or metastatic disease occurs in fewer than 20% of patients with superficial disease. However, in patients presenting with muscle invasive tumor, especially extravesical tumor, occult metastases are common and cure is possible in fewer than 50% of patients, even when radical locoregional therapy is applied.

Superficial Bladder Cancer (Ta, Tis, T1)

The majority of bladder tumors that are diagnosed are superficial papillary tumors. Most often, superficial lesions are solitary, but about one third of patients have multiple lesions at presentation. Approximately 50% of superficial tumors recur after the initial resection, often elsewhere in the bladder. It is not certain whether these recurrences occur as second primary events in a bladder mucosa with a "field defect" or as a result of tumor implants secondary to the initial resection. The fact that tumors can occur synchronously and metachronously throughout the urothelium suggests the former. The majority of patients who develop recurrence do so within the first year after primary treatment. The strongest predictive factors for recurrence are multifocality at presentation or positive cytology. Stage, grade, large size, solid configuration, and history of smoking have also been shown to predict recurrence in patients with superficial tumors. About 10% to 20% of patients with superficial tumors will eventually progress to muscle invasive or metastatic disease. The progression rate varies depending on the primary tumor characteristics. CIS, especially when diffuse, is associated with a rapid progression to muscle invasion. Grade and stage correlate well among superficial tumors, with most Ta tumors being grade 1 and most grade 2 and 3 tumors being T1 stage. The most widely used form of therapy for superficial tumors is transurethral resection (TUR) and fulguration of tumor. Once the patient undergoes primary therapy and is rendered disease free, close surveillance is essential. Typically this involves periodic cystoscopic evaluation with concomitant urine cytology. Although recurrences are common, the long-term disease-specific survival for patients with Ta–T1 disease ranges from 75% to 85%.

Other commonly used forms of treatment for superficial disease include segmental cystectomy, intravesical chemotherapy, or immunotherapy with Bacillus Calmette-Guerin (BCG). Radical cystectomy may be offered to selected patients. In patients who recur following the initial TUR, intravesical chemotherapy with Thiotepa, mitomycin, doxorubicin, or BCG is employed prior to forms of therapy other than transurethral resection. BCG is particularly effective in CIS, resulting in 70% complete response rate. However, approximately 50% of patients with CIS who achieve complete response with BCG will eventually relapse. Newer therapies, currently being investigated in superficial disease, include photodynamic therapy after administration of intravenous hematoporphyrin derivative and intravesical interferon α2B.

Muscle-Invasive Bladder Cancer (T2, T3, T4, N1–N3)

The definitive forms of treatment for muscle invasive disease (T2–T4A) include radical cystectomy, with or without preoperative radiation and external-beam radiation alone. The overall survival for patients with muscle invasion rarely exceeds 50% at 5 years. Patients with locally extensive tumors such as those invading the pelvic side wall have a median survival of 6 to 12 months.

Surgery

Patients with early superficial muscle invasion (T2) can occasionally be successfully treated with a TUR alone. However, the majority of patients require radical treatments such as cystectomy or RT. Radical cystectomy involves removal of the bladder, perivesical tissues, prostate, and seminal vesicles in men and the uterus, tubes, ovaries, anterior vaginal wall, and urethra in women, and may or may not be accompanied by pelvic node dissection. Recent studies indicate that radical cystectomy with preservation of sexual function can be performed in some men and new forms of continent urinary diversion can obviate the need for an external appliance. Although radical cystectomy is very effective treatment for patients with T2 disease (60% to 75% 5-year survival), it results in cure in only a small proportion of patients with extensive extravesical disease (20% to 30% 5-year survival).

Radiation Therapy

RT has been used in the management of transitional cell carcinoma of the bladder either alone as definitive therapy (radical RT) or as adjuvant treatment precystectomy (preoperative RT). The main benefit of radical RT is the opportunity to preserve normal bladder and male sexual function and the fact that such treatment is a viable alternative for patients who are not operative candidates. Radical radiation results in local tumor control in approximately 50% of patients. Further efforts to improve results are necessary to reduce the number of patients requiring salvage surgery. In some reports, radical RT, with salvage cystectomy when indicated, yields therapeutic results similar to those of radical cystectomy. Currently a combined chemotherapy and radiation therapy approach is being investigated to improve both local control and to reduce the risk of distant metastases. The main goal of preoperative RT has been to prevent local recurrence after cystectomy, but to date its benefit has not been documented in prospective clinical trials.

Chemotherapy

The pattern of failure in patients with muscle invasive disease includes local recurrence in the bladder in patients treated with RT, pelvic recurrence in patients with extravesical extension following treatment with either RT or radical surgery. The main pattern of failure, however, is that of distant metastases, with the main sites of distant spread including pelvic and para-aortic lymph nodes, bone, lung, liver, and brain. Because of this, it is estimated that any local form of therapy will not cure more than 50% of patients. To date there is no evidence that the use of systemic chemotherapy in patients with locally advanced disease improves the cure rate or survival, but several adjuvant studies have suggested that the use of adjuvant chemotherapy following cystectomy improves progression-free survival. Prospective trials are underway to test the role of neoadjuvant and adjuvant chemotherapy. The use of neoadjuvant chemotherapy and radiation offers the opportunity for bladder preservation in selected patients, and preliminary results indicate that such an approach does not compromise survival.

Metastatic Bladder Cancer (M1)

Only 5% to 10% of patients with bladder cancer have metastatic disease at presentation. The majority of patients who develop metastases do so following treatment for muscle invasive disease. The prognosis of patients with recurrent disease after local therapies is poor. Effective systemic chemotherapy, however, is available and treatment with combination chemotherapy such as MVAC (methotrexate, vinblastine, Adriamycin, cisplatin) or CMV (cisplatin, methotrexate, vinblastine) offers survival advantage as compared to treatment with single-agent cisplatin alone. It is important to note, however, that to date there is no evidence for cure and that a median survival of patients with metastatic bladder cancer treated with MVAC chemotherapy ranges from 8 to 12 months. Chemotherapy is toxic, with the majority of patients having significant gastrointestinal, hematologic, and neurotoxicity. Because of limited efficacy and toxicity chemotherapy may not be appropriate for elderly patients with poor performance status. In the last few years many new chemotherapeutic agents have been identified as useful in the management of bladder cancer. These include taxanes, gemcitabine, gallium nitrate, and ifosfamide. Trials to determine the optimal combinations of these drugs are currently ongoing.

Organ Preservation

Organ preservation is an important issue in the management of bladder cancer. Effective management of superficial cancer with TUR and intravesical therapy has improved local control and reduced the number of patients who progress and require cystectomy. Progress in the management of locally advanced bladder cancer has been less impressive. Although the acceptance of radical cystectomy and its morbidity has been reduced with the introduction of continent urinary diversion, little effort has been made to improve results of traditional bladder preserving methods of radiation therapy with and without chemotherapy. The latter have been reserved for elderly, or noncompliant patients, not the most suitable populations to study improved treatment methods. However, there is increasing evidence that definitive RT, with or without concurrent chemotherapy, achieves cure and organ preservation in patients with locally advanced bladder cancer.

Follow-Up for Local and Distant Recurrences

Superficial bladder cancer is a chronic disease with potential for many recurrences over 15 to 25 years. Optimal follow-up protocols continue to be defined. Currently follow-up with regular cystoscopic examinations and urine cytology is essential. In the future, other less invasive methods of disease assessment should become available.

Prevention

International efforts to reduce smoking and industrial exposure should result in a decreased incidence of bladder cancer. Further successful management of superficial bladder cancers has already reduced the number of patients who require treatment for locally advanced muscle invasive cancers. The remaining problem of the natural history of multiple recurrences in superficial bladder cancer is also being addressed. Although there is no firm evidence that recurrence can be uniformly prevented, there are currently ongoing chemoprevention trials for patients at high risk of bladder cancer recurrence using retinoids and megadose vitamins.

CANCER OF THE RENAL PELVIS AND URETER

Upper urinary tract urothelial tumors are relatively uncommon. The majority are transitional cell cancers. Renal pelvis tumors account for approximately 10% of all renal tumors and about 5% of all urothelial tumors. Ureteral tumors are even less common, occurring with one quarter of the incidence of renal pelvis tumors. The incidence of upper tract urothelial tumors is dramatically different in areas endemic for Balkan nephropathy. The etiology of Balkan nephropathy remains unknown. Cigarette smoking is the agent most strongly associated with an increased risk (up to 7.2-fold) of upper tract cancers. Analgesic abuse has also been associated with a higher risk of upper tract tumors (2.4- to 4.2-fold increase). The other etiologic factors are similar to those for cancer of the urinary bladder and include occupational factors, chronic infections, and cyclophosphamide. Bilateral involvement occurs in 2% to 5% of sporadic upper tract tumors. Upper tract cancers occur also in 2% to 4% of patients with bladder cancer. The interval between the bladder tumor and the upper tract tumor may be as long as 10 to 20 years. Approximately 30% to 75% of patients with upper tract tumors will have bladder tumor at some time. Ureteral tumors are most common in the lower ureter. The most common presentation is with hematuria, but renal colic due to ureteric obstruction can also be present. Diagnosis is usually made on intravenous pyelogram or retrograde urography, but CT is extremely valuable to assess soft tissue extent of disease and exclude metastases. Staging is according to the 1997 TNM classification (Table 29.4).

Treatment is dependent on stage and histologic grade. Patients with grade 1, low stage (TA, T1) tumors can be treated with conservative surgery, that is, partial ureterectomy. Patients with grade 2 and 3 tumors are best managed with total nephroureterectomy and resection of the bladder cuff.

TABLE 29.4. TNM Classification of Renal Pelvis and Ureter Cancers (1997 5th Edition)

Primary Tumor (T)

TX	Primary tumor cannot be assessed.
T0	No evidence of primary tumor
TA	Noninvasive papillary carcinoma
Tis	Carcinoma in situ
T1	Tumor invades subepithelial connective tissue.
T2	Tumor invades muscularis.
T3	(For renal pelvis only) Tumor invades beyond muscularis into peripelvic fat or renal parenchyma.
T3	(For ureter only) Tumor invades beyond muscularis into periureteric fat.
T4	Tumor invades adjacent organs or through the kidney into perinephric fat.

Regional Lymph Nodes (N)

NX	Regional lymph nodes cannot be assessed.
N0	No regional lymph node metastasis
N1	Metastasis in a single regional lymph node 2 cm or less in greatest dimension
N2	Metastasis in a single lymph node, more than 2 cm but not more than 5 cm in greatest dimension or multiple lymph nodes, none more than 5 cm in greatest dimension
N3	Metastasis in a lymph node more than 5 cm in greatest dimension

Laterality does not affect the N classification.

Distant Metastasis (M)

MX	Distant metastasis cannot be assessed.
M0	No distant metastasis
M1	Distant metastasis

Stage Grouping

0a	TA	N0	M0
0is	Tis	N0	M0
I	T1	N0	M0
II	T2	N0	M0
III	T3	N0	M0
IV	T4	N0	M0
	Any T	N1	M0
	Any T	N2	M0
	Any T	N3	M0
	Any T	Any N	M0

The 5-year survival rates are 85% to 95% for stage I disease, 40% to 60% for stage II disease, 20% to 30% for stage III, and less than 10% for stage IV disease. The role of radiation therapy is controversial. However, there is no role for RT in stage I and II disease. RT may be useful as adjuvant therapy following incomplete tumor resection in stage III disease, but to date there are no definitive data to support its use. Similar to bladder cancer, adjuvant systemic chemotherapy with MVAC has been used in patients with lymph node and distant metastases with some success, and is recommended in patients with a good performance status.

CANCER OF THE URETHRA

Cancer of the Male Urethra

Carcinoma of the male urethra is rare. Significant etiologic factors have not been identified, but chronic inflammation appears to play a role because many patients have history of prior urethritis, stricture, or sexually transmitted disease. The most frequent site of the tumor is the bulbomembranous urethra, which is also the most frequent site of urethral stricture. Cancers occur in the bulbomembranous urethra in 60%, penile urethra in 30%, and prostatic urethra in 10%. Histologically, 80% are squamous cell cancers, 15% are transitional cell cancers, and 5% have other histology. The spread is usually by direct invasion and extension to the perineal tissues. Metastatic spread is to the inguinal and external iliac lymph nodes. The 1997 TNM classification is used for staging (Table 29.5). Investigations include urethroscopy, examination under anesthesia, and CT or MRI imaging to determine soft tissue extent.

The primary mode of treatment is surgical excision. The superficial tumors may be managed by transurethral resection, with high potential for cure. In rare cases that involve mucosa only, stage Ta, Tis, resection and fulguration is justified as initial therapy. Infiltrating lesions require penile amputation for cancers of anterior urethra. The role of RT for tumors of the anterior urethra is not well defined, but cure with RT has been reported. Tumors involving bulbomembranous urethra require radical cystoprostatectomy and en bloc penectomy to achieve adequate margins of resection, minimize local recurrence, and achieve cure. There is little experience and data regarding the use of radiation therapy, but similar to the carcinoma of the female urethra RT may be useful in achieving local disease control. Five-year survival can be expected in only 15% to 20% of patients with the latter tumors.

Cancer of the Female Urethra

Urethral carcinoma is much more common in women than in men. Most patients are over the age of 50 years. The etiology is unknown, but similar to the relationship between male urethral cancer and chronic irritation, urinary tract infections have been reported. Most patients present with urinary frequency, obstruction, or palpable urethral lesion. Histology is that of squamous cell carcinoma in 60% of cases, transi-

TABLE 29.5. TNM Classification of Cancer of the Urethra (1997 5th Edition)

Primary Tumor (T) (Male and Female)

TX	Primary tumor cannot be assessed.
T0	No evidence of primary tumor
Ta	Noninvasive papillary, polypoid, or verrucous carcinoma
Tis	Carcinoma in situ
T1	Tumor invades subepithelial connective tissue.
T2	Tumor invades any of the following: corpus spongiosum, prostate or periurethral muscle.
T3	Tumor invades any of the following: corpus cavernosum, beyond prostatic capsule, anterior vagina, or bladder neck.
T4	Tumor invades other adjacent organs

Transitional Cell Carcinoma of the Prostate (Prostatic Urethra)

Tis pu	Carcinoma in situ, involvement of the prostatic urethra
Tis pd	Carcinoma in situ, involvement of the prostatic ducts
T1	Tumor invades subepithelial connective tissue.
T2	Tumor invades any of the following: prostatic stroma, corpus spongiosum, periurethral muscle.
T3	Tumor invades any of the following: corpus cavernosum, beyond prostatic capsule, bladder neck (extraprostatic extension)
T4	Tumor invades other adjacent organs (invasion of the bladder).

Regional Lymph Nodes (N)

NX	Regional lymph nodes cannot be assessed.
N0	No regional lymph node metastasis
N1	Metastasis in a single regional lymph node 2 cm or less in greatest dimension
N2	Metastasis in a single lymph node, more than 2 cm in greatest dimension or multiple lymph nodes

Distant Metastasis (M)

MX	Distant metastatis cannot be assessed.
M0	No distant metastasis
M1	Distant metastasis

Stage Grouping

0a	Ta	N0	M0
0is	Tis	N0	M0
	Tis pu	N0	M0
	Tis pd	N0	M0
I	T1	N0	M0
II	T2	N0	M0
III	T1	N1	M0
	T2	N1	M0
	T3	N0	M0
	T3	N1	M0
IV	T4	N0	M0
	T4	N1	M0
	Any T	N2	M0
	Any T	Any N	M1

tional cell carcinoma in 30%, and adenocarcinoma in 10%. Other tumors, melanoma, or sarcoma are rare. Staging classification and assessment are similar to those described previously for male urethral cancer.

Treatment may involve surgery or RT. For tumors of the anterior or distal urethra, local surgical excision or electroresection and fulguration may be sufficient for small distal tumors. Tumor destruction using Nd:YAG or CO_2 laser vaporization–coagulation represents an alternative option. RT for larger and invasive tumors may be used with external-beam radiotherapy, often with brachytherapy boost using interstitial or intracavitary techniques. Treatment results for early stage disease are good (65% to 80% survival), but more extensive disease is associated with poor survival probability (20% to 30%). Combined modality approaches with concurrent chemotherapy and RT are currently being explored in an attempt to improve local disease control and survival. Tumors of the posterior female urethra or entire urethra are usually invasive and are associated with a high incidence of lymph node metastases. Treatment involves exenterative surgery and urinary diversion, with adjuvant RT. For smaller tumors, RT alone or in combination with local tumor excision may be sufficient. Five-year survival is 60% if lesions are less than 2 cm in diameter, and 10% to 20% if larger than 4 to 5 cm in diameter.

CANCER OF THE TESTIS

Testis cancers are uncommon but constitute the most common group of malignancies in men ages 15 to 35 years. The vast majority are primary germ cell tumors (GCTs). Although the incidence of GCT has doubled in the past 30 years, the mortality associated with them has markedly declined. The introduction of tumor markers, CT imaging, and curative chemotherapy all contributed to improved outcomes. The identification of prognostic factors helped to refine management strategies and minimize treatment for those with favorable prognosis.

Etiology

Testicular cancer accounts for only 1% to 2% of all cancers in men. The cumulative lifetime risk of developing a germ cell tumor for an American Caucasian male is 0.2%. There is considerable geographic and ethnic variation in the incidence of GCT, with the highest incidence being reported from Denmark and Switzerland (6.2 to 8.84 per 100,000 per year). The incidence of testicular cancer is lower in nonwhites as compared to whites. The only factor definitely associated with testicular cancer is that of a history of testicular maldescent. Men with a history of cryptorchidism have an approximately fivefold increased chance of developing a testicular cancer. Familial clusters of testicular cancer have been reported, and patients with XY gonadal dysgenesis have an increased risk of developing testis cancer. Prior testicular cancer is a major risk factor for the development of a contralateral malignancy. The cumulative risk of developing a contralateral malignancy at 25 years after diagnosis is 5.2%. Other factors included mumps orchitis and a history of testicular trauma. Prenatal factors included threatened miscarriage, excessive maternal nausea, and delivery by caesarean section. It has been suggested that exposure of the germinal epithelium in utero to an elevated level of free unbound maternal estrogen could give rise to subsequent cryptorchidism and an elevated risk of developing a testicular tumor. However, the prenatal estrogen theory remains unproven.

Screening

There is insufficient evidence to establish that screening would result in a decrease in mortality from testicular cancer. Most testicular tumors are first detected by a patient, either unintentionally or by self-examination. No studies have been done to determine the effectiveness of testicular self-examination in reducing mortality from testicular cancer.

Diagnostic Measures

For clinical purposes, GCTs are classified into two major groups: seminomas and nonseminomatous germ cell tumors (NSGCTs). Approximately 45% of GCTs are pure seminoma, 40% are NSGCTs, and 15% are mixed tumors. Intratubular germ cell neoplasia, or carcinoma in situ (CIS), is felt to precede the development of all cases of seminoma and NSGCT with the exception of spermatocytic seminoma. In the general population the incidence of CIS is very low (0.2% to 0.5%), but it is somewhat higher in men with impaired fertility (0.5%) and in patients with cryptorchid testes (2% to 5%). Seminoma, the most common type of GCT, is usually seen in the fourth decade of life. NSGCTs comprise 40% of germ cell testicular cancers and occur most commonly in the third decade of life. In the WHO classification system, NSGCTs include embryonal carcinoma, teratoma (mature, immature, or with malignant differentiation), choriocarcinoma, yolk sac tumor, and mixed GCT (Table 29.6). Although some tumors have a component of seminoma, the association of seminoma within a histologically confirmed NSGCT has no major impact on the outcome.

TABLE 29.6. Histologic Classification of Germ Cell Testis Tumors

Intratubular germ cell neoplasia (carcinoma in situ)
Seminoma
Spermatocytic seminoma
Embryonal cell carcinoma
Teratoma
    Mature teratoma
    Immature teratoma
    Teratoma with malignant component
Yolk sac tumor
Choriocarcinoma
Mixed germ cell tumors
Polyembryoma

Local or direct extension of tumor into epididymis, through tunica vaginalis, into spermatic cord, and rarely into scrotum can occur, but the prognostic impact of such spread is small. In GCTs, lymphatic spread is the most common route of metastatic spread. In patients with NSGCTs, hematogenous spread also occurs early in the course of the disease. The lymphatic drainage of the testis is directly to the para-aortic lymph nodes. It is are often seen at the time of relapse. Pelvic and inguinal lymph node involvement is rare ($<3\%$). Factors predisposing to inguinal lymph node involvement include prior scrotal or inguinal surgery, scrotal orchiectomy with incision of the tunica albuginea, tumor invasion of the tunica vaginalis or lower third of the epididymis, and cryptorchid testis. In patients with NSGCTs, hematogenous spread occurs early in the course of the disease. The pulmonary parenchyma is the most common site of hematogenous spread but liver, bone, brain, kidney, and gastrointestinal metastases are also seen. In a recent review of more than 5000 patients with metastatic GCT, pulmonary metastases were present in 44% of cases, liver metastases were present in 6% of cases, and all other areas of hematogenous spread were present in 1% or less of patients. GCTs have a distinctive capacity for totipotential differentiation as demonstrated by the frequent finding of combinations of choriocarcinoma, embryonal carcinoma, and seminoma in a single tumor. They also can retain their ability to differentiate as displayed by the not infrequent identification of mature teratoma in residual posttreatment retroperitoneal masses. Cytogenetic analysis of GCTs has shown that chromosome numbers are more homogeneous in seminomas than in NSGCTs. Triploid and tetraploid chromosomal patterns are common in seminomas, and hyperdiploid to hypertriploid counts are common in NS-GCTs. A characteristic chromosome anomaly in GCTs of all histologic types is the presence of an isochromosome of the short arm of chromosome 12. It is present in more than 80% of cases, and in GCTs without 12p isochromosome extra copies of 12p segments are incorporated into other chromosomes. The 12p isochromosome is also found in testicular CIS. Isochromosome copies tend to be more numerous in NSGCTs than in seminoma.

Patients with testis tumors most commonly present with painless testicular enlargement. Up to 45% of patients have testicular pain. Less common presenting features include those related to the presence of metastases, for example, back pain and dyspnea. A radical orchiectomy is usually performed after the tumor is detected on physical examination and verified by ultrasonography. Serum tumor markers including (α-fetoprotein (AFP), human chorionic gonadotropin (β-hCG), and lactate dehydrogenase (LDH) should be obtained preoperatively to allow monitoring of decay with treatment. Staging investigations include chest X-ray film, CT of the abdomen and pelvis, CT of the thorax, and postoperative tumor markers in NSGCTs. CT of the thorax is of little value in patients with seminoma and no evidence of retroperitoneal lymph node involvement. Measurements of AFP, β-hCG, and LDH are essential in the diagnosis and management of patients with GCTs. hCG is a glycoprotein with a molecular weight of 45,000, composed of two subunits, of which the α-subunit is identical to that of luteinizing hormone (LH), follicle-stimulating hormone (FSH), and thyroid-stimulating hormone (TSH), and a distinct β-subunit. The half-life of β-hCG in human serum is approximately 22 hours. AFP is a glycoprotein of molecular weight 70,000. Besides NSGCTs, it is elevated in hepatocellular carcinomas, cirrhosis, hepatitis, and pregnancy. The half-life of AFP is approximately 5 days. AFP is not found in pure seminoma; its elevation in this setting implies the presence of NSGCT tumor elements. One or both of these markers are elevated in 85% of patients with NSGCTs. LDH is an independent prognostic factor in patients with GCT, being elevated in up to 60% of patients with NSGCTs, and in a high proportion of patients with advanced seminoma. Placental alkaline phosphatase (PLAP) is an isoenzyme of alkaline phosphatase and is normally expressed by placental syncytiotrophoblasts. It is also expressed by testis tissue and has been used as a tumor marker in seminoma. Although PLAP is often elevated in patients with seminoma, it has proven to be of little value in routine clinical management.

Staging

The 1997 UICC classification (Table 29.7), which combines anatomic and newly recognized nonanatomic prognostic factors, is the recommended staging system.

Multimodality Treatment

The initial management involves a radical inguinal orchidectomy in almost all cases. Postorchidectomy management is based on the histology and stage. The management policies for both seminomas and NSGCTs have evolved separately.

Surgery

Orchidectomy is both diagnostic and therapeutic and offers cure in a high proportion (60% to 90%) of patients with stage I disease. The role of orchidectomy has been recently questioned in patients with bilateral testis tumors. The possibility of organ-sparing surgery with tumor enucleation, or partial orchidectomy with or without postoperative low-dose RT, has been proposed. Preservation of hormonal function was achieved in 10 of 14 cases managed by tumor excision with low-dose (18 to 20 Gy) postoperative RT to the residual testis.

Seminoma

The majority of patients with seminoma present with clinical stage I disease, 15% to 20% have infradiaphragmatic lymph node involvement, and fewer than 5% present with distant disease. Treatment options in patients with stage I seminoma include adjuvant RT, surveillance, and adjuvant chemotherapy. The overall survival for stage I seminoma following retroperitoneal RT ranges between 92% and 99% at 5 to 10 years, with most deaths being due to intercurrent illness. With moderate RT dose (25 to 30 Gy), infield disease control is almost 100%. Approximately 5% of patients will relapse outside the RT treatment volume, most commonly in supraclavicular lymph nodes, mediastinum, lung, or bone. The second treatment option is surveillance with

TABLE 29.7. TNM Classification of Testis Tumors (1997 5th Edition)

Primary Tumor (pT)

The extent of primary tumor is classified after radical orchiectomy.

pT	Primary tumor cannot be assessed. (If no radical orchiectomy has been performed TX is used.)
pT0	No evidence of primary tumor (e.g., histologic scar in testis)
pTis	Intratubular germ cell neoplasia (carcinoma in situ)
pT1	Tumor is limited to testis and epididymis without vascular/lymphatic invasion. Tumor may invade into tunica albuginea but not tunica vaginalis.
pT2	Tumor is limited to testis and epididymis with vascular/lymphatic invasion, or tumor extends through tunica albuginea with involvement of tunica vaginalis.
pT3	Tumor invades spermatic cord with or without vascular/lymphatic invasion.
pT4	Tumor invades scrotum with or without vascular/lymphatic invasion.

Regional Lymph Nodes (N)

Clinical

NX	Regional lymph nodes cannot be assessed.
N0	No regional lymph node metastasis
N1	Metastasis with a lymph node mass 2 cm or less in greatest dimension; or multiple lymph nodes, none more than 2 cm in greatest dimension
N2	Metastasis with a lymph node mass more than 2 cm but not more than 5 cm in greatest dimension; or multiple lymph nodes, any one mass greater than 2 cm but none more than 5 cm in greatest dimension
N3	Metastasis with a lymph node mass more than 5 cm in greatest dimension

Pathologic Lymph Nodes (pN)

pNX	Regional lymph nodes cannot be assessed.
pN0	No regional lymph node metastasis
pN1	Metastasis with a lymph node mass 2 cm or less in greatest dimension and 5 or fewer positive nodes, none more than 2 cm in greatest dimension
pN2	Metastasis with a lymph node mass, more than 2 cm but not more than 5 cm in greatest dimension; or more than 5 nodes positive, none more than 5 cm; or evidence of extranodal extension of tumor
pN3	Metastasis with a lymph node mass more than 5 cm in greatest dimension

Distant Metastasis (M)

MX	Distant metastasis cannot be assessed.	
M0	No distant metastasis	
M1	Distant metastasis	
	M1a	Nonregional nodal or pulmonary metastasis
	M1b	Nonpulmonary visceral metastasis

(continued)

a crude relapse rate of 15% to 19%. The predominant site of relapse in all studies is in the para-aortic lymph nodes (82% to 89%). The median time to relapse ranged from 12 to 18 months, but late relapses (>4 years) have been reported. Adverse prognostic factors for relapse include large primary tumor size, the presence of lymphatic and/or vascular invasion, and younger age. At relapse, most patients are treated with

TABLE 29.7. (*continued*)

Serum Tumor Markers (S)

SX	Marker studies not available or not performed	
S0	Marker study levels within normal limits	
S1	LDH	< 1.5× N AND
	hCG (mIU/ml)	< 5000 AND
	AFP (ng/ml)	< 1000
S2	LDH	1.5–10 × N OR
	hCG (mIU/ml)	5000–50,000 OR
	AFP (ng/ml)	1000–10,000
S3	LDH	> 10× N OR
	hCG (mIU/ml)	> 50,000 OR
	AFP (ng/ml)	> 10,000

N indicates the upper limit of normal for the LDH assay

Stage Grouping

Stage 0	pTis	N0	M0	S0, SX
Stage I	pT1-4	N0	M0	SX
Stage IA	pT1	N0	M0	S0
Stage IB	pT2	N0	M0	S0
	pT3	N0	M0	S0
	pT4	N0	M0	S0
Stage IS	Any T	N0	M0	S1-3
Stage II	Any T	N1-3	M0	SX
Stage IIA	Any T	N1	M0	S0
	Any T	N1	M0	S1
Stage IIB	Any T	N2	M0	S0
	Any T	N2	M0	S1
Stage IIC	Any T	N3	M0	S0
	Any T	N3	M0	S1
Stage III	Any T	Any N	M1	SX
Stage IIIA	Any T	Any N	M1, M1a	S0
	Any T	Any N	M1, M1a	S1
Stage IIIB	Any T	N1-3	M0	S2
	Any T	Any N	M1a	S2
Stage IIIC	Any T	N1-3	M0	S3
	Any T	Any N	M1a	S3
	Any T	Any N	M1b	Any S

retroperitoneal RT. Chemotherapy is very effective in advanced seminoma and is an alternative to RT or surveillance in stage I seminoma. The use of one to two courses of carboplatin as adjuvant therapy after orchidectomy has been reported by Oliver et al. and Dieckman et al., with only two relapses reported in almost 200 patients treated. A single adjuvant carboplatin injection is an attractive treatment option for patients at moderate to high risk of relapse on surveillance protocols. However, before this approach can be generally adopted, further study is necessary. The MRC

UK group is presently conducting a phase III study comparing adjuvant carboplatin to retroperitoneal RT in stage I seminoma.

In summary, almost 100% of patients with stage I testicular seminoma are cured regardless of the choice of treatment. Adjuvant RT remains the most common treatment approach. One of the most attractive features of surveillance is the ability to limit treatment to orchidectomy alone. Although isolated occurrences of second nontesticular tumors following RT have been reported for decades, there are now convincing data indicating an increased risk of second malignancy. The largest study of second cancers showed excess of second cancers over the expected number (O/E = 1.43).

Stage II and III Seminoma   The most common presentation is with stage IIA disease. Treatment with retroperitoneal RT carries only a 10% risk of relapse. Chemotherapy is also curative, but is associated with increased short- and long-term toxicity. Patients with stage IIC, disease are at high risk of occult distant disease and should be treated with etoposide and cisplatin chemotherapy. The overall disease-specific survival of patients with stage II seminoma should approach 100%. Following treatment of stage II seminoma, especially stage IIC, patients may have a residual retroperitoneal mass after treatment and its management is controversial. In the Memorial Hospital experience, patients with residual mass less than 3 cm in diameter rarely had residual tumor (3%), whereas 27% of those with a mass >3 cm had viable tumor. Given this high proportion of persistent malignancy, resection or biopsy of masses of 3 cm or larger has been recommended. However, if residual retroperitoneal mass continues to decrease in size after treatment, observation is recommended. Periodic CT examinations are mandatory and treatment is indicated for residual masses that increase in size on follow-up. Stage III seminoma is uncommon (<5%), and has been shown to be exceptionally chemosensitive. In the International Germ Cell Cancers Collaborative Group study, two prognostic groups were identified in seminoma: a good prognosis group without nonpulmonary visceral metastases (NPVM) and a 5-year survival of 86%, and an intermediate prognosis group with NPVM and a 5-year survival of 72%. The Memorial Hospital results in 140 patients with advanced stage seminoma showed 93% complete response rate to chemotherapy and 88% 5-year survival. The current standard chemotherapy regimen is four courses of etoposide and cisplatin.

Nonseminomatous Germ Cell Tumors

Before the availability of cisplatin-based chemotherapy regimens, NSCGCTs were associated with very poor survival and rarely were cured. With current chemotherapy regimens, complete responses to treatment were frequent and cures were apparent in patients with metastatic disease.

Stage I NSGCT   Since the 1970s, RT has been recognized as ineffective in stage I NSGCT. Current treatment strategies for these patients include either a modified bilateral retroperitoneal lymph node dissection (RPLD) or surveillance. The clinical factors associated with a high risk of occult distant disease include the presence of vascular invasion, embryonal carcinoma, and the size of the primary tumor. In the Medical Research Council UK study of 259 patients managed by orchidectomy, four factors (presence of embryonal carcinoma, absence of yolk sac elements, invasion of blood vessels or lymphatics) were identified on multivariate analysis as predictive of relapse. Published studies of surveillance have shown a 30% risk of disease progression with up to 95% of patients progressing within 12 months of diagnosis; progression more than 24 months from diagnosis is extremely rare. Approximately 60% of patients progress in the retroperitoneal lymph nodes, with or without other evidence of disease. The other common sites of progression are lung metastases or tumor marker elevation alone. The critical factors for successful surveillance include regular imaging of the retroperitoneal nodes and patient compliance. At the time of progression patients are usually treated with chemotherapy, although RPLD is used in selected cases with small retroperitoneal lymph nodes. Most patients are cured at relapse and the cause-specific survival in most series is greater than 95%. RPLD is a recognized alternative to surveillance in clinical stage I disease. Surgical techniques have undergone considerable modification in the last 20 years. A modified unilateral infrahilar RPLD is now performed, with nerve-sparing techniques to preserve ejaculation. The relapse rate following surgery is approximately 10% for patients with clinical pathologic stage I disease. As with relapses on surveillance, most patients who relapse after RPLD are cured with subsequent chemotherapy. In some centers patients with stage I NSGCT at high risk of relapse on surveillance are offered adjuvant chemotherapy. Because the outcomes of surgery, surveillance, and adjuvant chemotherapy are similar, some patients and physicians favor immediate treatment over a wait-and-see approach.

Stage II NSGCT   Treatment options include RPLD, chemotherapy, or a combination of both. Patients with retroperitoneal disease nodes greater than 5 cm in diameter have a high relapse rate following RPLD and are usually approached with chemotherapy. The outcome is excellent. In North America patients with solitary nodal mass less than 3 cm in size are treated with RPLD. Patients with retroperitoneal disease between 3 and 5 cm in size may be treated with initial surgery or primary chemotherapy. Published data suggest that 8% to 44% of patients will relapse following RPLD if lymph nodes less than 6 cm are involved, with no node greater than 2 cm in diameter. For this group of patients close monitoring, with chemotherapy reserved for relapse, is the recommended approach for compliant patients. Almost all patients who relapse can be salvaged with chemotherapy. For patients with more than six nodes involved, or with any node greater than 2 cm in diameter, adjuvant chemotherapy should be considered. A number of trials using two to four cycles of chemotherapy have been reported. Williams et al. reported the results of a randomized trial of 195 patients with N1–3 disease who received two cycles of PVB chemotherapy, or observation with standard treatment at relapse. Equivalent survival was shown in this study with observation and two cycles of adjuvant chemotherapy.

Stage III NSGCT   Although the cure of many patients with metastatic NSGCT is one of the most remarkable advances in cancer therapy in the last 20 years, difficulty arose in comparing published results because of a lack of agreement on prognostic factors predictive for a favorable or unfavorable outcome. Different prognostic groupings made comparison of trial results impossible. Stage migration and other similar factors could have accounted for observed differences, rather than different treatment protocols. To promote greater uniformity in assigning patients to risk groups and interpreting results from different treatment centers, the IGCCCG analyzed data from 5168 patients with NSGCTs. Independent prognostic variables included tumor markers AFP, β-hCG, LDH, and the presence or absence of NPVM, for example, liver, gastrointestinal tract. Based on these, the IGCCCG recommended three prognostic groups. The 5-year survival for the good prognosis group was 92%; for the intermediate group, 80%; and for the poor prognosis group, 48%. For seminoma, only two prognostic groups were identified: a good prognosis group without NPVM with a 5-year survival of 86%, and an intermediate prognosis group with NPVM with a 5-year survival of 72%. At present, patients with low-risk disease are routinely treated with four cycles of BEP (bleomycin, etoposide, cisplatin). Patients with high-risk disease have durable complete response (CR) rates of 28% to 63% with four courses of BEP, or with a similar cisplatin-based regimen. About 25% to 30% of patients who present with high-risk disease will fail to achieve CR or relapse from CR following chemotherapy. For these patients further attempts at curative therapy include ifosfamide-based regimens and high-dose chemotherapy with autologous bone marrow transplantation. At present the latter approach is considered experimental. Durable complete responses are seen in up to 25% of patients with recurrent disease receiving combinations of ifosfamide and cisplatin. Patients with bulky retroperitoneal disease commonly have residual disease on CT scan after chemotherapy. Less frequently residual mediastinal or pulmonary metastases may be seen. It is recommended that residual disease be resected. Approximately 85% to 90% of patients will have necrosis or teratoma, and 10% of patients will have active cancer. In the latter group, two additional cycles of a platinum-based chemotherapy are recommended.

Salvage Therapy

Approximately 30% of patients with high-risk GCT relapse or fail to achieve a CR with first-line chemotherapy regimens. Complete responses can be achieved with second- and third-line regimens in 25% to 35% of cases and 15% to 25% of patients treated in this way can be cured. Many of the currently used second-line salvage regimens include ifosfamide, often combined with cisplatin and etoposide or vinblastine. High-dose intensive therapy with peripheral blood stem cell support is being investigated and preliminary reports indicate that up to 20% of heavily pretreated patients can achieve a durable complete response.

CNS Metastases

Approximately 2% to 3% of patients with stage III GCT will present with brain metastases and up to 40% of patients who die of progressive disease will have brain metastases at autopsy. Approximately 25% of patients presenting with brain metastases, or who develop metastases after a favorable response to chemotherapy, can achieve long-term disease control. Whole brain irradiation may be administered along with systemic chemotherapy. Patients who develop brain metastases during systemic chemotherapy have a very poor prognosis and should likely receive palliative RT only.

Toxicity

Testicular germinal epithelium is exquisitely sensitive to ionizing radiation. Although the contralateral testis is not located directly in the radiation field, scatter dose can be significant and may cause profound depression of spermatogenesis and compromise future fertility. A radiation dose between 20 and 50 cGy may produce temporary aspermia, and doses greater than 50 cGy may preclude recovery of spermatogenesis. The use of scrotal shielding reduces the scattered radiation dose to the testis, but cannot ensure protection of spermatogenesis in all patients. In men who recover spermatogenesis after RT for seminoma, there is no evidence of an increased incidence of genetic abnormalities among offspring. Limiting RT target volume to the para-aortic and common iliac area eliminates the concerns regarding RT-induced fertility.

Nausea and vomiting occur with chemotherapy, but are controlled effectively in most patients with 5-hydroxytryptamine$_3$ (5-HT$_3$) antagonists and steroids. Myelosuppression is frequent and febrile neutropenia is seen in about 10% to 15% of patients receiving etoposide and cisplatin, and such patients benefit from hematopoietic growth factors. Nephrotoxicity occurs with the use of cisplatin and ifosfamide. Raynaud phenomenon has been reported in 23% to 49% of patients. Chronic peripheral neuropathy is well recognized after treatment with cisplatin, vinblastine, and etoposide. Pulmonary toxicity is seen with the use of bleomycin and is dose related. Impaired fertility, which may precede the use of chemotherapy, may also continue after its use. Although chemotherapy also produces infertility, in the majority of patients, recovery of sperm counts has been observed.

Follow-Up

Follow-up is an integral part of the management of testis tumors. The patterns of failure are well defined, and follow-up investigations are focused on early detection of relapse, or treatment complications. Late relapse is rare, and its detection depends more on patient education than on close long-term follow-up in specialized centers.

CANCER OF THE PENIS

Penile cancer accounts for only 0.4% to 0.6% of all malignancies in males in North America, but it constitutes up to 10% of male cancers in some African and South American countries. The incidence of penile cancer varies greatly with hygiene standards and cultural and religious practices. Cancer of the penis is extremely rare in those with neonatal circumcision. In contrast, adult circumcision offers little or no protection from subsequent development of the disease. Penile tumors usually present with a visible lesion most commonly on the glans (50%) and prepuce (20%). At presentation, the majority of lesions are confined to the penis. Histology is usually a well-differentiated squamous cell carcinoma. The most common route of spread is local invasion and spread to the inguinal lymph nodes. The UICC TNM classification is used to describe anatomic disease extent (Table 29.8). Stage is the strongest prognostic factor.

TABLE 29.8. TNM Classification of Penis Tumors (1997 5th Edition)

Primary Tumor (T)

TX	Primary tumor cannot be assessed.
T0	No evidence of primary tumor
Tis	Carcinoma in situ
Ta	Noninvasive verrucous carcinoma
T1	Tumor invades subepithelial connective tissue.
T2	Tumor invades corpus spongiosum or cavernosum.
T3	Tumor invades urethra or prostate.
T4	Tumor invades other adjacent structures.

Regional Lymph Nodes (N)

NX	Regional lymph nodes cannot be assessed.
N0	No regional lymph node metastasis
N1	Metastasis in a single, superficial inguinal lymph node
N2	Metastasis in multiple or bilateral superficial inguinal lymph nodes
N3	Metastasis in deep inguinal or pelvic lymph nodes), unilateral or bilateral

Distant Metastasis

MX	Distant metastatis cannot be assessed.
M0	No distant metastasis
M1	Distant metastasis

Stage Grouping

0	Tis	N0	M0
	Ta	N0	M0
I	T1	N0	M0
II	T1	N1	M0
	T2	N0	M0
	T2	N1	M0
III	T1	N2	M0
	T2	N2	M0
	T3	N0	M0
	T3	N1	M0
	T3	N2	M0
IV	T4	Any N	M0
	Any T	N3	M0
	Any T	Any N	M1

   CIS of the penis is referred to by urologists and dermatologists as erythroplasia of Queyrat if it involves the glans penis, prepuce, or penile shaft and as Bowen's disease if it involves the remainder of the genitalia or perineal region. CIS of the penis may be treated similarly to skin cancers with topical 5-fluorouracil, laser, or liquid nitrogen with excellent control and cosmetic outcome. For early lesions conservative treatment with Moh's micrographic surgery (MMS) has been used. MMS is a method of removing skin cancer by excising tissue in thin layers and includes color coding of excised specimens with tissue dyes and microscopic examination of excised layers with frozen section techniques until all malignant tissues have been removed. Mohs reported excellent cure rates for tumors less than 1 cm in diameter using this technique.

   The standard treatment involves total or partial penectomy, although in patients with early tumors RT using brachytherapy with iridium implants is very successful in early stage lesions (80% to 90% local control) and offers the opportunity for organ preservation. Prophylactic or therapeutic inguinal lymph node dissection has been recommended for patients with T1 grade 2–3 tumors and T2–3 tumors. Chemotherapy has not been particularly useful in the management of this disease, and has been used only for palliation. The active agents include bleomycin, methotrexate, and cisplatin.

Organ Preservation

The standard treatment involves total or partial penectomy, although in patients with early tumors RT using brachytherapy with iridium implants is very successful in early stage lesions (80% to 90% local control) and offers the opportunity for organ preservation.

FURTHER READING

Kidney Cancer

Bukowski RM (1997) Natural history and therapy of metastatic renal cell carcinoma: The role of interleukin-2. *Cancer* 80:1198–1220.

deKernion JB, Huland H (1990) The operable renal cell carcinoma: Summary and conclusions. *Eur Urol* 2:48–51.

Elson PJ, Witte RS, Trump DL (1988) Prognostic factors for survival in patients with recurrent or metastatic renal cell carcinoma. *Cancer Res* 48:7310–7313.

Fyfe G, Fisher RI, Rosenberg SA, et al. (1995) Results of treatment of 255 patients with metastatic renal cell carcinoma who received high-dose recombinant interleukin-2 therapy. *J Clin Oncol* 13:688–696.

Montie J, El Ammar RR, Pontes J, et al. (1991) Renal cell carcinoma with inferior vena cava tumor thrombi. *Surg Gynecol Obstet* 173:107–115.

Motzer RJ, Russo P, Nanus DM, Berg WJ (1997) Renal cell carcinoma. *Curr Prob Cancer* 21:185–232.

Ritchie A, deKernion J (1987) The natural history and clinical features of renal cell carcinoma. *Semin Nephrol* 7:131–139.

Schmid HP, Szabo J (1997) Renal cell carcinoma—a current review. *Schweiz Rundsch Med Prax* 86:837–843.

Sobin LH, Wittekind Ch (1997) International Union Against Cancer (UICC). *TNM Classification of Malignant Tumors* 5th Edition. Wiley-Liss, New York, pp. 180–182.

Storkel S, Thoenes W, Jacobi GH, et al. (1990) Prognostic parameters of renal cell carcinoma. *Eur Urol* 2:36–37.

Cancer of the Urinary Bladder

Dalesio O, Schulman CC, Sylvester R, et al. (1983) Prognostic factors in superficial bladder tumors. A study of the European Organization for Research on Treatment of Cancer: Genitourinary Tract Cancer Cooperative Group. *J Urol* 129:730–733.

Evans CP, Swanson DA (1996) What to do if the lymph nodes are positive. *Semin Urol Oncol* 14:96–102.

Gospodarowicz MK, Quilty PM, Scalliet P, Tsujii H, Fossa SD, Horenblas S, Isaka S, Prout GR, Shipley WU, Wijnmaalen AJ, et al. (1995) The place of radiation therapy as definitive treatment of bladder cancer. *Int J Urol* 2:41–48.

Heney NM (1992) Natural history of superficial bladder cancer. Prognostic features and long-term disease course. *Urol Clin N Am* 19:429–433.

Herr HW, (1997) Natural history of superficial bladder tumors: 10- to 20-year follow-up of treated patients. *World J Urol* 15:84–88.

Kantoff PW (1990) Bladder cancer. *Curr Prob Cancer* 14:235–291.

Kryger JV, Messing E (1996) Bladder cancer screening. *Semin Oncol* 23:585–597

Kurth KH (1997) Diagnosis and treatment of superficial transitional cell carcinoma of the bladder: Facts and perspectives. *Eur Urol* 1:10–19.

Kurth KH, Schellhammer PF, Okajima E, Akdas A, Jakse G, Herr HW, Calais da Silva F, Fukushima S, Nagayama T (1995) Current methods of assessing and treating carcinoma in situ of the bladder with or without involvement of the prostatic urethra. *Int J Urol* 2:8–22.

Lamm DL (1995) BCG in Perspective: Advances in the treatment of superficial bladder cancer. *Eur Urol* 1:2–8.

Lamm DL, Riggs DR, Shriver JS, vanGilder PF, Rach JF, DeHaven JI (1994) Megadose vitamins in bladder cancer: A double blind clinical trial, *J Urol* 151:21–26.

Loehrer PS, Einhorn LH, Elson PJ, et al. (1992) A randomized comparison of cisplatin alone or in combination with methotrexate, vinblastine, and doxorubicin in patients with metastatic urothelial carcinoma: A Cooperative Group Study. *J Clin Oncol* 10:1066–1073.

Martinez-Pineiro JA, Martinez-Pineiro L (1997) BCG update: Intravesical therapy. *Eur Urol* 1:31–41.

Paulson D, Denis L, Orikasa S, Bartolucci A, Bouffioux C, Hirao Y, Jewett MA, Pagano F, Pontes JE (1995) Optimal staging procedures, including imaging, to define prognosis of bladder cancer. *Int J Urol* 2:1–7.

Richie JP (1992) Surgery for invasive bladder cancer. *Hematol Oncol Clin NA* 6:129–145.

Roth BJ (1996) Chemotherapy for advanced bladder cancer. *Semin Oncol* 23:633–644 .

Shipley WU, Prout GR, Kaufman DS (1990) Bladder cancer. Advances in laboratory innovations and clinical management, with emphasis on innovations allowing bladder-sparing approaches for patients with invasive tumors. *Cancer* 65:675–683.

Stadler WM, Kuzel TM, Raghavan D, Levine E, Vogelzang NJ, Roth B, Dorr FA (1997) Metastatic bladder cancer: Advances in treatment. *Eur J Cancer* 33:S23–26.

Sternberg CN (1996) Neoadjuvant and adjuvant chemotherapy in locally advanced bladder cancer. *Semin Oncol* 23:621–632.

Warde P, Gospodarowicz MK (1997) New approaches in the use of radiation therapy in the treatment of infiltrative transitional-cell cancer of the bladder. *World J Urol* 15:125–133.

Cancer of the Renal Pelvis and Ureter

Cozad S, Smalley S, Austenfeld M, Noble M, Jennings S, Reymond R. (1995) Transitional cell carcinima of the renal pelvis or ureter: Patterns of failure. *Urology* 46:796–800.

Das A, Carson C, Bolick D, Paulson D (1990) Primary carcinoma of the upper urinary tract. Effect of primary and secondary therapy on survival. *Cancer* 66:1919–1923.

Krogh J, Kvist E, Rye B (1991) Transitional cell carcinoma of the upper urinary tract: Prognostic variables and post-operative recurrences. *Br J Urol* 67:32–36.

Nielson K, Ostri P (1988) Primary tumors of the renal pelvis: Evaluation of clinical and pathological features in a consecutive series of 10 years. *J Urol* 140:19– 21.

Raabe N, Fossa S Bjerkhagen SB (1992) Carcinoma of the renal pelvis. Experience of 80 cases. *Scandin J Urol Nephrol* 26:357–361.

Seaman E, Slawin K, Benson M (1993) Treatment options for upper tract transitional-cell carcinoma. *Urol Clin NA* 20:349–354.

Cancer of the Urethra

Amin MB, Young RH (1997) Primary carcinomas of the urethra. *Semin Diagn Pathol* 14:147–160.

Dinney CP, Johnson DE, Swanson DA, Babaian RJ, von Eschenbach AC (1994) Therapy and prognosis for male anterior urethral carcinoma: An update. *Urology* 43:506–514.

Grigsby PW, Corn BW (1992) Localized urethral tumors in women: Indications for conservative versus exenterative therapies. *J Urol* 147:1516–1520.

Linn R, Moskovitz B, Munichor M, Levin DR (1990) Transitional Cell carcinoma of the distal female urethra. *Int Urol Nephrol* 22:275–277.

Micaily B, Dzeda MF, Miyamoto CT, Brady LW (1997) Brachytherapy for cancer of the female urethra. *Semin Surg Oncol* 13:208–214.

Ray B, Canto AR, Whitmore WF (1977) Experience with primary carcinoma of the male urethra. *J Urol* 117:591–594.

Sailer SL, Shipley WU, Wang CC (1988) Carcinoma of the female urethra: A review of results with radiation therapy. *J Urol* 140:1–5.

Zeidman EJ, Desmond P, Thompson IM, (1992) Surgical treatment of carcinoma of the male urethra. *Urol Clin NA* 19:359–372.

Cancer of the Testis

Bosl GJ, Motzer RJ (1997) Testicular germ-cell cancer. *N Engl J Med* 337:242–253.

Boyer M, Raghavan D (1992) Toxicity of treatment of germ cell tumors. *Semin Oncol* 19:128–142.

Cullen M, James N (1996) Adjuvant therapy for stage I testicular cancer. *Cancer Treat Rev* 22:253–264.

Dieckmann KP Krain J, Kuster J, et al. (1996) Adjuvant carboplatin treatment for seminoma clinical stage I. *J Cancer Res Clin Oncol* 122:63–66.

Doherty AP, Bower M, Christmas TJ, (1997) The role of tumor markers in the diagnosis and treatment of testicular germ cell cancers. *Br J Urol* 79:247–252.

Giwercman A, von der Maase H, Rorth M, Skakkebaek NE (1994) Current concepts of radiation treatment of carcinoma in situ of the testis. *World J Urol* 12:125–130.

Herr HW, Sheinfeld J, Puc HS, Heelan R, Bajorin DF, Mencel P, Bosl GJ, Motzer RJ (1997) Surgery for a post-chemotherapy residual mass in seminoma. *J Urol* 157:860–862.

Horwich A, Dearnaley DP (1992) Treatment of seminoma. *Semin Oncol* 19:171–180.

Jewett MA, Incze P (1996) Retroperitoneal lymphadenectomy: The traditional treatment option. *Semin Urol Oncol* 14:24–29.

International Germ Cell Cancer Collaborative Group (1997) International Germ Cell Consensus Classification: A prognostic factor-based staging system for metastatic germ cell cancers. *J Clin Oncol* 15:594–603.

Mencel PJ, Motzer RJ Mazumdar M et al. (1994) Advanced seminoma: Treatment results, survival, and prognostic factors in 142 patients. *J Clin Oncol* 12:120–126.

Motzer RJ (1996) Adjuvant chemotherapy for stage II nonseminamatous testicular cancer: What is its role? *Semin Urol Oncol* 14:30–33.

Sturgeon JF, Jewett MA, Alison RE, et al. (1992) Surveillance after orchidectomy for patients with clinical stage I nonseminamatous testis tumors. *J Clin Oncol* 10:564–568.

Travis L, Curtis R, Storm H, et al. (1997) Risk of Second malignant neoplasms among long-term survivors of testicular cancer. *J Natl Cancer Inst* 89:1429–1439.

Warde P, Gospodarowicz MK, Panzarella T, et al. (1995) Stage I testicular seminoma: Results of adjuvant irradiation and surveillance. *J Clin Oncol* 13:2255–2262.

Cancer of the Penis

Burgers JK, Badalament RA, Drago JR (1992) Penile cancer. Clinical Presentation, diagnosis, and staging. *Urol Clin NA* 19:247–255.

Delannes MN, Malavaud B, Douchez J, Bonnet J, Daly N (1992) Iridium 192 interstitial therapy for squamous cell carcinoma of the penis. *Int J Radiat Oncol Biol Phys* 21:178.

Gerbaulet A, Lambin P (1992) Radiation therapy of cancer of the penis: Indications, advantages, and pitfalls. *Urol Clin NA* 19:325–332.

McDougal WS, Kirchner FK Jr, Edwards RH, Killion LT (1988) Treatment of carcinoma of the penis: The case of primary lymphadenectomy. *J Urol* 136:38–41.

Mohs F, Snow SN, Larson PO (1992) Mohs micrographic surgery for penile tumors. *Urol Clin NA* 19:291–304.

Pizzocaro G, Piva L, Bandieramonte G, Tana S (1997) Up-to-date management of carcinoma of the penis. *Eur Urol* 32:5–15.

Sarin R, Norman AR, Steel GG, Horwich A (1997) Treatment results and prognostic factors in 101 men treated for squamous carcinoma of the penis. *Int J Radiat Oncol Biol Phys* 38:713–722.

Wiener JS, Walther PJ (1995) The association of oncogenic human papillomaviruses with urologic malignancy. The controversies and clinical implications. *Surg Oncol Clin NA* 4:257–276.

CHAPTER 30

TUMORS OF THE CENTRAL NERVOUS SYSTEM

CHARLES J. VECHT

Department of Neuro-Oncology
Daniel den Hoed Cancer Center
University Hospital
Rotterdam, The Netherlands

Primary brain tumors account for about 2% of cancer deaths . In children, they are the second most common type of cancer. Brain metastasis develops in more than 20% of all cancer patients.

Primary brain tumors are diverse and can be distinguished in a spectrum of about 50 different types, characterized by a wide variety of phenotypic and a diversity of genotypic abnormalities. Hereditary factors may play a role and about 15% of patients with brain tumors have a family history of cancer. Grossly, primary brain tumor can be divided into neuroepithelial tumors, tumors of the meninges, tumors arising from lymphatic cells, germ cell tumors, and cystlike tumors (see Table 30.1).

Genetic defects in brain tumors can consist of overexpression in oncogenes or deletion of tumor suppressor genes. Frequently, loss of heterozygosity in hereditary and nonhereditary tumors results in inactivation of tumor suppressor genes that normally counteract the function of proto-oncogenes. In gliomas, genetic loss frequently occurs on chromosomes 1p, 9p, 10q, 17p, 19q, and 22q.

As well as overexpression of *EGFR*, *PDGFR*, and *MDM-2*, *p53* mutations and *p16* deletions are all associated with malignant transformation in gliomas. Classic factors such as environmental changes, viral infections, or hormonal influences all contribute to the induction of central nervous system (CNS) tumors.

Manual of Clinical Oncology, 7th edition, Edited by Raphael E. Pollock
ISBN 0-471-23828-7, pages 607–619. Copyright © 1999 Wiley-Liss, Inc.

TABLE 30.1. Primary Brain Tumors

Tumors of Neuroepithelial Tissue	*Mesenchymal Nonmeningothelial Tumors*
A. Astrocytoma Anaplastic astrocytoma Glioblastoma Pilocytic astrocytoma	BENIGN Osteocartilagous tumors, lipomas
B. Oligodendroglioma Anaplastic oligodendroglioma	MALIGNANT Chondrosarcoma, rhanbdomyosarcoma,
C. Ependymoma Anaplastic ependymoma	hemangiopericytoma
D. Mixed oligoastrocytoma	
E. Choroid plexus tumor Neurononal and mixed Neuronoglial tumor Pineal tumors Pineocytoma Pineoblastoma	

Embryonal Tumors	*Primary CNS Lymphomas*
A. Medulloblastoma	GERM CELL TUMORS
B. Neuroblastoma	A. Germinoma
C. Ependymoblastoma	B. Embryonal carcinoma
D. Primitive	C. Endodermal sinus tumor
E. Neuroectodermal tumor (PNET)	D. Horiocarcinoma
	E. Teratoma
	F. Mixed germ cell tumor

Tumors of Cranial and Spinal Nerves	*Cysts and Tumorlike Lesions*
A. Schwannoma	A. Epidermoid cyst
B. Neurofibroma	B. Dermoid cyst
C. Malignant schwannoma	C. Colloid cyst of third ventricle
	D. Crainiopharyngioma

Tumors of the Meninges	*Pituitary Tumors*
A. Meningioma	
B. Anaplastic meningioma	

SIGNS AND SYMPTOMS

One feature of brain tumors is that neurologic symptoms develop gradually over time, in contrast to vascular (ischemic or hemorrhagic) lesions of the brain, which arise acutely. Nevertheless, more than 25% of patients with brain tumors present spontaneously, often in the form of seizures. For that reason, the appearance of one or more seizures in an adult patient requires a computerized tomography (CT) or preferably magnetic resonance imaging (MRI) scan. Acute presentation is also possible due to hemorrhage into the tumor.

The nature of signs and symptoms of brain tumors can usually be explained by both the localization of the tumor within the brain and the presence of increased intracranial pressure. The actual location of a brain tumor defines the focal neurologic signs caused by the tumor. A good working knowledge of neuroanatomy enables one to better understand and localize the appearance of neurologic signs and symptoms within the CNS. Frontal tumors lead to changes in personality, for example, loss of drive, poor social adaptation, indifference or loss of self-criticism, apathy, and occasionally outbursts of aggression. Temporal tumors lead to hemianopia and to aphasia if the left hemisphere is dominant. Parietal tumors lead to contralateral motor and sensory abnormalities and to apraxia. Occipital tumors lead to hemianopias and, if the tumor extends into the splenium, to visual agnosia.

In general, right-sided tumors, that is, in the nondominant hemisphere, take more time to become symptomatic and may present with apraxia or visuoconstructive agnosias. Cerebellar tumors may give rise to ataxia, dysarthria, and early signs of increased intracranial pressure by obstructive hydrocep and direct compression of the brainstem. Focal brainstem signs may exist with cranial nerve signs including Bell's palsy (peripheral seventh nerve dysfunction), bilateral pyramidal weakness of the extremities, and sensory abnormalities.

Increased intracranial pressure is caused by a space-occupying lesion within the rigid boundaries of the skull. The presence of a tumor in one cerebral hemisphere can lead to a horizontal shift of midline structures that can easily be seen on CT or MRI. Also, particularly with intraventricular or tumors in the brainstem or cerebellum, hydrocephalus by obstruction of cerebrospinal fluid (CSF) flow with signs of increased intracranial pressure may develop.

The space-occupying properties of the tumor will, if left untreated, lead to direct compression of the brainstem. This may also cause so-called false-localizing signs as in the form of a third or sixth cranial nerve palsy. The closed boundaries of the skull are responsible for a gradual increase in the volume of the tumor, and an exponential or disproportional increase in intracranial pressure may ensue. In physical terms, this phenomenon can be characterized by a shift to the right of the pressure–volume curve.

Increased intracranial pressure with or without disturbance of CSF flow or direct compression of the brainstem may lead to herniation of the brainstem. The clinical signs of increased intracranial pressure consist of headache, nausea, and vomiting. Impaired consciousness starts as drowsiness, followed by stupor and coma. Herniation of the brainstem is evident by ptosis and an ipsilateral enlargement of the pupil (third palsy), flexor spasms of the arms with extension spasms of the legs, and Cheyne–Stokes respiration. This may evolve into fixed pupils, extension spasms of the arms and legs, and hyperventilation (mid-brainstem or mesencephalic signs), followed by absent corneal and pupillary reflexes, pinpoint pupils, flaccid tetraparesis, hypoventilation (lower brainstem or pontine signs), and death.

IMAGING

Great progress has been achieved in imaging of the brain over the last 15 years. CT scanning of the brain can reliably delineate the contours of brain tumors located in the cerebral hemispheres. Use of iodinated contrast agents indicates the presence of blood–brain barrier disturbances. As a rule, MRI scanning is more sensitive than CT, particularly following contrast administration, and is required for accurate delineation of lesions of the posterior fossa, the leptomeninges, and the spinal cord. In fact, the use of CT and MRI has become indispensable in the diagnosis and reliable follow-up of brain tumors. It is likely that MRI will completely replace CT for the imaging of brain tumors. MRI spectroscopy may be used for differentiating tumor tissue from areas of radionecrosis. Positron emission tomography (PET) scanning can also be used for this goal.

GLIOMAS

The glioma group consist of astrocytomas, oligodendrogliomas, and ependymomas that together represent about 60% of all primary brain tumors with an incidence of ~5 per 100,000. The astrocytomas can be graded according to their degree of malignancy. The most commonly used grading systems are those of the WHO and of St. Anne–Mayo. Both systems use the presence of histologic criteria such as nuclear atypia, mitosis, endothelial cell proliferation, and necrosis as markers of malignancy. The WHO grading system divides the astrocytomas into grade 1 (pilocytic astrocytoma), grade 2 (astrocytoma, low-grade diffuse), grade 3 (anaplastic astrocytoma), and grade 4 (glioblastoma multiforme). The Daumas–Duport classification depends on the number of dedifferentiation features: with one histologic criterion an astrocytoma grade 2 is diagnosed, with two criteria as grade 3, and with three or four criteria as grade 4 astrocytoma (Table 30.2). In general, there is a good correspondence between both systems in the prognosis for grade 2, 3, and 4 astrocytomas. Of these, grade 4 tumors or glioblastomas are the most frequent type of primary brain tumors, constituting more than half of all gliomas.

TABLE 30.2. Astrocytoma Grading Systems

WHO Grade	WHO Designation	St. Anne-Mayo Designation	St. Anne-Mayo Histological Criteria
I	Pilocytic astrocytoma		
II	Astrocytoma	Astrocytoma	
	Low-grade diffuse	Grade 1	0 Criterion
		Grade 2	1 Criterion
III	Anaplastic astrocytoma	Astrocytoma	2 Criteria
		Grade 3	
IV	Glioblastoma multiforme	Astrocytoma	
		Grade 4	

Low Grade Gliomas

The astrocytomas or low-grade gliomas can be divided into pilocytic and nonpilocytic astrocytomas. The pilocytic or juvenile astrocytoma is a benign tumor and represents more than half of all low-grade gliomas in childhood. Histologically, pilocytic astrocytomas are characterized by Rosenthal fibers and thin elongated astrocytes (pilocytes). Diagnosis is based on CT or MRI showing an intensely enhancing mass with or without cyst formation or space-occupying features.

They are often located in the infratentorial compartment usually the cerebellum. Presenting signs and symptoms are those of increased intracranial pressure (headache, nausea and vomiting, impaired consciousness with or without third or sixth nerve palsy as a false localizing sign), secondary to obstructive hydrocephalus caused by compression fo the sylvian duct. A unilateral cerebellar syndrome may be concomitantly present, indicating the localization of the tumor. Supratentorially located pilocytic astrocytomas become manifest in the majority of cases by epileptic seizures and in the remainder by neurologic signs depending on the localization of the tumor. The preferred treatment is surgery alone and, when gross tumor resection can be achieved, the 10-year survival is 80% or more.

Nonpilocytic low-grade gliomas consist of diffuse, protoplasmic, and fibrillary astrocytomas. They may occur anywhere in the brain, but characteristic localizations include the supratentorial compartment including optic pathways, the cerebellum, and brainstem. About 60% of supratentorial tumors become manifest by epileptic seizures. The characteristic pattern on CT or MRI is a nonenhancing lesion that can be space-occupying and often shows an infiltrating and irregular pattern in the white matter. If the neuropathologist confirms a nonpilocytic low-grade glioma, the next question is whether these patients should have radiotherapy or not. One trial did not show a superior effect of 59 Gy radiation therapy over 45 Gy. Another trial has shown a longer progression-free period following surgery and radiotherapy in a dose of 54 Gy but without a longer overall survival as compared to surgery alone. The effect of age has not been studied in these trials. Retrospective studies have indicated that radiotherapy seems mainly effective inpatients 35 to 40 years and older. The overall median 5-year survival is 4 to 5 years. If patients have epilepsy only and are otherwise neurologically intact, the choice consists of either a wait-and-see policy or straightforward surgery. Younger patients, in particular <35 years of age, carry a much better prognosis, and these patients may be followed by CT or MRI as long as they have no symptoms or imminent signs. For symptoms other than epilepsy, surgery is the treatment of choice and depending on the localizaton, a gross tumor resection is the preferred therapy.

High-Grade Gliomas

Anaplastic astrocytoma and glioblastoma multiforme (GBM) constitute together the high-grade or malignant gliomas of which GBM represent 80%. Following standard treatment, the median survival with anaplastic astrocytoma is 18 months and with GBM 9 to 11 months. At 5 years, the survival rate with anaplastic astrocytoma is 10% to 35%, while the equivalent figure for GBM is 5% or less.

Prognostic Factors

The prognosis of high-grade glioma depends not only on the histologic diagnosis and grade of the tumor, but also on a number of other independent prognostic facts, including age and the performance status at the time of treatment. The presence of favorable or unfavorable prognostic factors determines the outcome of patients with malignant gliomas to a large extent. These consist of age (younger versus older than 50 years), performance status (Karnofsky over or under 70), histology (anaplastic astrocytoma versus GBM), and extent of surgery (extensive surgery versus limited surgery or biopsy).

The standard therapy for malignant gliomas is surgery followed by radiation therapy. Extensive resection of the tumor depends on the neuroanatomic localization of the tumor and when possible leads to a longer survival when compared with limited surgery or biopsy. Postoperative conventional radiation therapy in a cumulative dose of 60 Gy leads to a median survival with malignant gliomas of about 9 months. Doses over 60 Gy have not demonstrated an advantage in survival. Modifications in radiation therapy including concomitant boost, hyperfractionation, accelerated hyperfractionation, or use of radiation sensitizers have all not resulted in better outcome.

It is presently uncertain whether application of stereotactic or conformal radiation therapy for malignant tumors of small volume would give better results.

Chemotherapy

A number of randomized trials have been carried out on the efficacy of adjuvant chemotherapy in malignant gliomas. Most trials have concentrated on lipophilic agents which easily pass the blood-brain barrier. The alkylating agents lomustine (CCNU) and carmustine (BCNU) have shown a significant though modest improvement in median survival of 9 months following surgery while the addition of radiation therapy to BCNU or procarbazine is associated with survival of up to 11 months.

In contrast to anaplastic astrocytoma and GBM, anaplastic oligodenrogliomas (AOs) seem highly chemosensitive. A number of phase II trials in recurrent AO have shown response rates of 60% to 70% lasting 1 year or more in most cases. These results have been established by a combination of procarbazine, vincristine, and CCNG (PCV). Both in the United States and in Europe, two independent phase III trials are now being carried out on the efficacy of adjuvant chemotherapy with PCV in AO following surgery and radiotherapy.

In recurrent tumors, following surgery and radiation therapy, reoperation of gliomas can be useful after a remission-free period of 6 months or more. Subsequently systemic chemotherapy may be offered, preferably as part of phase II trials.

PEDIATRIC NEUROONCOLOGY

Ependymomas

Ependymomas are relatively frequent in children under 3 years of age and often arise in the posterior fossa around the fourth ventricle, although they may occur at any age and at any site in the CNS. The primary mode of therapy is surgery. Limited field irradiation is usually given for well-differentiated ependymomas. For anaplastic tumors, particularly posterior fossa ependymomas, whole neuraxis irradiation is often advised. The 5- to 10-year progression-free survival rate of ependymomas is 60% and 40%, respectively. Recurrence following surgery may necessitate reoperation, particularly when neurologic signs become imminent. Occasionally, a positive response following chemotherapy has been reported.

Brainstem Tumors

Brainstem tumors account for 10% to 20% of CNS tumors in childhood. Brainstem gliomas can be separated into focal brainstem tumors, which are often amenable to resection compared to diffuse or large pontine gliomas, which are usually irresectable. The latter are associated with a median survival of less than 1 year, a 2-year survival of 10% to 20%, and constitute the majority of brainstem tumors.

Primitive Neuroectodermal Tumors (PNETs)

Medulloblastoma and other PNETs are small-cell highly cellular tumors that stain positively with S-100. If present in the posterior fossa, these tumors are designated as medulloblastomas. In the supratentorial compartment, they are in general labeled as PNETs. Ependymoblastomas and pineoblastomas are other types of the PNET group.

Medulloblastoma

Medulloblastomas originate in the cerebellum or brainstem. These tumors occur mainly in children under 15 years of age. Treatment consists of surgery followed by craniospinal axis radiation with a cumulative dose of 54 Gy to the posterior fossa and 36 Gy in 20 fractions to the remaining part of the CNS, resulting in a 5-year survival of 50% to 60%. The use of adjuvant chemotherapy (regimens employing CCNU, cisplatin, and vincristine) gives better results in high-risk patients, that is, following an incomplete resection or in children younger than 3 years of age. In the latter group radiation therapy is usually delayed until the age of 36 months to spare cognitive development and to prevent growth retardation. Treatment consists of extensive resection, if possible, followed by neuraxis radiation with a boost to the tumor bed. Adjuvant chemotherapy in medulloblastomas may be indicated in partially resected tumors or in children younger than 2 years. In children younger than 3 years of age, radiation therapy is harmful to the developing CNS and therefore surgery plus adjuvant chemotherapy is favored in this age group.

Acoustic Schwannomas

These tumors are benign schwannomas that preferentially arise form the acoustic nerve and are located in the meatus acusticus internus or externus in the cerebellopontine angle. Presenting signs include unilateral hearing loss with or without signs of vestibular dysfunction. The treatment of choice is surgical excision, although radiosurgical treatment with focused high-dose radiation in a single fraction can be used as well.

Meningiomas

These tumors arise from arachnoidal cells of the meninges and can be distinguished in diverse types including syncytial, transitional, and desmoplastic meningiomas. They can be graded in four classes, but in more than 80% of cases the tumor is benign (grade 1 or 2). When feasible, treatment consists of surgical resection including the surrounding dura. For malignant, recurrent, or incompletely resected meningiomas, radiation therapy can be applied. Following surgical excision, the 20-year survival is more than 80%. After partial resection, radiation therapy improves the 10-year survival from 50% to 80%.

Primary Brain Lymphoma

These tumors seem to appear with increasing frequency, either within or outside the context of immunosuppression and/or HIV. Histologically, these are usually B-cell lymphomas and are purely restricted to the CNS although they may occur simulataneously in the vitreous part of the eye (uveitis). Although the precise frequency is unknown, the incidence worldwide is rising. Apart from a diagnostic biopsy, preferably without preceding use of glucocorticoids, the treatment of choice is radiotherapy (45 to 50 Gy). In recent years, phase II studies have shown that intensive chemotherapy including high-dose systemic methothexate and cytosine arabinoside (Ara-C) followed by radiation therapy may prolong the median survival from about 12 months to 24 to 36 months, although patient selection may have influenced these results.

Germ Cell Tumors

These tumors can be separated into germinatous (germinomas) and nongerminatous germ cell tumors (NGGCTs). The NGGCTs consist fo teratomas, endodermal sinus tumors, embryonal carcinomas, and choriocarcinomas. The presence of α-fetoprotein and β-human chorionic gonadotropin (β-hCG) in the serum may help in the diagnosis of NGGCT. The majority of patients are between 10 and 21 years of age, and the lesion occurs mainly as a midline tumor in the pineal or suprasellar area. As a rule, confirmation of histologic diagnosis is required, but may be difficult to obtain. As these tumors may spread through the leptomeninges, gadolinium-enhanced MRI and CSF cytology should be included in the work-up. For germinomas, radiation therapy is the standard treatment in a dose of $\sim$50 Gy. For NGGCT, craniospinal axis radiation is usually advised and may be followed by systemic chemotherapy. Alternatively, systemic chemotherapy may be given in a neo-adjuvant setting, that is, before the start of radiation therapy. The 5-year survival for germinomas is ~60% and the median survival for patients with NGGCT is less than 1 year.

Pituitary Adenomas

Pituitary adenomas arise from the anterior or posterior pituitary gland an can be divided into prolactin, growth hormone (GH), or adrenocorticotropic hormone (ACTH) producing tumors. Two thirds of pituitary tumors are nonsecreting and the remainder produce prolactin (prolactinomas) or GH, causing acromegaly. The incidence is about 2 per 100,000. Treatment consists mainly of administration of dopamine agonists that impair prolactin secretion or drugs that inhibit either GH or ACTH secretion. If ineffective, surgery and radiation therapy can be employed.

Spinal Cord Tumors

Tumors of the spinal cord are rare and consist mainly of astrocytomas and ependymomas. Patients present with signs of a myelopathy, and initial diagnosis depends on MRI. Often these tumors cannot be surgically removed and diagnosis is achieved by biopsy. Astrocytomas of the spinal cord may be divided into low-grade, anaplastic, or GBM. Radiotherapy is usually an indispensable part of the therapy. Ependymomas are usually low-grade tumors and are mostly confined to the lower part of the spine. Tumors located in the cauda equina can often be completely removed and, if so, do not require postoperative radiotherapy. Otherwise, following incomplete resection, radiotherapy is indicated. Extramedullary/intradural tumors of the spine consist mainly of meningiomas and neurinomas. Both may present with signs of radiculopathy and diagnosis depends on MRI. Complete resection, if possible, is the treatment of choice. Following incomplete resection or recurrence, radiation therapy may be indicated for meningiomas.

Brain Metastasis

Brain metastasis is the most frequent brain tumor and develops in about 20% of all cancer patients. The majority, more than 80%, originate from lung and breast cancer. About one third are single and two thirds are multiple brain metastases. If it is not known if a patient has cancer, surgery is required to obtain a tissue diagnosis. Occasionally, a diagnostic work-up may be indicated to see whether a space-occupying lesion in the brain represents a metastasis or a primary brain tumor. This can take too much time during which the patient may deteriorate neurologically. In patients known to have cancer, there is a 10% chance that the single enhancing lesion will not represent a metastasis, further substantiating the need for tissue diagnosis.

Prognostic Factors   The prognosis in patients with brain metastases is mainly determined by a number of independent prognostic factors. These include age (60-year cutoff), performance status (Karnofsky performance status under or over 70), and extent of systemic cancer (absent or controlled versus active extracranial cancer).

As a rule, patients with brain metastases cannot be cured, and the aim of treatment is preservation of a good quality of life for the remainder of the limited lifetime. For a single brain metastasis, combined therapy of surgery and radiotherapy is useful in patients with no progression of systemic disease over the preceding 3 months. Instead of surgery, radiosurgery can also be applied, producing similar results. In multiple brain metastases, whole brain irradiation therapy is the treatment of choice. For a single brain metastasis with good prognostic factors, the 1-year survival is 40% and the 2-year survival 20%. For multiple brain metastases and favourable prognostic factors, the 1-year survival is 20% and the 2-year survival 10%. In general, the appearance of brain metastases is a sign of progression of the tumor, and for that reason the median survival of patients with multiple brain metastasis is not more than 3 to 4 months overall.

Leptomeningeal Metastases

Leptomeningeal metastases occur as the consequence of the spread of tumor cells to the leptomeninges surrounding the brain and spinal cord. For that reason, patients may show signs of increased intracranial pressure and multiple cranial nerve or nerve root dysfunction. For diagnosis, CSF cytology and gadolinium-enhanced MRI is required. For chemoinsensitive tumors, radiotherapy alone to the symptomatic part of the CNS is indicated. For leptomeningeal leukemias and lymphomas, intrathecal or intraventricular methotrexate and/or Ara-C can be administered. Once the CSF is cleared of tumor cells, consolidation radiotherapy is applied. In breast cancer with leptomeningeal spread, similar schedules are in use.

Metastatic Spinal Cord Compression

Vertebral metastasis is the most common form of osseous metastasis. Symptoms consist of local pain, radiculopathy, and when left untreated may lead to epidural compression of the spinal cord. A complete transverse lesion of the spinal cord may develop rapidly and essentially consists of painless weakness in both legs. This is a dreaded complication of cancer, and impending spinal cord compression is an emergency. Diagnosis depends on MRI. Therapy is initiated with high-dose dexamethasone 10 mg IV bolus, followed by 16 mg/d. The standard therapy is radiotherapy to the involved part of the spine. Occasionally when there is one metastatic vertebra involved without systemic cancer elsewhere in the body, surgical resection of the tumor with implantation of artificial material and stabilization of the spine may be considered. Presently, a laminectomy for metastatic spinal cord compression is considered obsolete, although it may be useful for tissue diagnosis or occasionally for removal of a metastatic deposit to the posterior arch of the spine.

ISSUES OF THERAPY IN NEUROONCOLOGY

In general, brain tumors often lead to changes in personality, cognitive abnormalities, and severe handicap interfering with the normal activities of daily life. In the early stages, prompt diagnosis and therapy are often necessary to prevent irreversible damage to the brain. The main options for therapy are surgery and radiotherapy, and for some tumors systemic chemotherapy can be applied. Although radical surgery is often impossible with malignant brain tumors, as a rule extensive resection of the tumor may have important benefits. It is virtually impossible to acquire prospective data on the influence of the extent of surgery in a randomized fashion, but most studies indicate that larger resections lead to longer periods of progression-free survival. The most reliable data show that the postoperative volume of the tumor strongly correlates with survival. Although counterintuitive, extensive surgery on patients with brain tumors and neurologic deficit leads to improvement rather than deterioration in postoperative neurologic function. In general, lesions that are either deep-seated or are located in vital areas of the brainstem are often difficult or impossible to excise, and under these circumstances, stereotactic or open biopsy can be the best approach. Radiotherapy is of crucial importance for the control of brain tumors. The last decade has seen great advances in techniques that enable more accurate radiation of the tumor with the sparing of surrounding normal brain tissue. This factor had also made it possible to deliver higher doses of radiation limited to the tumor with better chances of cure or long-standing progression-free survival. One of these recent developments is the application of brachytherapy. By this technique, one implants stereotactically placed radioactive iodine-125 or iridium-192 seeds into the tumor tissue. With computer software, one can calculate the number and deliver precisely the exact desired radiation dose. Another development is the application of radiosurgery or conformal radiation therapy. The gamma-unit or Leksell frame consists of multiple cobalt sources and a collimator that concentrate the gamma beams into a sphere. With this technique, tumor volumes of less then 30 mm diameter can be radiated with the sparing of healthy surrounding brain tissue. Similar dose distributions can be achieved with a linear accelerator using a multiple beam technique by use of rotating arcs. This technique is also known as stereotactic or conformal radiation, and it enables precise radiation of various tumor shapes and volumes.

SYMPTOMATIC CONTROL OF BRAIN EDEMA AND INCREASED INTRACRANIAL PRESSURE

Use of Glucocorticoids

Brain edema usually accompanies brain tumors because of damage to the blood–brain barrier and is to a large extent responsible for the appearance of neurologic symptoms. Glucocorticoids effectively counteract vasogenic brain edema and diminish the rate of transcapillary water and albumin flow into the peritumoral tissue. This is caused by a stabilizing effect on the endothelial cell membrane with an ensuing decrease in the permeability of the blood–brain barrier. The therapeutic effects become apparent within 24 to 48 hours and neurologic symptoms generally resolve to a greater or lesser extent. Dexamethasone is often chosen because of lower mineralocorticoid activity and of lesser binding to albumin that prednisone. The generally prescribed dose is 16 mg/day, but if there is no increased intracranial pressure, doses of 4 mg/day are equally effective. In patients with impaired consciousness or impending herniation including posterior fossa tumors, a dose of 16 mg/d is usually recommended. Because radiation of the brain causes brain edema, one usually continues the use of dexamethasone until the end of the radiation in a dose of 4 mg/d.

Side effects of glucocorticoids are dose and time dependent, and for that reason one aims to prescribe the smallest effective dose. Apart from direct side effects including Cushing face, steroid myopathy, or ankle edema, one should be well aware of adrenocortical insufficiency and of steroid withdrawal following discontinuation or tapering off of glucocorticoids, particularly after long-term therapy in high dosage. Mannitol can be given to counteract acutely raised intracranial pressure, before any other therapy is commenced. The dose of mannitol is 1 to 1.5 q/kg IV bolus, followed by 0.5 g/kg every 4 to 6 hours. Glycerol can be given orally to control increased intracranial pressure when steroids are not tolerated or are insufficient. Glycerol is diluted with water or juice at a 50:50 ratio and administered at a dose of 0.25 g/kg every 6 to 8 hours. Unpleasant side effects of glycerol are its taste and marked diuresis.

Anticonvulsants

Seizures of partial type epilepsy are frequent in patients with benign and malignant brain tumors. For that reason, in patients with one or more seizures due to brain tumors, one may choose the anticonvulsants phenytoin, carbamazepine, or natrium-valproate. Often, particularly with low-grade tumors located in the gray matter, surgical resection of the tumor results in disappearance of seizure activity. Prophylactic use of antiepileptics is not a common practice. The disadvantage of phenytoin is its small therapeutic window of efficacy. Suboptimal serum concentrations may result in poor seizure control, and too high levels in phenytoin toxicity. A second factor is the interaction with glucocorticoids resulting in a faster metabolism of both phenytoin and steroids. A severe, and not infrequent, side effect is the Stevens–Johnson or erythema multiforme syndrome. Occasionally this may appear during or after the combined therapy of radiation, glucocorticoid, and phenytoin. This dramatic drug toxicity results in severe swelling of the mucosa, with or without bullae, redness, and epidermolysis of the skin.

NEUROTOXICITY

Following radiation therapy and chemotherapy of brain tumors, toxicity of the nervous system may develop. Cerebral atrophy is commonly observed on neuroimaging following radiotherapy and chemotherapy, although this does not necessarily imply neurologic dysfunction. Brain necrosis in adults is rarely noted blow 60 Gy in conventional radiation. However, neurocognitive effects are observed at lower doses, especially in children. A more pronounced volume effect is believed to exist for the brain than for the spinal cord.

FURTHER READING

Black P McL, Loeffler JS (eds) (1997) *Cancer of the Nervous System*. Blackwell Science.

Kaye AH, Laws ER (eds) (1995) *Brain Tumors*. Churchill Livingstone, Edinburgh.

Levin VA (ed) (1996) *Cancer in the Nervous System*. Churchill Livingstone, Edinburgh.

Posner JB (1995) *Neurologic Complications of Cancer*. Davis, Philadelphia.

Vecht Ch J (ed) (1997) Neuro-Oncology Part 1. Brain Tumors: Principles of Biology, Diagnosis and Therapy. Part 2. Gliomas and other Primary Tumors of Brain and Spinal Cord. Part 3. Neurological Disorders in Systemic Cancer. *Handbook of Clinical Neurology* by Vinken PJ, Bruyn GW. Volumes 67–69, (Revised Series 23–25) Elsevier, Amsterdam.

CHAPTER 31

SOFT TISSUE SARCOMAS

PETER W.T. PISTERS

Department of Surgical Oncology
The University of Texas M.D. Anderson Cancer Center
Houston, TX, USA

BRIAN O'SULLIVAN

Department of Radiation Oncology
The Princess Margaret Hospital
University of Toronto, Toronto, Canada

RAPHAEL E. POLLOCK

Department of Surgical Oncology
The University of Texas M.D. Anderson Cancer Center
Houston, TX, USA

Soft tissue sarcomas are a group of rare, anatomically and histologically diverse malignant neoplasms. These tumors account for 1% of adult malignancies and 15% of pediatric malignancies. Although the overall mortality rate approaches 50%, a substantial proportion of patients can be cured with careful selection of single- or combined-modality treatment strategies.

ETIOLOGY

No specific etiologic agent is identified in the majority of patients with soft tissue sarcoma. There are, nevertheless, a number of recognized associations between environmental factors and the subsequent development of sarcoma. These factors include therapy with ionizing radiation; exposure to alkylating chemotherapeutic agents; occupational exposure to phenoxyacetic acids, chlorophenols, vinyl chloride, or arsenic; or exposure to the previously employed intravenous contrast agent Thorotrast.

Manual of Clinical Oncology, 7th edition, Edited by Raphael E. Pollock
ISBN 0-471-23828-7, pages 621–639. Copyright © 1999 Wiley-Liss, Inc.

In addition, chronic lymphedema of congenital, infectious (filariasis), postsurgical, or postirradiation etiology has been implicated in the development of lymphangiosarcoma.

In clinical practice, the most commonly observed nongenetic predisposing factors are previous radiation and chronic lymphedema. By definition, radiation-induced sarcomas arise no sooner than 3 years after completion of therapeutic radiation and often decades later. The vast majority of these sarcomas are of high grade, and the predominant histology of radiation-induced sarcomas is osteosarcoma, possibly owing to the greater absorption of orthovoltage radiation by bone than by soft tissue prior to the era of megavoltage radiation. In women treated for breast cancer with radical mastectomy, chronic lymphedema of the arm may contribute to the development of lymphangiosarcoma.

A number of genetic conditions are also associated with an increased risk for development of soft tissue sarcoma. These conditions include neurofibromatosis, Li–Fraumeni syndrome, familial retinoblastoma, and Gardner's syndrome. Genetically related soft tissue sarcomas occur most commonly in patients with neurofibromatosis or Gardner's syndrome. Patients with neurofibromatosis have a 7% to 10% lifetime risk of developing a malignant neurofibrosarcoma. Desmoid tumors occur in 8% to 12% of patients with the Gardner's variant of familial polyposis.

Apart from the diagnostic dilemma in distinguishing additional neurofibromata from metastatic lesions in patients with neurofibromatosis, the precise etiology of an individual sarcoma is of little clinical significance because it does not affect therapeutic decision-making beyond the obvious fact that patients who have sarcomas arising in a previously irradiated field usually cannot receive further external-beam radiotherapy.

PATHOLOGY

Anatomic Distribution

Soft tissue sarcomas have been found in virtually all anatomic sites. Approximately half of all soft tissue sarcomas occur in the extremities (lower, 38%; upper, 15%), where the most common histopathologies are liposarcoma (30%) and malignant fibrous histiocytoma (22%). Retroperitoneal and intraabdominal sarcomas constitute 15% of all soft tissue sarcomas, with liposarcoma being the predominant histologic subtype (41%). Visceral sarcomas account for 13% and head and neck sarcomas for approximately 5% of all soft tissue sarcomas.

Histologic Classification

The most common classification for soft tissue sarcoma is based on histogenesis, as outlined in the recent World Health Organization (WHO) classification of sarcomas (see Bibliography). This classification is reproducible for the better differentiated tumors. However, as the degree of histologic differentiation declines, the determination of cellular origin becomes increasingly difficult. In particular, despite advanced immunohistochemical techniques and electron microscopy, determining the cellular origin for many spindle cell and round cell soft tissue tumors is difficult, occasionally arbitrary, and sometimes impossible.

In general, the specific histologic diagnosis is usually of secondary importance because histologic subtype is not generally directly related to biologic behavior. However, specific histologic subtypes such as epitheliod, clear cell, and embryonal rhabdomyosarcoma may have a greater risk of regional lymph node metastasis ($\leq 15\%$) and thus treatment strategies may differ for these specific histologies.

Histologic Grading

Biologic aggressiveness can be best predicted based on histologic grade. The spectrum of grades varies among histologic subtypes (Fig. 31.1). In comparative multivariate analyses, histologic grade is uniformly identified as the most important prognostic factor in assessing the risk for distant metastasis and tumor-related death. Several grading systems have been proposed, but there is no consensus regarding the specific morphologic criteria that should be employed in the grading of soft tis-

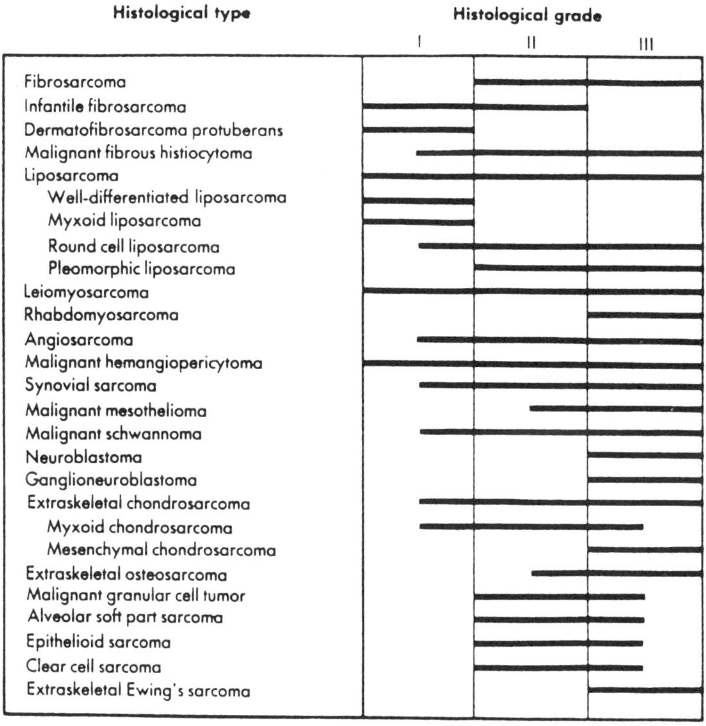

Histological type	Histological grade I	II	III
Fibrosarcoma		II	III
Infantile fibrosarcoma	I		
Dermatofibrosarcoma protuberans	I		
Malignant fibrous histiocytoma	I	II	III
Liposarcoma			
Well-differentiated liposarcoma	I		
Myxoid liposarcoma	I	II	
Round cell liposarcoma			III
Pleomorphic liposarcoma			III
Leiomyosarcoma	I	II	III
Rhabdomyosarcoma			III
Angiosarcoma	I	II	III
Malignant hemangiopericytoma	I	II	III
Synovial sarcoma		II	III
Malignant mesothelioma		II	III
Malignant schwannoma		II	III
Neuroblastoma			III
Ganglioneuroblastoma			III
Extraskeletal chondrosarcoma		II	III
Myxoid chondrosarcoma		II	
Mesenchymal chondrosarcoma			III
Extraskeletal osteosarcoma		II	III
Malignant granular cell tumor	I	II	
Alveolar soft part sarcoma	I	II	
Epithelioid sarcoma	I	II	
Clear cell sarcoma	I	II	
Extraskeletal Ewing's sarcoma			III

FIGURE 31.1. Spectrum of histologic grades observed among histologic subtypes of soft tissue sarcoma. (From Soft tissue sarcoma. In *Soft Tissue Tumors*, 3rd edition. Enzinger FN, Weiss SW [eds] Mosby-Year Book, St. Louis, 1995. With permission.)

sue sarcomas. Two of the most commonly employed grading systems are the US National Cancer Institute (NCI) system and the Federation Nationale des Centres de Lutte Contre le Cancer (FNCLCC) system developed by the French Federation of Cancer Centers Sarcoma Group. The NCI system is based on the tumor's histologic type or subtype, location, and amount of tumor necrosis, but cellularity, nuclear pleomorphism, and mitosis count are also considered in certain situations. The FNCLCC system employs a score generated by evaluation of three parameters: tumor differentiation, mitotic rate, and amount of tumor necrosis. Recent comparative evaluation of these grading systems suggests that the FNCLCC system may stratify patients more precisely for probability of overall and metastasis-free survival.

CLINICAL PRESENTATION

The clinical presentation of patients with soft tissue sarcoma is highly variable, reflecting the anatomic heterogeneity of these lesions. The majority of patients with extremity sarcomas present with a painless soft tissue mass. Delay in diagnosis is common, with the most common misdiagnoses including intramuscular hematoma ("pulled muscle"), sebaceous cyst, and benign lipoma. Symptoms are often not experienced until these tumors grow large enough to press directly on nearby neurovascular structures, causing pain, numbness, or swelling.

Patients with intraabdominal or retroperitoneal sarcomas commonly present with vague, nonspecific abdominal pain or a palpable abdominal mass. Retroperitoneal and intraabdominal tumors can also produce symptoms of nausea, vomiting, abdominal distention, or early satiety. Sarcomas arising from specific viscera may produce symptoms or signs related to the organ involved. For example, patients with gastrointestinal or uterine leiomyosarcomas may present with symptoms related to gastrointestinal or uterine bleeding.

DIAGNOSTIC EVALUATION

Physical examination should include an assessment of the size and mobility of the mass. The relationship of the mass to the investing muscular fascia (superficial versus deep) and to nearby neurovascular and bony structures should be noted. A site-specific neurovascular examination and assessment of regional lymph nodes should also be performed.

The diagnostic evaluation of patients with suspected soft tissue sarcoma involves appropriate biopsy and imaging of the primary tumor together with complete staging evaluation. The following comments focus primarily on patients with extremity sarcomas, as the extremities are the site of the majority of soft tissue sarcomas.

Biopsy

Biopsy of the primary tumor is essential for most patients presenting with primary soft tissue masses. In general, any soft tissue mass in an adult that is asymptomatic or enlarging, is larger than 5 cm, or persists beyond 4 to 6 weeks should undergo biopsy. The preferred biopsy approach is generally the least invasive technique required to allow a definitive histologic diagnosis and assessment of grade. In most centers, core needle biopsy permits satisfactory tissue diagnosis. Biopsy of superficial lesions can commonly be guided by direct palpation, but less accessible sarcomas may require an image-guided (sonography or computed tomography [CT]) biopsy to safely sample the most heterogeneous component of the mass. In some centers, fine-needle aspiration (FNA) may be an acceptable biopsy technique provided that an experienced sarcoma cytopathologist is available. However, because of the frequent difficulty in accurately diagnosing these lesions even when adequate tissue is available, the major utility of FNA in most centers is in the diagnosis of suspected recurrent sarcoma.

Incisional or excisional biopsy is rarely required but may be performed when a definitive diagnosis cannot be achieved by less invasive means. Several technical points merit comment. Relatively small, superficial masses that can easily be removed should be completely excised with microscopic assessment of surgical margins. Incisional and excisional biopsies should be performed with the incision oriented longitudinally (for extremity lesions) to facilitate subsequent wide local excision and/or to permit radiation treatment volumes to adequately encompass the volume at risk while maximally sparing limb circumference. The incision should be centered over the mass at its most superficial point. Care should be taken not to raise tissue flaps. Meticulous hemostasis should be ensured to prevent dissemination of tumor cells into adjacent tissue planes by hematoma. All excisional biopsy specimens should be sent anatomically oriented for pathologic analysis. At definitive resection of a previously biopsied sarcoma, the biopsy scar should be excised en bloc with the tumor.

When radiologic assessment indicates that a presumed primary retroperitoneal (extravisceral) mass is resectable, FNA and core needle biopsy are not indicated. This is because the overall therapeutic plan is rarely altered by preoperative histologic diagnosis and the histologically heterogeneous nature of individual lesions precludes a plan of "observation" when biopsy findings are "benign" or indeterminant. Preoperative image-directed biopsy is invasive, expensive, and rarely modifies treatment for patients in whom surgical exploration is planned. However, there are specific circumstances for which biopsy of primary retroperitoneal masses should be performed. These include (1) clinical suspicion of lymphoma or germ cell tumor, (2) tissue diagnosis for preoperative treatment, (3) tissue diagnosis of radiologically unresectable disease, and (4) suspected retroperitoneal or intraabdominal metastasis from another primary tumor. In the main, however, for patients for whom exploratory laparotomy is planned, surgical resection is the best means of establishing a tissue diagnosis of a resectable retroperitoneal mass; intraoperative incisional biopsy is appropriate if the lesion proves to be unresectable. Given the poor long-term outcome for patients with retroperitoneal sarcoma (see Treatment of Primary Soft Tissue of the Retroperitoneum), preoperative evaluation and subsequent treatment may be best accomplished in a referral center involved in combined-modality trials for these patients.

Radiologic Staging

Optimal imaging of the primary tumor is dependent on anatomic site. For extremity sarcomas, magnetic resonance imaging (MRI) has been regarded as the imaging modality of choice for soft tissue masses. This is because MRI enhances the contrast between tumor and muscle and between tumor and adjacent blood vessel and provides multiplanar definition of the lesion. However, a recent study by the Radiation Diagnostic Oncology Group that compared MRI and CT showed no specific advantage of MRI over CT. For pelvic lesions, the multiplanar capability of MRI may provide superior single-modality imaging. In the retroperitoneum and abdomen, CT usually provides satisfactory anatomic definition of the lesion. Occasionally, MRI with gradient sequence imaging can delineate the relationship of the tumor to midline vascular structures, particularly the inferior vena cava and aorta. More invasive studies such as angiography or cavography are almost never required for evaluation of soft tissue sarcomas.

Cost-effective imaging to exclude the possibility of distant metastatic disease is dependent on the size, grade, and anatomic location of the primary tumor. In general, patients with low- and intermediate-grade tumors or high-grade tumors smaller than 5 cm require only a chest X-ray film for satisfactory evaluation for thoracic disease. This directly reflects the comparatively low risk for pulmonary metastases at presentation in these patients. In contrast, patients with high-grade tumors larger than 5 cm should undergo more thorough staging by chest CT. Patients with retroperitoneal and intraabdominal visceral sarcomas should undergo MRI or CT of the liver to exclude the possibility of synchronous hepatic metastases as the liver is a common site of first metastasis for these lesions.

STAGING

The relative rarity of soft tissue sarcomas, the anatomic heterogeneity of these lesions, and the presence of more than 30 recognized histologic subtypes of variable grade have made it difficult to establish a functional system that can accurately stage all forms of this disease. The recently revised TNM staging system (5th edition) of the American Joint Committee on Cancer (AJCC) and UICC is the most widely employed staging system for soft tissue sarcomas. This staging system is a revision of the AJCC system, which was first published in 1977, that incorporates histologic grade into the conventional TNM system (Table 31.1; Fig. 31.2). All soft tissue sarcoma subtypes are included except dermatofibrosarcoma protuberans, a condition considered to have only borderline malignant potential. Four distinct histologic grades are recognized, ranging from well-differentiated to undifferentiated. Histologic grade and tumor size are the primary determinants of clinical stage (Table 31.1). Tumor size is further substaged as "a" (superficial tumor arising outside the investing fascia) or "b" (a deep tumor that arises beneath the fascia or invades the fascia). At this time, data validating this revised staging system have not been published. The original data used to validate the 1977 version of this staging system with stage-specific survival are plotted in Fig. 31.2.

TABLE 31.1. UICC/AJCC Staging System (5th Edition) for Soft Tissue Sarcomas

T1	≤5 cm		
T1a	Superficial to muscular fascia		
T1b	Deep to muscular fascia		
T2	>5 cm		
T2a	Superficial to muscular fascia		
T2b	Deep to muscular fascia		
N1	Regional nodal involvement		
M1	Distant metastatic disease		
G1	Well differentiated		
G2	Moderately differentiated		
G3	Poorly differentiated		
G4	Undifferentiated		
Stage IA	G1, 2	T1a, b	N0	M0
Stage IB	G1, 2	T2a	N0	M0
Stage IIA	G1, 2	T2b	N0	M0
Stage IIB	G3, 4	T1a, b	N0	M0
Stage IIC	G3, 4	T2a	N0	M0
Stage III	G3, 4	T2b	N0	M0
Stage IV	Any G	Any T	N1	M0
	Any G	Any T	Any N	M1

(Modified from *UICC TNM Classification of Malignant Tumors*, 5th edition, 1997. With permission.)
Note: For the majority of sarcoma patients, in whom regional lymphadenectomy is not performed owing to the low overall incidence of lymph node involvement for sarcomas in general, a case should still be considered as pathologic stage N0 and not pNx.

A major limitation of the present staging system is that it does not take into account the anatomic heterogeneity of these lesions. The present staging system is optimally designed to stage extremity tumors but is also applicable to torso, head and neck, and retroperitoneal lesions. It should not be used for sarcomas of the gastrointestinal tract. Anatomic site, however, is an important determinant of outcome. Patients with retroperitoneal and visceral sarcomas have a worse overall prognosis than do patients with extremity tumors. Although site is not incorporated as a specific component of any present staging system, outcome data should be reported on a site-specific basis.

TREATMENT OF LOCALIZED PRIMARY SOFT TISSUE SARCOMA

A general stage-specific treatment algorithm for patients with primary sarcomas of the extremity and superficial trunk is outlined in Fig. 31.3. The evidence supporting this general stage-specific treatment approach is outlined below. The treatment of patients with retroperitoneal sarcomas is discussed separately.

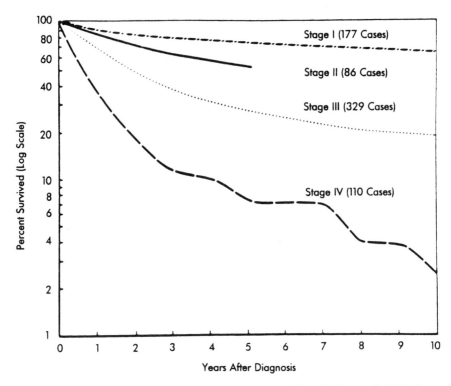

FIGURE 31.2. Overall survival by AJCC stage (From Russell et al. *Cancer* 40:1562. Copyright © [1977] American Cancer Society. Reprinted by permission of Wiley-Liss, Inc., a subsidiary of John Wiley & Sons, Inc.)

Surgery

Surgical resection remains the cornerstone of therapy for localized disease. Over the past 20 years, there has been a marked decline in the rate of amputation as the primary therapy for extremity soft tissue sarcoma. With application of multimodality treatment strategies, fewer than 10% of patients presently undergo amputation. There is clear evidence that for patients for whom limb-sparing surgery is an option, a multimodality approach employing limb-sparing surgery combined with pre- or postoperative radiotherapy yields disease-related survival rates comparable to those of amputation while preserving a functional extremity.

Satisfactory local resection involves resection of the primary tumor with a margin of normal tissue around the lesion. It is clear that dissection along the tumor pseudocapsule (enucleation) is associated with local recurrence rates of at least 50%. In contrast, wide local excision that includes a margin of normal tissue around the lesion is associated with local recurrence rates in the range of 12% to 31%, as observed in the control arms (surgery alone) of the randomized trials evaluating adjuvant radiotherapy. Unlike for other diseases such as malignant melanoma, there are no available

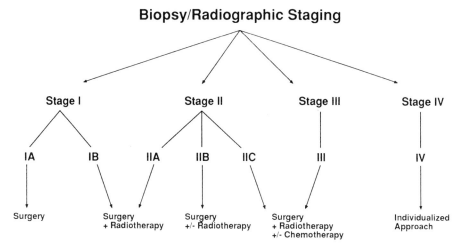

FIGURE 31.3. Treatment algoritm for patients with extremity or superficial trunk sarcomas based on UICC clinical stage. See Table 31.1 for UICC/AJCC Staging System. Surgery, wide local resection with assessment of microscopic surgical margins. Radiotherapy, pre- or postoperative (50 or 65 Gy, respectively) external-beam radiotherapy or brachytherapy (42 to 50 Gy) for suitable patients with G3/4 sarcomas. Chemotherapy, doxorubicin- and/or ifosfamide-based pre- or postoperative chemotherapy, optimally as part of a clinical trial.

randomized data to address what constitutes a satisfactory gross resection margin for a sarcoma.

Although the majority of patients with extremity soft tissue sarcoma should be treated with pre- or postoperative radiotherapy, there is evidence to suggest that radiotherapy may not be required for selected patients with completely resected, small primary soft tissue sarcomas. Surgical resection without radiotherapy may be considered for lesions that are smaller than 5 cm (T1), and located superficially in a portion of the extremity or superficial trunk where it is not difficult to obtain a satisfactory gross surgical margin. Treatment of patients with category T2a and T2b (>5 cm) primary sarcomas by surgery alone is generally not recommended and should not be done outside the confines of a clinical trial.

Pre- or Postoperative Radiotherapy

Radiotherapy has been combined with conservative (limb-sparing) surgery to optimize local control for patients with localized soft tissue sarcoma. Radiation can be administered preoperatively or postoperatively by external-beam techniques or by interstitial techniques (brachytherapy). A randomized trial of postoperative brachytherapy (extremity or superficial trunk sarcomas) and a randomized trial of postoperative external-beam radiotherapy (extremity sarcomas) have confirmed several retrospective reports suggesting that surgery combined with radiotherapy results in superior local control compared to surgery alone (see Bibliography). Although both random-

TABLE 31.2. Local Control with Surgery and Radiotherapy for Localized Soft Tissue Sarcoma

Radiotherapy Approach	First Author	Radiation Dose (Gy)	Study Design	No. Patients	Local Failure (%)	
Preoperative EBRT	Suit	50–56	Retrospective	89	17	
	Barkley	50	Retrospective	110	10	
	Brant	50.4	Retrospective	58	9	
Brachytherapy	Pisters	42–45	Prospective (RCT)	119	9	(High-grade)
				45	23	(Low-grade)
Postoperative EBRT	Lindberg	60–75	Retrospective	300	22	
	Karakousis	45–60	Retrospective	53	14	
	Suit	60–68	Retrospective	131	12	
	Yang	45+18	Prospective (RCT)	91	0	(High-grade)
				50	5	(Low-grade)

ized studies demonstrated an improvement in local control for patients treated with combined-modality therapy, this improvement did not translate into any detectable survival difference between the treatment (surgery plus radiotherapy) and control (surgery alone) arms.

Local failure rates with combined-modality regimens incorporating surgery and radiotherapy are generally less than 15% (Table 31.2). Despite theoretical advantages that may favor preoperative external-beam radiation, brachytherapy, or postoperative external-beam radiation, there does not appear to be a major difference in local control rates among these radiation techniques, although no presently available data directly compares the techniques. However, a phase III trial comparing preoperative external-beam radiotherapy to postoperative external-beam radiotherapy for patients with localized extremity soft tissue sarcoma (Protocol SR-2) is presently nearing completion under the direction of the National Cancer Institute of Canada Clinical Trials Group (NCIC CTG)/Canadian Sarcoma Group (CSG). This important study is designed to provide insight into the comparative efficacy, functional outcome, economic costs, and complication rates of these two options for external-beam radiotherapy.

In the absence of a clear local control advantage with any specific radiation technique, clinicians have considered other factors in formulating standards of care. Such factors have included wound complication rates, financial costs, and patient convenience. While field size and radiation dose may be minimized with preoperative radiotherapy, major wound complications following preoperative radiotherapy and surgery have been reported to be in the 20% to 30% range. This fact alone has caused some groups to favor postoperative radiotherapy. On the other hand, with brachytherapy, the patient's entire local treatment (surgery plus radiation) can be completed within 10 to 14 days. Allowing for the fact that some case selection for brachytherapy versus external-beam radiotherapy may exist, brachytherapy has significant cost advantages and significant implications in terms of overall patient convenience. In the absence of comparative data addressing the efficacy of these techniques in achieving local control, these additional considerations assume increased importance. Until data from the NCIC CTG phase III comparative study are available, it appears reasonable to treat most patients with postoperative external-beam radiotherapy because local control rates are comparable to preoperative techniques but major wound complication rates are significantly lower. Where the necessary expertise is available for brachytherapy, this technique provides an excellent, cost-effective alternative for appropriate patients with high-grade lesions. Brachytherapy should not be used for patients with low-grade sarcomas, which may be better treated with external-beam radiotherapy (see Table 31.2).

Postoperative Chemotherapy

The role of postoperative chemotherapy in the management of localized soft tissue sarcoma remains controversial. The results of 12 randomized trials evaluating adjuvant chemotherapy in patients with extremity soft tissue sarcomas have been published. Each of these trials had a control arm that received no adjuvant therapy and a treatment group that received postoperative systemic therapy with doxorubicin alone or in combination with other drugs. Four of the trials reported prolonged improved relapse-free survival but only 1 of the 12 trials found a statistically significant improvement in overall survival.

All of the published randomized trials of postoperative chemotherapy have recognized deficiencies in design and conduct. The most commonly cited deficiencies of these trials as a group relate to the relatively small sample size and to the fact that small differences in survival require relatively large numbers of patients to detect with sufficient statistical power. These deficiencies have been addressed to an extent in the Sarcoma Meta-Analysis Collaboration (SMAC) group's recent meta-analysis of the individual data in these randomized trials. This meta-analysis demonstrated statistically significantly higher local recurrence-free survival and disease-free survival rates in patients who received doxorubicin-containing postoperative chemotherapy (Table 31.3). However, there was no statistically significant improvement in

TABLE 31.3. Sarcoma Meta-Analysis Collaboration Group's Meta-Analysis of Randomized Doxorubicin-Based Postoperative Chemotherapy (versus Local Therapy Alone) in Soft Tissue Sarcoma

Endpoint	Hazard Ratio	Absolute Benefit	p Value
Local recurrence-free interval	0.74	6% (75% → 81%)	0.024
Distant recurrence-free interval	0.69	10% (60% → 70%)	0.0003
Overall recurrence-free interval	0.69	13% (45% → 58%)	0.000008
Overall recurrence-free survival	0.74	11% (40% → 51%)	0.00008
Overall survival	0.87	5% (50% → 55%)	0.087

Adapted from Tierney et al. (1996) *Proc Am Soc Clin Oncol* 15:2024. With permission.

overall survival rates. Because a significant improvement in survival with postoperative chemotherapy has not been detected with these advanced statistical techniques, it appears reasonable to conclude that if such a benefit exists, it must be quite small. Indeed, the meta-analysis suggests that if a survival benefit exists, it may be 5% or less (Table 31.3). Moreover, the local control rates in these trials fall short of the levels achieved in current outcome analyses evaluating the results of combined modality treatment. This observation may be confirmed in the NCIC CTG SR2 trial, which includes high-quality real-time radiotherapy quality assurance.

Recent investigations have focused on the possible benefits of newer agents in the postoperative treatment of localized soft tissue sarcomas. A recently reported randomized trial of five cycles of epirubicin (120 mg/m^2) and ifosfamide (9 g/m^2) following definitive local therapy versus local therapy alone showed a significant survival advantage in favor of the group receiving postoperative chemotherapy (see Bibliography). This study was reported with a relatively short 21-month median follow-up and has been criticized for the unexplained comparatively poor outcome in the group treated with local therapy alone (median survival, 13 months). Indeed, comparison of the outcome of the control group in this study with the aggregate control group in the SMAC meta-analysis or the treatment groups in the existing randomized trials of adjuvant radiotherapy (i.e., other groups treated with local therapy alone) reveals significantly worse outcome for the patients treated with local therapy alone in this postoperative chemotherapy trial. The preliminary observations are noteworthy, but longer follow-up and additional studies are needed. At this time, given the overall results of the SMAC meta-analysis and the preliminary nature of this recent positive trial of adjuvant epirubicin and ifosfamide, postoperative chemotherapy cannot be considered standard therapy for patients with localized soft tissue sarcoma. Potentially toxic postoperative chemotherapy should be optimally provided within the context of a clinical trial and should be reserved for selected patients who present with adverse prognostic factors for overall survival. These factors include large tumor size, deep tumor location, and high histologic grade (TNM stage 3, see Table 31.1).

Preoperative Chemotherapy

Proposed theoretical advantages to preoperative chemotherapy include (1) early treatment of occult micrometastatic disease, (2) in vivo evaluation of chemosensitivity, and (3) possible cytoreduction to an extent that less morbid local therapies might be applicable. There are only a few reports of long-term results with doxorubicin-based preoperative chemotherapy for patients with high-grade localized soft tissue sarcomas. These studies have revealed variable response rates ranging from 3% to 27%. The reasons for this variability in reported response rates are unknown but may include differences in patient populations, differences in chemotherapeutic drug dosing and number of cycles, and differences in the definition of major response. Long-term rates of local recurrence-free survival, distant metastasis-free survival, disease-free survival, and overall survival appear comparable to those reported for similarly staged patients treated with postoperative chemotherapy. At present, no studies have directly compared pre- versus postoperative chemotherapy.

Recently, isosfamide-containing combinations have been used in the preoperative setting. Selected patients treated with aggressive doxorubicin- and ifosfamide-based regimens have had major responses, and preliminary results suggest that response rates may be higher than in historic controls treated with non-ifosfamide-containing regimens. A randomized trial of preoperative chemotherapy (50 mg/m^2 doxorubicin; 5 g/m^2 ifosfamide) versus local therapy alone has recently been completed by the European Organization for the Research and Treatment of Cancer (EORTC) Bone and Soft Tissue Sarcoma Group (protocol 62874). Toxicity results of this trial have been presented, but data on event-free outcome have not yet been formally reported.

Combined Preoperative Chemotherapy and Radiotherapy

There has been recent interest in combined-modality preoperative treatment (concurrent or sequential chemotherapy and radiation) for patients with localized soft tissue sarcomas. Investigators from the Massachusetts General Hospital have employed sequential chemotherapy and radiation in the treatment of patients with localized, high-grade, large (>8 cm) extremity soft tissue sarcomas. This treatment protocol involved alternating courses of chemotherapy and radiotherapy: three courses of doxorubicin, ifosfamide, mesna, and dacarbazine and two 22-Gy courses of radiation for a total preoperative radiation dose of 44 Gy. This was followed by surgical resection with careful microscopic assessment of surgical margins. An additional 16-Gy radiation boost was delivered postoperatively for microscopically positive surgical margins. The outcomes of 26 patients treated with this regimen have been compared to those of matched historical controls. With a short 13-month median follow-up, 5-year actuarial local control, disease-free survival, and overall survival rates for the sequential chemoradiation group are 100%, 84%, and 93%, respectively. For the matched historic controls, these rates are 97%, 45%, and 60%, respectively. These preliminary results will require longer follow-up and additional studies for confirmation. An ongoing Radiation Therapy Oncology Group protocol (RTOG-95-14) is further investigating this treatment approach.

Concurrent doxorubicin-based chemoradiation has also been employed extensively by investigators at the University of California, Los Angeles. The treatment involved concurrent intraarterial doxorubicin with unusual high dose per fraction radiotherapy (35 Gy of external-beam radiotherapy delivered in ten daily fractions that was reduced to 17.5 Gy in five daily fractions to minimize local toxicity). A subsequent prospective randomized trial compared preoperative intraarterial doxorubicin to intravenous doxorubicin, both followed by 28 Gy of radiation in eight daily fractions followed by surgical resection. No differences in local recurrence or survival were noted. At this time, combined preoperative concurrent or sequential chemotherapy and radiotherapy regimens remain investigational and should not be provided outside the context of a clinical trial.

TREATMENT OF PRIMARY SOFT TISSUE SARCOMA OF THE RETROPERITONEUM

Surgical resection with negative margins remains the primary treatment for patients with retroperitoneal sarcoma. Overall resectability rates in recent series combining patients with primary and recurrent retroperitoneal sarcomas range from 53% to 59%. For patients with primary retroperitoneal soft tissue sarcomas, grossly complete resection may be possible in 80% to 90% of patients. The most common reasons for unresectability are the presence of major vascular involvement (aorta or vena cava), peritoneal implants, or distant metastases. In many cases, resection of adjacent retroperitoneal or intraabdominal organs may be necessary to facilitate complete resection. Partial resections or debulking procedures have been performed, but there is no evidence that partial resection improves survival. In general, deliberate partial resection of retroperitoneal sarcomas should be reserved for relief of bowel obstruction or palliation of other critical manifestations of advanced disease. Results from recent series demonstrate 5-year actuarial survival rates in the range of 54% to 64% for patients with completely resected retroperitoneal sarcomas. Recurrent disease remains a significant problem, with local and/or distant recurrences developing in the majority of patients (53% to 68%).

Although postoperative radiotherapy has been shown to reduce local recurrence rates for extremity and superficial trunk sarcomas, gastrointestinal and neurologic toxicities frequently limit the delivery of sufficient radiation doses to the retroperitoneum. Several retrospective reports have suggested that postoperative external-beam radiotherapy improves local control or at least prolongs the time to local failure after surgical resection of retroperitoneal sarcomas. No randomized trials have addressed this specific question. A randomized trial from the NCI demonstrated that surgical resection with intraoperative and subsequent postoperative external-beam radiotherapy resulted in improved local control versus treatment with resection and postoperative high-dose external-beam radiotherapy. However, intraoperative radiotherapy was associated with significant neurotoxicity (47%). This technique remains investigational and is generally limited to specialty centers because of the need for a dedicated operating room.

Retrospective studies have not demonstrated any benefit to preoperative or postoperative doxorubicin-based chemotherapy for retroperitoneal sarcomas. Thus, at present, no data from randomized trials support pre- or postoperative chemotherapy as standard treatment for retroperitoneal sarcomas. Because of the disappointing results in these patients, they should be encouraged to enter clinical trials investigating novel multimodality treatment strategies and are probably best referred to centers involved with these protocols.

TREATMENT OF LOCALLY RECURRENT SOFT TISSUE SARCOMA

Despite optimal multimodality therapy, local recurrence develops in a substantial number of patients. Treatment approaches for patients for locally recurrent soft tissue sarcoma need to be individualized based on local anatomic constraints and the limitations on present treatment options imposed by prior therapies. In general, all such patients should be evaluated for reresection of their local recurrence. The results of such "salvage surgery" are good, with two thirds of patients experiencing long-term survival. For patients who have not had prior radiotherapy to the area of recurrence, optimal treatment of the local recurrence includes surgery and pre- or postoperative radiotherapy. Few data have been published on the use of additional radiotherapy in patients who develop local recurrence in or at the margin of a previous external-beam radiation field. Brachytherapy may be an option for such patients. In addition, it may be reasonable to consider pre- or postoperative chemotherapy for patients with locally recurrent high-grade tumors because of the adverse prognostic significance of local recurrence and the fact that the SMAC meta-analysis of randomized postoperative chemotherapy trials suggests a local control advantage for patients receiving doxorubicin-based postoperative chemotherapy.

TREATMENT OF METASTATIC SOFT TISSUE SARCOMA

The most common site of metastasis from soft tissue sarcoma is the lung. Primary visceral and gastrointestinal sarcomas also commonly metastasize to the liver. For most nongastrointestinal or visceral sarcomas, extrapulmonary metastases are uncommon forms of first metastasis and usually occur as a late manifestation of widely disseminated disease. Median survival from the time of development of metastatic disease is 8 to 12 months. Prospective studies have demonstrated an 11% 3-year survival rate among all patients presenting with pulmonary metastases. Optimal treatment of patients with metastatic soft tissue sarcoma requires an understanding of the natural history of the disease and individualized selection of treatment options based on specific patient factors, disease factors, and limitations imposed by prior treatment.

Surgical Resection of Metastatic Disease

Carefully selected patients may benefit from complete surgical resection of metastatic sarcoma. Unfortunately, this treatment approach benefits only a small fraction of patients who develop pulmonary metastases. Among patients who are able to undergo complete resection of their pulmonary metastatic diasease (50% of all patients with pulmonary metastases), median survival from the time of complete resection is 18 to 27 months, and the 3-year survival rate is 23% to 42% (Table 31.4).

The rather disappointing overall treatment results for patients with metastatic disease underscore the importance of careful patient selection for resection of pulmonary metastases. The following criteria are generally agreed upon: (1) the primary tumor is controlled or is controllable, (2) there is no extrathoracic disease, (3) the patient is a medical candidate for thoracotomy and pulmonary resection, and (4) complete resection of all disease appears possible. With careful patient selection, the morbidity from thoracotomy can be limited to the subset of patients who are most

TABLE 31.4. Survival Following Complete Resection of Pulmonary Metastases from Soft Tissue Sarcoma in Adults

First Author(s)/ Institution (Year)	No. of Patients			Complete Resection (%)	Median Survival (mo)	3-Year Survival (%)
	Total	Pulmonary Metastases	Resection of Pulmonary Metastases			
Cregan/Mayo (1979)	112	112	112	64 (57%)	18	29
Putnam, Roth/NCI (1984, 1985)	487	93	68	51 (75%)	23	32
Jablons/NCI (1989)	74	57	57	49 (86%)	27	35
Casson/MDACC (1992)	68	68	68	58 (85%)	25	42
Verazin/Rosell (1992)	78	78	78	61 (78%)	21	21.5 (5-year)
Gadd/MSKCC (1993)	716	135	78	65 (83%)	19	23
van Geel/EORTC (1996)	255	255	255	255 (100%)	NR	54

Mayo, Mayo Clinic; Roswell Park Cancer Institute; NCI, US National Cancer Institute; MDACC, M.D. Anderson Cancer Center; MSKCC, Memorial Sloan–Kettering Cancer Center; EORTC, European Organization for the Research and Treatment of Cancer.

likely to benefit from this aggressive treatment approach. The role of perioperative chemotherapy with complete resection of pulmonary metastases is unknown and is presently under investigation in an EORTC randomized trial (Protocol 62933).

Chemotherapy for Metastatic Soft Tissue Sarcoma

Systematic treatment remains the only therapeutic option for the majority of patients with metastatic soft tissue sarcoma. A detailed review of the single-agent and combination chemotherapeutic approaches for advanced sarcoma is beyond the scope of this text but is available in the general reviews referenced in the Bibliography. The combination of cyclophosphamide, vincristine, doxorubicin, and dacarbazine (CyVADIC) has been considered the standard of care for well over a decade. Response rates in excess of 40% have been observed with this regimen. However, a randomized trial comparing CyVADIC to doxorubicin alone revealed no significant difference in response or survival rates. On the basis of these data, many investigators now consider single-agent doxorubicin to be the present standard of care against which new combinations should be evaluated.

Ifosfamide, an analogue of cyclophosphamide, has been reported to produce significant response rates in the range of 30% to 40% in patients with advanced soft tissue sarcoma. The most comprehensive comparative study performed to date was reported by the EORTC. In that study, 663 eligible patients were randomly assigned to receive doxorubicin (75 mg/m^2) (arm A); CyVADIC (arm B); or ifosfamide (5 g/m^2) plus doxorubicin (50 mg/m^2) (arm C). There was no statistically significant difference detected among the three study arms in terms of response rate (arm A, 23.3%; arm B, 24.4%; and arm C, 28.1%), remission duration, or overall survival (median 52 weeks for arm A, 51 weeks for arm B, and 55 weeks for arm C). The degree of myelosuppression was significantly greater for the combination of ifosfamide and doxorubicin than for the other two regimens. Cardiotoxicity was also more frequent in arm C. This study and others suggest that single-agent doxorubicin is still the standard against which more intensive or new drug treatments should be compared.

FURTHER READING

General Reviews

Brennan MF, Casper ES, Harison LB (1996) Soft tissue sarcoma. In: DeVita VTJ, Hellman S, Rosenberg SA (eds) *Cancer: Principles and Practice of Oncology*, 5th edition. JB Lippincott, Philadelphia, pp. 1738–1788.

Pisters PWT, Brennan MF (1995) Sarcomas of soft tissue. In: Abeloff M, Armitage J, Lichter A, Niederhuber J (eds) *Clinical Oncology*. Churchill Livingstone, New York.

Histopathology, Grading, and Biopsy

Enzinger FM, Weiss SW (1995) *Soft Tissue Sarcoma*, 3rd edition. Mosby-Year Book, St. Louis.

Guillou L, Coindre J, Bonichon F, et al. (1997) Comparative study of the National Cancer Institute and French Federation of Cancer Centers Sarcoma Group grading systems in a population of 410 adult patients with soft tissue sarcoma. *J Clin Oncol* 15:350.

Heslin MJ, Lewis JJ, Woodruff JM, Brennan MF (19xx) Core needle biopsy for diagnosis of extremity soft tissue sarcoma. *Ann Surg Oncol* 4:425–431.

Trojani M, Contesso G, Coindre JM, et al. (1984) Soft-tissue sarcomas of adults: Study of pathological prognostic variables and definition of a histopathological grading system. *Int J Cancer* 33:37.

Weiss SW, Sobin L (1994) *Histologic Typing of Soft Tissue Tumors*. Springer-Verlag, Berlin, pp. 7–14.

Staging and Prognostic Factors

Coindre JM, Terrier P, Bui NB, et al. (1996) Prognostic factors in adult patients with locally controlled soft tissue sarcoma: A study of 546 patients from the French Federation of Cancer Centers Sarcoma Group. *J Clin Oncol* 14:869.

Panicek DM, Gatsonis C, Rosenthal DI, et al. (1997) CT and MR imaging in the local staging of primary malignant musculoskeletal neoplasms: Report of the Radiology Diagnostic Oncology Group. *Radiology* 202:237.

Pisters PWT, Leung DHY, Woodruff J, Shi W, Brennan MF (1996) Analysis of prognostic factors in 1041 patients with localized soft tissue sarcomas of the extremities. *J Clin Oncol* 14:1679.

Author? (1997) Tumours of bone and soft tissues. In: Sobin LH, Wittekind C (eds) *TNM Classification of Malignant Tumours*, 5th edition. Wiley-Liss, New York, p. 101.

Surgical Treatment of Extremity Sarcoma

Williard WC, Collin C, Casper ES, Hajdu SI, Brennan MF (1992) The changing role of amputation for soft tissue sarcoma of the extremity in adults. *Surg Gynecol Obstet* 175:389.

Rosenberg SA, Tepper J, Glatstein E, et al. (1982) The treatment of soft-tissue sarcomas of the extremities: Prospective randomized evaluations of (1) limb-sparing surgery plus radiation therapy compared with amputation and (2) the role of adjuvant chemotherapy. *Ann Surg* 196:305.

Yang JC, Rosenberg SA (1989) Surgery for adult patients with soft tissue sarcomas. *Semin Oncol* 16:289.

Pre- and Postoperative Radiotherapy

Pisters PWT, Harrison LB, Leung DHY, Woodruff JM, Casper ES (1996) Long-term results of a prospective randomized trial of adjuvant brachytherapy in soft tissue sarcoma. *J Clin Oncol* 14:859.

Suit HD, Mankin HJ, Wood WC, et al. (1988) Treatment of the patient with stage M0 soft tissue sarcoma. *J Clin Oncol* 6:854.

Yang JC, Chang AE, Baker AR, et al. (1998) A randomized prospective study of the benefit of adjuvant radiation therapy in the treatment of soft tissue sarcomas of the extremity. *J Clin Oncol* 16:197–203.

Pre- and Postoperative Chemotherapy

Bramwell V, Rouesse J, Steward W, et al. (1994) Adjuvant CYVADIC chemotherapy for adult soft tissue sarcoma-reduced local recurrence but no improvement in survival: Study of the European Organization for Research and Treatment of Cancer Soft Tissue and Bone Sarcoma Group. *J Clin Oncol* 12:1137-1149.

Frustaci S, Gherlinzoni F, De Paoli A, et al. (1997) Preliminary results of an adjuvant randomized trial on high risk extremity soft tissue sarcomas (STS). The interim analysis. [Abstract]. *Proc Am Soc Clin Oncol* 16:1785.

Pisters PWT, Patel SR, Varma DGK, et al. (1997) Preoperative chemotherapy for stage IIIB extremity soft tissue sarcoma: Long-term results from a single institution. *J Clin Oncol* 15:3481–3487.

Tierney JF (1997) Adjuvant chemotherapy for localised resectable soft-tissue sarcoma of adults: meta-analysis of individual data. *Lancet* 350:1647–1654.

Combined Preoperative Chemotherapy and Radiotherapy

Eilber F, Giulano A, Huth JH, Mira J, Rosen G, Morton D (1988) Neoadjuvant chemotherapy, radiation, and limited surgery for high grade soft tissue sarcoma of the extremity. In:

Ryan JR, Baker LO (eds) *Recent Concepts in Sarcoma Treatment*. Kluwer, Dordrecht, The Netherlands, p. 115.

Spiro IJ, Suit H, Gebhardt M, et al. (1996) Neoadjuvant chemotherapy and radiotherapy for large soft tissue sarcomas. *Proc Am Soc Clin Oncol* 1689.

Treatment of Metastatic Sarcoma

McCormack P (1990) Surgical resection of pulmonary metastases. *Semin Surg Oncol* 6:297.

Santoro A, Tursz T, Mouridsen H, et al. (1995) Doxorubicin versus CYVADIC versus doxorubicin plus ifosfamide in first-line treatment of treatment of advanced soft tissue sarcomas: A randomized study of the European Organization for Research and Treatment of Cancer Soft Tissue and Bone Sarcoma Group. *J Clin Oncol* 13:1537.

Treatment of Retroperitoneal Sarcomas

Catton CN, O'Sullivan B, Kotwall C, Cummings B, Hao Y, Fornsier V (1994) Outcome and prognosis in retroperitoneal soft tissue sarcoma. *Int J Radiat Oncol Biol Phys* 29:1005–1010.

Heslin MJ, Lewis JJ, Nadler E (1997) Prognostic factors associated with long-term survival for retroperitoneal sarcoma: Implications for management. *J Clin Oncol* 15:2832.

Jaques DP, Coit DG, Hajdu SI, Brennan MF (1990) Management of primary and recurrent soft-tissue sarcoma of the retroperitoneum. *Ann Surg* 212:51.

Sindelar WF, Kinsella TJ, Chen PW, Delaney TF, Tepper JE, Rosenberg SA, et al. (1993) Intraoperative radiotherapy in retroperitoneal sarcomas. Final results of a prospective, randomized, clinical trial. *Arch Surg* 128:402–410.

CHAPTER 32

LYMPHOMAS

M.A. GIL-DELGADO, D. KHAYAT

Salpetriere Hospital
Medical Oncology Department
Paris, France

S.A.N. JOHNSON

Taunton and Somerset Hospital
Department of Haematology
Taunton, Somerset, England

The malignant lymphomas are a highly complex group of neoplasms. Attempts to classify these disorders have tried to relate the malignant proliferation to the equivalent normal cells, and with increasing sophistication of morphology, cytology, immunohistochemistry, and molecular biology methods it has become apparent that almost all non-Hodgkin's lymphomas are clonal proliferations in which all the cells arise from the same source. In contrast, Hodgkin's Disease is not usually associated with strong proof of clonality and the broad morphologic criteria used to establish the diagnosis may lead to problems in differentiating between Hodgkin's disease (HD), non-Hodgkin's lymphomas (NHL), and reactive lesions.

The wide distribution of lymphoid tissue within the body results in a range of clinical presentations and also produces a variety of sources for diagnostic material; lymph node biopsy may be replaced by or supplemented with tumor cells obtained from the blood, bone marrow, and a number of other extranodal sites that will together lead to accurate classification of the tumor.

Manual of Clinical Oncology, 7th edition, Edited by Raphael E. Pollock
ISBN 0-471-23828-7, pages 641–659. Copyright © 1999 Wiley-Liss, Inc.

NON-HODGKIN'S LYMPHOMAS

Epidemiology, Etiology, and Pathogenesis

The overall incidence of NHL is 10 to 15 cases per 100,000 population with a male preponderance; however, there are very considerable geographic variations in prevalence of the specific subtypes.

A viral etiology has been established for Burkitt's lymphoma (BL) by studies that emerged from its restricted geographic distribution; the high incidence of BL in tropical Africa and Papua New Guinea was shown to be associated with infection by the Epstein–Barr virus (EBV) at an early age. In vitro studies of EBV have shown that it is a potentially oncogenic virus that immortalizes B cells and it is proposed that this is the initial event in a multistep model for the pathogenesis of African BL. Subsequent events consist of stimulation of the immortalized B cells to proliferate (by malarial infection or other immunosuppressive factors), then chromosomal translocation results in irreversible c-*myc* activation and true malignant transformation. The pattern of lymphoma incidence in Japan is also dictated by the association between infection by human T-cell lymphotropic virus type I (HTLV-1) and a distinct form of T-cell lymphoma, adult T cell lymphoma–leukemia (ATLL); the Caribbean basin is also an endemic area for HTLV-1. In recent years acquired immunodeficiency syndrome (AIDS) following infection with human immunodeficiency virus (HIV) has resulted in a significant increase in the susceptibility to lymphoproliferative disorders mostly of high or intermediate grade and B-cell origin although Hodgkin's disease may also occur. A recently described subset of AIDS-related NHL in which the tumor grows predominantly in the pleural, pericardial, and abdominal cavities appears to be strongly associated with the presence of Kaposi's sarcoma-associated herpes virus (human herpesvirus 8) in the malignant cells, implying a causative role for the virus in producing these "primary effusion lymphomas." The incidence of NHL, however, appears to have been increasing over the last 30 years independent of the rise in HIV-related cases and the causative agents for most cases are not established.

A number of conditions that result in anomalies of the immune response are associated with an increased risk of developing NHL. Inherited conditions such as ataxia–telangiectasia and combined immunodeficiency syndrome are often accompanied by cytogenetic abnormalities but the relationship between these changes and the nonrandom translocations involving genes responsible for immunoglobin synthesis are not clear. In the X-linked immunoproliferative syndrome an expanded pool of immortalized cells is created as a result of EBV infection, and this may result in an unusual polyclonal malignant proliferation of B cells. Disease states that result in aberrant immunity as a secondary process such as rheumatoid arthritis, celiac disease, immunosuppressive therapy, and hypogammaglobulinaemia are also associated with an increased incidence of NHL. Neither the aforementioned mechanisms nor the involvement of specific viruses can account for the majority of cases of NHL; common subtypes such as follicular lymphoma (FL), although they are associated with well-defined nonrandom chromosomal translocation, do not appear to result from processes with an established sequence of steps leading to a malignant state.

The development of malignant lymphomas is assumed to result from the uncontrolled expansion of cells that have a normal counterpart in the immune system and it is therefore not surprising that lymphoma cells share morphologic and immunophenotypic characteristics with normal T and B cells in various states of activation and proliferation. The subsequent biologic characteristics of the malignant cells may be governed by additional genetic "hits" that confer more aggressive behavior and independence from the normal control mechanisms that regulate the response to antigen and contribution to the immune response.

Lymphomas of mucosa-associated lymphoid tissue (MALT lymphoma) are a particularly instructive example of the initiation of a malignant process from a reactive one. The association of MALT lymphoma with *Helicobacter pylori* infections of the stomach was followed by the observation that early-stage and low-grade disease could be induced to regress in response to anti-*Helicobacter* therapy (i.e., to withdrawal of antigenic stimulation) without the use of cytotoxic agents. It is models of disease behavior such as this that should encourage clinicians to treat each subtype of lymphoma as a different disease with its own distinctive genotypic and biologic pattern of behavior and that require its own specific approach to therapy.

Clinical Presentation, Investigation, and Staging

The majority of patients with NHL have generalized disease at presentation; however, it is important to identify those with only local involvement who may be primarily managed with radiotherapy. The course of the disease, prognosis, and treatment are influenced less by stage than by the cytologic type and bulk of the disease, so the most important initial management is designed to obtain an accurate tissue diagnosis and confidently exclude a reactive process.

Peripheral lymph node enlargement is present in 60% to 70% of patients, allowing an excision biopsy of a whole node to be taken so that both the nodal architecture and cytology can be assessed. If the lymphadenopathy is predominantly intraabdominal, adequate tissue may be obtained by computerized tomography (CT)-guided needle biopsy but representative material is not guaranteed by this approach. Other tissues may be the source of the primary site of NHL and so biopsy material from Waldeyer's ring, skin, gastrointestinal mucosa, liver, testis, and brain may prove to be involved by NHL. The incidence of bone marrow involvement is high, especially in a number of low-grade lymphomas; bone marrow aspiration may provide material for cytology, immunophenotyping, and molecular studies, while trephine biopsy may reveal the presence of focal or patchy involvement. It may be appropriate to retain part of the biopsy without fixation to permit immunocytochemical stains and extraction of DNA for gene rearrangement studies, using the remainder for conventional histology such as H&E- and Giemsa-stained sections together with immunohistochemical techniques with antibodies suitable for use on paraffin-embedded tissue.

Assessment of the patient at presentation should document the anatomic extent of the disease by physical examination, and measurements by lymph nodes should be clearly recorded in the patient's records in a reproducible format such as this:

	R	L
Cervical	$a \times b$ cm	—
Axillary	—	$c \times d$ cm
Inguinal	—	—
Tonsil	Enlarged	—

Liver = cm below costal margin

Spleen = cm below costal margin

This should be supplemented by radiological investigations including at least chest X-ray film and abdominal computerized tomography (CT) scan; gallium isotope scanning may be a useful additional means of documenting involved areas.

HD \
NHL —

Initial laboratory tests should consist of a full blood count (FBC), erythrocyte sedimentation rate (ESR), measurement of renal and hepatic function, serum lactate dehydrogenase (LDH), protein immunoelectrophoresis, and β_2-microglobulin.

Specific examination of extranodal sites is dictated by clinical signs, so although almost all patients will require bone marrow biopsy, fewer will need liver biopsy, gastrointestinal endoscopy, or detailed assessment of the central nervous system (CNS) by CT scan or lumbar puncture.

Although the Ann Arbor Staging System that is still used for the assessment of Hodgkin's disease helps define those patients who may be suitable for local therapy, treatment is more appropriately decided on the basis of risk stratification such as that proposed by the International Prognostic Index Project for patients with high-grade NHL (Table 32.1).

The problems of adequately staging extranodal lymphomas have resulted in alternative systems being proposed. For gastrointestinal lymphomas, the definition of

TABLE 32.1. International Index for Lymphoma

	0	1
Age	≤ 60	> 60
Performance status	0 or 1	2, 3, 4
Stage	I or II	III or IV
Extranodal involvement	< 2 sites	≥ 2 sites
LDH	Normal	High

	Risk
Low	0 or 1
Low/int	2
High/int	3
High	4 or 5

TABLE 32.2. Modified Blackledge Staging System for Primary Gastrointestinal Lymphomas

Stage I:	Tumor confined to gastrointestinal (GI) tract Single primary site or multiple, non-contiguous lesions
Stage II:	Tumor extending into abdomen from primary GI site Stage II_1 = local nodal involvement (paragastric or paraintestinal) Stage II_2 = distant nodal involvement (mesenteric, retroperitoneal, pelvic, inguinal)
Stage II_E:	Penetration of serosa to involve adjacent organs, or tissues (Enumerate actual sites of involvement, e.g., II_E (pancreas), II_E (post-abdominal wall) Where there is both nodal involvement and penetration to involve adjacent organs, stage should be denoted using both a subscript ($_1$ or $_2$) and E, for example II_{1E} (pancreas)
Stage IV:	Disseminated extranodal involvement or concomitant supradiaphragmatic nodal involvement

local disease by careful endoscopy is important, but extension of involvement into regional lymph nodes or distant sites must also be carefully assessed (Table 32.2).

Cutaneous T-cell lymphoma is frequently managed by local treatment in its early stages and a modified TNM system is used to guide treatment decisions (Table 32.3).

TABLE 32.3. TNM Classification of Cutaneous T-Cell Lymphoma

T—Skin	
T0	Clinical/histologically suspicious lesions
T1	Plaques/eczematous lesions $< 10\%$ skin surface
T2	Plaques/eczematous lesions $> 10\%$ skin surface
T3	Tumors
T4	Erythroderma
N—Lymph nodes	
N0	No clinically abnormal peripheral nodes
N1	Clinically abnormal peripheral nodes/pathology negative
N2	No clinically abnormal peripheral nodes/pathology positive
N3	Clinically abnormal peripheral nodes/pathology positive
B—Blood	
B0	Atypical peripheral blood mononuclear cells $< 5\%$
B1	Atypical peripheral blood mononuclear cells $> 5\%$
M—Visceral Organs	
M0	No visceral organ involvement
M1	Confirmed histological visceral involvement

Classification and Diagnostic Methods

Since the 1970s, different lymphoma classifications have been used in different parts of the world; the lack of agreement between the different systems has caused problems for practicing clinicians and created difficulties in interpreting published studies. The recent publication of the Revised European–American Lymphoma (REAL) classification and the anticipated publication of the updated World Health Organization (WHO) classification for hematologic malignancies represent serious attempts to establish an international consensus that takes account of current concepts of the biology of lymphomas.

Before immunophenotyping and molecular analyses were available, it was generally assumed that NHL was a single disease entity with a range of cytologic appearances and varying degrees of clinical aggressiveness; it was on this basis that the Working Formulation divided lymphomas into three prognostic groups (clinical grades) reflecting the survival prospects of the patients. Subsequently the use of immunologic reagents to assign lymphoma cells to either the B- or T-cell lineage and to a level of differentiation within the system (as reflected in the Kiel system) was extended by the realization that nonrandom chromosomal translocations are responsible for defining the biologic features of many lymphomas (Table 32.4). Many of these translocations result in the alignment of an oncogene with the gene responsible for either immunoglobin or T-cell receptor expression and produce specific abnormalities that favor the growth of the malignant clone. In addition to their use in establishing the diagnosis of an individual lymphoma, the detection of these

TABLE 32.4. Chromosomal Tumor Translocations Associated with NHL

	Chromosomal Translocation	Protooncogene	Partner Gene
B-Cell NHL			
LPL	t (9;14) (q13;q32)	*PAX-5*	*IgH*
FL, DLCL	t (14;18) (q32;q11)	*BCL-2*	*IgH*
	t (2;18) (q11;q11)	*BCL-2*	*IgK*
	t (18;22) (q11;q11)	*BCL-2*	*Igλ*
DLCL	t (3;?) (q27;?)	*BCL-6*	*IgH,IgL*
BL	t (8;14) (q24;q32)	*c-myc*	IgH
	t (2;8) (p11;q24)	*c-myc*	*IgK*
	t (8;22) (q24;q11)	*c-myc*	*IgK*
MCL	t (11;14) (q13;q32)	*BCL-1*	*IgH*
T-Cell NHL			
CD30+	t (2;5) (q23;q35)	*ALK*	—
ALCL	der (10) (q24)	*Lyt-10*	*X*
CTCL			

LPL, Lymphoplasmacytoid lymphoma; MCL mantle cell lymphoma; FL, follicular lymphoma; DLCL, diffuse large cell lymphoma; BL, Burkitt's lymphoma; ALCL, anaplastic large cell lymphoma; CTCL, cutaneous T-cell lymphoma.

translocations by sensitive polymerase chain reaction (PCR)-based assays may be utilized to monitor the presence of very low levels of "minimal residual disease" after treatment.

The REAL classification depends mainly on a combination of morphologic (and cytologic) criteria combined with the use of immunologic reagents to define cellular phenotype, a system that is aided by the availability of reliable reagents that can be used with paraffin-embedded tissue. Both lymphomas and lymphoid leukemias are included in this classification, as the distinction is an artificial one, and in addition Hodgkin's disease and plasma-cell myeloma are also included (Table 32.5).

Although it would appear that the large number of disease entities defined by the REAL classification will make clinical interpretation more difficult, it seems likely that real differences in the biology of lymphomas are being defined and as a consequence treatment decisions will be affected.

TABLE 32.5. Comparison of the REAL Classification with the Kiel Classification and Working Formulation

Kiel Classification	Revised European American Lymphoma Classification	Working Formulation
B-lymphoblastic	Precursor B-lymphoblastic lymphoma/leukemia	Lymphoblastic
B-Lymphocytic, CLL B-lymphocytic, prolymphocytic leukemia	B-cell chronic lymphocytic leukemia/prolymphocytic leukemia/small lymphocytic lymphoma	*Small lymphocytic consistent with CLL* Small lymphocytic, plasmacytoid
Lymphoplasmacytoid immunocytoma	Lymphoplasmacytoid lymphoma	*Small lymphocytic, plasmacytoid* Diffuse, mixed small and large cell
Centrocytic Centrobastic, centrocytoid subtype	Mantle cell lymphoma	Small lymphocytic *Diffuse, small cleaved cell* Follicular, small cleaved cell Diffuse, mixed small and large cell Diffuse, large cleaved cell
Centroblastic– Centrocytic Follicular	Follicular center lymphoma, follicular -Grade I -Grade II	*Follicular, predominantly small cleaved cell* *Follicular, mixed small and large cell*

(continued)

TABLE 32.5. Comparison of the REAL Classification with the Kiel Classification and Working Formulation *(continued)*

Kiel Classification	Revised European American Lymphoma Classification	Working Formulation
Centroblastic, follicular	-Grade III	Follicular, predominantly large cell
Centroblastic–centrocytic, diffuse	Follicular center lymphoma, diffuse, small cell [provisional]	*Diffuse, small cleaved cell* Diffuse, mixed small and large cell
—	Extranodal marginal zone B-cell lymphoma (low-grade B-cell lymphoma of MALT type)	*Small lymphocytic* Diffuse, small cleaved cell Diffuse, mixed small and large cell
Monocytoid, Including Marginal Zone	Nodal marginal zone B-cell lymphoma [provisional]	*Small lymphocytic*
Immunocytoma	—	Diffuse, small cleaved cell Diffuse, mixed small and large cell Unclassifiable
—	Splenic marginal zone B-cell lymphoma [provisional]	*Small lymphocytic* Diffuse small cleaved cell
Hairy cell leukemia	Hairy cell leukemia	—
Plasmacytic	Plasmacytoma/myeloma	*Extramedulary plasmacytoma*
Centroblastic (Monomorphic, polymorphic, and multilobated subtypes)	Diffuse large B-cell lymphoma	*Diffuse large cell* Large cell immunoblastic
B-Immunoblastic		Diffuse, mixed small and large cell
B-large cell anaplastic (Ki-l)		
—	Primary mediastinal large B-cell lymphoma	*Diffuse, large cell* Large cell immunoblastic
Burkitt's lymphoma	Burkitt's lymphoma	Small noncleaved cell, Burkitt's
—	High-grade B-cell lymphoma, Burkitt-like [provisional]	*Small noncleaved cell, non-Burkitt's*
? Some cases of centroblastic and immunoblastic	—	Diffuse, large cell Large cell immunoblastic
T-lymphoblastic	Precursor T-lymphoblastic lymphoma/leukemia	Lymphoblastic

TABLE 32.5. Comparison of the REAL Classification with the Kiel Classification and Working Formulation *(continued)*

Kiel Classification	Revised European American Lymphoma Classification	Working Formulation
T-Lymphocytic, CLL type	T-cell chronic lymphocytic, leukemia	Small lymphocytic Diffuse small cleaved cell
T-lymphocytic, prolymphocytic leukemia	prolymphocytic leukemia	—
T-lymphocytic, CLL type	Large granular lymphocytic leukemia -T-cell type -NK-cell type	*Small lymphocytic* Diffuse, small cleaved cell
Small-cell cerebriform (mycosis fungoides, Sezary syndrome)	Mycosis fungoides/Sezary syndrome	Mycosis fungoides
T-zone Lymphoepithelioid Pleomorphic, small T-cell	Peripheral T-cell lymphomas, unspecified [including provisional subtype: subcutaneous panniculitic T-cell lymphoma	Diffuse, small cleaved cell *Diffuse, mixed small and large cell large cell* Diffuse, large cell
Pleomorphic, Medium-Sized and Large T-Cell T-immunoblastic	Hepatosplenic γ-δ T-cell lymphoma [provisional]	*Large cell immunoblastic*
Angioimmunoblastic	Angioimmunoblastic T-cell	*Diffuse, mixed small and large cell*
(AILD, LgX)	lymphoma	*large cell* Diffuse, large cell *Large cell immunoblastic*
—	Angiocentric lymphoma	Diffuse, small cleaved cell *Diffuse, mixed small and large cell* Diffuse, large cell *Large cell immunoblastic*
—	Intestinal T-cell lymphoma	Diffuse, small cleaved cells Diffuse, mixed small and large cell Diffuse, large cells *Large cell immunoblastic*
Pleomorphic small T-cell HTLV1+	Adult T-cell lymphoma/leukemia	Diffuse, small cleaved cell
Pleomorphic Medium-Sized and Large T-Cell, HTLV1+		*Diffuse, mixed small ad large cell* Diffuse, large cell *Large cell immunoblastic*
T-large cell anaplastic (Ki-1+)	Anaplastic large cell lymphoma T- and null-cell types	Large cell immunoblastic

Treatment

A clinical schema can be derived from the REAL classification based on the clinical course of the respective entities and the results that can be expected from presently available treatment and modalities. Although this allows a broad guide to therapy there are considerable variations in treatment with respect to both individual disease and prognostic groupings (Table 32.6).

TABLE 32.6. Proposed Clinical Schema for Malignancies of the Lymphoid System

B-Cell Lineage	T-Cell Lineage
I. Indolent lymphomas (low risk)	I. Indolent lymphomas (low risk)
Chronic lymphocytic leukemia/small lymphocytic lymphoma	Large granular lymphocytic leukemia, T and NK cell types
Lymphoplasmacytic lymphoma/immunocytoma Waldenstrom's macroglobulinemia	Mycosis fungoides/Sezary syndrome Smoldering and chronic adult T-cell leukemia/lymphoma
Hairy cell leukemia	
Splenic marginal zone lymphoma	
Marginal zone B-cell lymphoma Extranodal (MALT-B-cell lymphoma) Nodal (monocytoid)	
Follicle center lymphoma/follicular, (small cell)—grade 1	
Follicle center lymphoma/follicular, (mixed small and large cell)—grade II	
II. Aggressive lymphomas (intermediate risk)	II. Aggressive lymphomas (intermediate risk)
Prolymphocytic leukemia	Prolymphocytic leukemia
Plasmacytoma/multiple myeloma	Peripheral T-cell lymphoma, unspecified
Mantle cell lymphoma	Angioimmunoblastic lymphoma
Follicle center lymphoma/follicular, (large cell)—grade III	Angio centric lymphoma
Diffuse large B-cell lymphoma (includes immunoblastic & diffuse large & centroblastic lymphoma)	Intestinal T-cell lymphoma Anaplastic large cell lymphoma (T- and null cell type)
Primary mediastinal (thymic) large B-cell lymphoma	
High-grade B-cell lymphoma, Burkitt-like	
III. Very aggressive lymphomas (high risk)	III. Very aggressive lymphomas (high risk)
Precursor B-lymphoblastic lymphoma/leukemia	Precursor T-lymphoblastic lymphoma/leukemia
Burkitt's lymphoma/ B-cell acute leukemia	Adult T-cell lymphoma/leukemia
Plasma cell leukemia	

INDOLENT (LOW RISK) LYMPHOMAS

Chronic Lymphocytic Leukemia/Small Lymphocytic Lymphoma

These conditions have been traditionally managed by observation only in the early stages. Alkylator (chlorambucil or cyclophosphamide) therapy is used for later stages, and anthracycline-based combinations for advanced disease. There is strong recent evidence to suggest that purine analogues (fludarabine, cladribine) are more active as both second line treatment and initial therapy, but they are contraindicated in patients with concurrent autoimmune hemolytic anemia. Combination purine analogue/alkylator therapy may be used as salvage therapy.

Waldenstrom's Macroglobulinemia

Purine analogues are considerably more active than alkylating agents in this condition.

Hairy Cell Leukemia

The use of interferon-α has largely been supplanted by short courses of pentostatin or single 5 to 7 day infusions of cladribine.

Marginal Zone Lymphoma

Gastric MALT lymphoma at early/localized stages and with low-grade histology may regress with anti-*Helicobacter* therapy alone but requires close endoscopic surveillance; alkylator based cytotoxic treatment may be needed for more extensive or unresponsive lesions.

Follicle Center Lymphoma

The pattern of response to therapy followed by repeated relapse with an increasing risk of transformation to higher grade disease at each recurrence has resulted in the view that not all patients benefit from therapy immediately after they are diagnosed. When treatment is required, initial therapy usually consists of alkylator-based approaches although patients with true stage I or II disease may be cured by involved field radiotherapy. The duration of response may be increased by inteferon-α maintenance. Later recurrences associated with transformation to higher grade disease are usually managed by anthracycline-containing combinations (e.g., CHOP). Purine analogues are active as single agents and extremely active in combination therapy. The role of high-dose therapy with hemopoietic stem cell support is being evaluated in younger patients and there is also early evidence of active immunotherapeutic agents (e.g., anti-CD20).

Mycosis Fungoides/Sezary Syndrome (CTCL)

Localized disease is managed with topical therapy (steroids, mustine) while more extensive involvement may respond to psoralen ultraviolet radiation (PUVA). In disease refractory to the above approaches but still localized total skin electron beam irradiation (TSEB) may still be curative; however, this does not apply to more extensive cutaneous involvement. Once the condition has progressed to tumor stage or erythrodermic forms it is likely to require a combination of cytotoxic chemotherapy and either retinoids or interferon. Single agents with activity include methotrexate, chlorambucil, cyclophosphamide, fludarabine, cladribine, and pentostatin while conventional combinations such as CHOP have also been used. When the disease has progressed to the point where cells are found in the circulation (Sezary syndrome) responses may still be obtained by the use of extracorporeal photochemotherapy.

Smoldering/Chronic ATLL

Disease which is truly clinically unaggressive may be treated with a combination of Zidovudine and interferon, while immunotherapeutic agents (anti-Tac) may also be active. The majority of patients treated in this way relapse and require more conventional cytotoxic therapy in conjunction with treatment to the CNS and aggressive control of hypercalcemia.

AGGRESSIVE (INTERMEDIATE RISK) LYMPHOMAS

Prolymphocytic Leukemias (B or T Cell)

These are generally refractory to alkylating agents but may respond to purine analogues. Immunotherapeutic agents (anti-CD52) appear promising.

Mantle Cell Lymphoma (MCL)

Even with modern therapy MCL is probably the NHL associated with the worst survival 10 years after diagnosis. Most patients are initially managed with alkylator-based combinations and the contribution of anthracyclines is uncertain. Trials are currently evaluating the early use of high-dose therapy with stem cell transplantation. Maintenance therapy with interferon-α may prolong the duration of response.

Follicle Center Cell Lymphoma (Large Cell Type)

Studies suggesting that initial cyclophosphamide/anthracycline-based combination chemotherapy can achieve high response rates with long remission durations have not been confirmed by all investigators. The prognosis of these patients may prove to be more reliably predicted by the criteria of the International Prognostic Index than by histologic selection alone.

TABLE 32.7. Standard CHOP for High-Grade NHL

Cyclophosphamide	750 mg/m^2 IV		
Doxorubicin	50 mg/m^2 IV	Day 1	Repeated every 21 days
Vincristine	1.4 mg/m^2 (max 2 mg IV)		
Prednisolone	100 mg PO daily	Days 1–5	

Diffuse Large B-Cell Lymphoma (DLCL)

For those with no strong risk of spread to the CNS, combination chemotherapy is the initial approach to treatment, and the large number of combinations promoted over the last 15 years have failed to produce results that are consistently better than those that can be achieved with CHOP for patients with low or low/intermediate risk disease (Table 32.7).

Patients with identifiably worse prognostic features are being evaluated to see whether they will benefit from intensified but conventional chemotherapy or high-dose therapy with stem-cell transplantation. Once a patient has failed initial chemotherapy, the outlook is poor; salvage therapy with etoposide- or cisplatin-based combinations may be effective but high-dose treatment is likely to benefit only those who are still at least partially sensitive to conventional-dose treatment.

Primary Mediastinal (Thymic) Large B-Cell Lymphoma

The initial management with conventional anthracycline-based combination chemotherapy commonly results in residual radiologic abnormalities that may or may not represent active disease. Consolidation therapy with radiotherapy is frequently given.

Peripheral T-Cell Lymphoma/Angioimmunoblastic Lymphoma/Angiocentric Lymphoma

These high-grade T-cell lymphomas are generally accepted to respond less well to conventional chemotherapy than the equivalent B-cell tumors.

Intestinal T-Cell Lymphoma

Conventional combination chemotherapy should be supplemented by gluten withdrawal for those patients whose disease arises on a background of celiac disease.

Anaplastic Large-Cell Lymphoma (CD30$^+$)

Although initially considered to be a very aggressive form of lymphoma, this is not the case. Childhood disease has a better prognosis than that in adults and isolated cutaneous lesions are more responsive than those with nodal presentation.

Primary CNS Lymphoma (HIV+)

The differential diagnosis of AIDS-related CNS lymphoma involves careful exclusion of infection (e.g., toxoplasmosis) and even when biopsy material is available the prognosis is poor. Good symptom control can be achieved with cranial irradiation but survival is short; meningeal involvement may be treated with intrathecal methotrexate and/or cytosine arabinoside. Systemic cytotoxic agents with the capacity to cross the blood–brain barrier include idarubicin, high-dose methotrexate, high-dose cytosine arabinoside, nitrosoureas, and dexamethasone.

VERY AGGRESSIVE (HIGH RISK) LYMPHOMAS

Lymphoblastic Lymphomas (LL)/Acute Lymphoblastic Leukemia (ALL)/Burkitt's Lymphoma

These conditions are neoplasms arising from precursor cells at various stages of differentiation in both T- and B-cell lineages. Particular management problems at presentation may include anatomic complications of the presence of a large mediastinal mass and metabolic consequences of uric acid nephropathy. Induction therapy tends to follow the pattern of treatment used for ALL with full CNS prophylaxis involving intrathecal therapy and cranial irradiation. Consolidation with autologous bone marrow transplantation has been widely used, and the prognosis for disease associated with t(9;22) and t(4;11) is so poor that allogeneic transplantation is felt to offer the only chance of cure.

HODGKIN'S DISEASE

Epidemiology, Etiology, and Pathogenesis

HD is an uncommon malignancy with incidence rates ranging between 1 and 4/100,000 except in Asian countries, where it is much less common. There is an unusual age pattern with a bimodal curve showing peaks at ages 15 to 40 and over 55 years. Overall, HD is more common in males than females but there is little difference for the nodular sclerosing subtype which also lacks the association with EBV infections of Reed–Sternberg cells, which is a feature of cases in children from lower socioeconomic groups. Considerable effort has gone into exploring an infectious etiology for HD, but despite strong circumstantial evidence a direct causative relationship has not been established.

Although HD classically has a low proportion of the clonal, malignant Reed–Sternberg cells (RS) the immunophenotype of lymphocyte predominant (LP) HD is frequently associated with B-cell markers and the RS cells may show rearrangements of the *IgH* locus, implying a B-cell germinal-center origin for these cases. The classic features of the other types of HD are variably associated with impaired immune response, sclerosis, T-cell activation and proliferation, plasmacytosis, and eosinophilia, all of which suggest a condition of abnormal cytokine production; there are proposals that the tissue eosinophilia may contribute to unregulated growth by providing ligands for CD30 and CD40 that can stimulate the RS cell.

Clinical Presentation, Investigation, and Staging

The diagnosis of HD is made after peripheral lymph-node biopsy in more than 90% of cases; the characteristic symptoms consist of weight loss, fever, sweats, and itching but are much less common in patients with localized disease (8% in stage I, 29% in stage II) than in extensive disease (41% in stage III, 71% in stage IV).

Investigations are designed to define the anatomic extent of disease so that the appropriate treatment decision can be taken in relation to radiotherapy for localized disease or chemotherapy for more extensive disease. Although the detailed information provided by staging laparotomy contributed greatly to knowledge of the natural history of HD it is not now felt to be justified. Radiologic investigation with lymphangiography has also been replaced by the use of CT imaging of the abdomen and thorax although this approach may fail to detect splenic involvement. The yield of bone-marrow biopsy in localized disease is very low but it is advisable in patients with extensive (stage III or IV) involvement by other criteria. Laboratory investigations are principally of use in following the response to treatment where correction of abnormal ESR or LDH may confirm resolution of disease while persistence of elevated levels may prompt a careful search for residual disease.

The well-established Ann Arbor system has been revised to clarify some aspects relating to the distribution of disease and the implications of large areas of involvement (Table 32.8).

Classification and Diagnostic Methods

The Rye Classification graded HD according to the content of lymphocytes as either Lymphocyte Predominant (LP) or Lymphocyte Depleted (LD), accounting together for about 5% to 10% of total HD with larger groups of Nodular Sclerosis (NS) and Mixed Cellularity (MC), but the recent REAL classification has also identified a provisional entity called lymphocyte-rich classic HD.

REAL Classification

- Lymphocytic predominance nodular (with or without diffuse areas)
- Lymphocyte rich, classic disease

- Nodular sclerosis
- Mixed cellularity
- Lymphocyte depletion

Rye Classification

- Lymphocyte predominance, nodular (most cases)
- Lymphocyte predominance diffuse + lymphocyte predominant mixed cellularity
- Nodular sclerosis
- Mixed cellularity (most cases)
- Lymphocyte depletion

TABLE 32.8. The Ann Arbor Staging System/Cotswold's Revision

Stage	Characteristics
I	Involvement of a single lymph node region or of a single extranodal organ or site (IE)
II	Involvement of two or more lymph node regions on the same side of the diaphragm or localized involvement of an extranodal organ or site (IIE) and one or more lymph node regions on the same side of the diaphragm. R and L hilum regarded as one area, each independent of mediastinum
III	Involvement of lymph node regions on both sides of the diaphragm that may be accompanied by involvement of the spleen (IIIS) or by localized contiguous involvement of only one extranodal organ site (IIIE) or both (IIIES)
III1	With involvement limited to spleen, hilar portal, or celiac nodes
III2	With involvement of para-aortic, iliac, or mesenteric nodes.
IV	Diffuse or disseminated involvement of one or more distant extranodal sites with or with or without associated lymph node involvement
Bulky disease	Mediastinum/thoracic ratio > 1:3 at the T5–6 level; mass > 10 cm
Subclassification	
A	No symptoms
B	Fever, night sweats, weight loss >10% of body weight over 6 months.

Although LP HD is a rare entity, its B-cell origin, high initial response rate, and occasional capacity for very late relapse are characteristic of the natural history. The distinction from T-cell-rich B-cell lymphoma (a form of NHL) may be very difficult. The natural history of LD HD is also established as being more aggressive than other types of HD and differentiation between this subtype and anaplastic large cell lymphoma may cause problems unless the t(2;5) translocation characteristic of that form of NHL is detected. Nodular Sclerosis histology is strongly correlated with young age, female gender, and clinical presentation with mediastinal involvement and has a favorable prognosis, especially in early stage disease, where Mixed Cellularity is more frequently associated with extralymphatic spread and has a worse prognosis.

Treatment

The early experience of successful treatment of patients with HD by either radiotherapy or combination chemotherapy has been affected by the appreciation that increases in the aggressiveness of management were causing immediate and delayed toxicities that were not balanced by an improvement in survival. It also became clear that the efficacy of salvage therapy, especially in patients initially treated with radiotherapy alone, would achieve durable responses in many patients with relapsed disease.

Stage I and II patients without additional adverse prognostic factors (B symptoms; bulky disease, including mediastinal involvement; large number of sites) have

TABLE 32.9. Standard ABVD for Hodgkin's Disease

Doxorubicin	25 mg/m^2	
Bleomycin	10 mg/m^2	Days 1 and 14 repeated every 28 days
Vinblastine	6 mg/m^2	
Dacarbazine	375 mg/m^2	

a low risk of occult abdominal disease and may be treated with radiotherapy to a mantle field alone. Although up to 40% of those staged clinically (i.e., without laparotomy) may relapse eventually, many of these will obtain further complete remissions with chemotherapy, whereas those continuing to be free of disease after radiotherapy alone will have preserved their fertility and have a low risk of secondary malignancy. Second solid tumors (e.g., lung, stomach, breast) are more common after extended field radiotherapy.

Patients with stage IA or IIA disease and adverse prognostic factors require combined chemoradiotherapy, and in a typical presentation such as the young woman with bulky mediastinal NS HD treatment will consist of four cycles of combination chemotherapy followed by radiotherapy to 40 Gy to *at least* the area of bulky disease.

The nature of the chemotherapy administered to patients with either symptomatic or more extensive disease (IIB, III, IV) now generally reflects a compromise between effective eradication of HD and severe late toxicity. The association of older alkylator-based (MOPP type) chemotherapy with infertility and the induction of secondary acute leukemias has led to the wider use of anthracycline-containing single, alternating or "hybrid" combinations (Table 32.9).

An analysis of the pattern of recurrence after chemotheapy has led many groups to follow chemotherapy by radiotherapy to initial sites of bulky disease.

Salvage therapy after failure of initial chemotherapy exploits the steep dose–response curve that HD has for many chemotherapeutic agents. Cytoreduction using non-cross-reactive agents (such as combinations with etoposide and/or vinorelbine) can be followed by high-dose chemotherapy (e.g., BCNU etoposide ara-C Melphalan (BEAM) supported by hemopoietic stem cells. As with the salvage of NHL, retention of some degree of response to conventional-dose chemotherapy is a prerequisite for achieving worthwhile responses.

FURTHER READING

The text has been prepared from a large number of published sources; the following list contains key articles that form a reading list for those wishing to extend their knowledge.

1. Bartlett NL, Rosenberg SA, Hoppe RT, et al. (1995) Brief chemotherapy, Stanford V, and adjuvant radiotherapy for bulky or advanced-stage Hodgkin's disease: A preliminary report. *J Clin Oncol* 13:1080–1088.

2. Biti GP, Cimino G, Cartoni C, et al. (1992) Extended-field radiotherapy is superior to MOPP chemotherapy for the treatment of pathological stage I-IIA Hodgkin's disease: Eight-year update of an Italian prospective randomised study. *J Clin Oncol* 10:378–382.

3. Chopra R, McMillan AK, Linch DC, et al. (1993) The place of high-dose BEAM therapy and autologous bone marrow transplantation in poor-risk Hodgkin's disease. A single-centre eight-year study of 155 patients. *Blood* 81: 1137–1145.

4. Deangelis LM (1995) Current management of primary central nervous system lymphoma. *Oncol Huntingt* 9:63–71.

5. Diamandidou E, Cohen PR, Kurzrock R (1996) Mycosis fungoides and Sezary syndrome. *Blood* 88:2385–2409.

6. Fisher RI, Gaynor ER, Dahlberg S, et al. (1993) Comparison of a standard regimen (CHOP) with three intensive chemotherapy regimens for advanced non-Hodgkin's lymphoma. *N Engl J Med* 328:1002–1006.

7. Gribben JG, Saporito L, Barber M, et al. (1992) Bone marrows of non-Hodgkin's lymphoma patients with a *Bcl-2* translocation can be purged of polymerase chain reaction-detectable lymphoma cells using monoclonal antibodies and immunomagnetic bead depletion. *Blood* 80:1083–1089.

8. Haluska FG, Brufsky AM, Cannellos GP (1994) The cellular biology of the Reed–Sternberg cell. *Blood* 84:1005–1019.

9. Harris NL, Jaffe ES, Stein H, et al. (1994) A Revised European-American classification of lymphoid neoplasms: A proposal from the International Lymphoma Study Group. *Blood* 84:1361–1392.

10. Hiddemann W, Longo DL, Coiffier B, et al. (1996) Lymphoma classification—the gap between biology and clinical management is closing. *Blood* 88:4085–4089.

11. International Non-Hodgkin's Lymphomas Prognostic Factors Project. (1993) A predictive model for aggressive non-Hodgkin's lymphoma. *N Engl J Med* 329:987–994.

12. Johnson SA (1996) Purine analogues in the management of lymphoproliferative diseases. *Clin Oncol* 8:289–296.

13. Jox A, Rohen C, Belge C, et al. (1997) Integration of Epstein-Barr virus in Burkitt's lymphoma cells leads to a region of enchanced chromosome instability. *Ann Oncol* 8 (Suppl 2):S131–S135.

14. Mac-Manus MP, Hoppe RT (1996) Is radiotherapy curative for stage I and II low-grade follicular lymphoma? Results of a long-term follow-up study of patients treated at Stanford University. *J Clin Oncol* 14:1282–1290.

15. Mauvieux L, MacIntyre EA (1996) Practical role of molecular diagnostics in non-Hodgkin's lymphomas. *Baillieres Clin Haematol* 9:653–667.

16. McLaughlin P, Hagemeister FB, Romaguera JE, et al. (1996) Fludarabine, mitoxantrone and dexamethasone: An effective new regimen for indolent lymphoma. *J Clin Oncol* 14:1262–1268.

17. Morel P, Lepage E, Brice P, et al. (1992) Prognosis and treatment of lymphoblastic lymphoma in adults: A report on 80 patients. *J Clin Oncol* 10:1078–1085.

18. Morgan G, Vornanen M, Puitinen J, et al. (1997) Changing trends in the incidence of non-Hodgkin's lymphoma in Europe. *Ann Oncol 8* (Suppl 2):S49–S54.

19. Nador RG, Cesarman E, Chadburn A, et al. (1996) Primary effusion lymphoma: A distinct clinicopathological entity associated with the Kaposi's sarcoma associated herpes virus. *Blood* 88:645–656.

20. Rohatiner A (1994) Report on a workshop convened to discuss the pathological and staging classifications of gastrointestinal tract lymphoma. *Ann Oncol* 5:397–400.

21. Zucca E, Stein H, Coiffier B on behalf of the European Lymphoma Task Force. (1994) Report on the workshop on Mantle Cell Lymphoma. *Ann Oncol* 5:507–511.

CHAPTER 33

THE LEUKEMIAS

FREDERICK R. APPELBAUM

The Fred Hutchinson Cancer Research Center
and
The University of Washington School of Medicine
Seattle, WA 98109 USA

DEFINITION AND CATEGORIZATION

Normal hematopoiesis requires the controlled proliferation and orderly differentiation of pluripotent hematopoietic stem cells to become mature peripheral blood cells. Leukemia is the result of a genetic event or series of events occurring in a hematopoietic precursor causing the affected cell and its progeny to no longer proliferate and differentiate normally.

The leukemias are broadly categorized according to the normal cell population they most resemble (i.e., myeloid versus lymphoid) and according to their clinical aggressiveness (see Table 33.1). In the case of the acute leukemias, the malignant event occurs in a very early hematopoietic precursor. The altered cells continue to proliferate but fail to differentiate, resulting in the rapid accumulation of immature myeloid (in acute myeloid leukemia) or lymphoid (in acute lymphoid leukemia) cells in the marrow. These cells replace normal bone marrow, resulting in the diminished production of normal red cells, white cells, and platelets which, in turn, gives rise to the usual manifestations of acute leukemia, including anemia, infection, and bleeding. The leukemic cells also escape into the bloodstream and occupy the lymph nodes, spleen, and other vital organs. The acute leukemias are rapidly fatal if left untreated, with most patients dying within several months of diagnosis. The chronic leukemias are also clonal malignancies of hematopoietic cells, but the malignant cells are able to differentiate in a more nearly normal manner. Accordingly, these

Manual of Clinical Oncology, 7th edition, Edited by Raphael E. Pollock
ISBN 0-471-23828-7, pages 661–687. Copyright © 1999 Wiley-Liss, Inc.

TABLE 33.1. The Leukemias

  I. Acute leukemia
     A. Acute myeloid leukemia
     B. Acute lymphocytic leukemia

 II. Chronic leukemia
     A. Chronic myeloid leukemia
     B. Chronic lymphocytic leukemia

III. Myelodysplastic syndromes

 IV. Chronic myeloproliferative disorders
     A. Polycythemia vera
     B. Essential thrombocythemia
     C. Agnogenic myeloid metaplasia

  V. Hairy cell leukemia

disorders are characterized by the overproliferation of relatively mature cells that resemble normal neutrophils (in chronic myeloid leukemia), normal lymphocytes (in chronic lymphocytic leukemia), normal red cells (in polycythemia vera), or normal platelets (in essential thrombocythemia). Even untreated, patients can live for several years with these disorders. However, with time, the accumulation of abnormal cells results in lack of production of normal cells. In addition, the malignant clones are genetically unstable and accumulate additional genetic abnormalities, resulting in the eventual progression to a disorder that more closely resembles acute leukemia.

ETIOLOGY AND EPIDEMIOLOGY

Epidemiology

The annual incidence of leukemia is approximately 8 to 10 new cases per 100,000. The relative incidences of the four most common forms of leukemia are acute lymphocytic leukemia (ALL), 11%; chronic lymphocytic leukemia (CLL), 29%; acute myeloid leukemia (AML), 40%; and chronic myelogenous leukemia (CML), 14%. Males are more commonly affected than females. These incidence rates have been fairly stable over the last 30 years. ALL is the most common leukemia seen in childhood and shows the least increase with age. All other forms of leukemia are relatively uncommon in children and increase in incidence with age, particularly beyond age 50. In general, there are not marked variations in leukemic incidence among countries, although CLL is reported to be less frequent in the Asian population.

In the large majority of cases, no cause of leukemia can be found, but in occasional cases, a likely reason can be identified.

Genetic Predisposition

There is an approximately one in five chance that a child will develop leukemia if he or she has an identical twin with leukemia diagnosed before age 10. Several families have been identified without other known genetic diseases in which multiple members have developed similar forms of leukemia. An increased incidence of leukemia exists in patients with the autosomal recessive disorders associated with chromosomal instability including Fanconi's anemia, Bloom's syndrome, and ataxia–telangiectasia. Also, patients with congenital immunodeficiency disorders, including infantile X-linked agammaglobulin anemia and Down's syndrome, have a higher than expected incidence of leukemia.

Viruses

An uncommon form of leukemia, adult T-cell leukemia (ATL), is associated with human T-cell lymphotrophic virus type 1 (HTLV-1). The virus is common in southwestern Japan, the Caribbean basin, and Africa and can be spread by sexual contact, blood transfusions, and from mother to fetus. Approximately 1% to 2% of those infected with HTLV-1 will develop ATL, usually after a very long latency period of 10 to 30 years. Blood banks in the United States now routinely screen for HTLV-1. Rare cases of an unusual chronic lymphoid leukemia have been linked with a second human retrovirus, HTLV-2.

Radiation

Previous studies showed that the incidences of AML, ALL, and CML, but not CLL, were increased in patients given radiation therapy for ankylosing spondylitis, in radiologists practicing when shielding was inadequate, and in survivors of the atomic bomb in Hiroshima and Nagasaki. The increased incidence of leukemia starts several years after exposure, appears to peak at 5 to 10 years, and then diminishes. A number of studies have asked whether exposure to low-frequency nonionizing electromagnetic fields increases the risk of leukemia and most have failed to find any association.

Chemicals and Drug Exposure

Heavy exposure to benzene and benzene-containing solvents such as kerosene can cause marrow damage leading to myelodysplasia or AML. There is a suggested link between heavy exposure to pesticides and an increased chance of developing CLL. Prior exposure to alkylating agents such as chlorambucil, nitrogen mustard, and melphalan increases the risk of developing AML. Such secondary leukemias often present initially as a myelodysplastic syndrome 4 to 7 years after exposure and are associated with abnormalities of chromosomes 5 and 7. Exposure to the epipodophyllotoxins teniposide or etoposide increases the risk for developing AML with abnormalities of 11q23. These cases develop after a shorter period, 2 to 3 years, lack a myelodysplastic prodrome, and often have a monocytic morphology.

ACUTE MYELOID LEUKEMIA

Biology

Pathophysiology AML, like all leukemias, is a clonal disorder with all leukemic cells developing from a single precursor. The precise molecular events causing malignant transformation in AML are not completely understood but result in the uncontrolled proliferation of immature hematopoietic cells that have lost the ability to differentiate. Several lines of evidence suggest that the development of overt leukemia is a multistep process, including the fact that in many cases AML is preceded by a prolonged myelodysplastic disorder, and the observation that, following chemotherapy, some patients enter a complete remission devoid of obvious malignant cells but with clonal hematopoiesis. The level of differentiation at which AML becomes evident is variable. In some cases, the malignancy occurs in a very early hematopoietic precursor and all red cells and platelets along with all myeloid cells originate from the malignant clone. In other cases, only myeloid cells derive from the malignant clone and red cells and platelets do not. As the malignant clone expands, normal hematopoiesis fails. The reasons for this are complex, but both actual physical replacement of normal precursors as well as release of soluble substances by leukemic cells that suppress normal hematopoiesis are thought to play important roles.

Classification AML is generally classified according to cell morphology but is also classified according to cell-surface markers and cytogenetics. AML is usually classified according to the French–American–British (FAB) system, which subdivides AML into eight subtypes according to morphology and histochemistry (see Table 33.2). AML cells are typically 12 to 15 μm in diameter with discrete nuclear chromatin, multiple nucleoli, and cytoplasmic azurophilic granules. Subtypes M0 through M3 reflect increasing degrees of maturation; M4 and M5 AMLs have some degree of monocytic differentiation; M6 leukemia has features of erythroid lineage; and M7 is acute megakaryocytic leukemia. FAB types M1 to M4 contain myeloperoxidase whereas M4 and M5 have the monocytic enzyme nonspecific esterase. These morphologic subtypes have some, but only limited, clinical relevance. The most distinct subgroup is M3 AML (also called acute promyelocytic leukemia), which is usually associated with the t(15;17) and responds well to all-*trans*-retinoic acid. Complete response rates and overall survival are best with M2, M3, and M4 AML. Patients with M6 AML may have a smoldering course. Antibodies reactive with cell-surface antigens can be used to help diagnose and classify AML. Most cases of AML react with antibodies specific for CD13, CD14, CD33, and CD34. M6 AML reacts with antibodies against glycophorin, whereas M7 AML cells react with antibodies against CD41, also known as GpIIb/IIIa.

TABLE 33.2. Classification of AML

Subtype	Morphology	Histochemistry			Monoclonal Reactivity	Cytogenetic Abnormalities
		Myeloperoxidase	Nonspecific Esterase	PAS		
M0 Acute undifferentiated leukemia	Uniform, very undifferentiated	—	—	—	For subtypes M0–M5b, approximately 90% of cases will react with at least one of the following antimyeloid antibodies:	Various
M1 Acute myeloid leukemia with minimal differentiation	Very undifferentiated, few azurophilic granules	+/-	+/-	—		Various
M2 Acute myeloid leukemia with differentiation	Granulated blasts predominate; Auer rods may be seen.	+++	+	+	Anti-CD13	Various
M3 Acute promyelocytic leukemia	Hypergranular promyelocytes predominate.	+++	+	+	Anti-CD14 Anti-CD33	t(15;7)
M4 Acute myelomonocytic leukemia	Both monoblasts and myeloblasts present. Like M4 but with eosinophils	++	+++	++	Anti-CD34	Various inv/del(16)
M5 Acute monocytic leukemia M5a M5b	Monoblasts predominate. Type a >80% monoblasts Type b >20% promonocytes	+/-	+++	++		Various, including t(9;11)
M6 Acute erythroleukemia	Erythroblasts and megaloblastic red cell precursors seen.	—	—	++	Antiglycophorin, antispectrin	Various
M7 Acute megakaryocytic leukemia	Undifferentiated blasts	—	+/-	+	Antiplatelet GpIIb/IIIa	Various

AML can also be characterized by the clonal chromosomal abnormality seen in each case. The most frequent abnormalities are a gain of chromosome 8 or a loss of part or all of chromosomes 7 or 5. Each of these changes is seen in 5% to 10% of cases of AML and are associated with a poor prognosis. In contrast, several translocations are associated with a favorable prognosis in AML, including t(8;21) and inv(16), the latter being seen in M4 AML with abnormal eosinophils. As noted earlier, acute promyelocytic leukemia (APL) is virtually always associated with t(15;17). In addition to providing diagnostic and prognostic information, the identification of specific cytogenetic abnormalities associated with particular leukemias has aided in the identification of the particular oncogenes involved. For example, the t(15;17) associated with APL has been found to result in the fusion of a transcription factor (PML) on chromosome 15 with the α-retinoic acid receptor gene (RARα) on chromosome 17. The t(8;21) abnormality involves the fusion of a gene termed *ETO* with one termed CBF-α (for core binding factor-α) resulting in the production of a chimeric protein generated by the t(8;21) that inhibits the function of genes normally stimulated by CBF-α.

Clinical Features

The signs and symptoms of AML are the result of decreased production of normal blood cells and invasion of leukemic blasts into normal organs. Most patients are anemic and thrombocytopenic at diagnosis, resulting in fatigue and pallor, and in at least one third of patients there is clinically evident bleeding, usually in the form of petechiae, ecchymoses, and bleeding gums. Most patients are also granulocytopenic, and approximately one third will have a significant infection at diagnosis. Occasional patients will present with extramedullary leukemic masses, termed chloromas, which are rubbery and fast growing. Also, cutaneous involvement (leukemia cutis) and central nervous system (CNS) involvement are occasionally seen.

Laboratory Manifestations

Anemia is seen in most patients at diagnosis, as is thrombocytopenia. Approximately 25% of patients have severe thrombocytopenia ($<20,000/mm^3$). Most are granulocytopenic, but the total white cell count may be very high ($>50,000/mm^3$) in 25%, moderately elevated (between 5000 and $50,000/mm^3$) in 50%, or low ($<5000/mm^3$) in 25%. Blasts are usually present in peripheral blood. The bone marrow is usually hypercellular and contains from 30% to 100% blasts. Sometimes other findings are also present including marrow fibrosis (in M7 AML) or, rarely, marrow necrosis.

Differential Diagnosis

Although there are sometimes difficulties in subclassifying leukemia, usually the diagnosis is straightforward. Aplastic anemia and myelodysplasia can result in peripheral pancytopenia, but in neither are large numbers of blasts seen on marrow exam. Other small round cell neoplasms can infiltrate the marrow and sometimes mimic leukemia, but immunologic and cytogenetic markers now make these distinctions usually relatively easy. Leukemoid reactions can be seen in certain infections including tuberculosis but, although young myeloid cells may be seen in the peripheral blood in some settings, they virtually never reach 30%.

Treatment

Remission Induction   AML is a rapidly progressive disease and, without treatment, most patients will die within several months of diagnosis. With appropriate therapy, however, many patients can now be cured. The first goal of treatment is to achieve an initial remission. Treatment with a combination of an anthracycline (daunomycin or idarubicin) and cytarabine can induce complete remissions in 60% to 80% of patients. In randomized studies, use of additional drugs such as etoposide or high-dose instead of conventional dose cytarabine have failed to improve the complete response rate. Profound myelosuppression is always seen following induction chemotherapy. The period of myelosuppression can be shortened by several days with the use of myeloid growth factors, but their use has not been found to improve overall complete response rates.

Postremission Chemotherapy   If no therapy is given after induction, the duration of remission will be short and most patients will relapse within 6 months. If, after achieving a complete remission, patients are treated with two to four courses of consolidation chemotherapy using an anthracycline and cytarabine at doses similar to those used for initial induction, the median survival in AML can be extended to approximately 18 months and 15% to 20% of patients can be cured. The best results achieved to date with postremission chemotherapy involves treating patients with repeated cycles of high-dose cytarabine. In one large randomized trial, approximately 40% of patients treated with four cycles of high-dose cytarabine, 1.5 g/m^2 every 12 hours on days 1, 3, and 5, were alive and disease-free at 3 years. In a second trial, approximately 35% of patients treated with two cycles of high-dose cytarabine, 1 g/m^2 q12 hours days 1 to 6 were alive and disease-free at 3 years. If patients are treated with intensive postremission chemotherapy, there is no clear role for the addition of low-dose maintenance or late intensification chemotherapy, or CNS prophylaxis.

Risk Factors   A number of factors correlate with the likelihood of achieving an initial complete remission and with remission duration (Table 33.3). Younger patients, those with a low white cell count at diagnosis, without a prior hematologic disorder, and with blasts with t(8;21), inv(16) or t(15;17) do relatively well. Older patients, patients with high white cell counts at diagnosis, a prior history of myelodysplasia and with blasts that express the multidrug resistance gene-1 (*MDR-1*) or with abnormalities of chromosomes 5, 7, and 8 do worse.

Chemotherapy for Relapsed Patients   Patients who relapse following chemotherapy can, in approximately 30% to 50% of cases, achieve a second remission, but the duration of such remissions tends to be short, on average, 6 months. The longer

TABLE 33.3. Prognosis in Acute Myeloid Leukemia.

Unfavorable	Favorable
Advanced age	Younger age
High WBC at diagnosis	Low WBC at diagnosis
Prior myelodysplasia	No prior myelodysplasia
MDR-1 positive	MDR-1 negative
Cytogenetics:	Cytogenetics:
Abnormalities of 5,7	t(8;21)
t(9;11)	t(15;17)
Trisomy 13	inv(16)

the initial remission, the better the chance of achieving a second complete remission (CR).

Bone Marrow Transplantation   High-dose chemotherapy with or without total body irradiation (TBI) followed by matched sibling bone marrow transplantation is being increasingly used to treat AML in patients age <55 years. For patients who fail to achieve an initial complete remission, allogeneic marrow transplantation offers the only realistic chance for a cure. Prior studies have shown that approximately 15% to 20% of such patients can be saved. Similarly, patients who have relapsed after chemotherapy and have failed reinduction can be cured with allogeneic transplantation in 15% to 20% of cases. The results improve if transplantation is carried out earlier in the course of disease, with success in approximately 30% to 35% of patients transplanted in first relapse or second remission and with 50% to 60% cure rates with matched sibling transplantation in first remission. Only about one third of patients have matched siblings. For those without such donors, the use of autologous transplantation is being increasingly explored. The results of autologous transplantation have generally been slightly inferior to those achieved with matched sibling transplantation owing to a considerably higher risk of posttransplant relapse, although the immediate risks with autologous transplantation are less. In a large prospective randomized trial, the 4-year disease-free survival with matched sibling transplantation was 55% versus 48% for autologous transplantation and 30% with high-dose chemotherapy. Studies using matched unrelated donor transplantation are also being conducted.

Acute Promyelocytic Leukemia   Acute promyelocytic leukemia deserves special mention because of its increased sensitivity to therapy with all-*trans*-retinoic acid (ATRA). ATRA alone induces complete responses in 75% of patients with APL. Unlike conventional chemotherapy, ATRA appears to work, at least in part, by inducing terminal differentiation of leukemic blasts. Within several days of starting ATRA, the coagulation disorders associated with APL begin to improve and the number of both abnormal and normal granulocytes begins to increase. Morphologic analysis of bone marrow over the first weeks of ATRA therapy shows progressive differentiation of malignant cells without hypoplasia. Complete remissions using ATRA alone generally take 2 to 3 months. Although ATRA alone can induce complete responses, virtually all patients treated with ATRA as a single agent will subsequently relapse. The combination of ATRA with chemotherapy appears more effective in inducing complete remissions than the use of either agent alone. The best form of postremission therapy in APL is not entirely defined. Studies suggest that APL is particularly sensitive to anthracycline treatment and thus most experts recommend its inclusion during consolidation, whereas the role of high-dose cytarabine is more questionable. At least one randomized study suggests that ATRA maintenance prolongs disease-free survival.

A potentially dangerous side effect of ATRA is the development of a syndrome characterized by pulmonary infiltrates and shortness of breath. This ATRA syndrome is more commonly seen in patients who develop leukocytosis on ATRA and can be fatal. In patients who develop evidence of the ATRA syndrome, ATRA should be temporarily discontinued and they should be treated with Decadron. In the majority of patients, the syndrome will resolve and ATRA can be restarted. Other adverse effects of ATRA include skin and mucosal membrane dryness, headache, and bone pain.

ACUTE LYMPHOCYTIC LEUKEMIA

Biology

Like AML, ALL is a clonal proliferation of an early hematopoietic progenitor, but in contrast to AML, the ALL blasts resemble very early lymphoid cells. The FAB schema classifies ALL cases as being L1, L2, or L3 (see Table 33.4). L1 blasts are uniform in size with scanty cytoplasm, indistinct nucleoli, and few, in any, granules. L2 blasts are larger and more heterogeneous in size and may have nucleoli. L3 blasts are quite distinct with deeply basophilic cytoplasm containing vacuoles and with prominent nucleoli. ALL cases can also be categorized according to cell surface antigens. Approximately 60% of cases express CD10, also known as the common ALL antigen or CALLA. Such cases usually coexpress early B-cell antigens such as CD19 and thus are thought to represent a very early B-cell differentiation state (a pre-pre-B cell). About 20% of CALLA-positive cases also have intracytoplasmic immunoglobulin, suggesting a slightly greater differentiative state (pre-B cell). Approximately 5% of cases express surface immunoglobulin, thus representing a more differentiated state (B-cell ALL). Approximately 20% of cases of ALL are of T-cell origin and express CD5, CD3, or CD2. Finally, approximately 15% of cases express neither B- nor T-cell antigens and are termed null cell ALL. Myeloid antigens, such as CD13, CD14, or CD33 can be found on the surface of as many as 25% of ALL cases, and in some but not all studies, the coexpression of myeloid markers on ALL blasts has been associated with a poor outcome.

The cytogenetic changes most often seen in adult ALL include t(9;22) (the Philadelphia chromosome) seen in 15% to 20% of cases; t(8;14), an abnormality associated with the L3 variant of ALL; and t(1;19), a translocation commonly seen

TABLE 33.4. Classification of ALL

Subtype	Morphology	Histochemistry			Monoclonal Reactivity	Cytogenetic Abnormalities
		Myeloperoxidase	Nonspecific Esterase	PAS		
L1 Acute lymphoid leukemia Childhood variant	Small, uniform blasts, nucleoli indistinct	—	—	+++	65% react with anti-CD10 (anti-CALLA)	Various
L2 Acute lymphoid leukemia Adult variant	Larger, more irregular nucleoli present	—	—	++	20% react with anti-CD5, 3, or 2 (anti-T cell)	Various, including t(1;19)
L3 Burkitt-like acute lymphoid leukemia	Large with strongly basophilic cytoplasm and vacuoles	—	—	—	Antisurface immunoglobulin, anti-CD19, anti-CD20	t(8;14).

in pre-B-cell ALL. All of these abnormalities suggest a poor prognosis. In about 20% of cases, the leukemia cells gain chromosomes, often reaching more than 50 per cell. Patients with so-called hyperdiploid ALL tend to have a better prognosis. Some of the chromosomal abnormalities seen in ALL suggest their pathogenesis. For example, in ALL, cases characterized by t(8;14), t(8;11), and t(8;22), the c-*myc* gene is translocated with the heavy or light chain immunoglobulin gene. In such cases, immature B cells could be driven to expand in an unregulated fashion by the presence of high and unregulated levels of the c-*myc* transcription regulatory protein.

Clinical Features

The clinical features of ALL, like AML, are usually the result of a diminished production of normal red cells, white cells, and platelets. Thus, signs of anemia, infection, and bleeding are common presenting symptoms. ALL tends to infiltrate normal organs more often than AML and thus enlargement of lymph nodes, liver, and spleen is common at diagnosis, being seen in approximately 50% of cases. Thymic enlargement is commonly seen in cases of T-cell leukemia. At the time of diagnosis, in approximately 5% of cases, ALL cells may infiltrate the leptomeninges, causing headache and nausea. In occasional cases, testicular involvement with leukemic cells may also be seen.

Laboratory Features

At the time of presentation, anemia is virtually always seen; most patients have at least mild thrombocytopenia and most also granulocytopenic. The white cell count is elevated in approximately 50% of cases, usually due to presence of circulating leukemic blasts. The bone marrow is almost always hypercellular and largely replaced by leukemic blasts. Many patients have an increased serum lactate dehydrogenase level, and in some cases, serum uric acid is elevated. Lumbar puncture with cytocentrifuge evaluation reveals leukemic cells in 5% to 10% of cases.

Differential Diagnosis

Clinically, the signs and symptoms of ALL may resemble those of any other marrow failure state. Infectious mononucleosis and other viral illnesses can sometimes resemble ALL, particularly when large numbers of atypical lymphocytes are present in the peripheral blood and when the disease is accompanied by hemolytic anemia or immune thrombocytopenia, but once a marrow exam is performed and current immunologic and molecular techniques are applied, the diagnosis is rarely in doubt.

Treatment

In childhood ALL, complete responses are achieved in better than 90% of cases and cures can be expected in 60% to 70% of children. Results in adults are not as favorable, with complete response rates averaging 75% and cure rates closer to 30% to 40% in most studies.

Remission Induction Standard remission induction usually includes vincristine, prednisone, an anthracycline, and often L-asparaginase. With such regimens, complete responses can be expected in 65% to 85% of cases. Other regimens, for example, the VAD regimen, employing continuous infusion vincristine and anthracycline along with dexamethasone, also yield high CR rates, but none have been shown to be superior to the more conventional regimens when tested in randomized trials. As in the case of AML, ALL induction therapy is followed by marked pancytopenia and, as in AML, the use of myeloid growth factors can shorten the period of myelosuppression, but does not improve overall complete response rates or survival.

Postremission Chemotherapy If patients receive only induction chemotherapy, remissions are invariably short lived, demonstrating the need for some form of postremission chemotherapy. The best results have been achieved using intensive consolidation chemotherapy, often using various combinations of cytarabine, cyclophosphamide, and an anthracycline followed by some form of maintenance chemotherapy using, for example, 6-mercaptopurine and methotrexate. Neither the optimal intensity nor duration of maintenance therapy has been precisely determined. Although CNS disease is less common in adults than in children, without CNS prophylaxis, at least 35% of adults relapse with CNS disease. Patients with a very high white cell count at diagnosis or with an elevated serum LDH appear to be particularly at risk. With CNS prophylaxis using intrathecal methotrexate with or without CNS radiation, the incidence of CNS relapse can be reduced to less than 10%. With current chemotherapeutic regimens, 30% to 40% of adults can be cured.

Risk Factors Younger patients, those with a low leukocyte count at diagnosis, with leukemic blasts with L1 morphology, with hyperdiploidy, and those who enter an initial remission early after induction appear to have the best prognosis. In contrast, older patients, those with a high white cell count at diagnosis, with an L2 morphology, and those who require additional chemotherapy to achieve remission do worse (see Table 33.5). In addition, patients with t(9;22), t(8;14), and t(1;19) have a poor prognosis.

Bone Marrow Transplantation Allogeneic transplantation is the only form of therapy that offers a realistic chance for cure to patients who fail to achieve an initial remission or who relapse with disease resistant to chemotherapy, curing approximately 10% to 20% of cases in both circumstances. If allogeneic transplantation is carried out earlier, while patients are in second remission, the results improve, with a 5-year disease-free survival of 35% being reported. The best results with allogeneic transplantation are seen in patients transplanted during first remission, with cure rates from 40% to 65% being reported. Whether these results are superior to what could be achieved adopting a strategy of first using chemotherapy and saving allogeneic transplantation for patients who relapse is untested in randomized trials. At present,

TABLE 33.5. **Prognosis in Acute Lymphocytic Leukemia**

Unfavorable	Favorable
Advanced age	Younger age
High WBC at diagnosis	Low WBC at diagnosis
Late achievement of CR	Early achievement of CR
Cytogenetics:	Cytogenetics:
t(9;22)	Hyperdiploidy
t(4;11)	
t(8;14)	
t(1;19)	

there is general agreement that patients with ALL with unfavorable prognostic characteristics such as t(9;22) or t(8;14) should be transplanted in first remission if a matched sibling is available. Results with autologous transplantation are harder to evaluate. Patients with multiple relapsed disease rarely benefit, owing to a very high posttransplant relapse rate. Autologous transplantation in second remission results in long-term survival in 20% to 30% of cases, which appears to represent a significant improvement over results achieved with conventional salvage chemotherapy. The role of autologous transplantation for patients in first remission is a subject currently being studied in prospective randomized trials. The use of matched unrelated donor transplantation is also currently under study.

CHRONIC MYELOGENOUS LEUKEMIA

Biology

Chronic myelogenous leukemia is characterized by the overproduction and accumulation of cells of the myeloid series, leading to marked splenomegaly and very high peripheral white blood cell counts. The circulating white cells are usually made up of normal-appearing granulocytes or bands, some earlier appearing myeloid cells, and occasional blasts. These cells retain most of their normal function and so patients can survive, often for several years, with active CML if treated with relatively nonspecific therapy such as busulfan or hydroxyurea to prevent the white cell count from reaching dangerously high levels. With time, however, the leukemic clone becomes less stable, and the disease progresses to a disorder that more closely resembles acute leukemia.

Studies of the biology of CML have found that the disease results from the clonal expansion of a very primitive pluripotent hematopoietic stem cell. Thus, although the clinical manifestation of the disease largely reflects overproduction of granulocytes, the erythrocytes, megakaryocytes, macrophages, and even B lymphocytes in patients with CML derive from the malignant clone.

In greater than 90% of cases, the Ph chromosome is found in marrow cells from patients with CML. The Ph chromosome results from the balanced translocation between the long arm of chromosomes 9 and 22, and was the first chromosomal abnormality to be identified with a specific disease. This translocation involves the movement of the majority of the *ABL* proto-oncogene from chromosome 9 to become contiguous with the 5′ portion of the *BCR* gene on chromosome 22. The breakpoint in the *BCR* gene occurs within one of two relatively short sequences. One sequence, the major breakpoint cluster region (M-*bcr*), is the one involved in all cases of CML and about half the cases of Ph+ ALL. The chimeric protein produced by this transcript is a hybrid p210 protein. The other sequence, the minor breakpoint cluster region (m-*bcr*), results in a p190 hybrid protein and is responsible for the other 50% of Ph+ ALL cases. Recent studies have found a molecular *BCR/ABL* translocation in most of those cases with clinical evidence of CML but with normal conventional cytogenetics. It is now generally concluded that true *BCR/ABL*-negative CML does not exist. The *BCR/ABL* translocation is more than just a marker of CML. Insertion of a retrovirus that produces the p210 protein into hematopoietic cells of mice leads to the development of a syndrome resembling CML.

Clinical Features

CML is normally characterized as being in chronic phase, accelerated phase, or blast crisis. More than 90% of cases are diagnosed while in chronic phase. As many as 25% of patients are diagnosed serendipitously when a routine blood count reveals an elevated granulocyte count. More often, however, patients present with fatigue, weight loss, night sweats, or complaints of fullness in the left upper abdomen due to splenomegaly. Rarely, bleeding associated with thrombocytosis is seen. Neutrophil function is usually normal, so infection as a presenting sign is uncommon. Leukostatic symptoms, such as dyspnea, drowsiness, confusion, or diminished visual acuity, which are due to sludging in the pulmonary, cerebral, or retinal vessels, are uncommon, although sometimes seen when the presenting white count exceeds 400,000/mm^3. Splenomegaly is, by far, the most common physical sign of CML, being present in more than 60% of cases and may be marked, extending down as far as the pelvic brim. Lymphadenopathy is uncommon during the chronic phase. Rarely, patients with CML present in blast crisis at diagnosis. These patients have clinical manifestations similar to those seen in acute leukemia.

Laboratory Features

Virtually all patients have an elevated white cell count at diagnosis, with counts ranging from 10,000 to greater than 1,000,000/mm^3. The majority of cells are in the neutrophil series, with cells ranging from myeloblasts to normal mature-appearing neutrophils. Eosinophilia is sometimes seen and basophilia is common. Platelets are often increased and mild anemia is sometimes present. Bone marrow examination shows marked myeloid hyperplasia and, occasionally, increased marrow fibrosis. Blasts usually make up less than 5% of the marrow cells in most cases. The peripheral blood neutrophils show a markedly decreased leukocyte alkaline phosphatase score. Vitamin B$_{12}$ levels are often very high due to increased levels of transcobalamin I and III. Serum LDH and uric acid levels are sometimes increased. The diagnosis of CML is made by the finding of the Ph chromosome on cytogenetic analysis of marrow.

Differential Diagnosis

Usually, the diagnosis of CML is straightforward. Any patient with a sustained unexplained increase in the peripheral neutrophil count, particularly if splenomegaly is present, should be suspected of having CML. The diagnosis is generally made by bone marrow exam with cytogenetic analysis. In those cases where the clinical picture resembles CML but cytogenetics are read as normal, molecular studies looking for the presence of the hybrid *BCR/ABL* gene product should be undertaken. Diseases that may resemble CML include the various myeloproliferative disorders (polycythemia vera [P-vera], agnogenic myeloid metaplasia, and essential thrombocythemia) as well as chronic myelomonocytic leukemia.

Therapy

Patients usually tolerate the chronic phase of CML well but, over time, the clinical behavior of the disease changes. Approximately two thirds of patients transform into an accelerated phase characterized by an increase in blasts greater than 15% or basophils greater than 20% in blood or marrow, thrombocytopenia less than 100,000/mm^3 not due to therapy, documented extramedullary leukemia, or the finding of a new chromosomal change in addition to the Ph chromosome. The other one third of patients abruptly develop blast crisis, with more than 30% blasts in marrow or peripheral blood.

Conventional Therapy   The traditional therapy for newly diagnosed chronic phase CML consists of either busulfan starting at a dose of 2 to 4 mg/m^2 per day or hydroxyurea starting at a dose of 1 to 2 g/m^2 per day. These agents are generally used to control patients' symptoms and keep the peripheral blood count under 20,000/mm^3. With these therapies, the duration of the chronic phase is often quoted as 3.5 years and once blast crisis occurs, survival averages no more than 6 months. Sokol et al. studied 625 patients aged 5 to 50 and identified five variables that predicted survival for patients treated with conventional chemotherapy including sex, spleen size, platelet count, hematocrit, and percent circulating blasts. Since the studies by Sokol, randomized trials comparing busulfan with hydroxyurea have documented that both the duration of the chronic phase as well as overall survival are prolonged with the use of hydroxyurea.

Interferon   More recently, studies have found that interferon used either as a single agent or, more often, after counts are first controlled with hydroxyurea, can also control peripheral counts in CML. In addition, anywhere from 5% to 20% of patients have a partial or complete cytogenetic response with interferon therapy, something that is rarely seen with hydroxyurea. The effectiveness of interferon is dose dependent and best results are seen at doses of 5×10^6 units/m^2/day or above. Several randomized trials have now been completed comparing hydroxyurea with either interferon alone or interferon plus hydroxyurea. In most of these studies, the duration of the chronic phase and overall survival was improved with interferon. A recent meta-analysis of these studies found a 15% improvement in 5-year survival (57% versus 42%) with the use of interferon-containing regimens. Those patients who achieved a complete cytogenetic response appear to do particularly well.

Interferon is associated with considerably more toxicities than hydroxyurea, including fever, chills, malaise, anorexia, myalgia, and, rarely, autoimmune disorders. These complications can be lessened by increasing the dose slowly and adding acetaminophen. In most patients, these symptoms diminish after 2 to 3 months.

Bone Marrow Transplantation Bone marrow transplantation is the only known cure for CML. Approximately 15% of patients transplanted from HLA-matched siblings for CML in blast crisis can be cured. Results are improved if transplantation is carried out during the accelerated phase, where cure rates of approximately 40% are reported. The best results are seen if transplantation is carried out during the chronic phase. Data from several thousand patients reported to the International Bone Marrow Transplant Registry, as well as large single institution experiences, such as those reported from Seattle, show that transplantation from an HLA-identical sibling can cure 65% to 70% of patients. The probability of relapse is approximately 20%, and 15% die from transplant-related complications.

In most studies of allogeneic transplantation for CML, age has been found to be an important prognostic factor. However, long-term survival in better than 50% of patients age 50 to 60 has recently been reported. In most studies, the interval from diagnosis to transplant has also influenced outcome, with the best results seen in patients transplanted within 1 year of diagnosis. Most transplant studies have used either busulfan plus cyclophosphamide or cyclophosphamide plus total body irradiation as the preparative regimen, and in controlled randomized trials, the two appear equivalent. Graft-versus-host disease (GVHD) prophylaxis with cyclosporine and methotrexate is the most widely used approach.

The use of matched unrelated donor transplantation for patients with CML is being increasingly reported. Recent registry summaries report a 50% chance of long-term disease-free survival. The somewhat worse outcome with matched unrelated donors is almost completely accounted for by an increase in GVHD and related infections. Several pilot studies of autologous transplantation for CML have been reported. As yet, there is no convincing evidence that autologous transplantation prolongs survival or cures patients with CML.

CHRONIC LYMPHOCYTIC LEUKEMIA

Biology

Chronic lymphocytic leukemia (CLL) defines a group of chronic B-cell diseases characterized by the abnormal proliferation and/or accumulation of mature-appearing lymphocytes. The clonality of CLL is best demonstrated by the finding of identical (i.e., clonal) rearrangements of the immunoglobulin gene in all malignant cells in individual cases of CLL. The fundamental abnormality in CLL is not well understood. Some investigators believe that CLL is the result of the overproliferation of mature B cells, whereas others argue that CLL is more a disease of accumulation with CLL lymphocytes living for long periods. In either case, the end result is the existence of increased numbers of lymphocytes originating from the malignant clone with accumulation in blood, bone marrow, lymph nodes, and spleen, resulting in organomegaly and abnormal bone marrow function. In addition, the clonal expansion of one population of B cells is at the expense of other B-cell populations, so that normal B-cell immunity is diminished. If untreated, CLL ultimately proves fatal in one of three general ways. In some patients, the relentless accumulation of mature B cells leads to marrow failure and fatal granulocytopenia or thrombocytopenia. In some patients, there are further mutations in the CLL clone, leading to a more aggressive ALL-like disease, termed Richter's syndrome. In others, the diminished B-cell function leads to fatal infectious complications.

The malignant B cell in CLL, in contrast to normal B cells, only weakly expresses surface immunoglobulin (sIg) and also expresses CD5, an antigen normally largely restricted to T cells or fetal lymphoid tissue. Otherwise, the B cells of CLL are similar to normal B cells expressing CD19, CD20, and CD24. CLL is usually staged according to the modified Rai system (Table 33.6). Patients with early-stage disease have immediate survival better than 10 years, whereas those with intermediate stage and advanced stage have median survivals of 5 to 7 and 1.5 to 3 years, respectively. Other factors that influence survival include advanced age, diffuse marrow involvement, lymphocyte doubling time, and cytogenetic abnormalities. The most common cytogenetic abnormalities are trisomy 12, which is present in up to 40% of cases, 14q+ present in 25%, and abnormalities of the long arm of chromosomes 6 and 11. Patients with cytogenetic abnormalities seem to have a shorter survival than patients with a normal karyotype, and those with a single cytogenetic abnormality appear to do better than those with complex chromosomal abnormalities.

TABLE 33.6. The Modified Rai Strategy System for CLL

Rai Stage	Risk	Clinical Features	Median Survival (years)
0	Low	Lymphocytosis only in blood and marrow	>10
I	Intermediate	Lymphocytosis and lymphadenopathy	7
II	Intermediate	As in stage I plus splenomegaly and/or hepatomegaly	
III	High	Lymphocytosis and anemia	1.5
IV	High	Lymphocytosis and thrombocytopenia	

Clinical Features

Many patients with CLL are asymptomatic and are diagnosed when an elevated lymphocyte count is noted during a routine examination or during evaluation for another unrelated problem. Some patients present with nonspecific symptoms including fatigue, lethargy, reduced exercise tolerance, or loss of appetite. Others present with enlarged lymph nodes, most often cervical, as their chief complaint. Infectious complications, including bacterial, fungal, and viral infections, although common during later stages of the disease, are uncommon at diagnosis. Occasionally, patients present with signs associated with immune thrombocytopenia or autoimmune hemolytic anemia and, on further evaluation, are found to have CLL.

The usual physical findings at diagnosis include lymphadenopathy, which is present in two thirds of patients. Approximately 50% of patients will have splenomegaly, but hepatomegaly is much less common, seen in less than 10% of cases. Although massive adenopathy can cause dysfunction of other organs causing, for example, obstructive jaundice, obstructive uropathy, or partial bowel obstruction, these complications are rare at diagnosis and usually only seen late in the disease course. Similarly, unilateral or bilateral leg edema can occur, but is usually a late event.

Laboratory Features

The hallmark of CLL is a peripheral lymphocytosis, usually in the range of 40 to 150,000/mm^3. The lymphocytes are indistinguishable from normal small B lymphocytes on light microscopy but, as noted earlier, have abnormal immunophenotyping, including expressing CD5 on their surface and also are clonal and therefore exhibit either κ or λ light chain excess or a consistent immunoglobulin gene rearrangement. Also, as noted earlier, the cells may show a consistent cytogenetic abnormality. Bone marrow biopsy usually demonstrates a lymphocytic infiltrate, which amounts to more than 30% of cells and may be in a diffuse or nodular pattern. A diffuse pattern is felt to carry a somewhat worse prognosis. Anemia is present in approximately 20% of patients at diagnosis and thrombocytopenia in 10%. The anemia is usually mild and the direct cause uncertain but, in some patients, autoimmune hemolytic anemia, confirmed by a positive Coombs test, reticulocytosis, elevated bilirubin level, and low serum haptoglobin is found. Similarly, autoimmune thrombocytopenia with antiplatelet antibodies is seen in some patients. The antibodies associated with red cell and platelet destruction are not a direct product of the malignant clone, but both autoimmune hemolytic anemia and thrombocytopenia usually respond to treatment of the underlying CLL. Hypogammaglobulinemia is seen in 25% of newly diagnosed CLL patients and becomes a more frequent problem as the disease progresses, being seen in 50% to 70% of patients with more advanced disease.

Differential Diagnosis

The diagnosis of CLL is generally straightforward. Occasionally, lymphocytosis can be caused by an infection such as mononucleosis, cytomegalovirus, pertussis, or tuberculosis, but in these cases, signs of the infection predominate and the lymphocytosis is not persistent. The more difficult problem is differentiating CLL from other indolent lymphoproliferative disorders including hairy cell leukemia, Waldenstrom's macroglobulinemia, large granular lymphocytosis, prolymphocytic leukemia, and the leukemic phase of nodular lymphomas. These distinctions are largely made by histopathology and cell surface immunophenotyping.

Treatment

Except for the uncommon application of allogeneic transplantation to treat the occasional younger patient, CLL is incurable with available therapies. Further, there is no evidence that treatment of early stage patients improves survival. Therefore, deciding when to initiate therapy in CLL is an important issue. Generally, treatment can be safely withheld until patients develop disease-related symptoms, progressive bone marrow failure, significant autoimmune anemia, or thrombocytopenia or recurrent infections. Radiation can be used to treat splenomegaly or bulky lymphoid masses in occasional cases, but chemotherapy is required for most patients. The greatest experience has been with chlorambucil, which is effective in controlling manifestations of the disease in most patients. Chlorambucil can be given at 6 to 8 mg daily, 15 to 20 mg/m^2 every 2 weeks, or 20 to 40 mg/m^2 monthly, with subsequent doses adjusted according to clinical response and myelotoxicity. Cyclophosphamide and combinations of cyclophosphamide with vincristine and prednisone (CVP) are approximately equivalent to chlorambucil with respect to response rates, time to progression, and survival. More intensive combinations, for example, CVP plus an anthracycline, appear to result in higher response rates than chlorambucil, but it is less clear if survival is improved by their use.

The purine analogues fludarabine, 2-chlorodeoxyadenosine (2-CDA), and 2-deoxycoformycin (DCF) have been found to have considerable activity in CLL. Fludarabine, at a dose of 25 mg/m^2 for 5 consecutive days each month for approximately 6 months, is often effective in patients who no longer are responding to alkylating agents, resulting in 15% complete responses and 45% partial responses. When compared to chlorambucil as initial therapy for CLL, fludarabine results in a significantly higher incidence of complete and partial remissions and a longer remission duration. However, there is not yet evidence that use of fludarabine as initial therapy prolongs survival compared to a strategy of first using chlorambucil and reserving fludarabine to treat patients after progression. 2-CDA appears to produce response rates very similar to that achieved with fludarabine. Responses have also been seen with DCF but the experience with this drug is limited. Unfortunately, there is little evidence for non-cross-resistance among the three purine analogues, and resistance of leukemic cells to one usually means resistance to the other two. All three purine analogues are myelosuppressive and immunosuppressive. The myelosuppression is short lived but the immunosuppressive effects may be cumulative and render patients susceptible to opportunistic infections for considerable periods.

A major problem associated with CLL and its treatment is the risk of opportunistic infection. High-dose intravenous immunoglobulin therapy decreases the frequency of bacterial infections in patients with CLL. Although expensive, its use should be strongly considered for patients with documented recurrent bacterial infections. Use of purine analogues has increased the risk of infections with *Pneumocystis carinii*, candida, and other opportunistic agents, and so prophylaxis with trimethoprim–sulfamethoxazole and fluconazole might be considered during their use.

Long-term disease-free survival has been reported in a small number of patients with CLL treated with allogeneic marrow transplantation. The best preparative regimens and GVHD prophylaxis for this indication are uncertain. There does appear to be a potentially important role for a graft-versus-leukemia effect in this disease given the observation that following transplantation, it may take from months to years for the disease to entirely disappear, and that donor lymphocyte infusions are sometimes effective in reestablishing a complete response.

The median survival of patients with CLL is 4 to 5 years following initiation of therapy but is heavily influenced by the stage of disease at diagnosis. Younger patients usually eventually die of progressive CLL with associated marrow failure and infectious complications. Older individuals often die of other intercurrent illnesses. In a small proportion of patients, CLL evolves into a more aggressive disease, commonly termed Richter's syndrome, which closely resembles a diffuse large-cell lymphoma. In approximately half of the cases of Richter's syndrome, the malignant cells display the same cytogenetic and molecular features of the original CLL. Response to therapy is poor, with a median survival of 4 months.

OTHER LEUKEMIA-LIKE DISORDERS

Myelodysplastic Syndromes

The myelodysplastic syndromes (MDS) describe a group of clonal hematopoietic disorders characterized by impaired maturation of hematopoietic precursors with the development of progressive peripheral cytopenias. MDS is the result of the neoplastic transformation of a cell at a level of differentiation close to that of the hematopoietic stem cell. Unlike the acute leukemias, the abnormal clone in MDS retains the ability to differentiate, albeit not entirely normally. With time, the abnormal clone suppresses all normal hematopoiesis and becomes increasingly abnormal. The final result is the development of either progressive severe pancytopenia or progression to an acute leukemia-like state. The cause of the defect in MDS is usually unknown but the disease is seen more often in patients with DNA repair deficiency syndromes, in those exposed to irradiation or other marrow toxins, and in patients previously exposed to alkylating agents. The disorder is much more common in the elderly, with a median age at onset of approximately 60 years. Symptoms are usually a direct result of impaired marrow function, with the most common presenting complaints being fatigue, pallor, and, less commonly, recurrent infections. Occasionally, bruising or bleeding is the presenting symptom.

The laboratory features of MDS include peripheral pancytopenia and marrow dysplasia including dyserythropoiesis, often with ringed sideroblasts, dysgranulopoiesis with hypogranulation, and dysmegakaryocytopoiesis with micromegakaryocytes. Five distinct forms of MDS have been defined by the French–American–British Cooperative Group (see Table 33.7). Clonal chromosomal abnormalities are found in 50% to 70% of MDS patients, most commonly loss of part or all of chromosome 7, trisomy 8, isochrome 17, 5q-, and 20q-. These abnormalities appear to carry independent prognostic significance, with abnormalities of chromosome 7 being particularly unfavorable. Even after FAB and cytogenetic classification, MDS remains a heterogeneous disease, particularly concerning prognosis. Accordingly, a number of scoring systems have been developed to help further categorize patients. Recently, a system based on an international study of 816 cases was published. This international prognostic scoring system uses marrow, blast percentage, cytogenetic data, and peripheral counts to categorize patients as being low, intermediate, or high risk.

The category of MDS dictates the appropriate therapy. Except for allogeneic transplantation, there is no proven curative treatment for MDS. Patients with low-risk disease can generally be followed without treatment unless they have a single severe cytopenia requiring therapy. Erythropoietin has been studied in patients with low-risk MDS with anemia as their major problem and results in 20% to 30% of patients becoming red cell transfusion independent. Use of granulocyte-macrophage-colony stimulating factor (GM-CSF) or granulocyte-colony stimulating factor (G-CSF) to treat granulocytopenia is associated with improved granulocyte counts in the majority of patients and should be considered in infected neutropenic patients. Whether long-term use of myeloid growth factors in MDS is warranted has not been determined. Differentiating agents, especially 13-*cis*-retinoic acid, have been tested in patients with MDS and were not found to improve progression-free or overall survival. Pilot studies of low-dose cytarabine suggested response rates of 15% to 20%, but randomized trials failed to show any improvement in overall survival. Intensive combination chemotherapy, similar to that used in AML, has been studied in younger patients with intermediate or high-risk disease and results in complete response rates of 40% to 60%. The highest complete response rates occur in younger patients. The average response duration is less than 12 months and few patients are cured, results that are inferior to those seen using similar chemotherapeutic approaches in patients with de novo AML.

The only curative therapy for MDS is allogeneic bone marrow transplantation, which results in long-term disease-free survival in 40% to 50% of transplanted patients. Results appear best for younger patients transplanted for early-stage disease using HLA-matched sibling donors.

Chronic Myeloproliferative Diseases

The chronic myeloproliferative diseases are clonal disorders affecting cells of myeloid lineage, resulting in overproduction of relatively mature cells. These disorders are usually subdivided on the basis of the predominant phenotype of the abnormal cell's population. Red cell production is categorized as "polycythemia vera" and platelet excess as "essential thrombocythemia." A third category of chronic

TABLE 33.7. FAB Classification of Myelodysplastic Syndromes

Classification	Marrow blasts (%)	Peripheral blood blasts (%)	Ringed sideroblasts >15% of bone marrow	Monocytes >1000/μL
Refractory anemia	<5	≤1	–	–
Refractory anemia with ringed sideroblasts	<5	≤1	+	–
Refractory anemia with excess blasts	5–20	<5	–/+	–
Refractory anemia with excess blasts in transition	20–30	>5	–/+	–/+
Chronic myelomonocytic anemia	≤20	<5	–/+	+

myeloproliferative syndrome is "agnogenic myeloid metaplasia," a disease characterized by bone marrow fibrosis and extramedullary hematopoiesis. Chronic myeloid leukemia conceptually fits as a fourth syndrome, but because of its frequency and clinical uniformity, it is usually considered as a separate entity.

Polycythemia Vera   Polycythemia vera is a clonal hematopoietic disorder resulting in an increased red cell mass. The disease has a peak incidence at age 60 and affects both genders equally. Patients are often asymptomatic, with the diagnosis initially being suspected following routine screening tests. Common symptoms include generalized pruritus, especially after showering or bathing, fatigue, paraesthesias, headache, and epigastric distress. As many as one third of patients present following thrombotic or hemorrhagic events. Patients often have a ruddy complexion and both splenomegaly and hepatomegaly are common. Most patients have an elevated hematocrit, but it is important to remember that a hematocrit may be elevated without an increase in red cell mass, for example, if the plasma volume is decreased and conversely, that the red cell mass can be increased without a marked increase in the hematocrit. The peripheral white cell count and platelet count are often mildly elevated, and bone marrow examination usually shows trilineage hypercellularity. Iron stores are usually low while vitamin B_{12} levels are frequently elevated, in part due to an increase in B_{12} binding capacity.

The major concern in making a diagnosis of P-vera is distinguishing primary P-vera from secondary erythrocytosis. Secondary erythrocytosis is usually the result of increased erythropoietin levels that result from a physiologic demand, as in patients living at high altitudes, with chronic lung disease, or with arteriovenous shunts. Rarely, pathologic erythropoietin overproduction occurs from tumors, uterine fibroids, or as a result of renal disorders. Whereas in the past the diagnosis of P-vera required measurement of the red cell mass, currently the easiest way to distinguish between primary and secondary erythrocytosis is to measure erythropoietin levels. An autonomous proliferation of erythrocytes, as in P-vera, is associated with low erythropoietin levels.

The cornerstone of therapy for P-vera is phlebotomy. Maintenance of a hematocrit of approximately 42% or less is recommended, which may require weekly phlebotomies of 500 ml. Therapy with phlebotomy alone is associated with an increased risk of thrombosis and so many experts recommend the use of hydroxyurea at 1 to 2 g/day to keep the platelet count below 500,000/mm^3. Chlorambucil and radiophosphorus are not, in general, recommended for treatment of P-vera because of their leukogenic effects.

The average survival from diagnosis is greater than 10 years. Approximately 50% of patients develop thrombotic or hemorrhagic complications that can be generally controlled with therapy. In 5% to 10% of patients, the disease evolves into an acute myeloid leukemia-like syndrome while in another 20%, the disease transforms into a picture resembling that seen with agnogenic myeloid metaplasia.

Essential Thrombocythemia   Essential thrombocythemia is a clonal hematopoietic disorder characterized by the autonomous overproduction of platelets and platelet precursors. Most patients are asymptomatic and the disease is generally diagnosed incidentally. However, approximately 25% of patients present with either thrombotic or hemorrhagic events. Splenomegaly is present in 50% of patients but hepatomegaly and lymphadenopathy are rare. The platelet count is usually greater than 600,000/mm^3 but other peripheral counts are generally normal. Marrow examination usually shows increased numbers of megakaryocytes, often appearing in clusters, and an increase in marrow reticulin fibrosis is sometimes seen.

Essential thrombocythemia is the least aggressive of the myeloproliferative syndromes, and patients with this disease can have, on average, a nearly normal life expectancy. The disease rarely transforms into an acute leukemia. However, more than one third of patients will suffer a major thrombotic or hemorrhagic event. The risk of thrombotic events is increased with a previous history of a thrombotic event, with inadequate control of thrombocytosis, and in patients with other cardiovascular risk factors. The risk for hemorrhage is increased when platelet counts exceed 2,000,000/mm^3 and in patients using nonsteroidal anti-inflammatory agents. Most experts recommend therapy to keep platelet counts less than 600,000/mm^3 for all patients over age 50 and in those with cardiovascular risk factors or a previous history of thrombosis. The appropriate management of younger patients without risk factors is unsettled, but some experts recommend treatment to keep the counts less than 600,000/mm^3 in these individuals, as well. The two most commonly used agents are anagrelide, 0.5 mg/qid and hydroxyurea 1 g/day. Both are highly active, are administered orally, and are generally well tolerated.

Agnogenic Myeloid Metaplasia Agnogenic myeloid metaplasia (AMM) is characterized by substantial bone marrow fibrosis, peripheral blood leukoerythroblastosis, and marked splenomegaly. In this disorder, the marrow fibroblasts are polyclonal, whereas a population of hematopoietic cells is clonal and, therefore, the marrow fibrosis is thought to be a reactive process caused by the clonal cell population. Current studies suggest that abnormally high levels of transforming growth factor-β (TGF-β) and, perhaps, platelet-derived growth factor produced by the clonal cell population are the predominant causes for the fibroblast proliferation.

Most patients with AMM present with symptoms related to anemia, approximately 25% present because of the mechanical effects of an enlarged spleen, while occasional patients have signs of bleeding or hypermetabolism (weight loss, night sweats) as their initial complaint. Usual laboratory findings include a peripheral leukoerythroblastosis, with teardrop red cells and immature myeloid elements being present. Bone marrows are usually not aspirable and bone marrow biopsy shows bone marrow fibrosis and osteosclerosis. Large numbers of blasts are usually not seen in the marrow and, if present, suggest M7 acute myelogenous leukemia. Other diseases sometimes confused with AMM are CML with marrow fibrosis and hairy cell leukemia.

Survival with AMM is quite varied, ranging from 1 to 30 years but averaging around 5 years. A poor prognosis is associated with increasingly severe anemia, thrombocytopenia, hepatomegaly, and B symptoms. AMM, in general, is considered incurable, and therapy is aimed at treating the anemia and thrombocytopenia and the problems associated with an enlarged spleen, including pain, portal hypertension, and hypersplenism. Anemia is usually treated with transfusion therapy (with deferoxamine if long-term support is anticipated) although some patients respond to androgens plus steroids and a few to erythropoietin. Treatment of thrombocytopenia is difficult, with platelet transfusion support the usual approach. Splenectomy should be considered for patients with splenic pain, portal hypertension, or hypermetabolic symptoms not responsive to hydroxyurea. Approximately 50% of patients with low blood cell counts will improve following splenectomy. Splenic irradiation (200 to 300 cGy delivered in 10 to 15 daily fractions) can provide transient benefit for patients with symptomatic splenomegaly but rarely improves peripheral blood counts. Recently, the use of allogeneic marrow transplantation has been reported in younger patients with AMM. Complete engraftment with evident eradication of the disease has been reported, with some patients remaining continuously disease-free for prolonged periods, suggesting that cure is possible.

Hairy Cell Leukemia

Hairy cell leukemia is an uncommon B-cell disorder, occurring in approximately 500 patients per year in the United States. The clinical picture is characterized by pancytopenia with an inaspirable bone marrow, splenomegaly, and often lymphadenopathy. The malignant cells stain positively with tartrate-resistant acid phosphatase. They also express pan-B-cell antigens, such as CD19 and CD20, as well as the monocyte-related antigen CD11c. Hairy cell leukemia is an indolent disorder and as many as 10% of patients may never require treatment. Therapy is indicated for massive progressive splenomegaly, lymphadenopathy, worsening blood counts, or recurrent infections. Splenectomy, previously the traditional treatment, improves symptoms related to splenomegaly and, in most cases, peripheral blood counts, often for prolonged periods of time, but does not affect the disease itself. Because excellent results have been observed with interferon, 2-CDA, and DCF, splenectomy should be reserved for patients who do not respond to therapy with these agents. Therapy with interferon 2×10^6 units/m^2/day or 3×10^6 units three times per week produces responses in 80% of splenectomized or unsplenectomized patients; however, only 10% of responses are complete. Responses generally occur within 3 to 4 months, although up to a year of therapy may be required. The disease invariably recurs after interferon therapy is discontinued, but maintenance therapy is associated with excessive toxicity and expense. Therapy with DCF, 4 mg/m^2 intravenously every other week for 4 to 6 months, produces complete responses in 60% to 90% of previously treated or untreated patients, including those who failed to respond to interferon. Moreover, only 25% of patients relapse with more than 5 years of follow-up. Relapse is most often characterized by an increased number of hairy cells in the bone marrow without associated clinical indications for therapy. The drug is myelosuppressive and immunosuppressive with an increase in opportunistic infections even in the absence of neutropenia. However, the improved response rate makes DCF preferable to interferon as the initial therapy of hairy cell leukemia. A single 7-day continuous infusion of 2-CDA produces complete response rates of 65% to 85% and partial responses in another 10% of cases. Although follow-up is shorter than with DCF, the responses appear to be similar in their duration. Side effects of 2-CDA therapy include febrile neutropenia, immunosuppression, and myelosuppression with opportunistic infections as well as pulmonary, cutaneous, cardiac, and neurologic toxicity. Both DCF and 2-CDA provide excellent results in the treatment of hairy cell leukemia, and there has not been a prospective randomized study comparing the two.

ACKNOWLEDGMENT

This work is supported, in part, by Grant CA-18029 from the National Cancer Institute, National Institutes of Health, DHHS.

FURTHER READING

Anderson JE, Appelbaum FR, Schoch G, Gooley T, Anasetti C, Bensinger WI, Bryant E, Buckner CD, Chauncey TR, Clift RA, Doney K, Flowers M, Hansen JA, Martin PJ, Matthews DC, Sanders JE, Shulman H, Sullivan KM, Witherspoon RP, Storb R (1996) Allogeneic marrow transplantation for refractory anemia: A comparison of two preparative regimens and analysis of prognostic factors. *Blood* 87:51.

Appelbaum FR (1996) The acute leukemias. In: Bennett JC, Plum F (eds): *Cecil Textbook of Medicine*, WB Saunders, Philadelphia, p. 936.

Beelen DW, Graeven U, Elmaagacli AH, Niederle N, Kloke O, Opalka B, Schaefer UW (1995) Prolonged administration of interferon-α in patients with chronic-phase Philadelphia chromosome-positive chronic myelogenous leukemia before allogeneic bone marrow transplantation may adversely affect transplant outcome. *Blood* 85:2981.

Cline MJ (1994) The molecular basis of leukemia. [Review]. *N Eng J Med* 330:328–336.

Copelan EA, McGuire EA (1995) The biology and treatment of acute lymphoblastic leukemia in adults. [Review] *Blood* 85:1151-1168.

Degos L, Dombret H, Chomienne C, Daniel MT, Miclea JM, Chastang C, Castaigne S, Fenaux P (1995) All-*trans*-retinoic acid as a differentiating agent in the treatment of acute promyelocytic leukemia [Review] *Blood* 85:2643–2653.

Greenberg P, Cox C, LeBeau MM, Fenaux P, Morel P, Sanz G, Sanz M, Vallespi T, Hamblin T, Oscier D, Ohyashiki K, Toyama K, Aul C, Mufti G, Bennett J (1997) International scoring system for evaluating prognosis in myelodysplastic syndromes. *Blood* 89:2079.

Hehlmann R, Heimpel H, Hasford J, Kolb HJ, Pralle H, Hossfeld DK, Queiber W, Loffler H, Hochhaus A, Heinze B, Georgii A, Bartram CR, Griebhammer M, Bergmann L, Essers U, Falge C, Queiber U, Meyer P, Schmitz N, Eimermacher H, Walther F, Fett W, Kleeberg UR, Käbisch A, Nerl C, Zimmerman R, Mueret G, Tichelli A, Kanz L, Tigges F-J, Schmid L, Brockhaus W, Tobler A, Reiter A, Perker M, Emmerich B, Verpoort K, Zankovich R, Wussow Pv, Prümmer O, Thiele J, Buhr T, Carbonell F, Ansari H, German CML Study Group (1994) Randomized comparison of interferon-α with busulfan and hydroxyurea in chronic myelogenous leukemia. *Blood* 84:4064.

The Italian Cooperative Study Group on Chronic Myeloid Leukemia (1994) Interferon alpha-2a as compared with conventional chemotherapy for the treatment of chronic myeloid leukemia. *N Engl J Med* 330:820.

Kantarjian HM, Deisseroth A, Kurzrock R, Estrov Z, Talpaz M (1993) Chronic myelogenous leukemia: A concise update. *Blood* 82:691.

Larson RA, Dodge RK, Burns CP, Lee EJ, Stone RM, Schulman P, Duggan D, Davey FR, Sobol RE, Frankel SR, et al. (1995) A five-drug remission induction regimen with intensive consolidation for adults with acute lymphoblastic leukemia: Cancer and leukemia group B study 8811. *Blood* 85:2025–2037.

Leith CP, Chir B, Kopecky KJ, Godwin J, McConnell T, Slovak ML, Chen I-M, Head DR, Appelbaum FR, Willman CL (1997) Acute myeloid leukemia in the elderly: Assessment of multidrug resistance (MDR1) and cytogenetics distinguishes biologic subgroups with remarkably distinct responses to standard chemotherapy. A Southwest Oncology Group Study. *Blood* 89:3323.

Mayer RJ, Davis RB, Schiffer CA, Berg DT, Powell BL, Schulman P, Omura GA, Moore JO, McIntyre OR, Frei EI (1994) Intensive post-remission chemotherapy in adults with acute myeloid leukemia. *N Engl J Med* 331:896.

Radich JP, Gehly G, Gooley T, Bryant E, Clift RA, Collins S, Edmands S, Kirk J, Lee A, Kessler P, Schoch G, Buckner CD, Sullivan KM, Appelbaum FR, Thomas ED (1995) Polymerase chain reaction detection of the *BCR-ABL* fusion transcript after allogeneic marrow transplantation for chronic myeloid leukemia: Results and implications in 346 patients. *Blood* 85:2632.

Stone RM, Berg DT, George SL, Dodge RK, Paciucci PA, Schulman P, Lee EJ, Moore JO, Powell BL, Schiffer CA, for the Cancer and Leukemia Group B (1995) Granulocyte-macrophage colony-stimulating factor after initial chemotherapy for elderly patients with primary acute myelogenous leukemia. *N Engl J Med* 332:1671.

Thirman MJ, Gill HJ, Burnett RC, Mbangkollo D, McCabe, NR, Kobayashi H, Ziemin-van der Poel S, Kaneko Y, Morgan R, Sandberg AA, et al. (1993) Rearrangement of the *MLL* gene in acute lymphoblastic and acute myeloid leukemias with 11q23 chromosomal translocations. *N Engl J Med* 329:909–914.

Warrell RP, Jr., De The H, Wang Z, Degos L (1993) Acute promyelocytic leukemia. *N Engl J Med* 329:177.

Weick JK, Kopecky KJ, Appelbaum FR, Head DR, Kingsbury LL, Balcerzak SP, Bickers JN, Hynes HE, Welborn JL, Simon SR, Grever M (1996) A randomized investigation of high-dose versus standard-dose cytosine arabinoside with daunorubicin in patients with previously untreated acute myeloid leukemia: A Southwest Oncology Group Study. *Blood* 88:2841.

Zittoun RA, Mandelli F, Willemze R, De Witte T, Labar B, Resegotti L, Leoni F, Damasio E, Visani G, Papa G, Caronia F, Hayat M, Stryckmans P, Rotoli B, Leoni P, Peetermans ME, Dardenne M, Vegna ML, Petti MC, Solbu G, Suciu S (1995) Autologous or allogeneic bone marrow transplantation compared with intensive chemotherapy in acute myelogenous leukemia. *N Engl J Med* 332:217.

CHAPTER 34

PEDIATRIC MALIGNANCIES

RUBY KALRA and JUDITH K. SATO

Department of Pediatric Oncology
City of Hope National Medical Center
Duarte, CA 91010, USA

Great strides have been made in the treatment of childhood cancer over the past several decades. The overall 5-year survival rate of children with cancer is 60% to 70%; it is estimated that in the year 2000, one in 1000 young adults ages 20 to 29 in the United States will be a survivor of childhood cancer. Many combination chemotherapy regimens were first employed in the treatment of childhood cancers. The "two-hit" theory of carcinogenesis, that is, the loss of tumor suppressor gene function, was first described in retinoblastoma, a childhood eye tumor. The most predominant childhood cancers are described in this chapter.

WILMS' TUMOR

Wilms' tumor, also known as nephroblastoma, is the most common malignant renal tumor of childhood. This tumor needs to be distinguished from neuroblastoma which arises from the adrenal gland. Both tumors are common in children less than 5 years of age and can present as an abdominal mass. In addition to an abdominal mass, many children with Wilms' tumor present with abdominal pain, hematuria, anemia, hypertension, and fever. Over the past 70 years the cure rate has improved dramatically from less than 10% to an 85% to 90% overall cure rate.

Epidemiology

Approximately one child in 10,000 children under the age of 15 years will be diagnosed with Wilms' tumor in North America, Europe, and Australia. The incidence

Manual of Clinical Oncology, 7th edition, Edited by Raphael E. Pollock
ISBN 0-471-23828-7, pages 689–707. Copyright © 1999 Wiley-Liss, Inc.

of Wilms' tumor is approximately three times higher in those of African descent than in Caucasians or Asians. This tumor is only slightly less frequent in males than in females. Unilateral tumors present in boys at a mean age of 41.5 months and in girls at 46.9 months. The mean age in patients with bilateral tumors is significantly younger, with males presenting at a mean age of 29.5 months compared to females at 32.6 months. A number of associated anomalies are described including hemihypertrophy, aniridia, cryptorchidism, and hypospadias. Associated syndromes include the Denys–Drash syndrome consisting of renal disease and pseudohermaphroditism; the WAGR syndrome consisting of Wilms' tumor, aniridia, genitourinary malformations, and mental retardation; and the Beckwith–Wiedemann syndrome defined by hemihypertrophy, macroglossia, omphalocele, and visceromegaly. Only 7.6% of all cases of Wilms' tumor occur as part of one of these syndromes; however, identification of these syndromes is important for screening patients at risk for developing Wilms' tumor. Children with the Beckwith–Wiedemann syndrome have about a 5% risk of developing Wilms' tumor, but children with the WAGR syndrome have about a 30% risk of developing Wilms' tumor. Also, about one third of patients with aniridia are at risk of developing Wilms' tumor.

Genetics

The genetics of Wilms' tumor is quite complex and only recently has begun to be defined. The finding of losses on chromosome 11p13 in patients with the WAGR syndrome led to the identification of the Wilms' tumor-1 (*WT-1*) gene at that locus. Similarly, the 11p15.5 locus has been linked to the Beckwith–Wiedemann syndrome; loss of heterozygosity at this locus has been identified in Wilms' tumor samples. This locus is now identified as the site of the Wilms' tumor-2 gene (*WT-2*). In addition, recent reports suggest that there may be additional loci on chromosomes 16q, 17q12-q21, and 7p13, which are still being investigated for their prognostic significance.

Diagnosis

In a child being evaluated for an abdominal mass, it is important to note the presence or absence of aniridia, hemihypertrophy, genitourinary abnormalities, hypertension, or evidence of venous obstruction. A plain film of the abdomen in Wilms' tumor typically does not show calcifications, in contrast to neuroblastoma. However, in some cases of subcapsular hemorrhage, Wilms' tumor may show a typical pattern of calcification described as an "eggshell" pattern. A chest radiograph is used to identify pulmonary metastases; the role of chest computerized tomography (CT) scan is still controversial. An abdominal ultrasound is necessary to evaluate the tumor as well as the inferior vena cava for tumor thrombus. A CT scan of the abdomen helps to define the anatomy, detect regional lymphadenopathy and metastatic disease in the liver, as well as to visualize the other kidney. However, it should be noted that in patients enrolled in the fourth National Wilms' Tumor Study (NWTS-4), 7% of bilateral lesions were not detected by preoperative imaging studies. Therefore, it is strongly recommended that the surgeon visualize and palpate the other kidney at the time of nephrectomy. Laboratory studies should include a complete blood count, a urinalysis and serum creatinine, liver function tests, serum calcium, and potentially urine catecholamines to distinguish this tumor from neuroblastoma.

Pathology

The classic Wilms' tumor is composed of three cellular elements: blastemal, stromal, and epithelial. The tumors are classified as being either of favorable or unfavorable histology. The latter is identified by the presence of nuclei with greatest diameters at least three times the size of adjacent cells with increased chromatin content and the presence of multipolar or polypoid mitotic figures. These anaplastic changes can be either focal or diffuse. Focal anaplasia is restricted to a sharply demarcated area within the primary tumor. Other tumors initially thought to be variants of Wilms' tumor are now classified separately as clear cell sarcoma of the kidney (CCSK) and rhabdoid tumor of the kidney (RTK). It is very important to identify these tumors, as they carry a much more unfavorable prognosis and have a different pattern of spread. Congenital mesoblastic nephroma, a relatively benign renal tumor, occurs predominantly in young male infants with a median age of 2 months. It is curable by nephrectomy alone. However, if the tumor margins are positive or there is evidence of a high mitotic tumor in an older child, these patients should be followed closely for recurrence. In addition, nephrogenic rests have long been identified as "precursor" lesions to Wilms' tumor; their presence suggests the need for closer follow-up, especially if present in the contralateral kidney.

Staging

Wilms' tumor can spread to both local and distant sites. Evidence of local spread can be seen in the renal sinus, intrarenal blood vessels and lymphatics, and penetration through the renal capsule. The most common sites of distant spread include the lungs, lymph nodes, and liver. Metastatic disease to the lungs only is identified in 80% of patients with metastatic disease, and 15% of patients may have involvement of the liver with or without lung metastases.

The National Wilms' Tumor Study Group Staging is described as follows:

Stage I—   The tumor is limited to the kidney and is completely excised with negative margins. There is no evidence of renal capsule invasion, renal sinus vessel involvement, or rupture.

Stage II—   The tumor extends beyond the kidney but is still completely excised. Disease extending into the inferior vena cava is free floating and non-adherent to the vessel wall.

Stage III—   Residual tumor remains in the abdomen either due to involvement of lymph nodes, peritoneal implants, tumor spillage not confined to the flank, adherent tumor thrombus in the inferior vena cava, or gross or microscopic residual disease remaining due to inability to completely resect the tumor.

Stage IV— Distant hematogenous spread to lungs, liver, bone, or brain, etc.

Stage V— Bilateral renal disease

Treatment

Treatment is multimodal and involves surgery, chemotherapy, and occasionally radiation therapy. The surgical approach should be transperitoneal and allow for exploration of the contralateral kidney, liver, and regional lymph nodes. The goal is to perform a radical or modified nephrectomy. Chemotherapy is usually given first for 8 to 10 weeks and consists of vincristine and actinomycin D with the addition of doxorubicin and cyclophosphamide in certain higher risk patients. Chemotherapy continues postoperatively to complete 18 to 54 weeks of therapy depending on the stage/histology. Radiation therapy is utilized in patients with stage III disease to treat the tumor bed; it is also used to treat the lungs and sites of unresectable metastases in patients with stage IV disease. Overall, the prognosis for Wilms' tumor is excellent, with more than 85% of all children surviving. Recently, a subgroup of patients who are under 2 years of age, with stage I tumors weighing less than 550 g, have been identified as possibly requiring no additional therapy beyond surgery. These patients are closely being followed in the NWTS-5 to assess the need for further therapy. Despite receiving no chemotherapy, these patients must be followed closely for any evidence of disease recurrence.

Recurrent Disease

Children with favorable histology tumors who relapse have a better outcome if they relapse beyond 12 months from diagnosis, were never treated with doxorubicin, and had no prior abdominal radiation. Treatment should include cyclophosphamide, ifosfamide, etoposide, doxorubicin, and carboplatin. The prognosis is much worse in children who recur despite treatment with doxorubicin or radiation; these patients may be considered for high dose therapy with stem cell rescue.

NEUROBLASTOMA

Neuroblastoma is the most common extracranial solid tumor of childhood and is the most common malignant tumor of infants. During normal development neuroblastoma cells can be detected in the adrenal glands of all fetuses at a peak age of 17 to 20 weeks' gestation. This tumor is unusual because it can be widely spread throughout the body but still spontaneously regress in infants less than 1 year of age. In contrast, in older children, the metastatic form is difficult to treat. The tumor cells are derived from the primordial neural crest cells which develop into the sympathetic nervous system including the adrenal medulla and sympathetic ganglia. Owing to the wide distribution of the sympathetic nervous system in the body, the disease can present with a number of different symptoms depending on the site(s) of tumor involvement.

Epidemiology

Neuroblastoma accounts for one case per 7000 live births. This may be an underestimation of prevalence owing to the number of cases that can spontaneously regress without becoming clinically evident. The median age at diagnosis is 22 months, and the disease occurs slightly more frequently in males than in females. Seventy-nine percent of cases are diagnosed before the age of 4 years and 97% by the age of 10 years. Disease occurrence has been associated with the fetal hydantoin, alcohol, and phenobarbital syndromes.

Genetics

A few cases of familial neuroblastoma have been reported in which the median age at diagnosis is 9 months and at least 20% of the tumors are bilateral or multifocal. There is evidence to suggest that a tumor suppressor gene may be located on chromosome 1p36. There is also some suggestion that neuroblastoma may be associated with neurofibromatosis type 1 (NF-1) and with aganglionic megacolon (Hirschsprung's disease), but these associations may be by chance alone. Although there are not any consistent constitutional abnormalities in patients with neuroblastoma, there are many genetic disturbances in the tumor cells. The loss of heterozygosity at chromosome 1p, amplification of extrachromosomal double minutes and homogeneously staining regions of the distal short arm of chromosome 2 (N-*myc* gene), and hyperdiploidy have all been described in tumor tissues. The 1p loss and amplification of the N-*myc* gene are associated with higher disease stages and a poor outcome, whereas hyperdiploidy is associated with low-stage tumors and a good outcome. N-*myc* amplification occurs in 30% to 40% of patients with high-stage disease. Deletions of 1p are found in 70% to 80% of all near-diploid tumors, which are also found in patients with higher disease stages. There is a strong correlation between 1p loss and N-*myc* amplification and poor outcome. There are also some tumors that show allelic loss on chromosomes 14 and 11 that may result in the identification of future tumor suppressor genes.

Diagnosis

Because neuroblastoma arises from cells that form the sympathetic nervous system, the disease may be found throughout the body. Sixty-five percent of all primary tumors arise in the abdomen, but this is age dependent. Children less than 1 year of age are more likely to have a primary site in the thoracic and cervical regions. Disease can spread to the lymph nodes, bone, bone marrow, liver, and skin. Unlike most childhood tumors, neuroblastoma rarely metastasizes to the lungs. The symptoms vary depending on the site of disease but can include an abdominal mass, spinal cord compression, hypertension, bone pain, superior vena cava syndrome, Horner's syndrome (unilateral ptosis, myosis, and anhidrosis), proptosis, periorbital ecchymoses, skin involvement with nontender blue-tinged subcutaneous nodules, failure to thrive, and fever. There are also associated paraneoplastic syndromes including secretory diarrhea secondary to vasoactive intestinal peptide secretion, and the opsoclonus–myoclonus syndrome described as "dancing eyes and dancing feet." The diagnosis can be made by either definitive pathologic examination of the primary tumor or by documenting metastatic neuroblastoma cells in the bone marrow with the presence of elevated urine catecholamines, vanillylmandelic acid (VMA), and homovanillic acid (HVA). All children suspected of this diagnosis should be evaluated with CT scans of the chest, abdomen, and pelvis; technetium bone scan; plain skeletal films; bilateral bone marrow aspirates and biopsies; and urine catecholamines (VMA and HVA). When available, a nuclear imaging study using meta-iodobenzylguanadine (MIBG), as well as magnetic resonance imaging (MRI), are also very helpful. Laboratory tests should include a complete blood cell count, serum ferritin, lactate dehydrogenase (LDH), and neuron-specific enolase (NSE), as well as serum creatinine, liver function tests, calcium, and urinalysis.

Pathology

The pathology can range from benign ganglioneuroma to intermediate ganglioneuroblastoma and frank neoplastic neuroblastoma. The histology can be identified as favorable or unfavorable based on Shimada's classification utilizing three variables: neuroblast differentiation, mitosis–karyorrhexis index (MKI), and the patient's age. Joshi and colleagues modified the Shimada classification to also add the following favorable features: ganglion cells, tumor giant cells, low mitosis ratio with fewer than 10 mitoses per 10 high-power fields, and calcification. It is very important to obtain pathology from the primary tumor for this pathologic prognostic grading and for biologic studies such as detecting losses on chromosome 1p and amplification of the N-*myc* gene.

Staging

The International Neuroblastoma Staging System (INSS) is described as follows:

Stage I— Localized tumor confined to the area of origin, which is completely excised with no microscopic residual and no evidence of lymph node involvement

Stage IIA—Unilateral tumor with incomplete gross excision and negative lymph nodes microscopically

Stage IIB—Unilateral tumor with complete or incomplete gross excision with positive ipsilateral lymph nodes and negative contralateral lymph nodes

Stage III— Tumor that crosses the midline with or without regional node involvement, a unilateral tumor with contralateral lymph node involvement, or a midline tumor with bilateral node involvement

Stage IV— Distant spread of tumor to distant lymph nodes, bone, bone marrow, liver, or other organs

Stage IVS—A stage I or II primary tumor in an infant less than 1 year of age with dissemination limited to bone marrow, liver, and skin (no bone involvement)

Treatment

Treatment is multimodal involving chemotherapy, surgery, radiation therapy, and in some cases high-dose chemotherapy with autologous bone marrow transplantation. Treatment is based on risk factors; most patients with neuroblastoma can be divided into low-, intermediate- and high-risk groups. The low-risk group patients include children with INSS stage I and IIA disease, and infants less than 1 year of age with INSS stage IIB, III and IVS disease. After surgery alone, children with INSS stage I disease enjoy a greater than 90% disease-free survival. The other children in the low-risk group have an 85% to 89% disease-free survival with minimum chemotherapy. The intermediate-risk group includes children with INSS IIB and III disease, and infants with stage IV disease. Here, N-*myc* amplification is a very poor prognostic sign, but without amplification, patients continue to do quite well. The highest risk group of patients are those children with INSS stage IV disease, who continue to elude attempts to improve their survival. The active chemotherapy drugs most commonly used include etoposide, cyclophosphamide, doxorubicin, cisplatin, and vincristine. Additional analogs such as teniposide, carboplatin, and ifosfamide have also been used. Biologic modifiers such as retinoids have also been used in the setting of minimal residual disease to help differentiate the tumor to benign ganglioneuroma and ganglioneuroblastoma.

Recurrent Disease

In certain centers where it is available, MIBG can be used to deliver radioactive iodine directly to tumor cells in patients with minimal residual disease after a recurrence. Very few patients survive after a recurrence, especially if they have already received a bone marrow transplant. New modalities of treatment utilizing the immune system, and new agents such as topotecan and melphalan may bring new hope to future patients. The goal for the future is to identify those patients at high risk for recurrence and to continue to intensify their treatment. Current studies are evaluating multiple courses of high-dose continuous infusion chemotherapy with stem-cell support.

HEPATIC TUMORS

Primary liver tumors in childhood are rare. Fifty-seven percent of all hepatic tumors in children are malignant, with the majority of benign tumors consisting of hemangiomas and hamartomas.

Epidemiology

The median age at diagnosis of hepatoblastoma is 1 year, with a predominance of males. In contrast, the median age at diagnosis for hepatocellular carcinoma in children is 12 years. Hepatoblastoma, like Wilms' tumor, has been associated with the Beckwith–Wiedemann syndrome and cases have been described with synchronous occurrence of these two embryonal tumors. There are some associations of hepatoblastoma with maternal use of oral contraceptives and gonadotropins, the fetal alcohol syndrome, dysplastic kidneys, and Meckel's diverticulum. Hepatocellular carcinoma is very closely associated with hepatitis B infection, and many primary liver disorders that result in cirrhosis such as hereditary tyrosinemia, biliary cirrhosis, α_1-antitrypsin deficiency, glucose-6-phosphate deficiency, and the use of anabolic steroids. Associated syndromes also include neurofibromatosis, ataxia–telangiectasia, and familial adenomatous polyposis.

Genetics

Loss of heterozygosity at the Beckwith–Wiedemann locus on chromosome 11p15 has been described in hepatoblastoma tumor tissue. In addition, trisomy 20, trisomy 2, and the presence of double minutes have all been described.

Diagnosis

Children with malignant liver tumors often present with painless abdominal masses. Patients may also have anorexia, weight loss, vomiting, and occasionally abdominal pain. Clinical features of the Beckwith–Wiedemann syndrome including hemihypertrophy may be evident. Systemic complaints such as nausea, vomiting, fever, weight loss, abdominal pain, and anorexia are more common in patients with hepatocellular carcinoma who often present with a much shorter duration of symptoms. In addition, these patients more often have associated splenomegaly, jaundice, and polycythemia. Definitive diagnosis is made on tissue from a liver biopsy. Diagnostic imaging studies should include a computerized tomography (CT) scan of the chest, abdomen, and pelvis and bone scan evaluating for pulmonary and bone metastases. Laboratory tests should be directed toward finding evidence of anemia, thrombocytosis, elevated liver function tests and bilirubin, and elevation of serum α-fetoprotein (AFP) which occurs in 80% to 90% of patients with hepatoblastoma and in 50% of patients with hepatocellular carcinoma. AFP is normally present in high values at birth, especially in premature infants, and gradually declines to normal adult values by 8 months to 1 year of life. In these young infants, it can be difficult to determine if the AFP is elevated due to production by the tumor or just due to age. The half-life varies significantly during this first year of life and age-related normals are published for full-term and premature infants at various ages. Evaluation for hepatitis B infection is also important in cases of hepatocellular carcinoma.

Pathology

Hepatoblastoma is composed of embryonal cells, fetal cells, or a mixture of the two. Pure fetal histology tumors carry a better prognosis. Hepatoblastoma tends to be unifocal and involves the right lobe of the liver most commonly. Hepatocellular carcinoma, on the other hand, tends to be multicentric and locally invasive. Extramedullary hematopoiesis is frequently detected in hepatoblastoma compared to hepatocellular carcinoma.

Treatment

Surgery plays an integral role in the treatment of malignant hepatic tumors. As much as 85% of the liver can be removed with complete regeneration within 1 to 3 months. However, only 50% to 60% of all cases are amenable to complete resection. In patients with metastatic disease, a liver transplantation is not recommended. In inoperable cases, chemotherapy with cisplatin, doxorubicin, 5-fluoruracil, vincristine, cyclophosphamide, ifosfamide, or etoposide has been employed to treat hepatoblastoma. There is evidence to suggest that children who have a rapid rate of fall in their serum AFP level have a better prognosis than children with a delayed rate of fall. In contrast to patients with hepatoblastoma, only one third of hepatocellular carcinoma patients are able to undergo a complete resection and only one third of those patients actually are long-term survivors. The same chemotherapeutic agents have been used to treat hepatocellular carcinoma as in hepatoblastoma. There are no well-accepted regimens for the treatment of recurrent disease.

RHABDOMYOSARCOMA

Rhabdomyosarcomas arise from mesenchymal cells that normally would develop into skeletal muscle. They can also be found in areas where skeletal muscle does not normally exist, such as the bladder. Rhabdomyosarcoma is the most common soft tissue sarcoma of childhood.

Epidemiology

Rhabdomyosarcoma is the third most common extracranial solid tumor of childhood after neuroblastoma and Wilms' tumor. Two thirds of all cases are diagnosed in children less than 6 years of age. There is a slight male preponderance and it appears to be less frequent in Asians. In the United States, African-American females have much lower rates than their Caucasian counterparts although no such difference occurs in males. There is an increased incidence of rhabdomyosarcoma in children whose parents used either marijuana or cocaine in the year prior to the child's birth.

Genetics

The Li–Fraumeni syndrome was described in families with children with rhabdomyosarcoma and mothers who developed breast cancer. Other family members also develop adrenocortical carcinomas and brain tumors. This syndrome has been linked to germline mutations of the *p53* gene. In addition, like Wilms' tumor and hepatoblastoma, rhabdomyosarcoma has been linked to the Beckwith–Wiedemann syndrome with abnormalities on chromosome 11p15. Neurofibromatosis has also been associated with rhabdomyosarcoma. Important genetic findings have been described recently through molecular biology screening of tumors and can distinguish between the two major histologic types of rhabdomyosarcoma, the embryonal and alveolar histologic subtypes. Alveolar rhabdomyosarcomas typically have a translocation between chromosomes 2 and 13 or 1 and 13, whereas embryonal rhabdomyosarcomas have losses at chromosome 11p15. Also, embryonal tumors can have variable DNA content and range from diploid to hyperdiploid.

Diagnosis

Rhabdomyosarcoma can occur throughout the body, with the most common sites being the head and neck area, followed by genitourinary sites, extremities, and the trunk. Sites of metastatic disease most commonly involve the lungs, bone marrow, bones, and lymph nodes. Rhabdomyosarcoma often presents as a mass but can also produce various signs and symptoms depending on the site of origin. In the head and neck area, tumors may involve the orbit and result in cranial nerve palsies, nasal, aural or sinus obstruction, headaches, and vomiting. Tumors in genitourinary sites may cause hematuria, urinary obstruction, constipation, vaginal discharge, scrotal enlargement, or evidence of urinary tract infection. In the extremities, a mass that can be painful or painless is often palpated with the presence of lymphadenopathy. The primary mass should be biopsied regardless of site, and the metastatic work-up should include a CT scan of the chest, abdomen, and pelvis; bone scan; bilateral bone marrow aspirates and biopsies; and when necessary magnetic resonance imaging (MRI) of the involved areas. The cerebrospinal fluid should be examined in cases of parameningeal disease. Metastatic disease at diagnosis is present in about 20% of all patients.

Pathology

In evaluating this tumor, the pathologist seeks to identify cross-striations characteristic of skeletal muscle. Immunohistochemical stains can further identify skeletal muscle. The major histologic variants of rhabdomyosarcoma are the embryonal and alveolar subtypes. The identification of the characteristic associated genetic anomalies can help to distinguish these two subtypes. Another subtype known as the botryoid type is characteristically found in the vagina or bladder of young infants or in the nasopharynx of older children and resembles "grapelike clusters." The botryoid type is found in the patients with the most favorable prognosis, followed by the embryonal type and lastly the alveolar type.

Staging

The TNM (Tumor, Nodes, Metastasis) staging system relies upon the site of the primary disease, size of the primary tumor (< or >5 cm), involvement of regional nodes, and presence of metastases. Stage I tumors are confined to the orbit, head, and neck area excluding parameningeal tumors, and genitourinary tract (nonbladder/nonprostate). They can be either less than or greater than 5 cm in size. Regional nodes may or may not be involved, but no distant metastases are present. Stage II tumors are found in the bladder/prostate area, extremity, cranial parameningeal, or other sites and are <5 cm in size with negative nodes and no metastases. Stage III is similar to stage II except that these tumors are >5 cm in size or have involved nodes in the tumors that are <5 cm in size. Stage IV is any disease with distant metastatic involvement.

Treatment

If possible, complete surgical removal is strongly recommended except in the setting of metastatic disease with large primary tumors. Both chemotherapy and radiation therapy play a role in the multimodal approach to treating these aggressive tumors. The most active chemotherapy agents include vincristine, actinomycin, cyclophosphamide, etoposide, ifosfamide, cisplatin, doxorubicin, and most recently topotecan and melphalan. Radiation therapy is delivered to all sites of disease with evidence of microscopic or gross residual postoperatively.

Recurrent Disease

The survival for children with recurrent rhabdomyosarcoma continues to be poor; newer modalities of treatment include the use of high-dose chemotherapy with stem-cell rescue. Salvage is possible in some children with a local recurrence of rhabdomyosarcoma, especially if the disease is completely resected.

EWING'S SARCOMA

Ewing's sarcoma was first described as a tumor of long bones in 1921. It is now evident that this tumor is actually of neural origin and can be found in either the bones or soft tissues. In the latter case, the tumor is often referred to as a peripheral primitive neuroectodermal tumor (PPNET). These two tumors, initially thought to be quite distinct, have been shown to share a common chromosomal translocation that has now grouped these tumors into the same family.

Epidemiology

Ewing's sarcoma occurs most commonly in the second decade of life, which represents about two thirds of all cases. Only 27% of all cases present in the first decade of life and 9% in the third decade. There are slightly more males affected than females.

This tumor seems to be much more prevalent in Caucasians and is only rarely present in those of African descent.

Genetics

Much has been learned recently about this family of tumors after it was noted that the genetic material in the tumors was altered, resulting in a translocation between chromosomes 11 and 22. The Ewing sarcoma gene (*EWS*) is found on chromosome 22, and a gene from the *ets* family of transcription factors is located on chromosome 11 (*FLI-1*). The combination of these two genes results in a fusion gene that promotes growth of tumor cells. A similar effect occurs when a second translocation between chromosomes 11 and 21 is present. In this case, another member of the *ets* family of transcription factors, *ERG*, is involved in the fusion with *EWS*. Both the t(11;22) and t(21;22) have been described in these tumors.

Diagnosis

Ewing's sarcoma can be found in the extremities or the central axis equally. The extremity tumors are also evenly distributed between proximal and distal sites. Almost all patients present with pain, and over half with a palpable mass, 21% with fever, and 16% with a pathologic fracture. The symptoms usually are present for at least 3 months. Twenty-three percent of patients present with metastatic disease at diagnosis and the most frequent sites of metastasis include the lungs, bone, and bone marrow. The spine may often be involved with bone metastases. The regional lymph nodes and liver are very uncommon sites of metastatic spread. The diagnosis is usually obtained through a biopsy of the tumor, which should be done in a manner that allows for excision of the biopsy tract during the definitive surgery. The plain films in Ewing's sarcoma usually reveal a lytic lesion in the diaphysis of bone. As the cortex is eroded and the tumor spreads into the soft tissues, the periosteal reaction takes on the appearance of an "onion peel."

Pathology

Ewing's sarcoma can often be difficult to distinguish from the other "small round blue cell" tumors, which include rhabdomyosarcoma, lymphoma, and neuroblastoma. Ewing's sarcoma tends to stain positively with periodic acid–Schiff (PAS) staining but this alone does not distinguish it from the other childhood tumors. The presence of the t(11;22) or t(21;22) and staining for a glycoprotein encoded by a gene, *MIC-2*, present on the surface of Ewing's sarcoma cells with monoclonal antibodies solidifies the diagnosis.

Staging

There currently is no accepted international staging system for Ewing's sarcoma, and these tumors are referred to as being either local or metastatic.

Treatment

Ewing's sarcoma, unlike osteosarcoma, is a radiosensitive tumor, so that it is usually treated with surgery and/or radiation therapy in addition to chemotherapy. Surgery is recommended for "expendible bones" such as the fibula and ribs. The most difficult site to provide local control is the pelvis, which may require a combination of surgery and radiation therapy. The active chemotherapy agents used to treat this disease include vincristine, doxorubicin, cyclophosphamide, etoposide, and ifosfamide. Much attention has been paid over recent years to dose intensification either through increased drug doses or shortened intervals between therapy. With local control only, more than 90% of the patients eventually die of metastatic disease, whereas with chemotherapy, the overall survival is closer to 70% to 80%. Favorable prognostic factors include sites in distal bones or ribs, tumors smaller than 100 cc, younger age, normal serum lactate dehydrogenase levels, and good response to initial chemotherapy. However, patients with metastatic disease at diagnosis, especially to bones, continue to do poorly, and new strategies employing high-dose chemotherapy with agents such as melphalan, carboplatin, etoposide, thiotepa, and ifosfamide with or without total body irradiation and stem-cell rescue are being evaluated.

Recurrent Disease

Treatment of children with recurrent disease is often not succesful. Pulmonary metastases should be surgically resected if only a few nodules are present. Chemotherapy should be directed toward active agents the patient has not previously received or experimental agents. High-dose chemotherapy with stem cell rescue is also being evaluated in this group of patients.

OSTEOSARCOMA

Only half of all childhood bone tumors are malignant, and osteosarcoma is the most common, followed by Ewing's sarcoma. It is derived from primitive bone-forming mesenchyme, which is distinct from the neural origins of Ewing's sarcoma. It is often diagnosed on plain films by its ability to produce new bone or osteoid tisssue. The survival of patients with nonmetastatic osteosarcoma has increased dramatically over the past 30 years.

Epidemiology

Bone tumors tend to peak in adolescence and are the third most frequent malignancy identified in young adults after leukemia and lymphoma. Ewing's sarcoma is more likely in a child younger than 10 years of age, and osteosarcoma is more common in an older child. Both tumors have a male predilection. The development of osteosarcoma is often associated with "growth spurts" when there is rapid elongation of bones. This is supported by the fact that this disease occurs at an earlier age in girls than in boys, is present in the humerus in younger children corresponding with the earlier growth of the humerus compared to the femur, occurs in individuals taller than their unaffected peers, and is found in the metaphyseal portion of bones. Patients with chronic bone diseases, such as Paget's disease, osteochondromas, enchondromas, fibrous dysplasia, chronic osteomyelitis, and sites of bone infarcts or implants, have an increased risk of malignant degeneration to osteosarcoma. Ionizing radiation and use of alkylating agents also can predispose patients to developing osteosarcoma.

Genetics

The genetics of osteosarcoma has been very closely linked to another childhood tumor, retinoblastoma. In the familial form, patients with retinoblastoma are at a greatly increased risk of developing a secondary osteosarcoma either within or outside of the radiation field. Both tumors have been shown to have losses of chromosome 13q14, which is the locus for the retinoblastoma gene (*RB*). In addition, mutations in another gene, *p53*, located on chromosome 17p13.1, have been described in up to 25% of all osteosarcoma tumors, whereas germ line mutations of this gene are present in 3.5% of all patients. This gene is involved in cell cycle regulation, and in mutated form damaged cells will not undergo the normal mechanism of self-destruction (apoptosis). Another gene on chromosome 12q13–14 encodes for the *MDM-2* gene, which regulates *p53*. Twenty percent of osteosarcoma samples show evidence of *MDM-2* gene amplification, which is speculated to inactivate *p53*. Certain cancer families at risk of developing osteosarcoma, breast cancer, brain tumors, leukemia, and adrenocortical tumors have germline mutations of the *p53* gene and are described as having the Li–Fraumeni syndrome. These families also have an increased rate of developing rhabdomyosarcomas.

Diagnosis

Patients often present with pain, with or without an associated mass, of a minimum of 3 months' duration. In contrast to Ewing's sarcoma, systemic symptoms such as fever are rare. Some patients may come to medical attention for a pathologic fracture. Sites of metastases mainly include other bones and the lungs. Unlike Ewing's sarcoma, osteosarcoma does not metastasize to the bone marrow. Most osteosarcomas are found in the distal femur or the proximal tibia. Laboratory tests may show an elevated serum alkaline phosphatase and lactate dehydrogenase. The definitive diagnosis is made after a biopsy of the tumor, which should be performed in a manner such that the entire biopsy tract can be resected at the time of the final surgery. CT evaluation of the lungs, plain films of the primary site, and a bone scan are all part of the initial radiographic evaluation. On plain films, one may note an intense periosteal reaction with lifting of the cortex in what is described as a Codman's triangle and production of osteoid material in the adjacent soft tissue described as a "sunburst."

Pathology

The detection of osteoid formation in the tumor biopsy sample with sarcomatous cells is helpful in the diagnosis of osteosarcoma. There are three major histologic subtypes: osteoblastic, chondroblastic, and fibroblastic osteosarcomas. Sarcomas in general can be graded as high or low grade, and the majority of pediatric osteosarcomas are high grade and require aggressive management. In addition, the pathologist can give important prognostic information based upon the degree of tumor necrosis in the tumor sample after chemotherapy.

Staging

There is no accepted international staging system for osteosarcoma. These tumors are in general classified by their extent of disease involvement as either local or metastatic.

Treatment

Patients without metastatic disease at diagnosis have an overall survival of 70% currently with the combination of chemotherapy and surgery. Unlike Ewing's sarcoma, osteosarcoma is not a radiosensitive tumor. The active chemotherapy agents include cisplatin, doxorubicin, high-dose methotrexate, and ifosfamide. Surgical resection of disease is accomplished by either an amputation or a limb-salvage procedure. The local recurrence rates in most studies are felt to be equivalent for the two procedures in properly selected patients. Patients with pulmonary metastases should have their disease fully resected if at all possible. Patients with bony metastases usually have a dismal prognosis.

Recurrent Disease

Children with isolated recurrent pulmonary nodules can be treated with excision of pulmonary metastases and further chemotherapy and can hope to attain a long-term cure. Children with bone metastases continue to fare poorly. Investigational agents currently being evaluated in this setting include topotecan and carboplatin.

BRAIN TUMORS

There are a number of different brain tumors in children; together they comprise the second largest group of malignancies in childhood after leukemia. Treatment continues to be difficult and should be undertaken in centers with a multidisciplinary approach including oncologists, neurosurgeons, radiation oncologists, psychologists, physical and occupational therapists, ophthalmologists, and social services.

Epidemiology

In childhood brain tumors, the peak incidence is during the first decade of life and consists mainly of embryonal tumors as compared to glial tumors, which are more common in adults. Brain tumors have been associated with an exposure to ionizing radiation and certain industrial chemicals. There are a number of different brain tumors including: (1) Medulloblastomas, which are also known as primitive neuroectodermal tumors (PNETs) of the cerebellum. They account for 40% of all childhood posterior fossa tumors and present at a peak age of 5 years with a male predominance. (2) Ependymomas, which are tumors arising from ependymal cells lining the ventricles of the brain, usually the fourth ventricle. Half of all children with ependymomas are diagnosed before the age of 5 years, with about half of those cases occuring before the age of 2 years. The male-to-female ratio is equal. (3) Cerebellar or infratentorial astrocytomas, which are predominantly pilocytic or low-grade tumors and peak at the age of 6 to 9 years. (4) Cerebral or supratentorial astrocytomas, which account for about one third of all childhood brain tumors and have a strong male predominance in the low-grade tumors. About 10% of these tumors are high grade and present at a median age of 9 to 10 years with an equal sex predilection. (5) Brain stem gliomas, which account for 10% to 20% of all childhood brain tumors and peak at age 5 to 9 years. Almost 80% of these tumors arise in the pons and are highly aggressive based upon their location. (6) Pineal germ cell tumors, which are rare tumors and tend to occur in males between 10 and 14 years of age.

Genetics

Numerous syndromes are associated with an increased risk of developing certain brain tumors. Neurofibromatosis type 1 is associated with optic gliomas and neurofibromatosis type 2 is associated with acoustic neuromas. Tuberous sclerosis can predispose patients to the development of glial tumors, and the von Hippel–Lindau syndrome is related to cerebellar hemangioblastomas. The Li–Fraumeni syndrome, which is a hereditary cancer syndrome resulting from a germline mutation of the *p53* gene, carries a high frequency of astrocytomas in affected family members. Other syndromes include the nevoid basal cell carcinoma syndrome, Turcot syndrome, ataxia–telangiectasia syndrome, and the multiple endocrine neoplasm syndromes. Outside of the context of a syndrome, many of these brain tumors show loss of heterozygosity at various chromosomal locations including chromosomes 17, 22, 10, and 9p. Other brain tumors show a gain of chromosomal material at chromosome 7.

Diagnosis

Most tumors in pediatrics are infratentorial, whereas adult tumors tend to be supratentorial. The initial signs and symptoms depend upon the age of the child and the location of the tumor. Evidence of raised intracranial pressure may be defined by morning headaches, vomiting, and lethargy. In addition, children may present with cranial nerve findings, ataxia, hemiparesis, hyperreflexia, clonus, papilledema, seizures, change in personality or school performance, anorexia, and irritability. A younger child may show a rapidly enlarging head circumference or the "setting sun" sign, which is an impaired upward gaze secondary to increased intracranial pressure. The MRI scan is the preferred method of evaluating a brain tumor and should include the entire spine to evaluate for tumor dissemination. Most tumors will be amenable to a biopsy but brainstem gliomas are usually not biopsied owing to their location and grim prognosis. If there is a high likelihood of meningeal or distant spread, such as in medulloblastomas, a lumbar puncture and/or a bone marrow aspiration may be necessary.

Pathology

Medulloblastomas have characteristic Homer Wright rosettes and can have varying degrees of differentiation. Ependymomas can also have pseudorosettes as well as evidence of calcification, hemorrhage, and cyst formation. Cerebellar astrocytomas tend to be of the pilocytic type, which often carry a good prognosis, whereas cerebral astrocytomas can be low to high grade. Staining for AFP and β-human chorionic gonadotropin can be useful in the diagnosis of intracranial germ cell tumors.

Staging

There is no accepted international staging system for brain tumors. The tumors are often referred to as localized or metastatic. The tumors can be unifocal or multifocal.

Treatment

Treatment depends on histology and age at diagnosis, but generally involves surgery, radiation therapy, and/or chemotherapy. Surgery may also include inserting a ventriculoperitoneal shunt for relief of obstruction, prevention of herniation, and resolution of midline shift. Decadron and diuretics such as mannitol are often used to reduce cerebral edema. Chemotherapy agents used in the treatment of central nervous system malignancies include cisplatin, carboplatin, cyclophosphamide, etoposide, the nitrosoureas, vincristine, and melphalan. In a younger child, new chemotherapeutic agents are being tested in an attempt to delay radiation therapy and to avoid the late sequelae of radiation. Prognosis varies depending upon the age of the child, histology of the tumor, surgical resectability, presence or absence of spread, and evidence of brainstem invasion.

Recurrent Disease

In certain high-risk tumors such as medulloblastoma, strategies such as high-dose chemotherapy with stem cell rescue are being explored in patients with recurrent disease. In addition, new agents specifically targeting the central nervous system are being evaluated including newer modalities of delivering radiation. New agents administered intrathecally are also being investigated.

LONG-TERM FOLLOW-UP

As there are increasingly more survivors of childhood cancer, the long-term follow-up of these patients becomes increasingly relevant. Many of these effects are directly related to the tumor itself, in addition to the therapeutic modalities involved. The age of the child during treatment is also crucial. Long-term toxicities from chemotherapy can include hearing loss, renal tubular disease with development of hypophosphatemic rickets, hepatic fibrosis, avascular necrosis of bone (femoral and humeral heads especially), pulmonary fibrosis, cardiomyopathy, infertility, bladder scarring, peripheral neuropathy, and the development of secondary malignancies. Radiation therapy can contribute to the development of growth disturbances including scoliosis and short stature. In addition, cataracts, xerostomia, hypothyroidism, pituitary hormone deficiencies, secondary malignancies, infertility, and learning disabilities may result from radiation therapy. Certain surgeries such as amputations for bone tumors can be disfiguring and require intensive rehabilitation.

FURTHER READING

Black PMcL (1991) Brain tumors. *N Engl J Med* 324:1471–1476.

Black PMcL (1991) Brain tumors. *N Engl J Med* 324:1555–1564.

Bonilla MA, Cheung N-KV (1994) Clinical progress in neuroblastoma. *Cancer Invest* 12:644–653.

Brodeur GM, Castleberry RP (1997) In: Pizzo PA, Poplack DG (eds), Neuroblastoma. *Principles and Practice of Pediatric Oncology*. JB Lippincott, Philadelphia, pp. 761–797.

Castleberry RP (1997) Biology and treatment of neuroblastoma. *Pediatr Clin NA Pediatr Oncol* 44:919–938.

Coppes MJ, Ritchey ML (1995) The management of synchronous bilateral Wilms' tumor. *Hematol Oncol Clin NA* 9:1303–1315.

Crist WM, Kun LE (1991) Common solid tumors of childhood. *N Engl J Med* 324:461–471.

Gasparin M, Lombardi F, Ballerini E, Gandola L, Gianni MD, et al. (1994) Long-term outcome of patients with monostotic Ewing's sarcoma treated with combined modality. *Med Pediatr Oncol* 23:406–412.

Green DM (1997) Pediatric oncology update Wilms' tumor. *Eur J Cancer* 33:409–418.

Green DM, D'Angio GJ, Beckwith JB, Breslow NE, Grundy PE et al. (1996) Wilms' tumor. *CA Cancer J Clin* 46:46–63.

Greenberg M, Filler RM (1997) Hepatic tumors. In: Pizzo PA, Poplack DG (eds) *Principles and Practices of Pediatric Oncology*. JB Lippincott, Philadelphia, pp. 717–732.

Greir HE (1997) The Ewing family of tumors: Ewing's sarcoma and primitive neuroectodermal tumors. *Pediatr Clin NA Pediatr Oncol* 44:991–1004.

Heideman RL, Packer RJ, Albright LA, Freeman CR, Rorke LB (1997) Tumors of the central nervous system. In: Pizzo PA, Poplack DG (eds) *Principles and Practice of Pediatric Oncology*. JB Lippincott, Philadelphia, pp. 633-698.

Horowitz ME, Malawer MM, Woo SY, Hicks JM (1997) Ewing's sarcoma family of tumors: Ewing's sarcoma of bone. In: Pizzo PA, Poplack DG (eds) *Principles and Practice of Pediatric Oncology*. JB Lippincott, Philadelphia, pp. 831–864.

Kobrinsky NL, Talgoy M, Shuckett B, Gritter HL (1993) Wilms' tumor. *Hematol Oncol Ann* 1:173–185.

Kun LE (1997) Brain tumors: Challenges and directions. *Pediatr Clin NA Pediatr Oncol* 44:907–918.

Kushner BH, Cheung N-KV (1993) Neuroblastoma: An overview. *Hematol Oncol Ann* 1:189–201.

Link MP, Eilber F (1997) Osteosarcoma. In: Pizzo PA, Poplack DG (eds) *Principles and Practice of Pediatric Oncology*. JB Lippincott, Philadelphia, pp. 889-920.

Marina N (1997) Long-term survivors of childhood cancer: The medical consequence of cure. *Pediatr Clin NA Pediatr Oncol* 44:1021–1042.

Meyers PA, Gorlick R (1997) Osteosarcoma. *Pediatr Clin NA Pediatr Oncol* 44:973–990.

Niethammer D, Handgretinger R (1995) Clinical strategies for the treatment of neuroblastoma. *Eur J Cancer* 31A: 568–571.

O'Reilly R (1996) NCCN pediatric neuroblastoma practice guidelines. *Oncology* 10:1813–1822.

O'Reilly R (1996) NCCN pediatric osteosarcoma practice guidelines. *Oncology* 10:1799–1812.

Pappo AS, Shapiro DN, Crist WM (1997) Rhabdomyosarcome: Biology and treatment. *Pediatr Clin NA Pediatr Oncol* 44:953–972.

Petruzzi MD, Green DM (1997) Wilms' tumor. *Pediatr Clin NA Pediatr Oncol* 44:939–952.

Rubnitz JE, Crist WM (1997) Molecular genetics of childhood cancer: Implications for pathogenesis, diagnosis, and treatment. *Pediatrics* 100:101–108.

Tebbi CK (1993) Osteosarcoma in childhood and adolescence. *Hematol Oncol Ann* 1:203–228.

Wexler LH, Helman LJ (1997) Rhabdomyosarcoma and the undifferentiated sarcomas. In: Pizzo PA, Poplack DG (eds) *Principles and Practice of Pediatric Oncology*. JB Lippincott, Philadelphia, pp. 799–830.

Wexler LH, DeLaney TF, Tsokos M, Avila N, Steinberg SM, et al. (1996) Ifosfamide and etoposide plus vincristine, doxorubicin, and cyclophosphamide for newly diagnosed Ewing's sarcoma family of tumors. *Cancer* 78:901–911.

CHAPTER 35

AIDS-RELATED MALIGNANCIES

ANIL TULPULE and ALEXANDRA M. LEVINE

Department of Medicine
University of Southern California
Los Angeles, CA 90033, USA

In this chapter, the pathogenesis and treatment of Kaposi's sarcoma and the malignant lymphomas etiologically related to underlying infection with the AIDS virus are reviewed. Treatment programs for these malignancies have evolved significantly over the past decade and involve the use of interferon-α or liposomal formulations of the anthracyclines for AIDS-related Kaposi's sarcoma or low-dose combination chemotherapy for AIDS-related lymphomas.

AIDS-RELATED KAPOSI'S SARCOMA

Epidemiology

Kaposi's sarcoma (KS) is the most common tumor seen in AIDS and has been reported in 20% to 50% of AIDS patients. It is seen more frequently in homosexual and bisexual men than in populations with other risk factors for HIV infection. There has been a steady decline in the incidence of KS since the beginning of the epidemic. This decline may be related to changes in lifestyle that have occurred in the male homosexual population, such as a decrease in high-risk sexual behaviors, number of sexual partners, use of recreational drugs, and occurrence of other sexually transmitted diseases. Furthermore, the use of antiretroviral agents through inhibition of human immunodeficiency virus (HIV) may inhibit the growth of KS. These possibilities, however, remain speculative at present and need appropriate scientific investigation.

Manual of Clinical Oncology, 7th edition, Edited by Raphael E. Pollock
ISBN 0-471-23828-7, pages 709–721. Copyright © 1999 Wiley-Liss, Inc.

Pathogenesis

To understand the pathogenesis of KS a number of issues must be addressed, including the origin of the KS cell, the role of autocrine and paracrine growth modulators, and the roles of HIV and human herpes virus type 8 (HHV8). Extensive studies have been performed to define the origin of the KS tumor cell. The KS tumor cells (spindle cells) display features of mesenchymal cells, particularly endothelical cells. Markers shared with endothelial cells include lectin binding sites for *Ulex europeaus* agglutinin-1 (UEA-1), CD 34, EN-4, PAL-E, and endothelial cell-specific tyrosine kinases such as vascular endothelial growth factor (VEGF) receptors. The hallmark of KS is the aberrant and enhanced proliferation of vascular structures. Various angiogenic factors have been shown to enhance endothelial cell proliferation and migration in vitro. AIDS-related KS cells express basic fibroblast growth factor (bFGF) and VEGF. VEGF can induce capillary permeability which is a prominent feature of a subset of AIDS-related KS. Furthermore, several studies have shown that cytokines such as interleukin (IL)-1β, IL-6, and Oncostatin M are autocrine growth factors for AIDS-related KS. Both IL-1β and IL-6 are produced by KS cells, and inhibition of their effects whether through blocking the receptors (IL-1 receptor antagonist) or inhibition of gene expression through antisense oligonucleotides (for IL-6) can inhibit the growth of KS cells. Oncostatin M expressed in KS cells is also known to induce the growth of these cells. Furthermore, inhibition of Oncostatin-M expression through antisense oligonucleotides can reduce the proliferative potential of AIDS-KS cells. The role of glucocorticoids in KS is also well documented. Use of glucocorticoids may be associated with either development or progression of KS. The expression of glucocorticoids and their mitogenic effect on KS in vitro has been established. HIV may play an indirect role in the pathogenesis of KS via the aforementioned cytokines. Thus, IL-1β, tumor necrosis factor-α (TNF-α), and IL-6 are perturbed as a result of HIV infection. These cytokines could increase the rate of growth of KS lesions. Furthermore, although HIV is not known to infect the KS cell per se, transfection of fertilized eggs from transgenic mice expressing the HIV tat protein results in expression of the tat protein in skin alone in the offspring, with development of a tumor that appears identical to KS, of mouse origin, in 15% of the male offspring. The tumor cells, however, do not express the tat gene. In addition, HHV8-related DNA sequences have recently been identified within KS tissues using a newly developed method called representation difference analysis. Approximately 95% of AIDS-KS tissues contain HHV8 viral sequences. Similar viral sequences were subsequently identified in B-lymphoma cell lines derived from patients with a rare type of lymphoma called body cavity lymphoma and/or primary effusion lymphomas. Large-scale epidemiologic studies of KS have revealed that all forms of KS contain HHV-8 DNA sequences, including the classic form of KS, African form, and transplant-associated KS. Analysis of various other tissues have shown that HHV-8 sequences are present in peripheral blood B lymphocytes, but rarely in other tissues. Of interest, infection by HHV8 has been shown to precede the clinical development of KS. Although the current data would suggest that HHV8 infection is necessary for KS development, infection per se is not sufficient, as normal blood donors with evidence of HHV8 infection have also been described.

Pathology

In addition to the diagnostic spindle cells, the KS tumor also consists of small vascular spaces, numerous dilated abnormal lymphocytes. Blood vessels, and extravasated red cells present in slitlike vascular structures. A variety of mononuclear cells may also be present in these lesions, including T cells, plasma cells, and phagocytic macrophages. Often there is associated edema. Histologically, KS lesions are remarkably similar, regardless of anatomic location (skin, lymph nodes, respiratory tract, or gastrointestinal tract).

The cutaneous lesions of Kaposi's sarcoma are classified into patch, plaque, and/or nodular lesions. Early on, KS of the skin begins as a small, flat purple lesion (patch lesion). The lesion may broaden and become elevated to form a plaque. A plaque may enlarge progressively to become a nodule. Histopathologic studies show that earlier lesions are located in the reticular (upper) dermis, with subdermal involvement in some cases.

Clinical Manifestations

AIDS-related KS, seen most commonly in homosexual men, affects predominantly the skin in the form of multifocal purplish lesions. Other sites of involvement include the lymph nodes, gastrointestinal tract, oral mucosa, conjunctiva, and lungs. Initially these skin lesions are small and flat, but may progress to form purple nodules, which are generally painless and nonpruritic. The lesions may be associated with local edema, may coalesce to form large infiltrating lesions, and may even ulcerate and cause local pain. Interestingly, although the soles of the feet can be affected, the palms are rarely involved. Extracutaneous involvement represents advanced disease. The oral cavity is involved in nearly one third of cases, often the palate. Visceral involvement, particularly in the gastrointestinal tract, occurs in nearly 50% of cases with oral KS and may involve the esophagus, stomach, duodenum, colon, and rectum. Advanced gastrointestinal involvement may cause abdominal pain, early satiety, and gastrointestinal (GI) bleeding. Asymptomatic gastrointestinal involvement does not affect survival, and routine evaluation is not needed in the absence of symptoms. However, symptomatic gastrointestinal involvement should be evaluated with endoscopy, as barium contrast studies often produce false-negative findings.

Pulmonary involvement has also been reported with increasing frequency in the past several years, and has occurred in 20% to 50% of KS cases. Pulmonary involvement can often be diagnosed with bronchoscopy without biopsy, owing to the classic appearance of these lesions; further, biopsy is often complicated by bleeding. Patients with significant involvement often complain of exertional dyspnea, dry cough, and hemoptysis. Radiographic findings are nonspecific and may include diffuse interstitial infiltrates, mediastinal adenopathy, pulmonary nodules, and/or pleural effusions, in order of decreasing frequency. Patients with advanced pulmonary involvement have a poor prognosis, with a median survival of only 3 months.

Prognostic Features

Poor prognostic factors in AIDS-related KS include systemic B symptoms, prior or coexistent opportunistic infections, and a CD4 count of less than 300/mm^3. While the expected median survival of patients without any of these poor prognostic factors is 31 months, survival decreases to 15 months in patients with CD4 counts less than 300/mm^3 and the presence of B symptoms, while the expected median survival in patients with CD4 $< D$300 m^3, systemic B symptoms, and history of opportunistic infection is only 7 months. In addition, gastrointestinal involvement can cause bleeding associated with increased morbidity and mortality, while pulmonary involvement is also a poor prognostic sign.

Treatment

Treatment of KS may be either local or systemic. Decisions regarding treatment are based on prognostic factors including tumor bulk, systemic B symptoms, and the presence or absence of visceral involvement. For example, patients with extensive cutaneous disease/visceral involvement require systemic therapy. Patients with symptomatic pulmonary KS need immediate treatment with systemic chemotherapy. In addition, the patient's immune status can have an impact on treatment decision because, for example, patients with CD4 counts $\leq$ 400/mm^3 are more likely to respond to interferon-α than patients with CD4 counts less than 200/mm^3. Local therapies are appropriate options for patients with localized cutaneous disease and a slowly progressive course. Local therapies are usually used for cosmetic purposes and include radiation therapy or intralesional injections of vinblastine, vincristine, or interferon-α. In addition, other local therapies that have been useful include surgical excision, liquid nitrogen, cryotheraphy, sclerotherapy, and argon laser therapy.

Systemic therapies for AIDS-related KS include interferon-α, and, in more advanced viseral disease, cytotoxic chemotherapeutic agents. Interferon-α is an important agent in KS because of its immunoregulatory, antitumor, and antiviral activity, interfering with viral assembly at the cell membrane. Furthermore, in vitro, interferon-α acts synergistically with axidothymidine of zidovudine (AZT) in HIV inhibition. Interferon-α has been used at a dose of 1 mU to 52 mU per day. Response rates ranging between 25% and 50% have been shown at the higher dose levels. Upon analyzing CD4 lymphocyte counts as a parameter to predict response to interferon, it is clear that patients with CD4 counts above 400/mm^3 are most likely to achieve tumor response. In view of known synergistic effects of interferon-α and zidovudine on HIV-1 replication, combinations of AZT and interferon have been shown to be more efficacious than interferon alone. Thus, combining 8 to 10 million units SQ daily of interferon-α with 500 mg/day of AZT, a response rate of approximately 30% was seen in patients with poor prognostic factors, while those with good prognostic factors experience a response rate of 50 % to 60%. Studies evaluating combinations of interferon-α and protease inhibitors are in progress.

Chemotherapy

Systemic cytotoxic chemotherapy is warranted in patients with extensive or rapidly progressive cutaneous KS, symptomatic visceral involvement, pulmonary KS, and those with significant lymphedema. Single-agent chemotherapy has been associated with modest responses. Thus, vinblastine used alone has produced responses in fewer than one third of cases. Other agents used effectively as single agents include etoposide, doxorubicin, and alternating vinblastine and vincristine. As shown by Gill et al., "ABV," a combination of doxorubicin (20 mg/m^2), bleomycin (10 mg/m^2), and vincristine (2 mg) given every 2 weeks is well tolerated, with responses in over 80%, while doxorubicin alone at the same dose and schedule produced major responses in just under 50% of the cases. Combinations of bleomycin and vincristine at the above dosages and schedule can be administered, even when patients have compromised bone marrow function, and result in response rates of approximately 70%. Patients with symptomatic pulmonary KS have a predicted survival of approximately 3 months without therapy, but may respond to combination chemotherapy with improved survival. In a retrospective analysis, combinations of AZT with bleomycin and vincristine have been well tolerated with high response rates (Gill et al., 1990); predominant toxicity consists of anemia and neutropenia. Prospective studies of chemotherapy and AZT, with or without granulocyte-macrophage-colony-stimulating factor (GM-CSF) have shown that AZT is very difficult to administer, even with GM-CSF support. Use of G-CSF in this circumstance may be more effective with fewer side effects. Two liposomal formulations, liposomal daunorubicin (DaunoXome®) and liposomal doxorubicin (Doxil®) have recently been shown to be less toxic and more efficacious than the ABV combination in the treatment of AIDS/KS. Based on these studies, DaunoXome® has been approved for first line treatment of AIDS/KS, and Doxil® has been approved for second-line treatment of AIDS/KS. Neutropenia is the most significant toxicity of both these agents. More recently, paclitaxel has been approved in the treatment of this condition. Employing paclitaxel at a dose of 100 mg/m^2 IV every other week, a response rate of 59% was achieved; the dose-limiting toxicity in this setting is bone marrow suppression, primarily neutropenia.

AIDS-ASSOCIATED LYMPHOMA

Epidemiology

Since the early 1980s the incidence of high-grade B-cell lymphomas has steadily increased in the HIV-infected population, now comprising between 3% and 5% of all patients with AIDS. In 1985 sufficient epidemiologic data were available to indicate a statistical increase in systemic lymphoma resulting in the inclusion of intermediate and high-grade B-cell lymphoma as AIDS-defining illnesses in October of 1985. This delayed recognition of systemic lymphoma as a criterion for AIDS is consistent with the hypothesis that lymphoma is a relatively late manifestation of infection by HIV, a concept that has recently been supported by data from the National Cancer

Institute. The incidence of lymphoma in HIV-infected individuals is approximately 60 times greater than that expected in the general population. The risk of developing lymphomas in patients with symptomatic HIV infection appears to be approximately 1.6% per year. Further, the chance of lymphoma developing in patients with AIDS alive on antiretroviral therapy for 3 years is estimated to be approximately 19%. Unlike KS, in which the predominant group affected appears to be homosexual men, AIDS lymphoma occurs at similar rates in any group at risk for HIV infection (Levine, 1982, 1988).

Pathogenesis

Although the precise mechanisms of the pathogenesis of lymphoma in the setting of HIV infection are not yet fully elucidated, there are several possible mechanisms including the roles of HIV, cytokines/growth factors, EBV, and ongoing B-cell proliferation. HIV, per se, is not directly involved in the malignant transformation of B lymphocytes. However, HIV may play an indirect role via cytokine release, which may then be responsible for the development of milieu supportive of the proliferation and activation of B lymphocytes, and eventually of B-cell lymphoma. These cytokines include IL-4, IL-6, IL-10, lymphotoxin, and B-cell growth factors. Diffuse large cell and immunoblastic lymphomas have been shown to express high levels of IL-10 produced directly by the tumor cells, and IL-10 has been confirmed as an autocrine growth factor in AIDS lymphoma. In addition, IL-6 is thought to be relevant to both premalignant B cell expansion as well as malignant transformation in AIDS lymphoma. IL-6 gene expression is upregulated by growth factors/cytokines such as IL-1 and tumor necrosis factor (Birx et al. 1990). Hence, HIV infection with resultant stimulation of these inflammatory cytokines might allow increased IL-6 expression.

In addition to the permissive cytokine milieu, numerous studies have demonstrated that EBV may be involved in the pathogenesis of AIDS lymphoma. While EBV is present in almost 100% of AIDS-related primary central nervous system (CNS) lymphomas, the percentage of EBV in systemic lymphomas varies in different studies. For instance, whereas 66% of 59 patients with AIDS-related systemic lymphomas from the University of Southern California were found to be associated with EBV, EBV sequences were detected in only 38% of 16 AIDS lymphoma tissues tested by Subar et al. The prevalence of EBV expression also depends on the histology of the lymphoma. Hence EBV DNA has been found in 65% of systemic large-cell and immunoblastic lymphomas as compared to 21% of cases with Burkitt's-like small noncleaved lymphoma.

Rearrangement of the c-*myc* oncogene occurs in approximately 75% of all systemic lymphomas. The probability of c-*myc* rearrangement also varies among the different in different histologic types, seen more frequently in small noncleaved lymphoma and less frequently in immunoblastic and diffuse large-cell lymphomas. Overall, there appear to be multiple pathogenic mechanisms leading to the development of AIDS lymphoma, with different aberrations leading to different pathologic types of lymphomatous disease.

Pathology

AIDS-related lymphomas consist of high-grade and intermediate grade histologic types. Approximately 66% consist of either immunoblastic or small noncleaved types expected in only 10% to 20% of lymphomas in the general population. The remaining third of AIDS lymphoma cases consist of "intermediate grade," diffuse large-cell lymphoma. Although, some investigators have found certain clinico-pathologic correlates of disease in the intermediate versus high-grade types, these correlates have not been confirmed in other series (Jones et al. 1973), and at the present time it is probably justified to consider patients with either intermediate or high-grade disease similarly, with regard to prognosis and therapy. A small number of patients with underlying HIV infection have also been diagnosed with low-grade lymphomas, including chronic lymphocytic leukemia, multiple myeloma, and small cleaved lymphoma.

Clinical Manifestations

In contrast to the intermediate and high-grade lymphomas in HIV-negative individuals, AIDS-related lymphomas usually have extranodal lymphomatous involvement at presentation. Hence, while 39% of 405 HIV-negative lymphoma patients were found to have extranodel disease at diagnosis, approximately 90% of patients with AIDS-related lymphomas have such extranodal disease. Extranodal sites commonly affected in AIDS lymphomas include the CNS in 26%; bone marrow in 22%, gastrointestinal tract in 17%; and liver in 12%. Unusual sites of disease such as the scalp, popliteal fossa, earlobe, and rectum have also been reported. Systemic B symptoms are very frequent (70% to 80%) and may pose a diagnostic problem, as they may also suggest an underlying infectious process in an immunocompromised patient. The degree of immunosuppression in patients with AIDS lymphoma is variable. Sixty percent have not had an AIDS-defining illness prior to the diagnosis of lymphoma, and the median CD4 count in this group is approximately $200/mm^3$. In contrast, approximately 75% of patients with AIDS-related primary CNS lymphoma have had a prior AIDS-defining illness, and the median CD4 count is $30/mm^3$.

Staging of AIDS lymphoma, as in the non-HIV situation, includes a history and physical exam, computerized tomography (CT) of chest, abdomen, and pelvis; a gallium scan; and a bone marrow aspirate and biopsy. However, because of the propensity for CNS involvement in AIDS lymphomas, CT or magnetic resonance imaging (MRI) of the brain, as well as a lumbar puncture, for routine studies, cultures, and cytology is warranted as part of the initial staging evaluation. In addition, general assessment of HIV-related factors such as history of prior AIDS, number of CD4 cells, and HIV viral load, performance status, and presence or absence of B symptoms should be recorded.

Prognostic Factors

Poor prognostic features in AIDS lymphoma include the presence of AIDS prior to the diagnosis of lymphoma, CD4 count of less than $100/mm^3$, Karnofsky performance status (KPS) of 70% or less, and the presence of extranodal disease. In a retrospective study of 60 cases of systemic lymphoma in known HIV-seropositive individuals, all of whom were treated with curative intent, Levine defined three poor prognostic indicators on multivariate analysis, including a KPS less than 70%; an AIDS diagnosis prior to development of lymphoma; and the presence of bone marrow involvement. Lower CD4 counts, on a continuous scale, were also a significant predictor of shorter survival. A more recent report on 192 patients identified age > 35 years and IV drug use as factors associated with shortened survival, in addition to CD4 count <100 /mm^3 and stage III/IV disease.

Patients with primary CNS lymphoma have a very poor prognosis with median survival of only 2 to 3 months. However, leptomeningeal involvement in patients with systemic lymphoma does not adversely affect prognosis, if appropriate treatment is rendered.

Treatment

There have been reports of the efficacious use of intensive therapy in HIV-infected patients with lymphoma. The MACOP-B regimen was employed by Bermudez et al. in 12 patients, 8 of whom (67%) attained complete remission. It is noteworthy that 6/8 had a KPS of 100%, and only one had a KPS less than 80%. Furthermore, only one had a history of AIDS prior to the diagnosis of lymphoma. It is certainly possible, then, that selected individuals, without poor prognostic characteristics, may be able to tolerate such dose-intensive therapy with good response. However, in the majority of individuals with more severe HIV-related disease (history of prior AIDS; low CD4 cells; low KPS), such dose-intensive therapy is likely to be quite toxic, and inefffective. Currently, low-dose chemotherapy should be considered the treatment of choice.

Primary CNS Lymphoma

Primary CNS lymphoma presents with mass lesions in the brain; any parenchymal area may be involved. Symptoms include seizures, focal neurologic dysfunction, headache, and/or cranial nerve palsies. Interestingly, affected patients may present with altered mental status, even of a very subtle nature, as the only clinical manifestation of disease.

Radiographic evaluation usually reveals one or two relatively large (2 to 4 cm) homogeneous or heterogeneous lesions within the parenchyma. Ring enhancement may be seen on double-dose contrast studies, and in general, the lesions are enhancing. Although CT scans of the brain may be similar in patients with cerebral toxoplasmosis, these individuals often have multiple, smaller lesions than those seen in primary CNS lymphoma. It is not unusual for such patients to receive empiric therapy for cerebral toxoplasmosis, with repeat of the CT scan within 1 to 2 weeks. With definite improvement documented, the patient may be safely assumed to have cerebral toxoplasmosis. However, with similar or worsening disease parameters after this period of empiric therapy, a brain biopsy is indicated to confirm the diagnosis of primary CNS lymphoma or some other pathologic process.

The prognosis of the HIV-infected patients with primary CNS lymphoma is quite poor. In fact, the survival of these individuals, even when treated, was only in the range of 2 to 3 months. Interestingly, patients with primary CNS disease have significantly more severe underlying HIV-related disease, as reflected by the fact that 73% had a prior diagnosis of AIDS, and the median CD4 count at diagnosis of lymphoma was only 34/mm^3.

Although radiation therapy may be associated with complete remission in approximately 50% of these patients, median survival is only 2 to 3 months with death due to intercurrent opportunistic infections and the presence of multiple ongoing neuropathologic processes. Of importance, however, CNS radiation may be associated with significant improvement in the quality of life in approximately 75% of treated patients. Nonetheless, it is clear that alternative methods of treatment must be devised for these individuals.

FURTHER READING

Gill PS, Hamilton A, Naidu Y (1994) Epidemic (AIDS-related) Kaposi's sarcoma: Epidemiology, pathogenesis and treatment. *AIDS Updates* 7:1–11.

Fauci AS, Masur H, Gelman EP, et al. (1985) The acquired immunodeficiency syndrome. An update. *Ann Intern Med* 102:800–813.

Russel Jones R, Spaul J, Spry C, Wilson Jones E (1986) Histogenesis of Kaposi's sarcoma in patients with and without acquired immunodeficiency syndrome. *J Clin Pathol* 39:742–749.

Massod R, Cai J, Zheng T (1997) Vascular endothelical growth factor, vascular permeability factor (VEGF/VPF) is an autocrine growth factor for AIDS-KS. *Proc Natl Acad Sci USA* 94:979–984.

Miles SA, Rezai AR, Salazar-Gonzales JF, et al. (1990) AIDS-Kaposi's sarcoma derived cells produce and respond to interleukin-6. *Proc Natl Acad Sci USA* 87:4068–4072.

Louie S, Cai J, Law R, et al. (1995) The effect of interleukin-1 in AIDS-KS. *J AIDS Hum Retrovirol* 8:455–460.

Nair BC, DeVico AL, Nakamura S, et al. (1992) Identification of a major growth factor for AIDS-Kaposi's sarcoma cells as Oncostatin M. *Science* 255:1432–1434.

Miles SA, Martinez-Mala O, Rezai A, et al. (1992) Oncostatin M as a potent mitogen for AIDS Kaposi's sarcoma-derived cells. *Science* 255:1432–1434.

Cai J, Zhang T, Gill PS (1997) Glucocorticoids enhance AIDS-related Kaposi's sarcoma growth through inhibition of TGF-β. *Blood* 81:1491–1500.

Vogel J, Hinrichs SH, Reynolds RK, Luciu PA, Jay G (1988) The HIV *tat* gene induces dermal lesions resembling Kaposi's sarcoma in transgenic mice. *Nature* 335:606–611.

Chang Y, Cesarmen E, Pessin MS, et al. (1994) Identification of herpesvirus-like DNA sequences in AIDS-associated Kaposi's sarcoma. *Science* 266:1865–1869.

Cesarman E, Chang Y, Moore PS, et al. (1995) Kaposi's sarcoma-associated herpesvirus-like DNA sequences in AIDS-related body-cavity-based lymphomas. *N Engl J Med* 332:1186–1191.

Huang YQ, Li JJ, Kaplan MH, et al. (1995) Human herpesvirus-like nucleic acid in various forms of Kaposi's sarcoma. *Lancet* 345:759–760.

Moore PS, Chang Y (1995) Detection of herpesvirus-like DNA sequences in Kaposi's sarcoma in patients with and those without HIV infection. *N Engl J Med* 332:1181–1185.

Dupin N, Grandadam M, Calvez V, et al. (1995) Herpes-virus-like DNA sequences in patients with Mediterranean Kaposi's sarcoma. *Lancet* 345:761–762.

Facchetti F, Lucini L, Gavazzoni R, Callea F (1988) Immunomorphologic analysis of the role of blood vessel endothelium in the morphogenesis of cutaneous Kaposi's sarcoma: A study of 57 cases. *Histopathology* 12:581–593.

Friedman-Kien AE, Laubenstein LJ, Rubinstein P, et al. (1982) Disseminated Kaposi's sarcoma in homosexual men. *Ann Intern Med* 96:693–700.

Gill PS, Akil B, Colletti P, et al. (1989) Pulmonary Kaposi's sarcoma: Clinical findings and results of therapy. *Am J Med* 87:57–61.

Chachoua A, Krigel R, Lafleur F, et al. (1989) Prognostic factors and staging classification of patients with epidemic Kaposi's sarcoma. *J Clin Onc* 7:745–748.

DeWit R, Boucher CB, Veenhof KN, et al. (1988) Clinical and virological effects of high dose recombinant interferon-alpha in disseminated AIDS related Kaposi's sarcoma. *Lancet* 2:1214–1217.

Lane HC, Feinberg J, Davey V, et al. (1988) Anti-retroviral effects of interferon-alpha in AIDS-associated Kaposi's sarcoma. *Lancet* 2:1218–1222.

Hill DR (1987) The role of radiotherapy for epidemic Kaposi's sarcoma. *Semin Oncol* 14:19–22.

Chak LY, Gill PS, Levine AM, et al. (1988) Radiation therapy for acquired immunodeficiency syndrome related Kaposi's sarcoma. *J Clin Onc* 6:863–867.

Epstein JB (1989) Oral Kaposi's sarcoma in acquired immunodeficiency syndrome. *Cancer* 64:2424–2430.

Sulis E, Floris C, Luisa Serlis M, et al. (1989) Interferon administered intralesionally in skin and oral cavity lesions in heterosexual drug addicted patients with AIDS-related Kaposi's sarcoma. *Eur J Cancer Clin Oncol* 25:759–761.

Serling U (1991) Local therapies for cutaneous Kaposi's sarcoma in patients with acquired immunodeficiency syndrome. *Arch Dermatol* 127:1479–1481.

Groopman JE, Gottlieb MS, Goodman J, et al. (1984) Recombinant alpha-2 interferon for Kaposi's sarcoma associated with the acquired immunodeficiency syndrome. *Ann Intern Med* 100:671–676.

Fischl MA, Uttamchandani RB, Resnick L, et al. (1991) A phase I study of recombinant human interferon-α 2a or human lymphoblastoid interferon-α NL and concomitant zidovudine in patients with AIDS-related Kaposi's sarcoma. *J AIDS* 4:1–10.

Volberding PA, Abrams DI, Conant M et al. (1985) Vinblastine therapy for Kaposi's sarcoma in the acquired immunodeficiency syndrome. *Ann Intern Med* 103:335–338.

Laubenstein LJ, Krigel RL, Odajnk CM, et al. (1984) Treatment of epidemic Kaposi's sarcoma with etoposide or a combination of doxorubicin, bleomycin, and vinblastine. *J Clin Onc* 2:1115–1120.

Gill PS, Rarick MU, Espina B, et al. (1990) Advanced acquired immunodeficiency syndrome related Kaposi's sarcoma. Results of pilot studies using combination chemotherapy. *Cancer* 65:1074–1078.

Gill PS, Rarick M, Bernstein-Singer M et al. (1990) Treatment of advanced Kaposi's sarcoma using a combination of bleomycin and vincristine. *Am J Clin Onc* 13:315–319.

Gill PS, Wernz J, Scadden DT, et al. (1996) Randomized phase III trial of liposomal daunorubicin versus doxorubicin, bleomycin and vincristine in AIDS-related Kaposi's sarcoma. *J Clin Onc* 14:2353-2364.

Harrison D, Tomlinson D, Stewart S (1995) Lipsomal-entrapped doxorubicin: An active agent in AIDS-related Kaposi's sarcoma. *J Clin Onc* 13:914–920.

Geobel F-D, Goldstein D, Goos M, et al. (1996) Efficacy and safety of stealth liposomal doxorubicin in AIDS-related Kaposi's sarcoma. *Br J Cancer* 73:989–994.

Ross RK, Dworsky RL, Paganini-Hill A, et al. (1985) Non-Hodgkin's lymphomas in never married men in Los Angeles. *Br J Cancer* 52:785–797.

CDC (1985) Revision of the case definition of acquired immunodeficiency syndrome for national reporting—United States. *MMWR* 34:373–375.

Pluda JM, Yarchoan R, Jaffe ES, et al. (1990) Development of lymphoma in a cohort of patients with severe human immunodeficiency virus (HIV) infection on long term antiretroviral therapy. *Ann Intern Med* 113:276–282.

Monfardini S, Vaccher E, Tirelli V (1990) AIDS-associated non-Hodgkin's lymphoma in Italy: Intravenous drug users versus homosexual men. *Ann Oncol* 1:208–211.

Jelinek DF, Lipsky PE (1987) Enhancement of human B cell proliferation and differentiation by tumor necrosis factor-alpha and interleukin 1. *J Immunol* 139:2970–2976.

Hirano T, Yasukawa K, Harada H, et al. (1986) Complementary DNA for a novel human interleukin (BSF-2) that induces B lymphocytes to produce immunoglobulin. *Nature* 324:73–76.

Sharma S, Mehta S, Morgan J, Maizel A (1987) Molecular cloning and expression of a human B-cell growth factor gene in *Escherichia coli*. *Science* 235:1489–1492.

Saeland S, Duvert V, Pandrau D, et al. (1991) Interleukin-7 induces the proliferation of normal human B cell precursors. *Blood* 78:2229–2238.

Massod R, Zhang Y, Bond MW, et al. (1995) IL-10 is an autocrine growth factor for AIDS-related B-cell lymphoma. *Blood* 85:3423–3430.

Karp JE, Broder S (1992) The pathogenesis of AIDS lymphomas: A foundation for addressing the challenges of therapy and prevention. *Leukemia Lymphoma* 8:167–188.

Birx DL, Redfield RR, Tencer K, et al. (1990) Induction of interleukin-6 during human immunodeficiency virus infection. *Blood* 76:2303–2310.

MacMahon EM, Glass JD, Hayward SD, et al. (1991) Epstein–Barr virus in AIDS-related primary central nervous system lymphoma. *Lancet* 338:969–973.

Shibata D, Weiss LM, et al. (1993) Epstein–Barr virus-associated non-Hodgkin's lymphoma in patients infected with human immunodeficiency virus. *Blood* 81:2102–2109.

Subar M, Neri A, Inghirami G, et al. (1988) Frequent c-*myc* oncogene activation and infrequent presence of Epstein–Barr virus genome in AIDS-associated lymphomas. *Blood* 72:667–671.

Hamilton-Dutoit SJ, Pallensen G, Franzmann MD, et al. (1991) Histopathology, immunophenotype, and association with EBV phenotype as demonstrated by in situ nucleic acid hybridization. *Am J Pathol* 138:149–163.

Ballerini P, Gaidano G, Gong JZ, et al. (1993) Multiple genetic lesions in acquired immuno-deficiency syndrome-related non-Hodgkin's lymphoma. *Blood* 81:166–176.

Levine AM, Meyer PR, Begandy MK, et al. (1984) Development of B-cell lymphoma in ho-mosexual men: Clinical and immunologic findings. *Ann Intern Med* 100:7–13.

Levine AM, Gill PS, Meyer PR, et al. (1985) Retrovirus and malignant lymphoma in homo-sexual men. *JAMA* 254:1921–1925.

Knowles DM, Chamulak GA, Subar M, et al. (1988) Lymphoid neoplasia associated with the acquired immunodeficiency syndrome (AIDS): The New York University experience. *Ann Intern Med* 108:744–753.

Lowenthal DA, Straus DJ, Campbell SW, et al. (1988) AIDS-related lymphoid neoplasia: The Memorial Hospital Experience. *Cancer* 61:2325–2337.

Ziegler JL, Beckstead JA, Volberding PA, et al. (1984) Non-Hodgkin's lymphoma in 90 homo-sexual men: Relationship to generalized lymphadenopathy and acquired immunodeficiency syndrome (AIDS). *N Engl J Med* 311:565–570.

Lukes RJ, Parker JW, Taylor CR, et al. (1978) Immunologic approach to non-Hodgkin's lym-phomas and related leukemias. Analysis of the results of multiparameter studies of 425 cases. *Sem Hematol* 15:322–351.

Non-Hodgkin's Lymphoma Pathologic Classification Project (1982) National Cancer Institute sponsored study of classifications of non-Hodgkin's lymphomas: Summary and description of a working formulation for clinical usage. *Cancer* 49:2112–2135.

Levine AM (1982) Reactive and neoplastic lymphoproliferative disorders and other miscella-neous cancers associated with HIV infection. In: De Vita VT Jr, Hellman S, Rosenberg SA (eds) *AIDS: Etiology, Diagnosis, Treatment and Prevention*, JP Lippincott, Philadelphia, pp. 263–275.

Carbone PP, Kaplan HS, Musshoff K, et al. (1971) Report of the committee on Hodgkin's disease staging classification. *Cancer* Res 31:1860–1861.

Jones SE, Fulks Z, Bullm M, et al. (1973) Non-Hodgkin's lymphomas. IV. Clinicopathologic correlation of 405 cases. *Cancer* 31:806–823.

Chadburn A, Cesarman E, Jagirdar J, et al. (1993) CD30 (Ki-1) positive anaplastic large cell lymphomas in individuals infected with the human immunodeficiency virus. *Cancer* 72:3078–3090.

Levine AM (1988) HIV-related lymphoma: Prognostic factors predictive of survival. *Blood* 72:247a.

Strauss DJ, Huang J, Testa MA, et al. (1997) Prognostic factors in the treatment of HIV-associated non-Hodgkin's lymphoma (HANHL): Analysis of ACTG 142 (low dose vs. standard dose m-BACOD + GM-CSF). *J Acquired Immune Deficiency Syndrome and Hu-man Retrovirology* 14:A38.

Levine AM (1991) Human immunodeficiency virus-related lymphoma. *Cancer* 68:2446–2472.

Bermudez MA, Grant KM, Rodvien R, Mendes F (1989) Non-Hodgkin's lymphoma in a pop-ulation with or at risk for acquired immunodeficiency syndrome: Indications for intensive chemotherapy. *Am J Med* 86:71–76.

Levine AM, Tulpule A, Tessman D, et al. (1997) Mitoguazone therapy in patients with refractory or relapsed AIDS-related lymphoma: Results from a multi-center phase II trial. *J Clin Oncol* 15:1094–1103.

Gill PS, Graham RA, Boswell W, et al. (1986) A comparison of imaging, clinical and pathologic aspects of space occupying lesions within the brain in patients with acquired immunodeficiency syndrome. *Am J Physiol Imaging* 1:134–141.

So YT, Beckstead JH, Davis RL (1986) Primary central nervous system lymphoma in acquired immune deficiency syndrome: A clinical and pathological study. *Ann Neurol* 20:566–572.

Formenti SC, Gill PS, Lean E, et al. (1989) Primary central nervous system lymphoma in AIDS: Results of radiation therapy. *Cancer* 63:1101–1107.

Baumgartner JE, Rachlin JR, Beckstead JH, et al. (1990) Primary central nervous system lymphomas: Natural history and response to radiation therapy in 55 patients with acquired immunodeficiency syndrome. *J Neurosurg* 73:206–211.

Forsyth PA, Yahalom J, DeAngelis LM (1994) Combined modality therapy in the treatment of primary central nervous system lymphoma in AIDS. *Neurology* 44:1473–1479.

CHAPTER 36

CANCER IN THE ELDERLY

RICCARDO A. AUDISIO

General Surgery—MultiMedica
Milano, Italy

VITTORINA ZAGONEL

Division of Medical Oncology
Centro di Riferimento Oncologico, INRCCS
Aviano, Italy

LAZZARO REPETTO

Department of Medical Oncology 1
IST-National Institute for Cancer Research
Genova, Italy

Although there is no definition for "the elderly" it is obvious that, once an individual stops working, he or she will soon be seen as a dependent member of a society in which some authors consider active life expectancy a relevant parameter in addressing health care policy. Diagnosis and treatment can effectively be restricted (or even neglected) in elderly patients on the basis of these general assumptions. The elderly also represent a nonhomogeneous group of patients because different age subsets have been mixed when studying the problem, the cutoff between young and elderly ranging between the ages of 60 and 80 years, according to various authors. Age cannot be considered as the simple parameter to rely on when addressing medical practice; for this reason senescence was defined as the passage of biologic time, and aging as the passage of chronologic time. Associated comorbidity, representing a clinically relevant problem, should be investigated and better understood. Attitudes need to change when considering chemotherapy, radiotherapy, and surgery in the elderly; focus should be drawn on pretreatment understanding of those risk factors capable of influencing posttreatment course.

Manual of Clinical Oncology, 7th edition, Edited by Raphael E. Pollock
ISBN 0-471-23828-7, pages 723–729. Copyright © 1999 Wiley-Liss, Inc.

ETIOLOGY AND EPIDEMIOLOGY

No evidence supports a different cause of cancer in the elderly when compared with younger age groups—the longer lifetime cumulative exposure to cancer-causing agents seems to be the primary reason for an increased cancer incidence within the aged population. Some immunologic differences may be recognized as responsible for the impaired host defense, such as a decline in immune surveillance, decreased ability to repair DNA, oncogene amplification, or tumor suppressor gene inactivation. No conclusive result is presently available, but it is reasonable to believe that the increased incidence of cancer in the elderly is likely to be a multifactorial process, including the ones just mentioned and several others still to come.

It has been shown that the incidence rates tend to increase in nearly all countries over time in all age groups and in both sexes. Substantial variations were noticed in Europe with regard to mortality. An upward trend was recorded among elderly females in northern Europe and among elderly males in central and in southern Europe, in contrast to declining rates registered in males of all ages in the north and in females in the south.

Cancer is a growing problem, representing one of the major health care burdens of our time. An increasing amount of energy has been delivered in the battle against cancer and significant scientific advances are being reported. Nevertheless, cancer remains the second cause of death, and its incidence continues to rise. The greatest risk factor for developing cancer is age: more than 50% of newly diagnosed patients with cancer are over 65 years of age, while both incidence and mortality is increasing progressively through life. This may well be explained by the remarkable rise in the average life expectancy (33 years in the Middle Ages, 49 years by 1900, 75 years in 1990, 85 years by 2050). A critical appraisal of the modern approach to cancer treatment should accept the evidence that we are ill prepared to accurately prevent, diagnose, and treat the greatly increasing number of elderly cancer patients. The high mortality rate from cancer in the elderly, compared with younger adults, may in part be explained by the poor quality of the treatment delivered to this age group.

DIAGNOSIS

There is growing interest in the area of cancer management in the elderly, and several authors have reported on the inadequacy of diagnoses as well as the undertreatment of elderly subjects. Several underlying reasons have been identified for these factors, such as underestimation of life expectancy, lack of criteria for establishing suitable treatment for the elderly, lack of attention to this topic in the medical literature (textbooks, journals, conferences, articles), exclusion of subjects aged >70 from clinical trials and lack of specific results from clinical research on the elderly, the common misbelief that cancer is more indolent in the elderly, patient delay in reporting symptoms, physician delay, and hospital delay. Symptoms are also likely to be underevaluated or minimized in the elderly. Dyspnea, for example, is often present among older subjects, thus delaying the diagnosis of lung or mediastinal neoplastic disease. Hemorrhoids are more frequent in the elderly, and the same is true for fecal blood that is mainly due to diverticular disease, thereby introducing confusing signs specific to colorectal cancer in the elderly. Urinary dysfunction is a frequent complaint among elderly males, and as this is also a symptom of prostate cancer, the latter is potentially more likely to be missed in the elderly. Other similar examples include bone pain and asthenia due to osteoporosis, which are also symptoms of bone and liver metastatic disease; increased skin pigmentation may mimic skin malignancies such as epidermoid tumors or melanoma. Minor signs and symptoms should never be underestimated on the basis of advanced age alone.

Delayed diagnosis and consequently delayed treatment of malignant disease is a dramatic event especially in the older patient. Fragile electrolytic balance, decreased tolerance to extensive surgical procedures, and possible irreversible worsening of the general condition mandate a proper and rapid diagnosis. An obvious example is the insidious onset of colorectal cancer symptoms, frequently accompanied by anemia, which often ends in large bowel obstruction. Such patients will benefit from early diagnosis and elective therapeutic strategy, and an aggressive approach in diagnosis in the elderly will almost certainly have a beneficial effect in terms of morbidity and mortality.

The argument that those investigations that are not likely to modify the therapeutic strategy should not be done in elderly people is weak because this holds true whatever the age of the patient. Staging is an important step in the work-up of the neoplastic patient; it is needed to define the extent of the disease at diagnosis and to determine treatment strategies. This is also true for elderly patients, but due consideration must be given to staging procedures that are either exhausting or frustrating. Exams that are unlikely to modify the therapeutic strategy should be critically considered before being conducted on the elderly. An unnecessary laparotomy due to incomplete staging must be avoided as a rule, particularly in the elderly, in whom quality of life is such an important issue.

In certain cancers, the affected site varies according to the patient's age: right-sided colon carcinoma is most frequently found in older patients while rectal cancer is twice as common in younger subjects, the difference between the incidence in the elderly being statistically significant. Gastric cancer is more likely to affect the distal part of the stomach in the elderly, and squamous cell carcinoma of the lung is more frequently detected than in younger subjects. Differences in clinical presentation and symptomatology may therefore be expected between the two age groups.

In some countries, different cultural attitudes may also mean that aged patients are not told that they have cancer. This may rise from a social taboo about fatal diseases, although it most often represents a wish to protect elderly individuals from the burden of knowing that they have cancer. Although this attitude is changing, there are still areas where discussion is not always open, thereby limiting the individual's opportunities to take part in the decision-making process. It has been clearly shown that older patients have developed more effective skills to manage stress, tend to be less depressed than younger patients, and show a reduced vulnerability concerning mental health and psychological functioning.

TREATMENT

The decision-making process in treating an older cancer patient with cytotoxic drugs or aggressive surgery is complex and should take into account the balance between potential advantages and risk of side effects. As in all medical interventions, the ultimate goal is to deliver to the patient the best available treatment.

Central to this issue is the consideration that the actual life expectancy of most older individuals affected by cancer is greater than the cancer-related life span. Therefore, one of the primary objectives of the treatment is to maximize the chance of the patient to fully benefit from his *natural* life expectancy. Indeed, considerations on potential gain in life expectancy should be matched to the expected changes in quality of life associated with the different therapeutic options. Thus, tumor growth control generally represents the best achievement in terms of survival, although its effect on the quality of life in the elderly is questionable.

Unfortunately, there is little agreement on general guidelines in the elderly to select those who should receive either surgical or chemotherapic options. Many studies have shown that both general practitioners and medical oncologists tend to base their therapeutic choices simply on the chronologic age of the patients. For example, as far as surgical treatments are concerned, several data from the literature show that older patients affected by solid tumors (i.e., breast and lung cancer) are less likely to receive potentially curative treatments than the adults, despite the established fact that elderly subjects frequently present localized disease at diagnosis. Even though such a trend in older patients with lung cancer could be related to concerns for thoracotomy-related complications, there are no reasons justifying a similar attitude in patients affected by breast carcinoma which is often curable with a minor surgical procedure. These and many other observations provide evidence that chronologic age still represents an important barrier to adequate treatment of the elderly cancer patient.

The commonly held prejudice that chemotherapy for older patients should be more simple and mild is not based on clinical studies, although single-agent protocols are obviously to be preferred owing to better compliance and tolerability. As an example, oral etoposide has shown good results in the clinical control of small-cell lung carcinoma, leading to an overall survival competitive with that achieved with the most effective combination chemotherapy. It has conversely been shown that survival of elderly patients affected by aggressive non-Hodgkin's lymphoma improved when combination chemotherapy (i.e., the CHOP regimen) is administrated. Cytokines and recombinant human growth factors (HGFs) may be used in older patients to support many standard-dose (adult-like) chemotherapy regimens in chemosensitive tumors, and appear safe and cost effective in view of the peculiar clinical features of aged subjects. The purpose of growth factor therapy should be to allow full dosages of chemotherapy to be administered on time, to decrease chemotherapy-related morbidity and mortality, and subsequently to reduce the median number of days spent in the hospital.

Conclusive data on most other cancers are scarce; the recent trend to enroll elderly patients into prospective controlled phase II trials, with the aim of evaluating the efficacy and tolerance of new drugs, will provide more information. The inclusion of older patients into phase II trials will help test the true efficacy of a given regimen for the entire patient population, as dose intensity is an important therapeutic index.

Considerable additional information in the process of therapeutic decision making can be obtained by the evaluation of functional status of older cancer patients. Performance status provides a valid tool for the functional evaluation of adult subjects within a working age range, but it may not represent an adequate parameter for the elderly. Many studies have shown that in the elderly, impaired functional status is a common condition owing to medical and nonmedical factors, thus representing an excellent indicator of health-related quality of life. For this reason the functional status appraisal among the elderly should be based on a multidimensional approach: a comprehensive geriatric assessment (CGA) should investigate comorbid conditions, physical mobility, mental status, geographic location, and social situation. Functional status has also been shown to be an independent prognostic factor in old age, and may be used to estimate average residual life expectancy, a relevant issue in tailoring treatment change. Furthermore, a multidimensional evaluation may address specific treatment options, as in the case of memory impairments affecting a person living alone, thus advocating against self-treatment at home. A comprehensive geriatric assessment, capable of accurately evaluating the global status of the elderly cancer patient (physical, mental, and disease related), might replace the Karnofsky or WHO scales to optimize the choice of the therapeutic strategy.

The importance of offering all benefits of aggressive cancer treatment to older patients has been underlined, but it must be recognized that age-related conditions may decrease the advantages and expand the risks of anticancer therapy. Age-associated comorbidity can influence the overall physical status of the patients, and generate important interactions in the pharmacological disposition of both antineoplastic and ancillary drugs. Comorbidity may also dramatically affect *quoad vitam* prognosis in the aged cancer patient; it should therefore be accounted for in the process of clinical decision making.

The aforementioned general assumptions may also be expanded to elderly cancer patients who are candidates for surgery. Operating on the elderly for cardiac, orthopedic, or vascular diseases is increasingly accepted, while there is continued reluctance to recommend aggressive intervention for abdominal malignancies other than those arising in the colon. Recent advances in preoperative risk assessment and surgical technique have resulted in a significant decrease in operative mortality and morbidity for the aged, when compared to the results of the last decades. Careful preoperative evaluation, intraoperative monitoring, and postoperative care are presently achieved in almost every major hospital; if this is not the case, poor-risk subjects should be referred to more specialized centers.

Age-related changes are most evident physical/psychological stress, and elderly people are slower to react and recover. Although anesthesiologic guidelines for management of elderly people at high risk for surgery are to be further developed, detailed evaluation of major organ function helps in choosing anesthetic and pharmacologic agents. Despite this wide experience, only two risk factors for perioperative cardiac morbidity have been definitively identified: recent myocardial infarction and current congestive heart failure. In the past years, multivariate analyses have identified combinations of risk factors allowing the organization of scoring systems. These scores are generally based on costly clinical and laboratory tests, often referring to further investigations. Most recently it has been argued that routine clinical evaluation before surgery is neither sufficiently sensitive nor specific, and higher costs are justified if specialized testing provides otherwise unavailable and relevant information.

The area of elective surgery for gastrointestinal tumors in the elderly has been extensively reviewed, and it was shown that operative mortality is not reported to be significantly increased among most of the surgical series, with the exception of major liver resections. This observation helped in identifying hepatic failure as a prominent risk factor after major liver resection, thus allowing better patient selection. Complication rates and mean hospital stay do not differ between the two age groups, provided that the procedure is conducted with careful technique in expert hands. A drop in operative morbidity has occurred in the past 3 decades, as emphasized by several authors. Finally, the 5-year survival is often better for younger patients, but the difference is not statistically valid when nonmalignant deaths are excluded.

Interesting outcomes have also been shown with the surgical management of non-small-cell lung cancer: 5-year survival rates of 30% to 48% have been reported, and when early stages are considered separately, cure rates can be in the range of 50%. A morbidity rate in the range of 16% to 67% should not be enough to exclude patients from "state of the art" management, particularly when operative mortality has decreased to acceptable rates (3% to 15%).

Containment of potentially curative surgery on the basis of age alone is no longer an acceptable option, and the medical profession must confront this reality in an area where the percentage of the elderly population will rapidly increase.

Because a large part of elderly patients are strictly dependent on the support of family members as far as logistic, economic, and daily living problems are concerned, treatment is not uncommonly planned on the basis of the relatives' opinion, including their availability to participate as caregivers in the treatment program. The decision to treat elderly cancer patients should be discussed within the family context.

SUMMARY

Living patterns change considerably over the years as well as over socioeconomical development. Modern society is keen to reduce the number of large family houses hosting several generations, which are often replaced by small family units, meaning that the elderly will often be living with their partners. The problems encountered by a large proportion of our elderly people in reporting symptoms, visiting their physicians, undergoing diagnostic exams, and attending scheduled treatments might be exacerbated by loneliness, depression, and limited satisfaction with life.

No matter what excuse is given, it has been shown that the elderly cancer patient is not adequately cared for: a group of researchers in the Netherlands found that the elderly with breast, colorectal, and lung cancers were more often diagnosed only on clinical grounds, with less recourse to cytologic confirmation (83% for over 70 compared with 93% for the 50 to 59 age group). They also demonstrated that, among patients with common solid tumors and lymphomas, the proportion not given treatment rose from 7% in the 50 to 59-year-old group, to 12% in the 60 to 69-year-olds, and to 22% in those patients aged over 70. This trend was particularly strong for lung cancer as well as metastatic colorectal and ovarian cancers. Furthermore, whereas 90% to 99% of patients with lymphoma, breast, head and neck, or nonmetastatic colorectal cancers had multimodality treatment, elderly patients with these diseases were less likely to receive combination treatment.

A better understanding of specific prognosticators is required to avoid aggressive and unnecessary treatment in patients with an expected poor outcome. The use of laboratory tests and biologic markers should be targeted to the elderly in whom specific biologic and immunologic differences have been documented.

It is the responsibility of the physician to critically appraise the elderly on an evidence-based practice approach rather than on personal beliefs. It should be recognized that the attitude of underevaluating and undertreating the elderly cancer patients breaches ethical code, and every effort should be made to alert public opinion and politicians to the existence of this emerging problem.

These conclusions need integration with cost–benefit analysis: it is not surprising that no financial differences have been shown in delivering surgical treatment to the aged population when compared with younger subjects. The cost of individual procedures can be controlled by centralization of an aggressive approach to specific institutions devoted to and trained and equipped for cancer care in the elderly.

FURTHER READING

Audisio RA, Veronesi P, Ferrario L, et al. (1997) Elective surgery in gastrointestinal tumors in the aged. *Ann Oncol* 8:317–27.

Audisio RA, Cazzaniga M, Veronesi P, et al. (1997) Elective surgery for colorectal cancer in the aged: A clinical-economical evaluation. *Br J Cancer* 76:382–384.

de Rijke JM, Shouten LJ, Shouten HC, et al. (1996) Age-specific differences in the diagnostics and treatment of cancer patients aged over 50 years and older in the province of Limburg, The Netherlands. *Ann Oncol* 7:677–685.

Fentiman IS, Tirelli U, Monfardini S, et al. (1990) Cancer in the elderly: Why so badly treated? *Lancet* 335:1020–1022.

Yancik R, Ries LG (1991) Cancer in the aged. *Cancer* 68:2502–2510.

Monfardini S, Yancik R (1993) Cancer in the elderly: Meeting the challenge of an aging population. *J Natl Cancer Inst* 85:532–537.

Monfardini S (1996) What do we know on variables influencing clinical decision-making in elderly cancer patients? *Eur J Cancer* 32A-1:12–14.

Monfardini S, Ferrucci L, Fratino L, et al. (1996) Validation of a multidimensional evaluation scale for use in the elderly cancer patients. *Cancer* 77:395–401.

CHAPTER 37

ONCOLOGICAL EMERGENCIES

MARK R. OLSEN

University of Wisconsin Comprehensive Cancer Center
Madison, WI 53792, USA

H. IAN ROBINS

University of Wisconsin Medical School
Madison, WI 53792, USA

The complications associated with neoplastic disease are usually the result of the disease process itself or are secondary to therapy. Supportive measures for the patient with cancer are often the major focus of care. Such measures can be important, particularly when a cost–benefit assessment of specific cancer-directed therapy suggests that treatment is not warranted. At these times, it is often psychologically optimal for the patient to view his or her illness as chronic, and therefore incurable, but not beyond supportive measures. In such situations, the complexity of medical intervention should be defined in the context of the patient's disease progression. Obviously, quality-of-life issues become the focal points in this decision-making process. Individualization of treatment and supportive care is critical.

Inherent in the approach to such complications is the underlying emotional support the physician must provide to establish a firm therapeutic alliance. Both pain control and emotional support are required for a patient to tolerate other aspects of supportive care (which at times may be invasive, as the medical team addresses acute and palliative issues). Thus, the subjects of pain and psychological issues have been dealt with in separate chapters.

When a patient is undergoing surgical procedures, chemotherapy, or radiotherapy, the physician has an unwritten contract to see the patient through any complications of therapy. Thus, in addition to describing the possible side effects of therapy, the

Manual of Clinical Oncology, 7th edition, Edited by Raphael E. Pollock
ISBN 0-471-23828-7, pages 731–743. Copyright © 1999 Wiley-Liss, Inc.

physician should delineate, prior to the initiation of treatment, supportive measures that might become necessary.

We discuss here approaches to commonly encountered oncologic emergencies, measures effective with many of the chronic complications encountered by cancer patients, and nonspecific adjuvant supportive therapies.

ONCOLOGIC EMERGENCIES

Infection

Antineoplastic therapy affects both cell-mediated and the humoral immune systems, predisposing patients to infections. Furthermore, myelosuppression and mucositis (resulting from endothelial surface damage) are serious side effects of chemotherapy and increase patients' risks for potentially fatal infections. In immunocompromised hosts, infections usually disseminate rapidly, frequently resulting in shock and death. Thus, patient education regarding fevers higher than 38°C (in the setting of immunosuppressions or malignant states predisposed to infection) coupled with prompt initiation of treatment are critical in this patient group.

Fever with a temperature >38.5°C persisting for 2 to 6 hours in a patient with cancer most often represents infection. Other causes include the presence of neoplastic disease itself (often associated with hepatic involvement), fever-producing drugs (bleomycin and cytosine arabinoside [Ara C] during the first 24 hours after administration), blood-product transition reactions, and tumor necrosis. Prior to beginning antibiotic treatment, a careful "fever work-up" should be completed. This may include a chest X-ray film, blood and urine cultures, and other clinically indicated directed cultures and procedures (Fig. 37.1). Fever or rigors may be the only sign

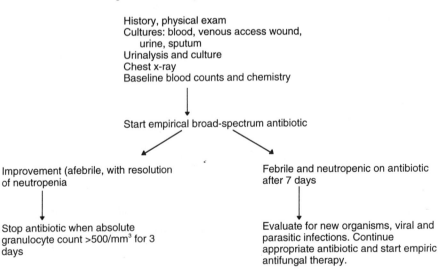

FIGURE 37.1. Algorithm for evaluation of fever in the neutropenic patient (<500 neutrophils/mm^3).

of infection; the other typical clinical signs and symptoms (e.g., erythema, swelling, abscess formation, purulent discharge) may be minimal or absent in an immunocompromised patient due to neutropenia. Thus, a careful history and physical examination (including the perianal area, for perirectal cellulitis) are mandatory to discover even limited signs of inflammation.

The chance that infection is present becomes significant when the absolute granulocyte (neutrophil) count drops below 100 per mm^3 and increases dramatically with a granulocyte count below 500 per mm^3. In the mid-1970s, a series of controlled clinical trials demonstrated the efficacy of prompt empiric antibiotic administration for patients who were neutropenic and then became febrile. In Europe and the United States, antibiotic treatment must cover gram-negative bacteria, with particular emphasis on *Pseudomonas aeruginosa*. Other organisms commonly encountered include *Escherichia coli* and *Klebsiella pneumoniae* as well as *Staphylococcus aureus* and *Bacteroides* species. Fungal infection with *Candida* accounts for less than 8% of positive blood cultures; other fungal infections are identified less often. The likelihood of fungal complication increases with the duration of time a patient is neutropenic. Typical combinations of antibiotics used for empiric antibacterial therapy include carbenicillin (ticarcillin or piperacillin) plus gentamicin (tobramycin or amikacin) or ceftazidine with or without an aminoglycoside. In addition, new fourth-generation cephalosporins (e.g., cefepime) as well as carbapenems (imipenem) are also now being utilized empirically in the setting of febrile neutropenia.

The empiric use of vancomycin had been reserved for clinical situations in which the risk for infection with resistant staphylococcus is high (e.g., in a patient with an indwelling central venous catheter). However, the recent emergence of vancomycin-resistant gram-positive organisms requires that one be very circumspect about this practice in the future. Obviously, specific culture results invariably dictate antibiotic selection.

In patients who have prolonged neutropenia and fever (for more than 1 week despite antibiotic treatment), empiric antifungal therapy with amphotericin B or fluconazole may be warranted.

Particular concern regarding anaerobic infections is usually justified only in special situations, such as disruption of the mucosal integrity of the gastrointestinal tract. Typhlitis (necrotizing colitis of the cecum) from infiltration of anaerobic species and gram-negative bacteria (*P. aeruginosa*, mainly) is another complication seen in oncologic patients who should be treated according to the antimicrobial guidelines outlined previously. In addition, surgical resection of the necrotic bowel is indicated. These patients usually present with right lower quadrant abdominal pain, which has a tendency to generalize over the next few hours, together with fever and diarrhea.

It should be noted that patients who have undergone splenectomy (e.g., as part of the staging for Hodgkin's disease) are always at risk for septicemia with encapsulated bacteria (e.g., *Streptococcus pneumoniae*, *Haemophilus influenzae*, *Neisseria meningitides*). This possibility must be considered when these patients present, and prompt antibiotic treatment should be given. (Presplenectomy immunization for such patients is strongly advised to help avert this complication.) Beyond splenectomy, clinicians should recognize that Hodgkin's disease patients may be inherently compromised immunologically (even in a remission state) and predisposed to infection.

Other considerations in the care of the immunocompromised patients include the use of acyclovir at the time of diagnosis of herpes zoster or cytomegalovirus, or the use of trimethoprim–sulfamethoxazole as a prophylactic measure (2 to 3 days per week) against *Pneumocystis carinii*, particularly in patients with acute leukemias or chronic steroids, for example, primary brain tumor patients. Beyond this, careful handwashing on the part of medical personnel has proven to be of significant value to reduce iatrogenic infections. The use of hematopoietic growth factors, which are also useful in controlling infection and fever, is discussed later in this chapter.

Until recently, febrile neutropenic patients were invariably treated on an inpatient basis as described previously. Studies completed during the past few years are consistent with the use of both parenteral and oral antibiotics in the ambulatory setting for low-risk febrile neutropenic patients. This has become realistic based on antibiotic advances including quinolones with oral antipseudomonal activity, as well as nursing and technical support for home drug therapy.

The use of fluoroquinolones in this setting raises the concept of their use prophylactically. The rationale for this is sound; currently, we reserve such an approach at our center for patients considered to be at high risk secondary to prolonged neutropenia, for example, allogenic bone marrow transplant patients. The use of cytokines is also relevant to this issue and is discussed later in this chapter. Antifungal prophylaxis is generally reserved for patients receiving prolonged courses of steroids, as well as for recipients for bone marrow transplants.

Metastases to Brain and Spinal Cord

Brain metastases occur in 25% to 35% of all cancer patients, more commonly in cancers of the lung and breast and in malignant melanoma. Common clinical signs and symptoms associated with brain metastases include headache, cranial nerve deficits, incoordination, muscle weakness, nausea, and change in mental status. Often a patient's first presenting symptom is a seizure. Generally, patients with a history of a seizure in this clinical setting are maintained on antiepileptic therapy, such as dilantin, for life.

Papilledema is an uncommon sign in patients with metastatic disease to the brain. If papilledema is visualized, intracranial pressure is usually elevated and, in addition to high-dose corticosteroids, measures such as mannitol or urea infusions should be considered. In high doses, corticosteroids such as dexamethasone are extremely effective in relieving symptoms for up to several weeks by decreasing edema around the metastases. Radiotherapy treatment to the entire brain is the usual additional treatment. On the completion of a course of radiotherapy, the steroids can usually be gradually tapered and stopped. If symptoms recur, steroids can be used again, often with a positive effect. A second course of radiotherapy is usually useful only if several months have gone by before symptoms recur. The prognosis for the patient with brain metastases depends on the extent of involvement (number and size of metastases) and the neurologic dysfunction present at diagnosis, treatment response, and control of the primary tumor. Generally, median survival ranges between 6 months and 1 year from the time of diagnosis of central nervous system (CNS) disease.

The advent of neurosurgical resection of patients with one to two brain metastases, as well as stereotactic radiosurgery, has resulted in the apparent increase in survival of selected patients.

Spinal cord compression is a medical emergency, as a delay in treatment can result in irreversible loss of neurologic function. Prompt diagnosis with immediate therapy will prevent further neurologic deterioration. Tumor types commonly associated with spinal cord compression include breast, lung, prostate cancers, malignant melanoma, multiple myeloma, renal cell carcinoma, and lymphoma. In the majority of adult patients, spinal cord compression is not the result of intradural metastases, but of metastases originating in a vertebral body. Primary involvement of paravertebral or epidural spaces is less frequent. When the metastases expand, the periosteum is extended, thus causing pain. Very localized pain is the first presenting symptom in more than 90% of patients. It is usually gradual in onset, present for weeks to months before the onset of neurologic dysfunction. Therefore, any history of neck and/or back pain should prompt consideration of this diagnostic possibility. The pain itself may be focal (localized, continuous bone pain), radicular (intermittent, unilateral or bilateral), or referred (occurring at a distant site, e.g., sacroiliac pain in L1 compression). In some cases, however, the syndrome develops rapidly and the patient presents with neurologic signs (e.g., weakness, sensory loss, ascending numbness in the lower extremities). Urinary retention and constipation are usually late signs. Progression to paraplegia over a period of hours to days is not an infrequent result. Sometimes a diagnosis can be made without special radiographic procedures, but myelography, or, if easily available, magnetic resonance imaging (MRI) or computed tomography (CT) scanning of the suspected area should be done promptly. Although corticosteroids can reduce the edema in a minority of cases, thus improving the neurologic function, radiotherapy is the mainstay of treatment. Surgery with decompressive laminectomy is usually reserved for patients whose neurologic status worsens rapidly. Surgery should be followed by radiotherapy as soon as possible.

Surgery is also utilized for situations in which a fragment of a vertebral body is retropulsed into the spinal cord, resulting in compression.

The use of intrathecal chemotherapy plays a significant role in the treatment of carcinomatous meningitis caused by lymphoma and leukemias. Intrathecal chemotherapy, however, is far less efficacious for solid tumors in this clinical setting.

Hypercoagulability

Laboratory evidence of coagulation abnormalities in cancer patients is a common finding. Hypercoagulable states occur when various pathologic processes, alone or in combination, disturb normal coagulation mechanisms. Typical processes include impairment of blood rheology, thrombocytosis with increased vascular reactivity, increase in fibrin/fibrinogen degradation products, and hyperfibrinogenemia. A hypercoagulable state may present as migratory thrombophlebitis (known also as Trousseau's syndrome), disseminated intravascular coagulation (DIC), and marantic (nonbacterial thrombotic) endocarditis. All three conditions can be seen together in the same patient. Solid tumors—including mucin-secreting adenocarcinomas of the gastrointestinal tract and cancers of the lung, breast, prostate, ovaries, and pancreas—are more commonly associated with thrombophlebitis, while DIC is frequently found in patients with acute leukemia (usually acute promyelocytic leukemia) and adenocarcinomas. At times, thrombosis and thrombophlebitis are related to hormonal therapy in breast cancer patients. Initial therapy for patients with hypercoagulable states is usually parenteral heparin, which can be followed by oral Warfarin®. Until recently, high-dose subcutaneous heparin has been the treatment of choice for these patients. The advent of low molecular weight heparin has given the clinician an added treatment option with an improved margin of safety. Complete control of this potential life-threatening complication requires control of the patient's underlying neoplastic process. Similarly, hyperviscosity syndromes associated with Waldenström's macroglobulinemia and, to a lesser extent, multiple myeloma, are best controlled with systemic chemotherapy. The symptoms and signs of hyperviscosity syndrome include hemorrhagic diathesis (epistaxis, purpura, and easy bruisability), neurologic disorders (stroke, seizures, peripheral neuropathy), and hypervolemia leading to congestive heart failure. Plasmapheresis, by removing selectively intravascular paraprotein, can provide only a temporary relief of the symptoms.

Hypercalcemia

Hypercalcemia is a common and potentially life-threatening metabolic emergency encountered in patients with cancer. Various circulating humoral factors released from, or induced by, neoplastic processes are summarized in Table 37.1. At times, hypercalcemia may be the result of hormonal therapy, such as in breast cancer patients with known bony involvement. Clinical symptoms are widespread with general and organ-specific presentations (Table 37.1). Initial therapy with intravenous normal saline coupled with furosemide diuresis is often effective. The use of the chemotherapeutic drug mithramycin (which inhibits osteoclastic activity) is usually of limited value after an initial dose or two, for the drug can cause significant thrombocytopenia. Bisphosphonates (i.e., pamidronate or etidronate) are effective in most patients. Therapy directed at the patient's underlying malignancy, if possible, remains a critical aspect of helping patients with this complication.

Gallium nitrate may be considered if bisphosphonates fail to control hypercalcemia, but this therapeutic option is generally more involved, requiring hospitalization for continuous infusion of the drug. In addition, gallium nitrate has the potential for serious nephrotoxicity and hypocalcemia.

Syndrome of Inappropriate Antidiuretic Hormone Secretion

Syndrome of inappropriate antidiuretic hormone secretion (SIADH) occurs predominantly in patients with small-cell carcinoma of the lung. Antidiuretic hormone is inappropriately released by tumor tissue, resulting in hyponatremia and water reten-

TABLE 37.1. Factors and Clinical Symptoms Associated with Tumor-Induced Hypercalcemia

Factors	Symptoms
Ectopic hyperparathyroidism, caused by parathyroid-like factors	Anorexia, polydipsia, polyuria
Prostaglandins: local release may activate osteoclasts	Nausea, vomiting, constipation
Osteoclast-activating factors (OAFs), stimulation of osteoclast-mediated bone resorption: the OAFs include a variety of cytokines with bone resorptive activities, such as IL-1,[a] TNF, transforming growth factors, and others.	Fatigue, lethargy, muscle weakness, confusion, seizures, coma ECG abnormalities

[a]IL-1, interleukin-1; TNF, tumor necrosis factor; ECG, electrocardiogram.

tion with an associated serum hypoosmolarity. The clinical symptomatology of this syndrome—including anorexia, nausea and vomiting, mental confusion, irritability, weakness, seizures, and coma—is derived from the water intoxication. Thus, SIADH has a presentation similar to CNS disease. In patients with small-cell carcinoma of the lung, chemotherapy is usually effective and will correct the plasma sodium levels. Currently, no drug will prevent tumor cells from producing and secreting antidiuretic hormone (ADH). Both demeclocycline hydrochloride and lithium carbonate, however, will interfere with the renal action of the ectopic ADH by inducing polyuria and can provide palliation to patients without resorting to fluid restriction.

Hyperuricemia and Tumor Lysis Syndrome

Hyperuricemia and tumor lysis syndrome (hyperuricemia, hyperkalemia, hyperphosphatemia, and hypocalcemia) can develop in patients with hematologic malignancies (acute and chronic leukemias), lymphomas (usually high-grade), and myeloproliferative diseases. When patients with these conditions are initially given chemotherapy, particularly those with bulky lymphomas or high cell numbers, they are at risk for developing hyperuricemia with associated acute renal failure (ARF). This is a result of breakdown of large numbers of tumor cells, which is associated with the release of massive amounts of purine precursors. The resulting hyperuricemia greatly increases the filtered load of uric acid; its solubility is exceeded and precipitation occurs in the renal tubules, resulting sometimes in ARF. During massive cell lysis, phosphate is also released in large amounts, and hyperphosphaturia with intrarenal deposition of calcium phosphate may be involved in the development of ARF. Hypocalcemia, related to hyperphosphatemia, can provoke cardiac arrhythmias, muscle cramps, and tetany. The observed hyperkalemia is caused by the release of intracellular potassium and can result in cardiac arhythmias as well. To prevent hyperuricemic states, patients should be well hydrated and should receive drug therapy with allopurinol before their systemic treatment is begun. In addition, urine alkalization (to achieve a pH greater than 7) should be sought with the use of intravenous sodium bicarbonate solution. Serum electrolytes, uric acid, phosphorus, calcium, and creatinine levels should be monitored during treatment to recognize and prevent further metabolic abnormalities.

Adrenal Insufficiency

Although metastatic involvement of the adrenals is not uncommon—particularly with breast and lung cancer—clinical symptoms such as nausea, vomiting, apathy, abdominal pain, and hyperthermia secondary to adrenal insufficiency are rare. When this diagnosis is suspected, however, steroid replacement should be instituted.

Ureteral and Urethral Obstruction

Ureteral obstruction occurs from pathologic involvement and enlargement of retroperitoneal lymph nodes in a variety of adult neoplasms including prostate, colon, ovarian and breast cancers, renal cell carcinoma, sarcoma, lymphoma, and malignant melanoma. Flank pain is the presenting symptom. Lower extremity edema and obstructive uropathy are often observed at presentation. Diagnosis is made by ultrasound and, if available, with retrograde radiographic studies or by CT scan. When the circumstances warrant, the placement of ureteral stents or a percutaneous nephrostomy tube can palliate this complication. In some situations, when patients are experiencing the uncomfortable side effects of the final stages of their disease process, no intervention may be the best course for the patient.

In children, urethral obstruction may develop with soft tissue sarcomas. This problem can be treated with catheterization. If this is not possible, a suprapubic cystostomy is performed until definitive therapy (e.g., radiation, chemotherapy, or surgery) is initiated.

Superior Vena Caval Syndrome

Clinically, superior vena caval syndrome (a result of blood flow obstruction through the superior vena cava caused by a pulmonary or mediastinal mass) presents a striking picture of dyspnea, dilated neck veins, and facial edema. A chest X-ray film, or, if available, CT scan will confirm the clinical diagnosis. Until a clear diagnosis is established, patients often have symptomatic relief following treatment with high-dose corticosteroids, although their use has never been rigorously evaluated. Bed rest with the head elevated and oxygen administered can reduce venous pressure. Treatment of the underlying disease with chemotherapy (in the case of small-cell lung cancer or lymphoma) or ionizing irradiation (in non-small-cell lung cancer) can often produce dramatic improvement, and the steroids should be rapidly tapered and stopped.

Catheter-induced superior vena caval syndrome is usually related to thrombosis. Heparin and oral anticoagulants may prevent progression of the thrombus, and thrombolytics may be utilized to bring about lysis. Catheter removal is an alternative as well.

Malignant Effusions

Malignant pleural effusions are evidenced by dyspnea, chest pain, cough, and/or shoulder pain. They result from pleural tumor growth with increased pleural fluid oncotic pressure or from impaired pleural lymphatic drainage secondary to metastatic involvement of the mediastinal lymph nodes. This usually causes an exudative effusion (protein content of more than 3 g/dl, specific gravity of more than 1.015). On cytologic examination, tumor cells are found in only about one third of cases. The primary cancers are often of the lung, breast, or ovary. The patient's comfort and respiratory status can often be improved on a short-term basis by thoracentesis. Diuretics are rarely effective. Repeated thoracentesis often results in fluid loculation; therefore, when the underlying disease is resistant to chemotherapy, a decision for early chest-tube drainage is often best followed by instillation of an antibiotic (e.g., tetracycline), talc, or an antineoplastic agent. (The beneficial effect when chemotherapy is used as a sclerosing agent results from mesothelial fibrosis and obliteration of small blood vessels, with adherence of the visceral and parietal pleurae, rather than an antineoplastic effect.) The prognosis of the patients with malignant pleural effusion is usually related to the prognosis associated with the primary tumor.

Malignant pericardial effusions can be caused by obstruction of the venous and lymphatic drainage of the heart. Common cancers presenting with pericardial involvement are lung, breast, leukemia, Hodgkin's and non-Hodgkin's lymphoma, melanoma, and sarcoma. The lymphatic drainage may be disturbed by metastatic involvement of mediastinal lymph nodes. Alternatively, the pericardium itself may be infiltrated with tumor. The increase in pericardial fluid results in cardiac tamponade with its related signs: cardiac enlargement, arrhythmias, distant heart sounds, pericardial friction rub, jugular venous distension, hepatosplenomegaly/ascites, paradoxic pulse, and dyspnea. The rapidity of the development of a pericardial effusion often has a direct relationship to the patient's symptomatology.

Pericardiocentesis can rapidly alleviate all clinical manifestations of cardiac tamponade. This is, however, only a temporary measure; long-term prognosis depends on the response to treatment of the primary cancer. In patients whose cancers are controlled by adjuvant therapies, and are thus expected to have long-term survival, a surgical resection of the pericardium—a pericardiectomy (window or complete)—should be considered. The use of "balloon" technology in the hands of a skilled cardiologist often simplifies this procedure. Instillation of antineoplastic agents (e.g., bleomycin) may also provide long-lasting control of pericardial effusion.

Malignant ascites is seen most commonly in patients with ovarian, colorectal, and gastric cancers. The increase of fluid can in part be related to drainage malfunction of the peritoneal cavity as a result of metastatic involvement of the lymphatics.

Neoplastic involvement of the liver can give cirrhotic-like symptoms also resulting in ascites. The clinical signs are related to the amount of intraperitoneal fluid. Difficulty in walking and breathing indicate the presence of a significant amount of ascites. A paracentesis often reduces the related symptoms and provides fluid for a complete evaluation. Repeated procedures, however, may have long-term sequelae for patients with ascites; protein depletion and risk of infection represent significant problems associated with this invasive maneuver. While diuretics appear to be ineffective in patients with malignant ascites, intraabdominal instillation of antineoplastic agents (e.g., cisplatin) benefits some patients. If the first-line treatment (e.g., chemotherapy, surgery) is no longer effective, a peritoneovenous shunt (i.e., a perforated tube implanted in the peritoneal cavity, which is connected to the superior vena cava with a manual pump for fluid flow) may palliate the problem and increase the patient's comfort.

Nausea and Vomiting

Patients experience chemotherapy-and-radiotherapy-induced nausea and vomiting as among the most unpleasant acute side effects of their therapies. The nausea and vomiting are not as self-limited as seen usually in gastrointestinal disease, but are often severe and of longer duration. Beyond this, the patient may develop anticipatory nausea and vomiting, which often requires time-consuming interventions (e.g., behavior modification, hypnosis) or the use of psychotropic medications. The distress experienced by patients can be so profound that they choose to discontinue their treatment.

The mechanism of this emesis is not completely understood. It is probably caused by the stimulation of receptors in a vomiting center of the brain. It is believed this area is located in the area postrema of the medulla and represents a chemoreceptor trigger zone sensitive to stimulation from the blood and the cerebrospinal fluid. Impulses generated there by antineoplastic agents are transported to the vomiting center, with nausea and vomiting occurring as a consequence.

The development of new, more effective antiemetic drugs and regimens in recent years reduces these difficulties. In general, the major tranquilizers or benzodiazepines (haloperidol and lorazepam), antihistamines (hydroxyzine), phenothiazines (prochlorperazine), antiserotonin agents (ondansetron, granisetron, and tropisetron), corticosteroids (dexamethasone), and dopamine antagonists (metaclopramide) have proven to be effective adjuncts to therapy with emetic potential. Rehydration of patients who present with nausea and vomiting is not only sound medically, but also helps in alleviating posttherapy emetogenesis. The addition of steroids to the antiserotonin agents has been shown to potentiate their effect.

When a cancer patient presents with non-therapy-induced nausea and/or vomiting, the clinician should consider bowel obstruction, severe constipation, hypercalcemia, renal failure (perhaps due to obstruction), and brain metastases as among the possible causes of these symptoms.

USE OF TRANSFUSIONS AND CYTOKINES (GROWTH FACTORS)

Anemia

Anemia in cancer patients is often caused by antineoplastic therapy. Other factors such as chronic disease or specific inhibitors of erythropoiesis may contribute to the anemia. Initially, anemia together with thrombocytopenia and granulocytopenia may be among the first signs leading to the diagnosis of a malignancy. This can be a result of the replacement of normal hemopoietic precursors by neoplastic cells.

Generally, patients become symptomatic with hematocrit levels below 24 vol % and hemoglobin levels below 8 g/dl. At this level, tissue oxygen delivery is suboptimal. Most patients begin to feel discomfort, fatigue, and/or dyspnea; the use of packed red cells will improve the cardiopulmonary status of such oncologic patients.

Thrombocytopenia

The pathophysiology of thrombocytopenia is similar to that of anemia. Other etiologic factors include sequestration by the spleen (hypersplenism) or dilution secondary to excessive fluid/transfusion replacement. In thrombopenic patients, severe hemorrhage is uncommon in those with a platelet count over $20,000/mm^3$. Bruising and petechiae represent common early findings with thrombocytopenia. The risk of a serious hemorrhage (e.g., intracranial bleeding) increases dramatically as the platelet count falls below $10,000/mm^3$. For this reason, platelet concentrates are first considered for empirical administration when the patient's platelet count falls below $20,000/mm^3$. Physicians treating patients with hematologic malignancies often have a lower threshold; those treating CNS malignancies may have a higher threshold owing to the irreversibility of the consequences of an intracranial bleed.

New growth factors now in development may change our approach to the problem.

Granulocytopenia

Whereas white blood cell (WBC) transfusions have been shown to be efficacious for the treatment of gram-negative infections (in neutropenic patients) as well as some fungal septicemias, their practical use is extremely limited because of cost, effort, and transfusion reactions. Furthermore, WBC activity declines rapidly as a function of time. Thus, WBC transfusions are no longer a standard practice.

Hematopoietic Growth Factors

Granulocyte colony-stimulating factor (G-CSF) and granulocyte-macrophage colony-stimulating factor (GM-CSF) are glycoproteins with various influences on myeloid hematopoietic cells, including survival, differentiation, and proliferation. Their use can improve hematopoietic recovery after chemotherapy. Over the past few years, the use of these recombinant cytokines has successfully decreased the morbidity of high-dose chemotherapy when given immediately following chemotherapy for

1 to 2 weeks (depending on the neutrophil count). Both duration and severity of neutropenia are markedly reduced, preventing severe febrile episodes and infections.

Erythropoietin is a glycoprotein produced in the kidney, responsible for the hormonal up-and-down regulation of erythrocyte production in the bone marrow. Several studies have shown that erythropoietin treatment improves the chemotherapy-related anemia by decreasing the need for transfusions. The costs of this treatment, however, are significant, and its use in cancer-related anemia is still limited and requires further evaluation.

Similarly, work on growth factors to stimulate platelet cell production (for example, the interleukins IL-1, IL-3, and IL-6 as well as thrombopoietin) remains an area of active research; no practical application of these biologic response modifiers has been defined to date.

SUMMARY

Numerous complications of therapy and disease processes confront any physician dealing with cancer patients. Among these many clinical problems, the medical practitioner can have a major impact on the treatment of infections associated with myelosuppression. The importance of prompt treatment in this setting cannot be overemphasized. Similarly, prompt diagnosis of spinal cord and brain metastases can have a significant impact on survival as well as on quality of life. Other conditions, including hypercoagulable states, SIADH, and hypercalcemia, can prove to be equally life threatening. Unfortunately, in many of these circumstances, the patient's underlying disease process at times may prove to be refractory to therapy.

Many major advances in pharmacologic and technologic approaches to the therapy and support of cancer patients have evolved through dedicated research. These achievements, however, become meaningless unless a physician approaches the individual patient during therapy with compassion and a sincere concern about the patient's physical and emotional well-being.

ACKNOWLEDGMENTS

Mark R. Olsen was supported by NIH Training Grant R25-CA47785. H. Ian Robins was supported by Cancer Research Institute, New York, NY; NIH GCRC Grant MO1-RR03186.

FURTHER READING

Abeloff MD, Armitage JO, Lichter AS, Niederhuber JE (1995) *Clinical Oncology.* Churchill-Livingstone, New York.

Byrne TN (1992) Spinal cord compression from epidural metastasses. *N Engl J Med* 327:613–619.

Chanock SJ, Pizzo PA (1996) Fever in the neutropenic host. *Infect Dis Clin NA* 10:777-796.

DeVita VT, Hellman S, Rosenberg S (eds) (1997) *Cancer—Principles & Practice of Oncology*, 5th edition, JB Lippincott, Philadelphia.

Escalante CP, Rubenstein EB, Rolston KV (1997) Outpatient antibiotic therapy for febrile episodes in low-risk neutropenic patients with cancer. *Cancer Invest* 15:237–242.

Hughes WT, Armstrong D, Bodey GP, et al. (1990) Guidelines for use of antimicrobial agents in neutropenic patients with unexplained fever. *J Infect Dis* 161:381–396.

Lifton R, Bennett JM (1996) Clinical use of granulocyte-macrophage colony-stimulating factor and granulocyte colony-stimulating factor in neutropenia associated with malignancy. *Hematol Oncol Clin NA* 10:825–839.

CHAPTER 38

PAIN MANAGEMENT

BETTY R. FERRELL

City of Hope National Medical Center
Duarte, CA 91010, USA

Pain is a complex and distressing symptom impacting quality of life for the patient with cancer. Definitions of pain have emerged, from simple explanations of this
symptom as a purely physiologic phenomenon to our current view of its multidimensional nature. The International Association for the Study of Pain (1986) provides a
definition of pain as "an unpleasant sensory and emotional experience associated
with actual or potential tissue damage, or described in terms of such damage." This
definition acknowledges the multidimensional view of pain as an individual experience that includes physical and psychosocial perspectives.

This chapter reviews recent progress in the assessment and management of cancer
pain with special considerations for chronic cancer pain management. Pain is viewed
as a multidimensional problem requiring an interdisciplinary approach. Essential
pharmacologic management is the cornerstone of pain relief. Fortunately, many recent advances in opioid pharmacology have improved our ability to greatly improve
the relief of pain.

THE PROBLEM OF PAIN

The problem of cancer pain has now emerged as a major health care concern. Pain
was identified by the World Health Organization (WHO) as an international priority in 1986 and continues as one of the WHO chief priorities. The National Cancer
Institute and other agencies in the United States have also designated the relief of
cancer pain as a priority area for professional education and research. A final impor-

Manual of Clinical Oncology, 7th edition, Edited by Raphael E. Pollock
ISBN 0-471-23828-7, pages 745–756. Copyright © 1999 Wiley-Liss, Inc.

tant advance in the United States has been the 1994 release of Chronic Cancer Pain guidelines developed by the Agency for Health Care Policy and Research (AHCPR). The cancer guidelines address the assessment and management of chronic cancer pain and recognize pain as an undertreated symptom impacting quality of life.

Many professional organizations throughout the world have begun assertive efforts to address the international problem of cancer pain. These efforts have resulted in clinical practice guidelines and a wealth of palliative care literature. The challenge for oncologists is to use this available knowledge to improve what has previously been a neglected area of cancer care. On a global scale, the WHO reports that of the 9 million new cancer cases each year, more than half are in developing countries and the majority of these patients have advanced disease at the time of diagnosis. Thus, improved pain management can result in benefit to a significant number of patients with cancer.

MECHANISMS OF PAIN

The physiology of pain is best explained by the perception and response of the individual to the noxious stimuli. There are several physiologic processes that result in the experience of pain. The first of these processes, transduction, begins when a noxious stimulus affects a peripheral sensory nerve ending that initiates the whole phenomenon of pain perception. Transmission, the next process, consists of the series of subsequent neural events that carry the electrical impulses throughout the nervous system, from peripheral to central. Modulation, the third process, is a neural activity that controls pain transmission neurons originating in the periphery and/or the central nervous system. The fourth process, perception, is the subjective correlate of pain that encompasses complex behavioral, psychological, and emotional factors that are little understood.

Pain in cancer is the result of multiple causes including direct tumor involvement, nerve compression or infiltration, or involvement of soft tissue. Pain also frequently results from treatments including chemotherapy, radiation therapy, and postsurgical syndromes such as postmastectomy pain. Pain resulting from stimulation of nerve receptors is nociceptive pain while pain resulting from damage to nerves is neuropathic pain. These classifications become important in selecting treatment options.

One of the most clinically important classifications of pain is the distinction between acute and chronic pain. Acute pain is defined as that of sudden onset and that generally has known cause and a limited duration. Acute pain, such as surgical or procedure related pain, is associated with activation of the autonomic nervous system. Patients in acute pain exhibit behaviors indicating their discomfort, and the pattern of this pain is predictable.

Chronic pain is characterized by adaptation of the autonomic nervous system that may result in the absence of outward behaviors in patients and/or the presence of other chronic illness behaviors such as depression. Chronic pain is quite a distinct phenomenon from acute pain as the individual often can no longer recall its onset and knows there may be no end, other than eventual death. Chronic pain becomes far more subjective an experience, and is also associated with suffering. The longer life span of patients with cancer has also meant that many patients live for months and years with cancer pain.

CANCER PAIN AS A MULTIDIMENSIONAL PHENOMENON

Current conceptualizations of pain have moved from basic physiologic theories to a broad view of the pain experience through the perspective of quality of life (QOL). Pain interrupts physical well-being and is related to other physical symptoms. Pain is closely associated with psychological well-being and symptoms such as anxiety and depression. Patients often report that they are fearful of a future with pain and see it as a sign of progressive disease.

Pain is also a symptom that impacts the family as well as the patient experiencing the cancer. Social well-being is diminished as pain interferes with roles and relationships, sexuality, and appearance. Spiritual well-being includes religious beliefs and the dimension of suffering as well as the meaning of illness and pain to the patient.

BARRIERS TO PAIN RELIEF

At the time of diagnosis and continuing through treatment, 30% to 45% of cancer patients experience moderate to severe pain. The prevalence increases to approximately 75% in advanced cancer. Of patients with pain, 40% to 50% describe it as moderate to severe and 25% to 30% report very severe pain. Unfortunately, pain is not only a common problem of cancer but is also seriously undertreated. The AHCPR pain guidelines estimate that 50% of surgery patients receive inadequate pain management and that this undertreatment escalates to approximately 80% of chronic cancer-related pain. Table 38.1 summarizes the many barriers to adequate pain relief including problems of health care professionals, patients, and those related to the health care system.

The first category of barriers, problems related to health care professionals, recognizes the importance of enhanced knowledge so that providers can improve the care provided to patients in pain. Previous studies have documented the deficiencies in the medical school curriculum and the need for improved formal and continuing education in palliative care. Beyond the barrier of knowledge, health care professionals also often have inappropriate fears of addiction and inadequate skills in pain assessment.

Frequently cited patient barriers to effective pain management include fears of respiratory depression, fear of drug tolerance, fear of drug addiction, and inability to communicate pain. Treatment side effects, such as opioid-induced constipation and nausea, are also major reasons for patient noncompliance with analgesic regimens. In several studies, cancer patients have been found to consume only 50% to 60% of medications ordered even when the patient is experiencing unrelieved pain. Patient noncompliance with pain medications is often due to fears of addiction, or respiratory

TABLE 38.1. Barriers to Cancer Pain Management

Problems Related to Health Care Professionals
  Inadequate knowledge of pain management
  Poor assessment of pain
  Concern about regulation of controlled substances
  Fear of patient addiction
  Concern about side effects of analgesics
  Concern about patients becoming tolerant to analgesics

Problems Related to Patients
  Reluctance to report pain
    Concern about distracting physicians from treatment of underlying disease
    Fear that pain means disease is worse
    Concern about not being a "good" patient
  Reluctance to take pain medications
    Fear of addiction or of being thought of as an addict
    Worries about unmanageable side effects
    Concern about becoming tolerant to pain medications

Problems Related to the Health Care System
  Low priority given to cancer pain treatment
  Inadequate reimbursement
    The most appropriate treatment may not be reimbursed or may be too costly for patients
      and families
    Restrictive regulation of controlled substances
    Problems of availability of treatment or access to it

From: Agency for Health Care Policy and Research (AHCPR). *Management of Cancer Pain. Clinical Practice Guideline* No. 9. AHCPR Publication No. 94-0592. Rockville, MD. U.S. Department of Health and Human Services, Public Health Service, March 1994.

depression, and a lack of understanding of principles of preventing pain through routine dosing of analgesics.

There are also many system barriers that inhibit adequate pain relief. The challenge to improve pain management occurs within a "just say no to drugs" social environment, often resulting in a lack of access to appropriate prescribing. The WHO has focused major efforts toward increased availability of opioids which has been a major problem in many countries. Aggressive pain treatment is also limited by reimbursement and access of patients to specialized pain services or palliative care systems.

Despite the challenges, there is growing evidence that cancer pain can be successfully treated in the vast majority of patients. Efforts at implementation of the guidelines developed by the WHO and other associations has demonstrated that approximately 90% of cancer pain can be controlled through relatively simple means. Application of basic pain management principles can provide a foundation for optimum comfort throughout the course of cancer.

PRINCIPLES OF PAIN ASSESSMENT

Assessment of cancer pain is critical for all health care professionals because failure to assess pain leads to its undertreatment. The role of cancer pain assessment was emphasized in a 1993 study of 897 United States oncologists who, collectively in the previous 6 months, had managed more than 70,000 cancer patients. According to these physicians, poor pain assessment was the greatest barrier to effective cancer pain management in their own practices.

The initial evaluation of pain should include a detailed history, including an assessment of the pain intensity and character; physical examination, emphasizing the neurologic examination; psychosocial assessment; and appropriate diagnostic workup to determine the cause of the pain.

One routine clinical approach to pain assessment and management was developed by the AHCPR cancer pain guideline panel and is summarized by the mnemonic "ABCDE":

A *A*sk about pain regularly.

A *A*ssess pain systematically.

B *B*elieve the patient and family in their reports of pain and what relieves it.

C *C*hoose pain control options appropriate for the patient, family, and setting.

D *D*eliver interventions in a timely, logical, and coordinated fashion.

E *E*mpower patients and their families.
   *E*nable them to control their course to the greatest extent possible.

The pain assessment begins with evaluating pain intensity. Pain intensity is the assessment of the severity of pain experienced. A great deal of research has focused on use of various scales to measure pain intensity. Clinicians are encouraged to use pain scales, such as an ordinal scale in which patients are asked to rate their pain on a scale of $0 =$ no pain to $10 =$ worst pain. Use of a pain rating scale assists in communicating pain and in evaluating changes in pain over time.

The assessment of the patients pain and the efficacy of the treatment plan should be ongoing, and the pain reports should be documented. Pain should be assessed and documented at regular intervals after starting the treatment plan and with each new report of pain. Reassessment or evaluation of pain relief is equally important. At a suitable interval after each pharmacologic or nonpharmacologic intervention, the patient should again provide a pain rating to evaluate effectiveness of the interventions. In addition, patients should be taught to report changes in their pain or any new pain so that appropriate reassessment and changes in the treatment plan can be initiated.

Pain assessment is not a one-time occurrence but rather it is an ongoing process requiring constant attention to new pain. Changes in pain or the development of new pain should not be attributed to preexisting causes but should instead necessitate diagnostic evaluation. New pain may signal treatable problems such as infection or pathologic fracture. A change in pain often signals advancing disease, and because pain management relies on the treatment of the underlying disease, establishing a medical diagnosis is critical. One study conducted in a pain center revealed that a comprehensive pain assessment identified new causes of pain in 64% of 270 oncology patients with new pain complaints; most of the new diagnoses were neurologic. Thus, the need to reassess persistent pain to identify new causes cannot be overemphasized.

PAIN MANAGEMENT

The WHO, AHCPR, and other organizations have emphasized that optimum pain management is based on a combined approach using nonsteroidal antiinflammatory drugs (NSAIDs), opioids, and adjuvant medications. These pharmacologic approaches are used in combination with other treatments such as radiation therapy or invasive procedures. The three major classes—NSAIDs, opioids, and adjuvants are described in the following sections.

Nonopioid Analgesics

paracetamol

The nonopioid analgesics include the NSAIDS, aspirin, and acetaminophen. They are useful for mild to moderate cancer pain and also are used in combination with opioids for moderate to severe pain. These drugs should not be used to replace the stronger opioid analgesics but are an important component of the pharmacologic regimen for optimum cancer pain relief.

Acetaminophen (paracetamol) has fewer side effects than other nonopioids and no effects on platelet function. The usual adult dose is limited to less than 6000 mg per day, as doses exceeding that limit may cause severe hepatic toxicity. Aspirin is also an excellent analgesic and works by inhibiting prostaglandin synthesis. Adverse effects such as nausea or other gastrointestinal effects limit its use as does its inhibition of platelet aggregation. Many patients get excellent pain relief from acetaminophen or aspirin when used alone and others receive increased analgesia from opioids from these drugs.

Ibuprofen is an NSAID that is also used extensively in this category. The usual dose of 600 to 800 mg of ibuprofen given every 6 to 8 hours for a maximum daily dose of 2400 mg is suggested. There are many other NSAIDs widely used for cancer pain. The nonacetylated salicylates including choline magnesium trisalicylate are often used because of a minimal effect on platelet aggregation. The NSAIDs are often limited in use with cancer patients because of their gastrointestinal and renal effects. NSAIDs can cause renal insufficiency and are of special concern for the elderly or those with chronic renal or hepatic disease.

There are many NSAIDs to consider for those patients for whom the above agents are not effective. Prior experience with analgesics and a thorough history of gastrointestinal or hepatic–renal effects is important in selecting NSAIDs. Longer acting NSAID analgesics can be important for patients to improve compliance, as it is well established that administering these drugs on a regular schedule for chronic pain helps to eliminate extreme episodes of pain when relief can be maintained in a steady state. Misoprostol has been used in conjunction with NSAIDs to minimize gastric ulcers, particularly for those who have been maintained on long-term administration of these analgesics. It is also important to assess the patient's overall drug regimen as many medications include NSAIDs and thus the combination of medications may exceed the dosage limits suggested for NSAIDs to avoid side effects. Patients should also be advised that use of NSAIDs, opioids, and adjuvants may often require several dosage titrations and several days of administration before benefits are seen.

Opioid Analgesics

Opioid analgesics reduce pain primarily through central mechanisms by binding to μ, δ, and κ receptors. The pure agonist opioids are preferred and morphine has been established as the gold standard for cancer pain analgesia. Other drugs from the pure agonist category recommended for cancer pain include hydromorphone, hydrocodone, oxycodone, methadone, and fentanyl. These drugs do have many adverse effects, the primary effects being nausea, constipation, and sedation. The selection and titration of an opioid requires a balance of pain relief with a minimum of side effects to truly enhance not only pain relief, but also quality of life.

There are many mixed agonist/antagonist opioids that are considered less appropriate for cancer pain management. Drugs such as pentazocine, butorphanol, and nalbuphine do not provide consistent analgesia like the agonists and also have a ceiling effect. These drugs often have side effects such as increased sedation, nausea, and confusion. The accepted standard of pain relief emerging over the past decade has been the use of a long-acting analgesic, morphine, along with short-acting opioids on an as-needed schedule for breakthrough pain. The WHO has established morphine as the standard of analgesia and many efforts are in place to increase the availability of morphine. Preparations that extend analgesia for 8 to 12 hours have been acknowledged as providing a much improved relief of pain and quality of life by reducing interruptions in sleep and enhancing consistent relief. Patients on long-acting analgesics will need a short-acting analgesic available for those episodes of breakthrough pain that may occur between long-acting doses. The usual recommendation is for doses of approximately 5% to 15% of their 24-hour dose equivalent of morphine to be given on a q 2-hour schedule for breakthrough pain.

Hydromorphone is an alternative to morphine and is often used for those patients who cannot tolerate morphine. In some countries it is also available as a long-acting preparation. Hydromorphone is often used in subcutaneous infusions and is widely used in the oral route with several dosage forms available. Fentanyl is an analgesic that was used earlier in its history primarily in the surgical setting but has been extensively used in recent years for cancer pain because of its availability in the transdermal route. The transdermal fentanyl patch is applied for 48 to 72 hours duration. Fentanyl is a potent analgesic and is also used intravenously or epidurally.

Oxycodone is a very good analgesic used for moderate to severe pain. It is now available in a noncompounded form and also in a long-acting preparation. This drug is often an excellent choice for patients who are reluctant to take morphine and yet who require significant amounts of analgesia. Oxycodone is also available in several compounded formulations, usually combined with acetaminophen or aspirin.

Many other strong analgesics are available. Methadone is a potent analgesic but its use is limited because of a long half-life which can cause accumulation and is of particular concern for the elderly or other patients for whom accumulation can create serious problems. Analgesics such as Levorphanol are not used as frequently in recent years as the availability of better analgesics such as morphine and oxycodone has offered advantages, particularly as long-acting formulations in higher doses are available.

Meperidine is an opioid analgesic that is strongly discouraged for use in cancer pain management. Normeperidine, the active metabolite of meperidine, can accumulate as the drug is metabolized and is of particular concern with higher doses for any patient who will receive the drugs for more than a few days. Accumulation of Normeperidine can result in central nervous system excitability, leading to seizures.

Table 38.2 includes dosing information for opioid analgesics. Knowledge of these key principles is important to provide the most aggressive pain relief possible.

Published tables vary in the suggested doses that are equianalgesic to morphine. Clinical response is the criterion that must be applied for each patient; titration to clinical responses is necessary. Because there is not complete cross-tolerance among these drugs, it is usually necessary to use a lower than equianalgesic dose when changing drugs and to retitrate to response.

Adjuvant Drugs

Adjuvant drugs are those medications used to enhance analgesic efficacy, treat concurrent symptoms, and provide independent analgesia for specific types of pain. The corticosteroids provide a range of effects including mood elevation, antiinflammatory activity, antiemetic activity, and appetite stimulation. They may be beneficial in the management of cachexia and anorexia. They also reduce cerebral and spinal cord edema and are used in the emergency management of epidural spinal cord compression or severe, acute bone pain, such as in pathologic fracture.

Anticonvulsants are also used to manage neuropathic pain, especially lancinating or burning pain. Those drugs are used with caution in cancer patients undergoing marrow-suppressant therapies, such as chemotherapy and radiation. Antidepressants are useful in pharmacologic management of neuropathic pain. These drugs have innate analgesic properties and may potentiate the analgesic effects of opioids. The most widely reported experience has been with amitriptyline, but other agents such as imipramine or doxepin are also used. Neuroleptics, particularly methotrimeprazine, have been used to treat chronic pain. Methotrimeprazine lacks opioid inhibiting effects on gut motility and may be useful for treating opioid-induced intractable constipation or other dose-limiting side effects. It also has antiemetic and anxiolytic effects.

Local anesthetics have also been used to treat neuropathic pain. Side effects for these may be greater than with other drugs used to treat neuropathic pain. Anxiety is a common symptom in patients with pain and hydroxyzine, a mild anxiolytic

TABLE 38.2. Dose Equivalents for Opioid Analgesics in Opioid-Naive Adults and Children ≥ 50 kg Body Weight[a]

Drug	Approximate Equianalgesic Dose		Usual Starting Dose for Moderate to Severe Pain	
	Oral	Parenteral	Oral	Parenteral
Opioid agonist[b]				
Morphine[c]	30 mg q 3–4 h (repeat around-the-clock dosing) 60 mg q 3–4 h (single dose or intermittent dosing)	10 mg q 3–4 h	30 mg q 3–4 h	10 mg q 3–4h
Morphine, controlled release[c,d] (MS Contin, Oramorph)	90–120 mg q 12 h	N/A	90–120 mg q 12 h	N/A
Hydromorphone[c] (Dilaudid)	7.5 mg q 3–4 h	1.5 mg q 3–4 h	6 mg q 3–4 h	1.5 mg q 3–4 h
Levorphanol 6–8 h (Levo-Dromoran)	4 mg q 6–8 h	2 mg q 6–8 h	4 mg q 6–8 h	2 mg q 6–8 h
Meperidine (Demerol)	300 mg q 2–3 h	100 mg q 3h	N/R	100 mg q 3 h
Methadone (Dolophine, other)	20 mg q 6–8 h	10 mg q 6–8 h	20 mg q 6–8 h	10 mg q 6–8 h
Combination Opioid/NSAID Preparations				
Codeine[f] (with aspirin or acetaminophen)	180–200 mg q 3–4 h	130 mg q 3–4 h	60 mg q 3–4 h	60 mg q 2h
Hydrocodone (in Lorcet, Lortab, Vicodin, others)	30 mg q 3–4 h	N/A	10 mg q 3–4 h	N/A
Oxycodone (Roxicodone, also in Percocet, Percodan, Tylox, others)	30 mg q 3–4 h	N/A	10 mg q 3–4 h	N/A

[a] **Caution**: Recommended doses do not apply for adult patients with body weight less than 50 kg.

[b] **Caution**: Recommended doses do not apply to patients with renal or hepatic insufficiency or other conditions affecting drug metabolism and kinetics.

[c] **Caution**: For morphine, hydromorphone, and oxymorphone, rectal administration is an alternate route for patients unable to take oral medications. Equianalgesic doses may differ from oral and parenteral doses because of pharmacokinetic differences.

[d] Transdermal fentanyl (Duragesic) is an alternative option. Doses above 25 μg/h should not be used in opioid-naive patients.

[e] **Caution**: Doses of aspirin and acetaminophen in combination opioid/NSAID preparations must also be adjusted to the patients body weight. Aspirin is contraindicated in children in the presence of fever or other viral disease because of its association with Reye's syndrome.

[f] **Caution**: Codeine doses above 65 mg often are not appropriate because of diminishing incremental analgesia with increasing doses but continually increasing nausea, constipation, and other side effects.

753

agent with sedating and analgesic properties, is useful in treating anxiety. This antihistamine also has antiemetic properties. Another common symptom in patients on opioids is sedation. This symptom can be treated by giving caffeine or caffeinated beverages, or psychostimulants may be useful in reducing opioid-induced sedation when opioid dose adjustment (i.e., reduced dose and increased dose frequency) is not effective. There are other drugs also in use for various pain syndromes for which limited empirical data are available yet offer promise for the future. The bisphosphonates and radiopharmaceuticals are becoming more frequently used and offer improved analgesia for metastatic bone pain. Other agents and novel drug delivery modes will continue to be added to the choices available for analgesia.

Nonpharmacologic Strategies

Optimum pain relief is achieved through a combination of drug and nondrug techniques. Most patients will benefit from a combination of pharmacologic approaches used with physical or cognitive pain relief strategies such as heat, cold, distraction, or relaxation. Pain management also requires patient education to overcome patient fears of addiction or drug tolerance and to involve the patient and family with the goals of pain assessment and treatment. Recognition of the multidimensional nature of pain as depicted in Fig. 38.1 also implies the need for an interdisciplinary approach to meet the complex physical and psychosocial needs of patients in pain.

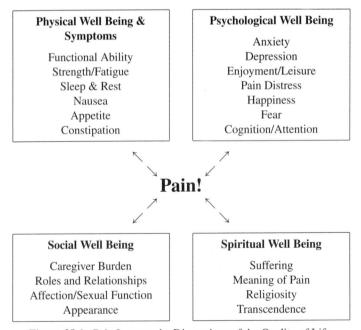

Physical Well Being & Symptoms	Psychological Well Being
Functional Ability	Anxiety
Strength/Fatigue	Depression
Sleep & Rest	Enjoyment/Leisure
Nausea	Pain Distress
Appetite	Happiness
Constipation	Fear
	Cognition/Attention

Pain!

Social Well Being	Spiritual Well Being
Caregiver Burden	Suffering
Roles and Relationships	Meaning of Pain
Affection/Sexual Function	Religiosity
Appearance	Transcendence

Figure 38.1. Pain Impacts the Dimensions of the Quality of Life.

SUMMARY

Cancer pain has been cited throughout the world as a seriously undertreated problem and one of enormous consequence for patients and their families. Advances in analgesia have provided the means to relieve the vast majority of pain using pharmacologic techniques and through recognition of the multidimensional nature of pain. Continued efforts are needed to eliminate barriers to adequate pain relief and to further close the gap between current practice and the potential for pain relief for all patients with cancer.

FURTHER READING

Agency for Health Care Policy and Research (AHCPR) (1994) *Management of Cancer Pain. Clinical Practice Guideline* No. 9. AHCPR Publication No. 94-0592. Rockville, MD. US Department of Health and Human Services, Public Health Service, March.

American Pain Society (APS) (1992) *Principles of Analgesic Use in the Treatment of Acute Pain and Chronic Cancer Pain*, 3rd edition. American Pain Society. Skokie, IL.

Cherny NI, Portenoy RK (1994) The management of cancer pain. *CA Cancer J Clin* 44:263–303.

Cleeland CS, Gonin R, Hatfield AK, et al. (1994) Pain and its treatment in out-patients with metastatic cancer. *N Engl J Med* 330:592–596.

Coyle N, Cherny N, Portenoy RK (1995) Pharmacologic management of cancer pain. In: McGuire DB, Yarbro CH, Ferrell BR (eds) *Cancer Pain Management*, 2nd edition. Jones and Bartlett, Boston.

Ferrell B (ed) (1995) *Suffering*. Jones & Bartlett, Boston.

Ferrell BR (1995) The impact of pain on quality of life: A decade of research. *Nurs Clin NA* 30:609–624.

Ferrell BR, Ferrell BA, Ahn C, Tran K (1994) Pain management for elderly patients with cancer at home. *Cancer* 74:2139–2146.

Ferrell BR, Rhiner M, Ferrell BA (1993) Development and implementation of a pain education program. *Cancer* 72:3426–3432.

Ferrell BR, Rivera LM (1997) Cancer pain education for patients. *Sem Oncol Nurs* 13:42–48.

Gonzales GR, Payne R, Foley KM, Portenoy RK (1992) Prevalence and characteristics of brachial plexopathy in a large cancer center: A retrospective study. In: *Third Annual Bristol-Meyers Pain Research Symposium*, Seattle.

International Association for the Study of Pain, Subcommittee on Taxonomy (1979) Part II. Pain terms: A current list with definitions and notes on usage. *Pain* 6:249–252 [updated 1982, 1986].

Levy MH (1996) Pharmacologic treatment of cancer pain. *N Engl J Med* 335:1124–1132.

Levy MH (1994) Pharmacologic management of cancer pain. *Sem Oncol* 21:718–739.

Melzack R, Wall P (1982) *The Challenge of Pain*. Basic Books, New York.

Patt RB (ed) (1993) *Cancer Pain*. JB Lippincott, Philadelphia.

Schug SA, Zech D, Door U (1990) Cancer pain management according to WHO analgesic guidelines. *J Pain Symp Manag* 5:27–32.

Twycross R (1994) *Pain Relief in Advanced Cancer*. Churchill Livingstone, London.

Ventafridda V, Caraceni A, Gamba A (1990) Field-testing of the WHO Guidelines for Cancer Pain Relief: Summary report of demonstration projects. In: Foley KM, Bonica JJ, Ventafridda V (eds) Proceedings of the Second International Contress on Pain. *Advances in Pain Research and Therapy*, Vol. 16. Raven Press, New York, pp. 451–464.

Von Roenn JH, Cleeland CS, Gonin R, Hatfield AK, Pandya KJ (1993) Physician attitudes and practice in cancer pain management: A survey from the Eastern Cooperative Oncology Group. *Ann Intern Med* 119:121–126.

World Health Organization (1996) *Cancer Pain Relief*, 2nd edition. WHO, Geneva, Switzerland.

■■■■■■ CHAPTER 39

NUTRITION

BRIAN I. LABOW

Department of Surgery,
Massachusetts General Hospital
Boston, MA 02114, USA

WILEY W. SOUBA

Division of Surgical Oncology and Nutrition Support Services
Massachusetts General Hospital
Boston, MA 02114, USA

Malnutrition is common in cancer patients and is an important cause of increased morbidity and mortality. The term *cancer cachexia* describes the clinical triad of weight loss, anorexia, and loss of lean body mass secondary to a growing malignancy. This condition is often accompanied by vitamin and trace mineral deficiencies and protein calorie malnutrition, the most common form of nutritional depletion, often results. Cachexia is often exacerbated by chemotherapy and/or radiation therapy along with surgery, which can further compromise an already fragile nutritional status.

Recent developments have increased our understanding of the relationship between nutrition and metabolism in cancer patients. Severe malnutrition has been shown to have adverse effects on immune function and treatment tolerance to anticancer regimens and is associated with increased postoperative complications in cancer patients who undergo surgery. In fact, weight loss itself is a predictor of therapeutic response and survival. Although limited weight loss in some cancer patients may be acceptable, many cancer patients develop significant malnutrition such that some form of nutrition support may be required. The rationale for such nutrition support is to prevent or reverse host tissue wasting, broaden the spectrum of therapeutic options, improve the clinical course, and ultimately prolong patient survival. Accordingly, oncologists should become familiar with the metabolic changes that develop

Manual of Clinical Oncology, 7th edition, Edited by Raphael E. Pollock
ISBN 0-471-23828-7, pages 757–777. Copyright © 1999 Wiley-Liss, Inc.

in response to malignancy and with the indications for and delivery of nutritional support to the cancer patient.

The purpose of this chapter is to examine the etiologies of and metabolic alterations that develop in cachectic patient and to establish a rationale for nutrition support in the malnourished cancer patient. In addition the indications for the various means of nutrition support are examined. Portions of this review have been previously published.[1-5]

CLINICAL MANIFESTATIONS OF CANCER CACHEXIA

Weight Loss

Most cancer patients develop weight loss at some point during the course of their disease and nearly half will have weight loss at the time of initial diagnosis. Published studies reported that patients who presented without weight loss had a significantly prolonged survival following therapy compared with similarly treated patients who had weight loss at presentation (Fig. 39.1).[6] These findings suggest that weight loss adversely affects survival following antineoplastic therapy and imply that appropriate nutritional therapy may be beneficial in certain patient groups. In addition, cancer patients with significant weight loss do not tolerate treatment regimens as well as the adequately nourished patient. Weight loss is dependent on the presence of the tumor, as curative surgical resection (or nonsurgical treatment) of the malignancy is almost invariably associated with a return to normal body weight. Although some weight loss following surgery may be expected because of postoperative ileus and increased metabolic demand, patients who do not regain their weight following surgical resection for cure should be investigated for metastatic or recurrent disease.

Anorexia

At some point during the course of their disease, most patients report a loss of appetite that includes alterations in taste and smell and a loss of appeal for most foods. Loss of appetite resulting in a reduction in voluntary food intake is a central component of cancer cachexia, and unfortunately oncologic therapies often initiate or worsen this anorexia. In some patients this is reflected by an increase in resting energy expenditure without a compensatory increase in calorie intake. This combination of increased energy demand without increased food intake exacerbates weight loss and negative calorie and nitrogen balance. Early satiety, mechanical obstruction, or nausea are common in patients with malignancies of the gastrointestinal tract which often produce profound anorexia. However, digestive tract dysfunction cannot solely explain this phenomenon, as significant anorexia is also noted in patients with cancers that originate outside the abdominal cavity as well. In fact, careful studies using animal models of cachexia have clearly documented a decline in food intake in response to cancer. Proposed mechanisms for this "anorexia of malignancy" include local effects of the tumor, alterations in taste or palatability, hypothalamic dysfunction, modification of satiety mechanisms, and learned food aversion.

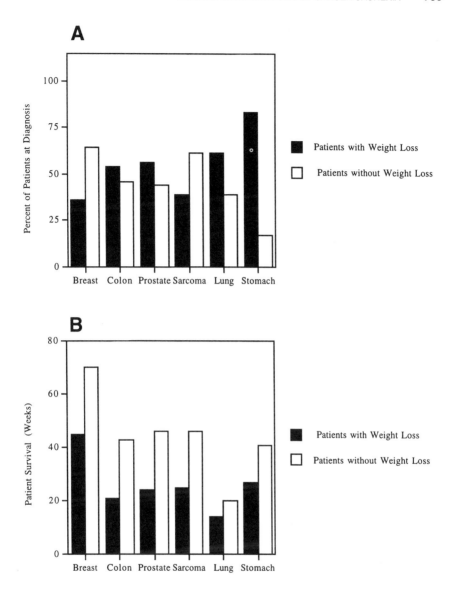

FIGURE 39.1. Prevalence of weight loss in cancer patients at the time of diagnosis (**A**) and its effect on survival following antineoplastic therapy (**B**), $p < 0.05$.[6]

Although tumors themselves may initiate or potentiate anorexia, many chemotherapeutic agents can also produce profound anorexia. Nausea, vomiting, mucositis, and/or gastrointestinal dysfunction often result from chemotherapy and radiation therapy. This "anorexia of therapy" may often contribute significantly to cachexia as well. Another important consideration for the clinician is that during diagnostic evaluation, hospitalized cancer patients are often restricted from taking adequate nutrition. As a result, the patient may become iatrogenically malnourished prior to the initiation of oncologic treatment.

Weakness

With a loss of body cell mass and because of the effects of treatment regimens, cancer patients almost invariably develop a reduction in strength and a diminished functional capacity for physical work. Evidence for a central role of the tumor in the etiology of this weakness is derived from the clinical observation that successful management of the tumor almost always results in a return to preillness strength and work capacity.

CAUSES AND CONSEQUENCES OF CANCER CACHEXIA

Because many cancer-related deaths are a consequence of malnutrition, an understanding of the metabolic mechanisms underlying cancer cachexia is imperative. Although the exact prevalence of cachexia is unknown, many studies have shown a high frequency of nutritional derangements in cancer patients. These studies have focused on findings such as weight loss or hypoproteinemia as indicators of cachexia. Consequently, the prevalence of cancer cachexia may be underestimated, as it is likely that subtle metabolic alterations precede these clinically apparent changes.

Many of the physiologic changes seen in cachectic patients resemble those of simple starvation, but it is clear that other derangements are also involved (Table 39.1). Instead of adapting to partial starvation by conserving lean body mass, the

TABLE 39.1. Metabolic Differences Between the Response to Simple Starvation and to Advanced Malignant Disease

	Simple Starvation	Advanced Malignant Disease
Basal metabolic rate	$-$ or $\downarrow$	$-$, $\uparrow$, or $\downarrow$
Presence of mediators	$-$	+++
Hepatic ureagenesis	+	+++
Negative nitrogen balance	+	+++
Gluconeogenesis	+	+++
Muscle proteolysis	+	+++
Hepatic protein synthesis	+	+++

$-$ indicates normal; + indicates slightly increased; +++ indicates a substantial increase.

host continues to deplete its own muscle mass, probably to provide amino acids for tumor growth and to support hepatic gluconeogenesis and protein synthesis. Unfortunately, few studies have documented that aggressive feeding of cachectic cancer patients restores lean body mass. Furthermore, no consistent or clear-cut association with duration of illness, stage of disease, or tumor histology has been demonstrated to correlate with the degree of cachexia. Although the demand for substrate may account in part for the loss of lean body mass, the actual energy and nitrogen demands of human tumors cannot account for the profound weight loss that is generally observed. For example, it is unusual for the total mass of the tumor to exceed 1% or 2% of total body weight, and yet patients with even much smaller tumors are often markedly cachectic. Many etiologies for cancer cachexia have been proposed, but no clear explanation exists, and the etiology is likely to be multifactorial. Studies over the last decade suggest that humoral factors such as cytokines may play a major role in mediating cachexia. Understanding the abnormalities in host intermediary metabolism and the effects of the mediators that produce them will hopefully allow the clinician to adopt a rational approach to therapy and will underlie efforts to develop better techniques to combat this devastating effect of malignancy.

ALTERATIONS OF INTERMEDIARY METABOLISM

Metabolic abnormalities affecting carbohydrate, protein and lipid utilization are characteristic of the tumor-bearing host. Although resting energy expenditure (REE) is variably affected by the presence of malignancy,[7] even patients with no increase in metabolic rate can develop weight loss and negative nitrogen balance despite a normal food intake and in spite of a small tumor burden. In fact, some studies demonstrated that in some in solid tumor-bearing patients whole body protein turnover was increased 50%, despite no change in REE.[8]

Glucose metabolism is often abnormal in cancer patients because of increased turnover. Furthermore, it has been shown that in patients with gastrointestinal malignancies hepatic gluconeogenesis increases in proportion to tumor burden.[9] Interestingly, patients with the largest tumors failed to suppress endogenous glucose production during glucose infusion, a response attributed to a reduction in insulin sensitivity. Other studies indicate that β-cell receptor sensitivity to glucose loading may also be diminished in the tumor-bearing host, in a manner similar to those with type II diabetes.[10] These effects could contribute significantly to depletion of energy stores and tissue wasting.

Protein and amino acid metabolism are also altered in the tumor-bearing host. The changes observed are not simply the results of starvation. This has been demonstrated by studies comparing tumor-bearing patients, malnourished non-tumor-bearing patients, and healthy controls; protein turnover was found to be elevated only in the cancer group.[11] In another study, patients with non-small-cell lung cancer were found to have increased whole-body protein turnover, elevated 3-methylhistidine excretion, and increased muscle proteolysis.[12] Tumor-bearing animal models also demonstrate increased whole body nitrogen turnover and increased liver protein fractional synthetic rates. In patients, studies measuring arterial and venous differences in amino acid content across a sarcoma-bearing limb, using the non-tumor-bearing limb as a control, have demonstrated that the tumor participates directly in augmenting protein metabolism.[13] Compared to the non-tumor-bearing extremity, the tumor-bearing limb released lesser amounts of all amino acids, suggesting increased demand for amino acids to support neoplastic growth.

Lipid metabolism is also altered in the host with cancer. Kinetics studies using radiolabeled glycerol and fatty acids found cancer patients with weight loss had increased glycerol and fatty acid turnover when compared to weight-stable patients.[9] These "cachectic" patients were incapable of oxidizing endogenous fatty acids or intravenous lipids at normal rates and failed to suppress lipolysis during glucose infusion.

GLUTAMINE AND CANCER CACHEXIA

Glutamine metabolism in the tumor-bearing host has been extensively studied for three principal reasons: (1) glutamine is the principal fuel used by many cancers, (2) it is the most abundant amino acid in the body and its stores are quite labile, and (3) glutamine is a conditionally essential amino acid. Glutamine is a good substrate for oxidation by tumor cell mitochondria and glutamine extraction by tumors may be quite high. In fact, tumor-bearing rats demonstrate a progressive fall in plasma glutamine concentrations that correlate with tumor size.[13] With time, blood glutamine levels may fall to less than 50% of normal, indicating an imbalance between rates of glutamine production and consumption. This reduction in circulating glutamine occurs despite increased muscle glutamine release, indicating either accelerated glutamine consumption by other tissues and/or tumor cells. Concomitantly, there are marked increases in tumor and hepatic glutamine uptake. Progressive tumor growth and glutamine depletion may accelerate muscle proteolysis, thereby exacerbating cachexia.[14]

CYTOKINES: MEDIATORS OF CANCER CACHEXIA

An understanding of the mediators that produce the metabolic changes described above would help derive nutritional strategies that optimize the metabolic integrity of the host and allow antitumor therapies to be maximally effective. Cytokines, a class of paracrine/autocrine proteins that produce a wide array of physiologic responses, have been implicated by a number of recent studies as important mediators of the host response to cancer. Cytokines can regulate both energy intake (i.e., appetite) and energy expenditure (i.e., metabolic rate) and thus play a pivotal role in determining the nutritional status of the tumor-bearing host.

Elevated concentrations of tissue and circulating cytokines have been demonstrated in the patients with cancer[15] and enhanced hepatic cytokine gene expression has been demonstrated in tumor-bearing animals. Administration of the cytokine tumor necrosis factor (TNF) to rodents and humans decreases food intake in a time- and dose-dependent manner.[16,17] In patients receiving exogenous TNF, food intake was also diminished as predicted. However, nitrogen losses were not accelerated, indicating that the resultant negative nitrogen balance was due to starvation alone. These effects of TNF on appetite may account in part for the anorexia observed in cancer patients.

The cytokine interleukin-1 (IL-1) also suppresses food intake and its effect, like that of TNF, appears to be a direct effect on appetite via the central nervous system. Further evidence for IL-1 and TNF as mediators of energy balance in cancer comes from studies that demonstrated that treatment of tumor-bearing mice with anticy- tokine antibodies improved food intake and attenuated weight loss[18] and that mice implanted with tumors that secreted TNF showed marked reductions in weight loss compared to animals with non-TNF-secreting tumors.[19]

In addition to their effects on appetite, cytokines also influence energy balance by stimulating basal metabolic rate (oxygen consumption). Studies indicate that patients receiving exogenous TNF may increase their metabolic rates by as much as 30%.[20] Furthermore, cytokines have also been shown to influence the metabolism of carbo- hydrates, proteins, and lipids and thus may contribute to cancer cachexia via both energy consumption and derangement of host metabolism.

Effects on Glucose Metabolism

Studies evaluating the effects of cytokine administration on the circulating glucose concentration indicate that the plasma glucose level will rise or fall depending on the dose administered, the temporal nature of the measurement, and on the specific cytokine given.

In rats, sublethal doses of TNF that did not produce hemodynamic changes re- sulted in the development of hyperglycemia within 1 hour of administration.[21] How- ever, plasma glucose concentrations rose only 20% and were associated with an increase in circulating glucagon, adrenocorticotropic hormone (ACTH), corticos- terone, and epinephrine all of which can cause hyperglycemia. When a lower dose of TNF was utilized, the plasma glucose did not change.[22] Similar alterations in blood glucose level were observed after IL-1 administration. Studies using relatively high IL-1 doses reported a 40% increase in plasma glucose concentration within 1 hour, with a return to basal levels by 2 hours.[23] Interestingly, this transient increase in plasma glucose was paralleled by a severalfold increase in hindquarter glucose con- sumption. Other studies examining tissue glucose utilization in vivo in rats showed that following infusion of a nonlethal dose of TNF, glucose uptake was increased by 80% to 100% in liver, kidney, and spleen, 60% in skin, 30% to 40% in lung and ileum, and 150% increase in diaphragm muscle.[24] No significant increase was ob- served in skeletal muscle, testis, or brain. These data indicate that TNF and IL-1 are capable of increasing whole body glucose utilization as well as plasma glucose concentration, and can certainly account in part for the alterations in carbohydrate metabolism seen in patients with cancer.

Effects on Protein/Amino Acid Metabolism

Marked changes in protein and amino acid metabolism are characteristic of cancer patients. A number of studies have evaluated the effects of cytokines on muscle protein metabolism and the results are conflicting. When recombinant TNF was infused into cancer patients, forearm amino acid efflux was accelerated, suggesting net skeletal muscle proteolysis, although this accelerated nitrogen release could also be accounted for by starvation effects.[25] Similarly, infused radiolabeled leucine into rats receiving TNF and/or IL-1 led to an increase in muscle protein degradation in cytokine-treated animals.[26] However, when IL-1 activity was blocked with specific anti-IL-1 antibodies, the accelerated protein breakdown was not attenuated.[27] Thus, although it is generally agreed that cytokine administration in vivo (at sufficient doses) stimulates net muscle proteolysis, it is unclear to what extent they act directly or via the effects of anorexia in cancer patients. In addition, in vitro studies[28] have failed to show a direct effect except in studies evaluating the effects of corticosterone on muscle protein breakdown. This glucocorticoid hormone, which accelerates protein degradation and diminishes protein synthesis, has a more potent effect in combination with TNF.[29] However, TNF alone did not alter protein turnover.

Impact on Fat Metabolism

Altered fat metabolism is apparent clinically in cachectic patients from the observation that fat stores are diminished in association with weight loss. This may be due in part to the ability of TNF and IL-1 to mobilize fat stores. Bolus administration of TNF to rats increased serum triglyceride levels within 2 hours.[20] The injection of IL-6 or TNF each reduced adipose tissue lipoprotein lipase (LPL) activity by more than 50% in tumor-bearing animals and both reduced heparin-releasable LPL activity in vitro in a dose-dependent manner by 50% to 70%.[30] Furthermore, TNF may also increase serum triglycerides via stimulation of hepatic lipid secretion in addition to its effects on adipocyte LPL activity.[31]

NUTRITIONAL SUPPORT OF THE CANCER PATIENT

Rationale

Although it seems obvious that the provision of nutritional support to the malnourished patient with cancer is essential, evidence indicating that currently available nutritional formulas can maintain or reverse malnutrition is lacking. The rationale behind the provision of specialized nutrition support, whether enteral or parenteral, is the belief that such support will preferentially benefit the patient rather than stimulate tumor growth. Nutrition support would not be indicated if it could be clearly demonstrated that it did not favorably impact the response to antineoplastic therapies, lengthen disease-free survival, and/or improve quality of life. Interestingly, a consensus opinion regarding the role and efficacy of nutrition support in patients with cancer is lacking. Nonetheless, several well-designed clinical studies have allowed us to generate guidelines for the use of enteral and parenteral nutrition in patients with cancer. Most physicians and surgeons who care for patients with cancer continue to use nutrition support aggressively under specific circumstances.

Nutritional Assessment of the Cancer Patient

The nutritional status of the cancer patient can usually be determined by a careful history and physical examination and should include inquiries about appetite, preferred foods, and weight loss. Anthropometric measurements including body weight, height, and skinfold thickness, as well as a 24-hour urine collection for nitrogen content are also useful. Peripheral blood lymphocyte count and assessment of cellular immunity via skin testing of delayed hypersensitivity to common antigens have been used as indicators of immunocompetence in the cancer patient. It should be noted that altered immunologic responses are not specific to nutritional deficiencies and are often observed in patients with advanced malignant disease who are adequately nourished. Serum albumin and transferrin are the most common serum proteins measured in nutritional assessment. Other laboratory studies that may be useful include red blood cell indices to determine iron and micronutrient deficiencies, plasma glucose to assess insulin resistance, blood urea nitrogen to determine renal status, and liver function tests.

The Use of Enteral Nutrition in Cancer Patients

Numerous clinical trials have evaluated the use of aggressive enteral nutrition support as adjunctive therapy during the administration of antineoplastic regimens to cancer patients. Unfortunately, well-designed studies comprise a small fraction of these. Although these trials do not demonstrate any consistent benefit to the use of routine enteral nutrition, most authorities would agree that when and if nutrition support is required, the enteral route is preferred whenever the gastrointestinal tract is functional. This preference is based primarily on studies in which animals receiving exclusively parenteral nutrition developed intestinal changes including villous atrophy, alterations in gut flora, and bacterial translocation from the intestinal lumen to mesenteric lymph nodes (Table 39.2). Enteral feedings can be supplied via a number of routes including transnasal–gastric or duodenal catheters or via permanently placed gastrostomy or jejunostomy tubes. Feedings may be supplied as between meal

TABLE 39.2. Proposed Benefits of Oral/Enteral Nutrition versus Parenteral Nutrition

1. Maintains gut mucosal mass
2. Maintains brush border enzyme activity
3. Supports gut immune function
4. Preserves gut mucosal barrier function
5. Maintains a balanced luminal microflora environment
6. Improves outcome after chemotherapy and radiation therapy

supplements or may replace meals altogether if eating becomes impossible. Some of the better enteral feeding clinical trials in cancer patients[32–44] are listed (Tables 39.3, 39.4, and 39.5).

Peripheral Intravenous Feedings

Although less commonly used as a means of nutrition support, indications for peripheral intravenous feeding include: (1) supplement to partially tolerated enteral feedings (2) as a method of nutritional support when the gastrointestinal tract must be kept relatively empty for short periods during diagnostic work-up and (3) as preliminary feedings prior to subclavian catheter insertion in patients requiring TPN. Peripheral veins may be used for infusion of glucose and amino acid solutions as well as fat emulsions. However, these solutions must be nearly isotonic to avoid peripheral vein sclerosis. Glucose solutions up to 10% by weight may be used and appear to increase the efficacy of amino acid utilization. Fat emulsions that provide an efficient fuel source can be administered simultaneously with glucose and amino acid infusions because they are isotonic. The major disadvantage of these peripherally administered mixtures is limited caloric delivery within tolerable fluid volumes.

Total Parenteral Nutrition in the Cancer Patient—General Recommendations

Although the initial enthusiasm for the use of total parenteral nutrition (TPN) in cancer patients was considerable, it is now clear that TPN should only be provided to selected patients. Because of the failure of numerous clinical trials to yield a consensus with regard to the efficacy of TPN in cancer patients[35,45–69] (Tables 39.3, 39.4, 39.5), recently published articles have used meta-analyses to review these studies collectively and generate feeding guidelines. The general conclusion has been that parenteral nutrition appears to be of little benefit in most cancer patients. However, the most important factor to consider when making decisions regarding TPN is the response of the tumor to antineoplastic therapy. If there is limited or no response to chemotherapy the potential complications of TPN therapy outweigh the benefits provided by the supplemental nutrition. However, there are certain patient populations that clearly benefit from the use of TPN and some guidelines for the use of TPN are listed (Table 39.6). These guidelines will likely undergo revision as more effective antitumor regimens become clinically available.

Specific Indications for the Use of Total Parenteral Nutrition in the Cancer Patient

Acute Radiation and Chemotherapy Enteritis   Cancer patients who receive abdominal/pelvic radiation or chemotherapy may develop severe and prolonged mucositis and enterocolitis that precludes the use of enteral feedings. Under these circumstances, TPN should be provided to malnourished patients until the enteritis resolves and enteral feeding can be resumed. Moreover, under circumstances where

TABLE 39.3. Results of Major Prospective Randomized Controlled Trials Evaluating Perioperative Nutrition

Author	Tumor Type	TPN Course	Number of Patients		Major Complications (%)		Perioperative Mortality (%)	
			TPN	Control	TPN	Control	TPN	Control
Parenteral Nutrition								
Holter and Fischer[45]	GI	3 d preop, 10 d postop	30	26	4 (13)	5 (19)	2 (7)	2 (8)
Heatley et al.[46]	Esophageal, gastric	7–10 d preop	38	36	2 (5), 3 (8), 9 (24)	3 (8), 11 (31), 16 (44)	6 (16)	8 (22)
Yamada et al.[47]	Gastric	18 d postop	18	16	1 (6)	5 (31)	0 (0)	1 (6)
Askanazi et al.[48]	Bladder	7 d postop	22	13	1 (5)	0 (0)	0 (0)	2 (15)
Muller et al.[49]	Esophageal	10 d preop	58	55	8 (14)	17 (31)	4 (7)	11 (20)
Bellantone et al.[50,51]	GI	7 d preop	49	51	13 (27)	18 (35)	1 (2)	2 (4)
Woolfson and Smith[52]	Oropharyngeal, esophageal, gastric, bladder	6 d postop	62	60	12	7	8(13)	8(13)
Buzby et al.[53]	GI, Lung	7–15 d preop, 3 d postop	192	203	49 (26)	50 (25)	16 (8)	12 (6)
Sandstrom et al.[54]	GI, bladder	postop	150	150	227	163	12 (8)	10 (7)
von Meyenfeldt et al.[35]	Gastric, colorectal	10 d preop	51	50	5 (10)	8 (16)	not reported	not reported
Sciafani, et al.[55]	Pancreas	5–20 d postop	24	27	9 (38)	12 (44)	2 (8)	
Enteral Nutrition								
ShuKla et al.[32]	GI, breast, oropharyngeal	10 d NG feeding preop	67	43	7 (10)	16 (37)	4 (6)	5 (12)
Smith et al.[33]	GI	10 d NCJ feeding postop	25	25	11 (44)	9 (36)	4 (17)	1 (4)
Foschi et al.[34]	Upper GI	12 d ND feeding postop	28	32	5 (18)	15 (47)	1 (4)	4 (13)
von Meyenfeldt et al.[35]	Gastric, colorectal	10 d preop	50	50	6 (12)	8 (16)	not reported	not reported

767

TABLE 39.4. Results of Prospective Randomized Controlled Trials in Patients Treated with Radiation Therapy

Author	Tumor Type	Number of Patients		Survival		Treatment Toxicity	
		NS	Control	NS	Control	Heme	GI
Parenteral Nutrition Trials							
Solassol et al.[5]	Ovarian	42	39	9 Month	8 Month (median)	Not reported	Better
Kinsella et al.[57]	Pelvic	17	15	47%	47%	Not reported	Not reported
Ghavimi et al.[58]	Childhood	14	14	27%	29%	Worse	Worse
Donaldson et al.[59]	Childhood	12	13	8%	8% (Posttherapy)	Not reported	Worse
Enteral Nutrition Trials							
Douglass et al.[36]	GI	13	17	62%	76%	No difference	Not reported
Brown et al.[37]	Pelvic	30	17	Not reported	Not reported	Better	No difference
Bounous et al.[38]	Abdomen/pelvic	9	9	Not reported	Not reported	Better	Better
Daly et al.[39]	Head and neck	22	18	Not reported	Not reported	Not reported	Worse
Moloney et al.[40]	Various	42	42	36%	38%	Not reported	Not reported

TABLE 39.5. Results of Prospective Randomized Controlled Trials Evaluating Nutritional Therapy in Patients Receiving Chemotherapy

Parenteral Nutrition

Author	Tumor Type	Number of Patients		Survival		Tumor Response (%)		Treatment Toxicity		Infection Rate (%)	
		TPN	Control	TPN	Control	TPN	Control	Heme	GI	TPN	Control
Nixon et al.[50,61]	Colorectal	20	25	79	308 (Mean)	15	12	Worse	No difference	5	4
Samuels et al.[62]	Testicular	16	14	72%	77% (2.5 y)	63	79	Better	No difference	17	4
Shamberger et al.[63,64]	Sarcoma	14	18	13%	44% (4 y)	14	50	No difference	No difference	42	33
Valdivieso et al.[65,66]	Small-cell lung	30	35	11 mo	12 mo (median)	43	66	No difference	Worse	27	18
Clamon et al.[67]	Small-cell lung	57	62	51%	57% (1 y)	48	43	Better	Not reported	35	5
Issell et al.[68]	Squamous cell lung	13	13	Not reported	Not reported	31	8	Better	Better	Not reported	Not reported
Jordan et al.[69]	Adenocarcinoma lung	19	24	22 wk (median)	40 wk	12	30	Worse	No difference	32	8

Enteral Nutrition

Author	Tumor Type	Number of Patients		Survival		Tumor Response (%)		Treatment Toxicity	
		EN	Control	EN	Control	EN	Control	Heme	GI
Elkort et al.[41]	Breast	24	23	84%	87% (1 y)	No difference		No difference	No difference
Evans et al.[42]	Non-small cell	30	36	8 mo	6 mo (median)	28	15	Not reported	Not reported
Evans et al.[42]	Lung	30		7 mo		20		Not	No
	Colorectal	21	33	9 mo	24 mo (median)	10	16	Not reported	Not reported
Tandon et al.[43]	GI	31	39	94%	85%	35	21	Not reported	Better
Bounous et al.[44]	Metastatic	9	12	Not reported	Not reported	56	64	No difference	No difference

TABLE 39.6. Indications for the Use of TPN in the Cancer Patient

A. TPN for brief, in-hospital periods (7–10 days)

    1. TPN is not indicated:
        (a) In well-nourished or mildly malnourished patients undergoing chemotherapy, radiation therapy, or surgery.
        (b) In patients with rapidly progressive malignant disease who fail to respond to treatment and in those patients who have evidence of terminal disease and are not candidates for further antitumor therapy.

    2. TPN is indicated:
        (a) In severely malnourished patients who are responding to chemotherapy or in those in whom gastrointestinal or other toxicities preclude adequate enteral intake for 7–10 days or a longer period. Available evidence would suggest that patients who are candidates for TPN under these circumstances should, when feasible, receive TPN prior to or in conjunction with the institution of therapy.

B. Prolonged periods of in-hospital TPN or home TPN

    1. TPN is not indicated:
        (a) In patients with rapidly progressive tumor growth that is unresponsive to therapy.

    2. TPN is indicated:
        (a) In those patients for whom treatment associated toxicities preclude the use of enteral nutrition and represent the primary impediment to the restoration of performance status. Such patients will usually respond to antitumor therapy.
        (b) In selected malnourished cancer patients where the natural history of the disease can be expected to permit a period of normal or near normal performance status. Such patients should be receiving antitumor therapy with a reasonable anticipation of response, or the natural history of the untreated tumor is such that a reasonable quality of life can be expected (survival greater than 6–12 months).

chemotherapy has been contraindicated secondary to severe malnutrition, TPN may improve nutritional status sufficiently to allow the initiation of chemotherapy.

Patients undergoing radiation treatment may also develop malnutrition secondary to inadequate caloric intake or from an inability to eat. The potential side effects from radiotherapy are numerous and include nausea, vomiting, malnutrition, mucositis, xerostomia, dysphagia, diarrhea, and anorexia. As stated previously, the enteral route is preferable for nutrition support whenever possible; however, in cases involving severe dysfunction of the gastrointestinal tract, TPN is indicated. TPN may allow the malnourished, high-risk patient to complete radiotherapy with less associated morbidity.

Perioperative TPN in Cancer Patients The use of preoperative TPN in cancer patients remains controversial and appears to depend highly on patient selection.

One large prospective randomized clinical study strongly suggested that preoperative TPN should be limited to only the severely malnourished patient and only if the gastrointestinal tract could not be used for tube feedings.[53] This study showed no difference in short-term or long-term survival and a higher rate of infectious complications including pneumonia, abscesses, and line sepsis in patients receiving TPN. Noninfectious complications (e.g., impaired wound healing) were significantly lower in those patients receiving TPN who were also severely malnourished (i.e., >15% weight loss and serum albumin < 2.8 mg%). In contrast, studies using perioperative TPN (starting 7 days prior to the planned procedure) for patients undergoing hepatectomy for hepatocellular carcinoma found that patients randomized to receive TPN had a statistically significant reduction in infectious complications and a decreased diuretic requirement compared to similar patients who did not receive TPN.[70]

Postoperatively, TPN is often required in the well-nourished cancer patient who develops a complication that precludes enteral support (e.g., prolonged ileus). In general, if the patient is unable to tolerate enteral feeding by the 7th postoperative day, TPN should be considered. Recent prospective studies have clarified both the indications for and contraindications to the use of TPN in the surgical patient with cancer.[71] The authors concluded that the routine use of postoperative TPN was not indicated and may in fact have harmful side effects following pancreatic resection. It should be noted that many surgeons would elect to place a feeding jejunostomy in such patients.

Composition of TPN Formulations

TPN solutions are hyperosmolar and calorie-dense (1 kcal/ml), and the infusion of 2.0 to 2.5 liters/day provides 2000 to 2500 kilocalories per day. The addition of minerals, vitamins, and electrolytes completes the basic composition of the solution. As a general rule, 20% of total calories should be provided in the form of an intravenous fat emulsion. The composition of a standard central venous solution is shown (Table 39.7). Solutions must be prepared under sterile condition and because of the hyperosmolarity of such solutions, they must be delivered into a high flow system to prevent venous sclerosis. Patients receiving TPN should be monitored regularly by measuring blood sugar, serum electrolytes, and liver function tests. The amounts of various electrolytes that are provided to cancer patients receiving TPN will vary depending on factors such as previous nutritional and hydration status.

Potential Complications of TPN

Advances in technology, monitoring, and catheter care have greatly reduced the incidence of complications associated with the use of TPN. The establishment of a nutritional support team (physician, dietitian, nurse, pharmacist) and the recognition of such a team as an important part of overall patient care have also been a key factor in reducing complications. Complications of TPN that occur in cancer patients can be divided into three types: (1) mechanical (e.g., pneumothorax, venous throm-

TABLE 39.7. Composition of a Standard Central Venous Solution[a]

Volume		
	10% Amino acid solution	500 ml
	50% Dextrose solution	500 ml
	Fat emulsion	—
	Electrolytes + vitamins + minerals	~ 50 ml
	Total volume	~ 1050 ml
Composition		
	Amino acids	50 g
	Dextrose	250 g
	Total N	50/6.25 = 8 g
	Dextrose kcal	250 × 3.4 kcal/g = 840 kcal
	mOsms/liter	~ 2000

[a] Intravenous fat emulsion can be administered simultaneously (via IV piggyback). A 500-ml bottle of 10% fat emulsion is given two or three times weekly. The fat solution should be infused over 6–8 hours to avoid hypertriglyceridemia.

bosis, air embolism); (2) metabolic (e.g., hyperglycemia, electrolyte abnormalities, abnormalities in liver enzymes); and (3) infectious (e.g., catheter sepsis).

Nutrition and Tumor Growth

With the introduction of specialized enteral and parenteral feeding regimens into clinical medicine, aggressive nutritional support can now be provided to cancer patients who previously could not or would not eat. However, concerns over the stimulation of tumor growth persist. Although there are some animal studies that indicate that tumor growth may be enhanced with a high-protein diet and diminished by low-protein diets, studies in cancer patients are unclear. Until more data are available, nutrition support should continue to be used for those patients in whom its use is clearly warranted.

Improving the Efficacy of Current Feeding Regimens

Hormonal Therapy   The potential beneficial effects of the administration of insulin, the primary anabolic hormone in the body, to the tumor-bearing host has been examined because of its role in stimulating amino acid uptake and protein synthesis in muscle. Studies indicate that treatment with insulin stimulates food intake and nitrogen retention without stimulating tumor growth. Likewise, administration of insulin in combination with the glutamine antimetabolite acivicin to tumor-bearing rats receiving TPN, preserved lean body mass, and retarded tumor growth. Whether these observations can be extrapolated to the clinical arena is unknown.

The recent availability of recombinant human growth hormone (GH) has led investigators to examine the role of this anabolic agent in cancer patients. Although studies show that GH is capable of promoting accrual of lean body mass in healthy individuals and in tumor-bearing rats, it is unknown whether this effect can be duplicated in cachectic cancer patients.

Glutamine   Glutamine has been classified as a nonessential or nutritionally dispensable amino acid because when absent from the diet, glutamine can be synthesized in adequate quantities from other amino acids and precursors. For this reason, and because of glutamine's relative instability compared to other amino acids, it has been eliminated from most TPN solutions and with few exceptions, and from oral and enteral diets except for the relatively low levels characteristic of its concentration in most dietary proteins.

Based on our knowledge of the changes in glutamine metabolism that are characteristic of the host with cancer, the categorization of glutamine as a nonessential amino acid may be misleading. Several studies in the tumor-bearing host suggest that supplemental glutamine may benefit the cancer patient. One study evaluated the effects of glutamine-enriched TPN in adults receiving allogeneic bone marrow transplants (BMTs) for hematologic malignancies for approximately 4 weeks after transplantation.[72] Patients receiving glutamine-supplemented TPN had improved nitrogen balance, a diminished incidence of clinical infections, less fluid accumulation, and a shortened hospital stay. In a more recent study, glutamine-enriched TPN prevented the increase in gut mucosal permeability that develops with the administration of commercially available glutamine-free TPN.[73] The investigators found no change in either villous height or gut permeability in the group receiving glutamine-enriched TPN whereas the control group showed both loss of villous height and increased gut permeability. This study provides evidence for a protective effect of glutamine on the gut. Similarly, arginine, because of its immunomodulatory properties, may be useful as a dietary supplement in cancer patients. However, further work is necessary to more clearly define the potential roles of these two amino acids in the nutritional care of the cancer patient.

Nutrition Support for Cancer Patients and Health Care Reform

The impact of corporate medicine on nutrition support has recently been addressed.[74] With the introduction of health care reform, nutrition support teams (NSTs) and the services they provide are now considered a cost center rather than a source of revenue. In the past, the cost required to pay the members of the nutrition support team have been more than offset by the reimbursements for the services provided, particularly for the delivery of TPN. However, this is no longer the case. The challenge to nutrition support professionals is to coordinate efficient and early intervention and to document its efficacy and outcome. Some techniques to ensure that nutrition support is cost effective have been suggested in the literature.[74] In this era of capitated health care, it is imperative that the team justify its importance to the hospital and convince the administration that withholding nutrition support from certain patients, particularly patients with cancer, may result in serious consequences.

FURTHER READING

1. Souba WW, Wilmore DW (1994) Diet and nutrition in the care of the patient with surgery, trauma, and sepsis. In: Shils M, Young V (eds) *Modern Nutrition in Health and Disease*, 8th edition. Lea & Febiger, Philadelphia, pp 1202–1240.

2. Souba WW (1993) Total parenteral nutrition. In: Copeland EM III, Levine BA, Howard RJ, et al. (eds) *Current Practice of Surgery*. Churchill Livingstone, New York.

3. Souba WW (1994) Cytokines: Key regulators of the nutritional/metabolic response to critical illness. *Curr Prob Surg* 31:577–652.

4. Hautamaki RD, Souba WW (1995) Principles and techniques of nutritional support in the cancer patient. In: Karakousis CP, Copeland EM, Bland KI (eds) *Atlas of Surgical Oncology* pp. 741–748.

5. Souba WW (1997) Nutrional Support. In: Rosenberg S., Helman S, Devita V. (eds) *Cancer Principles and Practice of Oncology*, 5th edition. Lippincott-Raven, Philadelphia, pp. 2841–2857.

6. DeWys WD, Begg D, Lavin PT, et al. (1980) Prognostic effect of weight loss prior to chemotherapy in cancer patients. *Am J Med* 69:491–497.

7. Knox LS, Crosby LO, Feurer ID, et al. (1983) Energy expenditure in malnourished cancer patients. *Ann Surg* 197:152–162.

8. Fearon KCH, Hansell DT, Preston T, et al. (1988) Influence of whole body protein turnover rate on resting energy expenditure on patients with cancer. *Cancer Res* 48:2590–2595.

9. Shaw JHF, Wolfe RR (1986) Glucose and urea kinetics in patients with early and advanced gastrointestinal cancer: The response to glucose infusion, parenteral feeding, and surgical resection. *Surgery* 101:181–191.

10. Lundholm K, Edstrom S, Karlberg I, et al. (1982) Glucose turnover, gluconeogenesis from glycerol, and estimation of net glucose cycling in cancer patients. *Cancer* 50:1142–1150.

11. Jeevanandam M, Lowry SF, Horowitz GD, et al. (1984) Cancer cachexia and protein metabolism. *Lancet* 1:1423–1426.

12. Heber D, Chlebowski RT, Ishibashi DE, et al. (1982) Abnormalities in glucose and protein metabolism in noncachectic lung cancer patients. *Cancer Res* 42:4815–4819.

13. Norton JA, Burt ME, Brennan MF (1980) In vivo utilization of substrate by human sarcoma bearing limbs. *Cancer* 45:29–34.

14. Souba WW (1993) Glutamine and cancer. *Ann Surg* 218:715–728.

15. Balkwill F, Osborne R, Burke F, et al. (1987) Evidence for tumor necrosis factor/cachectin production in cancer. *Lancet* 2:1229.

16. Michie HR, Sherman ML, Spriggs DR, et al. (1989) Chronic TNF infusion causes anorexia but not accelerated nitrogen loss. *Ann Surg*; 209:19–24.

17. Darling G, Fraker DL, Jensen C, et al. (1990) Cachectic effects of recombinant human tumor necrosis factor in rats. *Cancer Res* 50:4008–4013.

18. Sherry BA, Gelin J, Fong Y, et al. (1989) Anticachectin/tumor necrosis factor-α antibodies attenuate development of cachexia in tumor models. *FASEB J* 3:1956–1962.

19. Oliff A, Defeo-Jones D, Boyer M, et al. (1987) Tumors secreting human TNF/cachectin induce cachexia in mice. *Cell* 50:555–563.

20. Starnes HF, Warren RS, Jeevanandem M, et al. (1988) Tumor necrosis factor and the acute metabolic response to injury in man. *J Clin Invest* 82:1321–1325.

21. Darling G, Goldstein DS, Stull R, et al. (1989) Tumor necrosis factor: immune endocrine interaction. *Surgery* 106:1155–1160.

22. Arbos J, Lpoz-Soriano FJ, Carbo N, et al. (1992) Effects of tumor necrosis factor-α (cachectin) on glucose metabolism in the rat. *Mol Cell Biochem* 112:53–59.

23. Fischer E, Marano M, Barber AE, et al. (1991) Comparison between effects of interleukin-1α administration and sublethal endotoxemia in primates. *Am J Physiol* 261:R442–R452.

24. Meszaros K, Lang CH, Bagby GJ. (1987) Tumor necrosis factor increases in vivo glucose utilization of macrophage-rich tissues. *Biochem Biophys Res Commun* 149:1–6.

25. Warren RS, Starnes HF, Gabrilove JL, et al. (1987) The acute metabolic effects of tumor necrosis factor administration in humans. *Arch Surg* 122:1396–1400.

26. Flores EA, Bistrian BR, Pomposelli JJ, et al. (1989) Infusion of tumor necrosis factor/cachectin promotes muscle catabolism in the rat. *J Clin Invest* 83:1614.

27. Fong Y, Moldawer LL, Marano M, et al. (1989) Cachectin/TNF or IL-14α induces cachexia with redistribution of body proteins. *Am J Physiol* 256:R659–R665.

28. Moldawer LL, Svanninger G, Gelin J, et al. (1987) Interleukin-1 and tumor necrosis factor do not regulate protein balance is skeletal muscle. *Am J Physiol* 253:C766–C773.

29. Hall-Angeras M, Angeras U, Zamir O, et al. (1990) Interaction between corticosterone and tumor necrosis factor stimulated protein breakdown in rat skeletal muscle, similar to sepsis. *Surgery* 108:460–466.

30. Greenberg AS, Nordan RP, McIntosh J, et al. (1992) Interleukin 6 reduces lipoprotein lipase activity in adipose tissue of mice in vivo and in 3T3-L1 adipocytes: A possible role for interleukin 6 in cancer cachexia. *Cancer Res* 52:4113–4116.

31. Memon RA, Feingold KR, Moser AH, et al. (1992) Differential effects of interleukin-1 and tumor necrosis factor on ketogenesis. *Am J Physiol* 263:E301–E309.

32. Shukla HS, Rao RR, Banu N, et al. (1984) Enteral hyperalimentation in malnourished surgical patients. *Indian J Med Res* 80:339–346.

33. Smith RC, Hartemink RJ, Holinshead JW, et al. (1985) Fine bore jejunostomy feeding following major abdominal surgery: A controlled randomized clinical trial. *Br J Surg* 72:458–461.

34. Foschi, D. Cavagna G., Callioni, F, et al. (1986) Hyperalimentation of jaundiced patients on percutaneous transhepatic biliary drainage. *Br J Surg* 73:716.

35. von Meyenfeldt MF, Meyerink WJ, Soeters PB, et al. (1991) Perioperative nutritional support results in a reduction of major postoperative complications especially in high risk patients [Abstract]. *Gastroenterology* 100:A553.

36. Douglass HO, Milliron S, Nava H, et al. (1978) Elemental diet as an adjuvant for patients with locally advanced gastrointestinal cancer receiving radiation therapy: A prospectively randomized study. *JPEN* 2:682–686.

37. Brown MS, Buchanan RB, Karran SJ (1980) Clinical observations on the effects of elemental diet supplementation during irradiation. *Clin Radiol* 31:19–20.

38. Bounous G, LeBel E, Shuster J, et al. (1975) Dietary protection during radiation therapy. *Strahlentherapie* 149:476–483.

39. Daly JM, Hearne B, Dunaj J, et al. (1984) Nutritional rehabilitation in patients with advanced head and neck cancer receiving radiation therapy. *Am J Surg* 148:514–520.

40. Moloney M, Moriarty M, Daly L (1983) Controlled studies of nutritional intake in patients with malignant disease undergoing treatment. *Hum Nutr Appl Nutr* 37A:30–35.

41. Elkort RJ, Baker FL, Vitale JJ, et al. (1981) Long-term nutritional support as an adjunct to chemotherapy for breast cancer. *JPEN* 5:385–390.

42. Evans WK, Nixon DW, Dlay JM, et al. (1987) A randomized study of oral nutritional support versus ad lib nutritional intake during chemotherapy for advanced colorectal and non-small cell lung cancer. *J Clin Oncol* 5:113–124.

43. Tandon SP, Gupta SC, Sinha SN, et al.(1984) Nutritional support as an adjunct therapy of advanced cancer patients. *Indian J Med Res* 80:180–188.

44. Bounous G, Gentile JM, Hugon J. (1971) Elemental diet in the management of the intestinal lesion produced by 5-fluorouracil in man. *Can J Surg* 14:312–324.

45. Holter AR, Fischer JE (1977) The effects of perioperative hyper-alimentation complications in patients with carcinoma and weight loss. *J Surg Res* 23:31–34.

46. Heatley RV, Williams RH, Lewis MH (1979) Pre-operative intravenous feeding: A controlled trial. *Postgrad Med J* 55:541–545.

47. Yamada N, Koyama H, Hioki K, et al. (1983) Effect of postoperative total parenteral nutrition (TPN) as an adjunct to gastrectomy for advanced gastric carcinoma. *Br J Surg* 70:267–274.

48. Askanazi J, Hensle TW, Starker PM, et al. (1986) Effect of immediate postoperative nutritional support on length of hospitalization. *Ann Surg* 203:236–239.

49. Müller JM, Keller HW, Brenner U, et al. (1986) Indications and effects of preoperative parenteral nutrition. *World J Surg* 10:53–63.

50. Bellantone R, Doglietto GB, Bossola M, et al. (1988) Preoperative parenteral nutrition in the high risk surgical patient. *JPEN* 12:195–197.

51. Bellantone R, Doglietto, G, Bossola M, et al. (1988) Preoperative parenteral nutrition of malnourished surgical patients. *Acta Chir Scand* 154:249–251.

52. Woolfson AM, Smith JA (1989) Elective nutritional support after major surgery: A prospective randomized trial. *Clin Nutr* 8:15–21.

53. The Veterans Affairs Total Parenteral Nutrition Cooperative Study Group (1991) Perioperative total parenteral nutrition in surgical patients. *N Engl J Med* 325:525–532.

54. Sandstrom R, Drott C, Hyltander A, et al. (1993) The effect of post-operative intravenous feeding (TPN) on outcome following major surgery evaluated in a randomized study. *Ann Surg* 217:185–195.

55. Sclafani LM, Shike M, Quesada E, et al. (1991) A randomized prospective trial of TPN following major pancreatic resection or radioactive implant for pancreatic cancer. Presented at the Society of Surgical Oncology, March, Orlando, FL.

56. Solassol C, Joyeux J, Dubois JB (1979) Total parenteral nutrition (TPN) with complete nutritive mixtures: An artificial gut in cancer patients. *Nutr Cancer* 1:13–18.

57. Kinsella TJ, Malcolm AW, Bothe A, et al. (1981) Prospective study of nutritional support during pelvic irradiation. *Int J Radiat Oncol Biol Phys* 7:543–548.

58. Ghavimi F, Shils ME, Scott BF, et al. (1982) Comparison of morbidity in children requiring abdominal radiation and chemotherapy, with and without total parenteral nutrition. *J Pediatr* 101:530–537.

59. Donaldson SS, Wesley MN, Ghavimi F, et al. (1982) A prospective randomized clinical trial of total parenteral nutrition in children with cancer. *Med Pediatr Oncol* 10:129–139.

60. Nixon DW, Moffitt S, Lawson DH, et al. (1981) Total parenteral nutrition as an adjunct to chemotherapy of metastatic colorectal cancer. *Cancer Treat Rep* 65(Suppl 5):121–128.

61. Nixon DW, Heymsfield SB, Lawson DH, et al. (1981) Effect of total parenteral nutrition on survival in advanced colon cancer. *Cancer Detect Prev* 4:421–427.

62. Samuels ML, Selig DE, Ogden S, et al. (1981) IV hyperalimentation and chemotherapy for stage II testicular cancer: a randomized study. *Cancer Treat Rep* 65:615–627.

63. Shamberger RC, Brennan MF, Goodgame JT, et al. (1984) A prospective, randomized study of adjuvant parenteral nutrition in the treatment of sarcoma: results of metabolic and survival studies. *Surgery* 96:1–12.

64. Shamberger RC, Pizzo PA, Goodgame JT, et al. (1983) The effect of total parenteral nutrition on chemotherapy-induced myelosuppression. *Am J Med* 74:40–48.

65. Valdivieso M, Frankmann C, Murphy WK, et al. (1987) Long-term effects of intravenous hyperalimentation administered during intensive chemotherapy for small cell bronchogenic carcinoma. *Cancer* 59:362–369.

66. Valdivieso M, Bodey GP, Benjamin RS, et al. (1981) Role of intravenous hyperalimentation as an adjunct to intensive chemotherapy for small cell bronchogenic carcinoma. *Cancer Treat Rep* 65(Suppl 5):145–150.

67. Clamon GH, Feld R, Evans WK, et al. (1985) Effect of adjuvant central IV hyperalimentation on the survival and response to treatment of patients with small lung cancer: A randomized trial. *Cancer Treat Rep* 69:167–177.

68. Issell BF, Valdivieso MD, Zaren HA, et al. (1978) Protection against chemotherapy toxicity by IV hyperalimentation. *Cancer Treat Rep* 62:1139–1143.

69. Jordan WM, Valdivieso M, Frankman C, et al. (1981) Treatment of advanced adenocarcinoma of the lung with ftorafur, doxorubicin, cyclophosphamide, and cisplatin (FACP) and intensive IV hyperalimentation. *Cancer Treat Rep* 65:197–205.

70. Fan ST, Lo CM, Lai ECS, et al. (1994) Perioperative nutritional support in patients undergoing hepatectomy for hepatocellular carcinoma. *N Engl J Med* 331:1547–1552.

71. Brennan MF, Pisters PWT, Posner M, et al. (1994) A prospective randomized trial of total parenteral nutrition after major pancreatic resection for malignancy. *Ann Surg* 220:436–444.

72. van der Hulst RRWJ, van Kreel BK, von Meyenfeldt MF, et al. (1993) Glutamine and the preservation of gut integrity. *Lancet* 341:1363–1365.

73. Ziegler TR, Young LS, Benfell K, et al. (1992) Glutamine-supplemented parenteral nutrition improves nitrogen retention and reduces hospital mortality versus standard parenteral nutrition following bone marrow transplantation: a randomized, double-blind trial. *Ann Intern Med* 116:821–828.

74. Nelson, J (1995) The impact of health care reform on nutrition support—the practitioner's perspective. *Nutr Clin Prac* 4:1–7.

CHAPTER 40

REHABILITATION OF THE CANCER PATIENT

AILEEN M. DAVIS

Mount Sinai Hospital
Toronto, Ontario, Canada

MARLENE CARNO JACOBSON

Sunnybrook Health Science Centre
North York, Ontario, Canada

INTRODUCTION

Recent advances in the detection and treatment of cancer have resulted in prolonged survival even in the face of advanced disease. Consequently, cancer is now viewed as a chronic disease with a significant impact on patients, families, and communities. This impact is experienced within all realms of function including physical, social, and psychological domains. Rehabilitation interventions may reduce the effects of this chronic disease.

The purpose of cancer rehabilitation is to enhance quality of life by assisting individuals in achieving their maximum function within the limits imposed by their cancer and its treatment. The International Classification of Impairments, Disabilities, and Handicaps of the World Health Organization provides a model for identifying problems within the spheres of social, psychological, and physical function. Impairments are any loss or abnormality of psychological, physiologic, or anatomic structure or function and occur at the organ level. Hearing loss and reduced coordination are examples of impairments. Disability is any restriction or lack of ability (resulting from an impairment) to perform an activity within the normal range. Problems at the level of the person such as restrictions in activities of daily living or disordered communication represent disabilities. Handicap is a disadvantage resulting from an

Manual of Clinical Oncology, 7th edition, Edited by Raphael E. Pollock
ISBN 0-471-23828-7, pages 779–790. Copyright © 1999 Wiley-Liss, Inc.

impairment or disability that prevents the fulfillment of that individual's normal role in society (based on age, gender, social, and cultural factors). An individual with abnormal cosmesis following cancer surgery may experience social isolation resulting in a social handicap.

Impairments represent the simplest level of problem identified in the rehabilitation assessment. Disabilities are more complex and represent multifaceted tasks requiring coordination of multiple body systems. Disabilities include simple or complex functions. Activities of daily living such as bathing and shopping are complex activities. Execution of such tasks requires mastery of multiple simple functions (e.g., bending, transfers, walking). At the highest level of complexity are handicaps that represent functioning of the individual within a social context.

The specific goals of cancer rehabilitation depend upon the disease site(s), subsite(s), and stage, the prognosis, the treatment modality or combination and sequence of modalities (e.g., type of tumor resection and reconstruction, chemotherapy, radiotherapy, biological response modifiers), the age and medical condition of the patient, as well as the individual's wishes and desires.

The role of the treatment team is to prepare patients for functional and cosmetic changes and to assist in setting and achieving realistic rehabilitation goals. Within an interdisciplinary cancer care program, team members may include: the medical and radiation oncologists, surgeon, dentist, prosthodontist, nurse, physical therapist, occupational therapist, speech pathologist, prosthetist, chaplain, anaplastologist, clinical dietitian, social worker, psychiatrist and/or psychologist, and palliative care physician. Each team member has a unique role and, at any given time throughout the course of diagnosis, treatment, and follow-up, the degree of interaction between the patient and a specific team member may vary. Communication among team members is essential for each to understand the disease process, prognosis, and the proposed continuum of care and to assist patients in achieving their maximum functional potential.

IMPACT OF DISEASE SITE, STAGE, AND PROGNOSIS

Within the realms of psychological, physical, and social function, cancer patients may experience a vast range of potential impairments, disabilities, and handicaps. With disease progression, medications to relieve symptoms, and metastatic involvement, the number, nature, and severity of physical impairments may increase to incorporate symptoms not typically seen with less advanced disease within the same site. With certain oncologic sites, such as lymphoma, the physical deficits are highly variable, depending on the precise anatomical location of disease, whereas for other sites, such as lung, more predictable deficits are seen.

For example, head and neck cancer patients frequently experience difficulties in communication and swallowing. Following lobectomy or pneumonectomy for lung cancer, patients may experience exercise intolerance due to decreased lung capacity, particularly if they have a long history of smoking. Patients with bone or soft tissue tumors of the lower extremity may experience difficulty with mobility.

The psychological response to the diagnosis of cancer has been shown to be similar among types and sites of disease even though individual reactions may vary.

CANCER TREATMENT: IMPLICATIONS FOR REHABILITATION

For the newly diagnosed cancer patient, the proposed treatment plan may be curative or palliative. The primary goal of curative treatment is the eradication of disease even if a key structure is sacrificed (e.g., excision of the larynx during laryngectomy). Wherever possible, however, treatment strives for organ preservation and maximal function using either a single treatment modality or a combination of surgery, chemotherapy, radiation therapy, and biologic response modifiers. Palliative management strives for symptom control and optimum quality of life.

Different treatment modalities, that is, radiation therapy, chemotherapy, and surgery, require different precautions and contraindications. Both pre- and postoperative irradiation delay soft tissue healing and frequently result in abnormal sensation in the acute posttreatment period. Thus, the risk of burns from thermal or cold modalities is significantly increased. Irradiation also causes dry skin but moisturizers should not be used without the approval of the radiation oncologist, as these potentially affect radiation dose absorption. Deodorants containing aluminum may also be contraindicated if the irradiation field encompasses the axilla (e.g., in the treatment of breast cancer) because aluminum is a radiation enhancer.

Radiation therapy can produce devascularization of bone, osteoporosis, or osteoradionecrosis. When bony metastases of the lower extremity are irradiated, patients should be on a protected weight-bearing regimen to prevent fracture until X-ray films demonstrate that the bone is strong enough to permit full weight-bearing. If radiation therapy was used to treat a primary bone lesion, patients should be counseled against participating in contact sports that put them at risk of fracture. Downhill skiing and football are not recommended. Instead, patients should be encouraged to swim, cycle, or hike. Whereas irradiation of a limb may have minimal side effects, irradiation of the retroperitoneum may result in nausea and diarrhea, while head and neck irradiation may cause chronic xerostomia.

Chemotherapeutic agents delay bone healing such that bone ingrowth into a metal prosthesis used for limb reconstruction does not occur until approximately 6 weeks after completion of chemotherapy. Allograft bone does not have the same healing properties as normal bone (i.e., over approximately 3 months, a stable *fibrous* union develops; over the next 3 to 6 months a stable *bony* union generally occurs). When allograft bone has been used to reconstruct the lower limb, the physical therapist must be guided by the surgeon's interpretation of serial X-ray films in progressing the patient's weight-bearing. Hydrotherapy provides an ideal excrcise environment when protected weight-bearing is required, but is usually contraindicated in patients receiving chemotherapy. The immunosuppression imparted by chemotherapeutic drugs increases the risk of infection and the medical oncologist will usually advise against chemotherapy patients having hydrotherapy and using public whirlpools or swimming facilities.

In surgical cases, the rehabilitation clinician must appreciate the contribution of resected tissues and the properties of the reconstruction. During musculoskeletal surgery, muscles and tendons are separated and reattached to new sites while bones and joints may have been reconstructed with an endoprosthesis or allograft. The clinician's knowledge of the surgical procedure allows the development of treatment programs that provide protected weight-bearing and avoid stretching reconstructed soft tissues prematurely.

As the complexity of the treatment plan increases with multiple treatment modalities, more aggressive radiotherapy regimens, and more extensive reconstructive surgery (e.g., free tissue transfers), the potential problems experienced by the patient will vary. The risk of fibrosis in the subcutaneous tissues increases as radiation doses exceed 50 Gy such that swollen, shortened soft tissues and joint contractures may result. When wound complications arise or a soft tissue transfer is required for wound closure, it may be necessary to delay the start of exercise to stretch soft tissues and regain joint mobility. Knowledge of the treatment regimen and team communication is essential for the clinician to develop and progress the rehabilitation intervention.

For example, assessment of the head and neck cancer patient needs to be preceded by a thorough review of original disease extent and the treatment procedures. Operative notes identify excised, altered, or replaced anatomy, thus clarifying important physical changes. These may involve bone, soft tissue, complete organs, such as larynx or tongue, as well as muscles and nerves. The choice of reconstructive technique may significantly influence functional performance. Current technical advancements in surgical reconstruction are improving functional outcomes. The degree of radiotherapy-related impairment and disability in speech, voice, and swallowing may vary based on the parameters of total dose, fractionation, technique, treatment fields, and regimen (e.g., accelerated fractionation versus standard schedules). Functional changes contributing to postradiotherapy disability generally correspond with underlying structural features including edema, atrophy, altered salivation, fibrosis, and nerve damage. Successive or combined treatment modalities compound impairment and disability.

ASSESSMENT AND GOAL-SETTING

While a myriad of rehabilitation problems exist associated with cancer and its treatment, Lehman's (1978) study of 805 patients with cancers of varying sites identified that psychological and physical problems were most common. Usually, team members have *general* expectations about the nature of these psychological and physical problems and the likely rehabilitation outcomes based on knowledge of the disease site and the treatment plan. However, each patient needs to be counseled and assessed individually to identify specific problems and treatment goals. Assessment should cater to the patient's premorbid level of functioning, comorbidities, social supports, and wishes, as well as the disease process and proposed treatment plan.

The initial assessment consists of a patient interview and objective evaluation to establish a problem list. Interview specifics and objective assessment will depend on the clinician's discipline. For some disease sites, pretreatment assessment is necessary to obtain a functional baseline. Social work may be involved in the earliest stages of treatment planning to help the patient obtain financial assistance and to access support resources.

In assessing psychological functioning, knowledge of each individual's goals, values, needs, and lifestyle are critical. A person who is physically active may experience significant fatigue from treatment, preventing participation in usual activities. This may affect the individual's self-esteem, as he or she may no longer be able to perform activities requiring strength and endurance.

Altered body image has psychological and social significance. The diagnosis of cancer often results in feelings of loss of control of one's life *and* one's body. Furthermore, many cancer surgeries and adjuvant therapies result in body alterations (e.g., ostomy) which impact negatively upon self-concept and self-esteem, and cause concerns about social acceptance. Although an ostomy may not be visible, patients are concerned about odor and leakage should appliances malfunction. Thus, determining how patients feel about their cancer diagnosis *and* their physical selves is important.

Sexuality is integral for the rehabilitation of any person with a chronic disease. How sexuality is affected will depend on factors such as age, existing relationships, and type of treatment. Altered body image, mobility limitations, and the need for assistance with personal care will affect the patient's sexual confidence. Relevant team members need to convey to patients that sexuality is worth discussing. However, sexuality is personal and the privacy of patients who choose not to disclose such information must be respected.

The physical examination depends on the disease site. For example, examination of the oral cancer patient addresses key structures such as the tongue and palate. These are evaluated for their bulk, position, relative proportions, surface characteristics, symmetry, contour, range of motion, sensorimotor innervation, coordination, and control, and their contribution to complex processes such as oral–pharyngeal resonance and mastication. Instrumental evaluation procedures such as acoustic analysis may be essential in formulating a treatment plan that properly targets specific deficits.

Significant physical disability may result from treatment for bone or soft tissue sarcomas of the extremities. The patient needs to be assessed for impairments such as reduced motion at a joint or loss of muscle strength. However, for many patients, the whole extremity is involved such that the joints and muscles proximal and distal to the surgical site also require attention. In determining whether assessment findings are abnormal, the functional limitations imposed by the tumor excision and reconstruction must be considered. For example, removal of 50% of the quadriceps will prevent normal quadriceps strength being regained. When endoprostheses are used to reconstruct the knee joint many have flexion stops on the prosthesis such that greater than 100° of flexion is not possible.

For most patients, the motion of a joint or the strength of muscle groups is less important than their ability to perform activities of daily living such as personal hygiene, domestic chores, and work. Therefore, performance of such daily activities should be assessed. Frequently, fatigue and lack of endurance impair these functions.

Irrespective of the clinician's discipline, the assessment is undertaken using a problem-oriented approach. The interview records information from the individual's history including symptoms, home situation, work, leisure, and potential goals for rehabilitation. Objective tests are then performed (e.g., videofluoroscopic swallow study in a head and neck cancer patient, or gait analysis in a lower extremity cancer patient). Analysis of both subjective and objective information identifies problems to be addressed by the rehabilitation program. Together, the clinician and the patient establish treatment goals that correspond to the problem list. Goal-setting should be done for the short and long term. Treatment will vary depending on whether the patient is being treated with curative or palliative intent.

Irrespective of treatment intent, family members need to be included in the rehabilitation process because they play an important role in the level of adaptation achieved by the patient. Unless family members are involved in the rehabilitation process and the formulation of realistic treatment goals, they will not appreciate the implications for their own functioning within the family unit. For example, due to persistent posttreatment fatigue, an individual may be unable to assume his or her usual roles within the family unit and other members may need to assume more responsibilities.

The first assessment and treatment plan will form the basis of the rehabilitation program; however, ongoing assessment and reestablishment of short-term treatment goals need to occur throughout the rehabilitation process.

COMMON PROBLEMS AND THEIR MANAGEMENT

Evidence-based practice has become the standard for determining treatment interventions. However, within the field of rehabilitation, there is little supporting documentation of treatment efficacy based on randomized controlled trials (level one evidence). Friedenreich and Courneya (1996) published a structured literature review of 10 studies on the impact of exercise on the quality of life of cancer patients. Although the review was qualitative owing to heterogeneous study samples and variable study designs (e.g., randomized trials, quasi-experimental, cohort), the authors concluded that exercise improved the psychological and physiologic function of cancer patients. The remaining literature on rehabilitation in cancer patients comprises mainly functional outcomes reported in series of patients.

Rehabilitation interventions traditionally used with cancer patients are based on an understanding of the underlying physiology of tissue healing, muscle function, biomechanics (impairment level), and the component functions necessary to perform various activities and tasks (disability level). However, general patient factors such as age, general health, and cognitive status influence the range of rehabilitation options. Rehabilitation interventions include education, counseling, identification of compensatory strategies using intact mechanisms, exercise, physical modalities, and access to resources (e.g., technology, support groups, financial assistance, job retraining).

Patient Education

Patient and family education are perhaps the most important components of the rehabilitation program. Unless the patient has an understanding of his or her disease, his or her recovery potential, and the need for posttreatment adaptation, the rehabilitation process is unlikely to succeed.

Preoperative teaching is crucial to the patient's well-being and later adjustment. The clinician must establish what patients know about their disease and treatment, and then reinforce that understanding while correcting any misapprehensions. Educational aids such as videotapes, anatomic models, diagrams, and examples are useful. Frequently, meetings with carefully selected patients who have similar deficits provide peer support and complement the interventions of the multidisciplinary team.

Education is a component of all rehabilitation interventions; however, education may also be the *primary* intervention. For patients who experience significant fatigue, energy conservation techniques and pacing of activities need to be taught. Frequently, technical skills for self-care need to be taught to the patient and/or family members. Thus, the laryngectomee fitted with a tracheoesophageal voice prosthesis is taught to troubleshoot, insert, remove, and maintain the device. Similarly, acutely following surgery for bowel cancer, ostomy patients are taught to care for the stoma in preparation for discharge. This includes cleansing the stoma and fitting an appliance such that the patient is confident that there will not be leakage of stool. Use of an odorless appliance, appliance deodorant, and regular stoma irrigations results in a virtually odor-free appliance, which reassures the patient in social situations.

Expelling gas through the stoma may result in a gurgly sound that can be muffled by gentle pressure against the stoma. Gas cannot escape from the appliance and the patient will eventually need to open the appliance to allow the gas to escape. Certain foods such as cabbage and carbonated drinks may result in excessive gas. Such information provided in a timely manner prepares patients to cope better with their physical changes.

Patients with spinal cord tumors may also experience bowel and bladder dysfunction, where routine use of enemas and intermittent catheterzation may be required. Thus, the patient or a family member may be taught such procedures.

Physical Function

Physical impairments and disabilities are frequently experienced by cancer patients and certain disease sites are associated with specific deficits. For example, communication difficulties are common in patients with central nervous system (CNS) malignancies or head and neck cancer, and result in a variety of cognitive, linguistic, and speech disorders. These include loss of spoken and/or written comprehension and expressive language, unintelligible speech, altered voice quality, and changes in the relationships between articulatory, resonatory, respiratory, and phonatory mechanisms. The impact of a communication disorder may be profound with respect to a patient's occupational requirements and participation in social and familial activities. Thus, rehabilitation must address these broader contexts.

Interventions for impaired communication encompass many approaches and include teaching conversational strategies to significant others as well as patients, use of a supplementary modality (e.g., writing), or augmentative technology for communication. Speech intelligibility may be improved by intraoral or maxillofacial prostheses by altering the manner of articulation or speech rate. Range-of-motion exercises, biofeedback techniques, saliva substitutes, artificial larynges, surgical voice restoration, and minor surgical procedures for refining function (e.g., flap debulking) are further examples of the many options in developing a rehabilitation plan for such patients.

Swallowing disorders in patients with head and neck and CNS tumors vary widely in their structural features, physiology, and neurogenic origins. Thus, dysphagia may manifest as a diverse range of difficulties including problems with the oral preparatory, oral, pharyngeal, or esophageal stages of the swallow. Abnormal features include difficulties with oral containment of food or liquid, poor awareness of food location within the oral cavity, and a delayed, absent, or incoordinated reflexive pharyngeal swallow. Pharyngeal stage abnormalities include tracheopulmonary penetration and aspiration, impaired pharyngeal clearance, and poor transfer of material through the upper esophageal sphincter. Swallowing inefficiency across food consistencies is common and impacts nutritional status. A given treatment procedure (e.g., composite resection of the oropharynx) does not predict a particular type of swallowing disorder as subtle differences in anatomic site and surgical extent may result in markedly different impairments. Thus, each patient requires individualized assessment and systematic examination of findings.

Management of swallowing disorders usually requires multidisciplinary consultation involving the clinical dietitian, nurse, radiologist, and attending medical specialties. Rehabilitation may incorporate changing or supplementing the primary nutritional mode (e.g., primary use of a gastrostomy tube in conjunction with oral intake), diet modification for liquids or solid consistencies, and postural adjustments while eating. Further techniques include physiologic maneuvers for airway protection and pharyngeal clearance, adapted utensils for bolus delivery into the mouth, and strategies to enhance sensory input by cold or carbonation, thereby stimulating the swallow.

Swallow function may change dramatically during the posttreatment course and thus needs to be monitored until stable. Dysphagia may emerge months or years following treatment as the result of late, progressive effects of treatment, and will necessitate intervention only long after acute treatment.

Physical function is significantly impacted by general fatigue and lack of endurance. Patients who experience severe pain, weakness (perhaps due to weight loss), or immobilization *prior to treatment* will have increased difficulty mobilizing and regaining their physical function afterwards. An exercise program needs to be instituted during hospitalization to begin strengthening and improving cardiovascular function and mobility. Thus, a graduated exercise program including range-of-motion exercises and isotonic strengthening (within the bounds of the restrictions imposed by any reconstructive surgery) may begin while the patient is on bedrest and family members can be taught to assist. With prolonged bedrest, positioning to prevent muscle contractures, especially of the Achilles tendon, is imperative. Orthoses may be required to maintain positioning.

As the patient on prolonged bedrest begins to mobilize, postural hypotension may be experienced such that a tilt table is required to gradually aproximate the upright position. Progressively increasing periods for sitting, standing, and ambulating are gradually attained.

With excision of an extremity tumor involving either soft tissue or bone and re-section or undermining of muscle, selective strengthening of various muscle groups may be required. The potential for regaining strength will depend on the remaining volume of functioning tissue.

Postoperative pain and shortening of soft tissues may limit range-of-motion at specific joints. Once soft tissues are healed, gentle stretching will improve joint mo-bility. Range of motion exercises in conjunction with elevation and compression will also decrease edema. Edema is common in patients who have undergone axillary, neck, or inguinal lymph node dissection in combination with irradiation.

When a lower extremity tumor has been resected, assistive devices may be re-quired for ambulation. These may be temporary with the patient progressing from crutches to cane to no devices as bone heals. Sometimes, the volume of resected soft tissue results in instability and a cane is required in the long term. This may be the case in patients with a Trendelenberg lurch due to resection of the glutei, or in patients with an unstable knee due to total quadriceps resection. Most patients with quadriceps resection, however, are able to walk with a back-knee gait and do not require a cane.

Limb amputation has decreased with the advent of modern imaging techniques that allow surgeons to determine tumor extent more accurately. However, for those patients who do undergo amputation, special consideration needs to be given to ex-tended wound healing times which may delay the fitting of prostheses. Although early postoperative fitting of prostheses is encouraged, patients continuing on chemo-therapy or post-amputation radiotherapy will be slow to heal and may have signif-icant weight loss. Thus, a prosthesis may not fit in the months after completion of treatment and periodic adjustment may be required.

For patients with terminal disease, supportive care will be directed toward symp-tom control using heat and cold modalities and pain medications. For those with metastatic bone disease, walkers, crutches, or canes will limit weight-bearing through limbs and the spine. Exercise will maintain strength and cardiovascular status, decreasing fatigue.

Self-Care and Activities of Daily Living

The patient's ability to feed, bathe, dress, toilet, and move about within the home needs to be assessed and appropriate assistive devices and adaptations need to be prescribed. Devices may include a raised toilet seat, bath bench, or grab rails. Per-sonal assistance may be required to help with meal preparation. As the patient's level of function and independence improve, the need for home assistance may di-minish. Alternatively, for those receiving supportive care for terminal illness, the needs may increase significantly. Constant reassessment is necessary to reevaluate treatment plans and goals.

Return to Work

Malone et al. (1994) studied more than 200 cancer patients (multiple sites with breast, gastrointestinal, renal, and lung most common) with a mean age of 55 years. Their findings demonstrated that two thirds of patients were unemployed or had significantly reduced their hours or job demands as a result of their cancer. Forty-two percent of patients had retired early because of their disease.

Return to work following cancer treatment depends on many factors including the degree of residual disability, employer concerns about work performance or the inability to provide modified work, and co-worker and employer attitudes (or patient perceptions of their attitudes) toward the cancer patient. Employer attitudes may be influenced by institutional policy and state laws.

The role of the rehabilitation team is to assess the patient's capacity to return to his or her premorbid employment. If modified duties are required, the team should define the adaptations and limitations and assist patient and employer in accommodating the changes. When further education and job retraining are necessary, the team should assist in identifying vocational goals and in accessing retraining programs.

Psychological Support

Most patients experience fear and anxiety after their cancer diagnosis and should be assisted by the team in accessing the necessary resources for psychosocial support. Psychological problems also include a sense of disfigurement and altered body image following treatment as well as concerns about sexuality.

Either the cancer diagnosis or the treatment may result in sexual dysfunction. Fear of rejection due to altered body image, or impotence due to the resection of anatomic structures may occur. Symptoms such as fatigue, nausea, and weakness from treatment may also reduce interest. Sexuality should be addressed during rehabilitation; however, team members must be guided by the patient for the depth of information and the level of intervention undertaken. Interventions may vary from suggestions for altered positions to minimize pain, to optimal stomal protection and coverings, to intensive psychological counseling involving the sexual partner.

Hair loss following chemotherapy and radiation therapy may be dealt with by exploring available headgear or wigs. Other appearance-related side effects may be camouflaged using cosmetic products and beauty techniques. Prosthetic devices may be used to restore body contour following surgery. After mastectomy, the breast may be reconstructed by the plastic surgeon, or a commercially available external prosthesis may be used. If the gluteus maximus has been resected, a "buttock" can be made out of high-density foam. Similarly, shoulder pads may be fashioned if the deltoid and trapezius muscles have been resected. The anaplastologist may fashion a silicone prosthesis to replace a resected nose or ear. Where reconstructive procedures or devices do not exist, the rehabilitation team must help the patient deal with the altered body image.

Imagery, relaxation therapy, biofeedback, and supportive counseling are frequently used psychological techniques. Support groups provide a peer experience and help patients to understand how others have adapted to their disease and treatment sequelae.

Social and Leisure

For the cancer patient, previously comfortable interpersonal relationships may become strained. The patient may experience guilt about being unable to assume a usual role while family and friends may resent the need to assume extra responsibilities. Patient and family education are important so that all understand the effects of both the disease and the treatment. Social supports are a necessary component of the rehabilitation process.

For individuals who were active socially in volunteer work or recreational sports, the limitations imposed by fatigue, disordered communication, immobility, or prolonged lack of exercise can manifest psychologically. The rehabilitation team needs to help the patient to adopt alternate social activities and energy-conserving strategies that promote participation in important activities.

SUMMARY AND CONCLUSION

The purpose of cancer rehabilitation is to maximize patients' physical, psychological, and social health, thus enhancing quality of life. Rehabilitation outcomes depend on the disease site, treatment modalities, the prognosis, and the person. Rehabilitation problems range from generic symptoms such as fatigue to localized deficits such as nerve damage. These contribute to difficulties with complex functions such as ambulation, communication, and work. Altered body image and sexual function influence psychological and social function. The role of the multidisciplinary team is to educate the patient, assist in identifying problems, and establish realistic treatment goals and strategies for attaining maximum function.

The physical, psychological, and social problems faced by cancer patients vary depending on the disease site, individual personalities and coping styles, and the point along the trajectory of treatment and recovery. Early in the recovery process, it may be necessary to work on improving range-of-motion of a joint whereas further into recovery, more functional activities and teaching adaptations to the broader contexts of daily life will be more appropriate. The rehabilitation process is one of ongoing education, assessment, problem delineation, and treatment.

To assist cancer patients in achieving maximum outcomes for physical, psychological, and social health, members of the multidisciplinary team and the patient must work toward mutually defined goals reflecting the disease, its treatment, and the patient's needs. The ultimate result of successful rehabilitation is the enhancement of the patient's quality of life. The future challenge for rehabilitation is the evaluation of interventions under controlled conditions such that clinical decision-making reflects evidence-based care.

FURTHER READING

Blesch KS (1996) Rehabiliation of the cancer patient at home. *Semin Oncol Nurs* 12:219–225.

Dundas S (1991) Rehabilitation of the patient with cancer. *J Enterost Ther* 18:61–67.

Drause K (1991) Contracting cancer and coping with it. *Cancer Nurs* 14:240–245. 16:61–67.

Friedenreich CM, Courneya KS (1996) Exercise as rehabilitation for cancer patients. *Clin J Sport Med* 6:237–244.

Gudas ST (1992) Directives in cancer rehabilitation. *Oncology* 12:32–36.

Kronenberger MB, Meyers AD (1994) Dysphagia following head and neck cancer surgery. *Dysphagia* 9:236–244.

Lehman JF, DeLisa JA, Warren CG, DeLateur BJ, et al. (1978) Cancer rehabilitation: Assessment of need, development and evaluation of a model of care. *Arch Physi Med Rehab* 59:410–419.

Logemann JA (1994) Rehabilitation of the head and neck cancer patient. *Semin Oncol* 21:359–365.

Loveys BJ, Klaich K (1991) Breast cancer: Demands of illness. *Oncol Nurs Forum* 18:75–80.

Malone M, Harris AL, Luscombe DK (1994) Assessment of the impact of cancer on work, recreation, home management and sleep using a general health status measure. *Roy Soc Med* 87:386–389.

Mock V, Burke MB, Sheehan P, Creaton EM, Winningham ML, McKenney-Tedder S, Schwager LP, Leibman M (1994) A nursing rehabilitation program for women with breast cancer receiving adjuvant chemotherapy. *Oncol Nurs Forum* 21:899–908.

World Health Organization (1980) *International Classification of Impariments, Disabilities, and Handicap.* WHO, Geneva.

CHAPTER 41

QUALITY OF LIFE IN ONCOLOGY

VITTORIO VENTAFRIDDA

European Institute of Oncology
Milano, Italy

The majority of cancer treatments focus on the illness rather than on the patient and his or her subjective perceptions, such as quality of life (QOL). QOL evaluations are increasingly becoming an integral part of cancer care. The traditional endpoints, such as survival, disease-free survival time, response duration, treatment-associated toxicity, and tumor response, are beginning to include QOL as an outcome measure, because of the still limited results of therapies, and the physical and psychological burden related to disease and treatment. Different studies have shown that the concept of prolonging life for a few extra months is not sufficient in itself. It is therefore important to define success as prolongation of life while at the same time preserving its quality. In addition, the benefits from cancer treatments are often difficult to define because of the side effects, which also contribute to the QOL. Information about treatment toxicity and improvement in disease-related symptoms has generally come from the physician's perspective, whereas QOL concepts have the advantage of incorporating the patient's perspective as well. This aspect is particularly important in phase II and III studies, which often involve patients with advanced illness, and in which clinical decisions are often difficult. Even though QOL research material has been available, QOL evaluation is still often lacking in these studies.

Despite increasing interest, no consensus has been reached concerning the definition of QOL. Many definitions exist, for example, the WHO Quality of Life Group defines it as "an individual's perception of his position in life in the context of the culture and value systems in which he lives and in relation to his goals, expectations, standards and concerns."[2]

Manual of Clinical Oncology, 7th edition, Edited by Raphael E. Pollock
ISBN 0-471-23828-7, pages 791–803. Copyright © 1999 Wiley-Liss, Inc.

All authors agree that QOL is a subjective phenomenon. We can refer to a conceptual definition and to an operational one. With the former, we consider it an amalgam of satisfactory functioning in essentially four domains:

- Social
- Psychological and spiritual
- Occupational
- Physical

It is closely related to well-being, human values, and to the WHO concept of health as a global, multidimensional view of health status. Different authors have suggested evaluating the single components of QOL, but it still remains difficult to achieve an overview of these different parts.

The operational definition of QOL refers to a patient's evaluation of his or her health compared to what he or she thinks could be possible or ideal. It has been pointed out that in clinical studies QOL is not related to happiness, satisfaction, or living standards, but rather considers the impact of treatment, positive or negative, on some dimensions of life. Different approaches to define QOL have been recognized; some of them refer to psychological aspects; some to a patient's preference; and some are related to basic concepts of life or to reintegration to normal living, or to the gap between the hopes and the expectations of patients.

One relevant aspect of QOL of cancer patients is related to communication problems. A complete knowledge of the illness, stage, and planned treatment are important factors that allow a patient to decide about his or her future. This is extremely important in advanced and terminal phases of disease, when treatment is often of little benefit and QOL becomes the major issue. A patient-centered communication model should be used where patient's ideas can be explored and concerns about health and health care can be addressed. Sharing decisions and support to improve the patient's ability to take choices complete this approach. Doctors, nurses, and other professionals have a range of individual skills that can be used to achieve these tasks, while specific programs should be implemented to improve their ability to communicate.

MEASURING QOL

Two instruments can be used to measure QOL, which can be either disease specific or generic. Disease-specific instruments refer to measures used for one disease or for a narrow range of illnesses, whereas generic ones may be used for a wide range of goals. The instruments may be either designed specifically for a particular problem, or may be more general or specifically designed for measuring QOL in cancer patients. Broadly speaking, generic measures are less reliable in showing the particular effects of a treatment, although they may be more likely to detect unexpected effects. Generic measures may make comparisons between studies easier. It is of great importance to identify clearly which dimension of QOL is under evaluation and for which group of people it is used. Most QOL instruments rely upon visual analogue scales, where the patient is asked to mark a 10-cm line, according to the intensity of the symptom, or upon Likert scales, where values are related to discrete ranges of intensity. Likert scales are in general more easily understood by patients. Several instruments have been used for the measurement of QOL in cancer patients (Table 41.1).

An interesting approach has been made by the European Organization for Research and Treatment of Cancer (EORTC), by a modular assessment strategy.[3] The EORTC-QLQ-C30 is a generic questionnaire that can be completed by specific modules (e.g., lung, breast) to obtain more specific measures. Another example of this modular strategy is the Functional Assessment of Cancer-Therapy QOL questionnaire (FACT).[4] These questionnaires are suitable for study purposes, but are also adaptable to general clinical activities. A QOL questionnaire should investigate at least four dimensions: physical, psychological, social, and performance status. Physical functions, in particular including pain and other symptoms, mood, and social support should be evaluated from the time of diagnosis to terminal illness. Owing to the subjective nature of QOL, its evaluation should be obtained through a self-administered questionnaire. In a palliative care setting, where sometimes the patients may not be able to communicate, a rating on behalf of the patients (e.g., by relatives) should also be considered.

TABLE 41.1. Some QoL Instruments

Instrument	Administration	Items	Notes
EORTC–QLQ-C30 (3)	Self-report	30 Likert questions	Can be supplemented with site-specific questions. Cross-validated for different languages
Functional Assessment of Cancer Therapy (FACT) (4)	Self-report	29 Likert questions	Can be supplemented with site-specific questions. Cross-validated and available in different languages.
Functional Living Index Cancer (FLIC) (5)	Self-report	22 Likert/Analog scale	Especially suitable for physical and psychological factors. Indicated for outpatients. Site-specific questions not available.
Quality of Life— Cancer (6)	Self-report	30 Likert/Analog scale	Especially used in cancer nursing research. Some site-specific versions available.

PALLIATIVE CARE: GENERAL ASPECTS

Cancer is still a major worldwide problem. In 1996 there were an estimated 17.9 million persons with cancer surviving up to 5 years after diagnosis. Each year about 6 million deaths are due to this illness, and the percentage of cure remains still low, especially in developing countries.[7] For this reason a palliative approach is paramount. Palliative care can be defined as the active total care of patients whose disease is not responsive to curative treatment. Control of symptoms, especially pain, and of psychological, social, and spiritual problems is extremely important. A palliative care approach can be applied even during the early phases of disease, in conjunction with anticancer treatment. Specific antineoplastic therapies play a role in palliative care, provided that symptomatic benefits outweigh the disadvantages. More than 50% of cancer patients live in developing countries, but less than 10% of resources committed to cancer therapies are available to them. Most resources are devoted to curative (and usually expensive) treatments, with little attention given to training health personnel. For this reason a better allocation of resources is needed, especially in those countries where financial constraints are greater. (Fig. 41.1).[8]

Different palliative care programs have been developed, according to local resources and problems:

- *Home care*. Palliative care experts consider the home as the best place to take care of advanced cancer patients. Whenever possible a patient's autonomy and self-esteem, independent of an institution, should be sought and the presence of a primary health care team may greatly facilitate this model. However, existing funding does not always allow the equitable distribution of resources in many countries. Home care usually increases the costs for families, both financial and

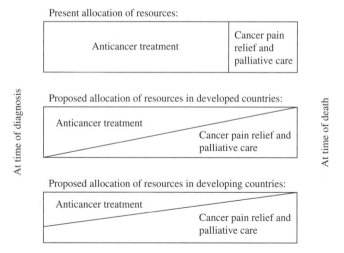

FIGURE 41.1. Proposed allocation of cancer resources. With permission, WHO, Technical Report Series 804, 1990 (8).

emotional. The dedicated caring for a relative at home should not be taken for granted, and expansion of home nursing services and provision for financial support are needed in many countries.

- *Inpatient care*. Hospice and Palliative Care Units represent this program. These settings are devoted to controlling pain and other manifestations of physical and social distress, and offer respite care for patients and families.
- *Consultation service*. Small teams, usually composed of nurses, a social worker, and a consulting physician, can provide specific consultation for different wards and hospitals. These programs also offer good educational opportunities for the health workers involved.
- *Day-hospice*. Day care programs may alleviate the burden of home care for relatives in offering therapy adjustments, physiotherapy, and social opportunity. Patients living alone may also benefit from these programs.
- *Bereavement support*. Trained health personnel, usually social workers and volunteers, may help relatives to cope with bereavement.

Continuity of care is the basis of palliative care. The aforementioned programs should pay great attention to this aspect. Palliative care also relies on prevention of distress related to symptoms. For this reason, members can be trained in different aspects of caring for their relative, such as administering analgesics, decubitus ulcer prevention, injection technique, and dealing with alimentary problems. Clear instructions for drug administration and for emergency problems should be explained and left at the patient's home. Ignorance concerning even small problems may be a cause of failure of an otherwise good program of care.

Palliative care aims to maintain or improve QOL of patients. We have already discussed this matter and how to measure it. In the palliative care setting methods to evaluate QOL should be very simple and should not increase the workload of health workers who have to support the patient and not spend their time administering questionnaires. The subjectivity of most measures of QOL is therefore important and does not mean its use is limited. Physical symptoms and performance, psychological state, and social interaction are the aspects usually evaluated. Some aspects often omitted include sexuality, spiritual aspects, the meaning of the illness, and its impact on the patient's family. A better knowledge of QOL in advanced and terminal phases could also help to convince policymakers to develop more balanced interventions in cancer care, with a different allocation of resources.

Several reports show that health professionals lack education in palliative care (e.g., cancer pain management). Education is a priority to guarantee successful implementation of a palliative care program. Different data indicate that palliative care knowledge can be transferred and integrated in existing health care systems. Education is concerned with the following:

- *Attitudes, values, and beliefs*. Philosophy of palliative care, attitude toward illness and death, and multidisciplinary teamwork are some of the topics related to this aspect.

- *Knowledge base*. Refers to the core of topics to be included, such as psycho-logical needs, pathophysiology of symptoms, or spiritual distress.
- *Skills*. Concerns the application of learned knowledge, through discussions, role-playing, and practice.

The educational program should be part of courses leading to basic professional qualification, university education, and be included in postgraduate programs. This effort should be made by joint public and private agencies, including health care associations. Also the public should be made aware of these topics, especially those concerning the meaning of the illness, and the relief of suffering. It is also important to ensure the availability of drugs needed for good palliative care; this is especially the case for opioids, such as morphine. These drugs should be widely available, together with the education on their use and easy prescription.

SYMPTOM MANAGEMENT: GENERAL STRATEGY

Cancer patients are affected by many varying types of symptoms.[9] These may range from pain to dyspnea, constipation, nausea, hiccups, and many others. As in other areas of cancer care the emphasis is on prevention and early diagnosis. Many problems, such as constipation due to opioids, pressure sores, and stomatitis, can be prevented if the care program includes prophylactic treatment and regular reassessment. Attention to detail is essential. Discussion with relatives is important: it allows evaluation of the level of cooperation and of participation of the family. During these talks it will possible to depict the main side effects of the therapies, explaining the strategy required to prevent them.[10] These aspects are extremely important when the patient is at home. Some principles for controlling symptoms should be underlined:

- A global evaluation
- An explanation of care for patient and family, checking to see if it has been understood
- Try to individualize therapies
- Attention to detail
- Reassess regularly.

It is especially important to administer drugs on a regular basis (e.g., for pain management or for constipation) while keeping specific drugs for rescue medication or for emergencies (e.g., sedatives for agitation or analgesia for breakthrough pain). Drugs should be kept to a minimum to ensure compliance and minimize the possibility of unexpected drug interactions. Standard doses do not exist and individualized titration of drugs is especially important (e.g., for pain management). Drugs may not be sufficient in themselves but should be administered in a manner that takes into account the physical and behavioral characteristics of the patient. It is often necessary to accept that some symptoms are not fully treatable (e.g., fatigue) and this fact should be accepted by the health care team provided that all efforts have been made. In this manner, continuity of care should remain the most important issue, thus reassuring the patient that he or she will not be abandoned. Eventually there comes a time when less technical skills are needed and psychosocial and spiritual aspects are paramount. Making the last hours of life more peaceful, and sustaining the family in their bereavement, are the major goals of this phase of the illness.

COMMON SYMPTOMS AND THEIR TREATMENT

In this section we deal with some of the most common symptoms affecting advanced and terminal cancer patients.[10] Pain, which is one of the most frequent and important, has been mentioned previously.

Dyspnea

Dyspnea is defined as an unpleasant awareness of difficulty in breathing. It is important to keep in mind such a definition, as the subjectivity of the symptom is especially important in patients who present with breathlessness. It can affect about 50% of terminal cancer patients, and up to 70% patients with lung cancer. Its incidence increases during the last weeks of life. This symptom may be related to cancer and its treatment, but often preexisting conditions such as COPD may be implicated. It is important to establish if the causes of this symptom are reversible or not. In the first instance specific measures such as radiotherapy, antibiotics, or thoracentesis may be used. Frequently, the causes of dyspnea are irreversible, as in advanced or terminal phases. It is then important to modify the way of life (e.g., correct positioning in the bed and/or the use of oxygen) and start respiratory sedatives, aimed at reducing the perception of breathlessness. Morphine is the main respiratory sedative in use. It has respiratory and analgesic properties, especially useful in those patients with concomitant pain (e.g., pathologic fracture of ribs), and it can be administered by different routes. Starting doses are usually 20 to 40 mg daily by mouth. In more acute situations, intravenous or subcutaneous routes are best. If the patient is already on morphine for pain, it may be sufficient to increase the dose by 50%. If the symptom is characterized by acute attacks, the use of nebulized morphine may be tried; normally 20 mg of morphine sulfate in 10 ml of saline solution is administered by a common nebulizer in air or oxygen. The rate of absorption of the drug is negligible and the action is mainly local. Oxygen by nasal prongs or mask is usually not helpful in most cancer patients, and a trial of therapy is the best way to determine benefit. Respiratory panic attacks benefit from regular oral morphine while additional measures include regular lorazepam or diazepam.

Constipation

This is a very common problem in advanced cancer patients, with a prevalence of approximately 40% in patients referred to hospices. Up to 90% of those receiving opioids complain of this symptom. There may be different causes and a preventive approach constitutes the best way of facing this symptom. The clinical history and examination help to identify concurrent problems related to this symptom such as bowel obstruction, presence of hard and impacted feces, and use of laxatives. Patients treated with opioids are almost always affected by constipation and prevention of this symptom should be quite aggressive. Prevention and management rely upon:

- Dietary measures: it is often not practical to prescribe a high-fiber diet. Fluid intake should be maximized.
- Whenever possible encourage activity and mobilization.
- Nursing measures, such as raising the toilet seat, privacy, warm bathroom, and the use of a commode are important.
- Treat with regular laxatives (especially when treated with opioids).
- If needed, measures such as suppositories, enemas, or even manual evacuation may be needed.

Different laxative regimens are available and it is usually advisable to start with a stool softener such as docusate and a bowel stimulant such as senna or bisacodyl at the same time.

Delirium

Delirium may be defined as an acute, organic global impairment of mental function. It differs from chronic, progressive loss of memory and intellectual functions, which is more typically dementia. The onset of delirium is typically within a few hours to days, its course fluctuates, and it is often worse at night. Hallucinations may be present while disorientation and agitation are common. Its prevalence ranges from 20% to 70% of advanced cancer patients, approaching more than 90% during the last days of life. Advanced age, hospitalization, and advanced disease are all risk factors for delirium. It generally constitutes a multifactorial problem. Sometimes a deaf or anxious patient might be interpreted as drowsy and confused. Common problems affecting advanced cancer patients such as hypercalcemia, severe anemia, sepsis, meningitis, and brain metastases must be ruled out prior to discussing specific therapy. In most cases, an empirical approach is required:

- If possible, stop or reduce as many drugs as possible, especially sedatives and analgesics. Withdrawal syndromes such as those following abrupt withdrawal of steroids should be kept in mind.
- Try to reassure the patient and his or her family and the patient should be kept in a quiet environment. Reorientating techniques may be useful (e.g., familiar objects, calendar, clock, some degree of physical activity).
- Correct metabolic imbalance and treat specific causes (e.g., steroids and anti-convulsants for brain metastases).

- Treat agitation with haloperidol, by oral or parenteral route. If more sedation is required, add midazolam or diazepam by continuous intravenous (IV) infusion. Midazolam can be also conveniently administered by the subcutaneous (SC) route.

Inform the family about the severity of the clinical picture and its likely natural history. In advanced cancer patients, acute confusional states are often a landmark of imminent death.

Nausea and Vomiting

These symptoms may be present in up to 60% of patients with advanced cancer. They are more common in breast, stomach, or gynecologic neoplasms. They can be frequent in patients requiring opioid treatment: tolerance to this side effect usually develops within 2 weeks. Whereas nausea is an expression of autonomic stimulation, vomiting is a complex reflex involving different muscles and functions. It is important to remember the existence of a vomiting center, located in the brainstem, receiving afferents from the chemoreceptor trigger zone. This region is very sensitive to different stimuli such as:

- Chemotherapeutic agents.
- Metabolic products (e.g., ammonium, uremia, acidosis)
- Radiotherapy
- Other drugs (e.g., digitalis)

Other stimulants reach the vomiting center from the upper gastrointestimal tract via sympathetic and vagal routes and are activated under various conditions (chemotherapy, gastrointestinal metastasis), whereas others come from cerebral and vestibular areas. A physical examination and evaluation are especially important. As a result of this varying etiology, the diagnostic work-up of nausea and vomiting may be complex. Some points should be stressed:

- Determine the pattern of nausea and vomiting (e.g., relationship with food ingestion).
- Check for neurologic symptoms suggestive of intracranial hypertension.
- Review the drug schedule.
- Make an accurate clinical examination, including rectal exam, where indicated.
- Laboratory studies may be needed (e.g., creatinine, calcium, albumin, some drugs level where appropriate)
- If gastrointestinal obstruction is present, have a surgical consultation. If not amenable to surgery treat it with conservative measures (see next paragraph).

Nondrug measures include frequent small meals and dietary advice, and a calm reassuring environment. Whenever possible reversible causes should be treated (e.g., hypercalcemia, gastritis, intracranial hypertension, and others).

The pharmacologic treatment of nausea and vomiting is most likely to succeed if given prophylactically, usually by the oral route. If the patient is already experiencing nausea and vomiting, a parenteral route is preferable. Continuous IV and SC administration are commonly used. In terminally ill patients, the following points may be useful:

- It is usual to start with metclopramide, 10 to 20 mg every 6 to 8 hours.
- If results are not satisfactory and brain metastases are present, add dexamethasone 16 to 36 mg/daily.
- If liver failure, uremia, or opiod-induced vomiting is present, haloperidol at a dose of 1 to 4 mg /daily should be added.
- In patients with nausea and vomiting unable to take oral medications, start a SC or IV continuing infusion with metclopramide 30 to 60 mg, haloperidol 2 mg in 24 hours.

Such infusions may be given by simple syringe-driver or, less expensively, by hypodermoclysis. Patients equipped with a permanent IV site, such as a Port-a-Cath, may easily utilize this approach.

Gastrointestinal Obstruction

Gastrointestinal obstruction may affect about 3% to 5% of hospice patients, but it is particularly common in advanced ovarian cancer and in colorectal cancer, ranging from 25% to 40% and 10% to 15%, respectively. Tumor is the main cause of obstruction in about 60% of patients, but nonmalignant causes and second tumors are also frequent in 25% and 10% of cases, respectively. It is important to distinguish between operable and inoperable bowel obstruction, and this is often very difficult, particularly in patients who have had previous surgery. If the patient is inoperable, then the level of obstruction will dictate management.

- High levels of obstruction (duodenum) may require a gastostomy or nasogastric tube to obtain relief of vomiting.
- Lower levels of obstruction generally do not require mechanical decompression, and can be satisfactorily managed only with pharmacologic agents as outlined below (indicated also for a high level of obstruction). Nasogastric intubation and IV fluids are recommended in the management of terminally ill patients only in the context of relief of the symptoms of dehydration. Such treatment is generally uncomfortable for the patient, interferes with social functions, and creates a barrier between the patient and the surrounding environment.

The principles of pharmacologic treatment of inoperable obstructions rely upon the following combined approaches:

- Control pain, both colicky and continuous.

- Reduce intraluminal fluids which will help to alleviate nausea and vomiting with antisecretive drugs.
- Reduce nausea and vomiting directly with antiemetics.

Pain control is easily obtained with opioids, mainly morphine. Nausea and vomiting can be relieved by haloperidol 2% to 6 mg/daily and antisecretory drugs such as hyoscine butilbromide 60 to 240 mg/daily or by the more recent and expensive synthetic somatostatin analogue octreotide 0.3 to 1 mg/daily. This last drug also increases the reabsorption of intraluminal fluids. All these different drugs may be mixed in the same solution and administered as a continuing SC/IV infusion, by syringe-driver or hypodermoclysis. Steroids may be added. Metclopramide and other prokinetic agents can be useful where intestinal continuity is maintained but in complete obstruction they can increase colicky pain and are not indicated.

The Terminal Phase

The main goals of care during the last days and hours of life can be as follows:

- Prepare the patient's family for the coming event and support them.
- Keep the dying person as comfortable as possible, maintaining his or her dignity.
- Respect the process of dying, do not try to shorten or prolong it.

It should be explained to relatives that antemortem symptoms such as changes in breathing are not distressing for the patient. Restlessness or agitation have to be prevented and emergency medications, usually parenteral haloperidol, provided. Unnecessary medications must be stopped, and drugs often need to be administered by SC or IV routes. Opioids, sedatives, and antiemetics are the drugs usually requiring administration during the last hours. Enteral and parenteral feeding should be stopped and parenteral fluids should not be given: hydration can increase cough, pulmonary congestion, peripheral edema, vomiting, and urinary problems. These aspects have to be clearly explained to the family. The death rattle may be reduced by adding, at the onset of this symptom, SC/IV hyoscine 60 to 120 mg/daily and correctly positioning the patient. If agitation or restlessness are present, continuing SC haloperidol (4 to 10 mg/daily) or midazolam (10 to 30 mg/daily) can be useful.

Ethical Aspects

Oncologists should always seek an acceptable balance between the advantages and the disadvantages of treatment, especially during the advanced and terminal phases of the illness. The ethical principles of doing good and minimizing harm reflect the correct approach. Three other principles apply:

- Respect for life

- Respect for patient autonomy
- Fairness in the use of limited resources

When facing situations of uncertainty, the totality of the patient is the utmost consideration. When the general condition of the patient deteriorates, freedom from pain and such symptoms are the pillars of a "good death." If, for example, shortening of life results from the use of adequate doses of analgesics, this is not the same as intentionally terminating life by overdose. Life-prolonging treatments also present ethical problems. Preservation of life at all costs is not always the right choice, especially if the burden of side effects and personal costs appears unacceptable to the patient. Moreover, life-supporting therapies often reduce the ability of the patient to communicate and to act as a complete human being. In many countries, health professionals have come to accept this notion, and the ethic of allowing cancer patients to die peacefully has become the rule. This approach involves withholding or discontinuing aggressive interventions, such as respiratory support, chemotherapy, or parenteral nutrition. The patient's will should be considered first and respected. Three other ethical principles are relevant:

- The principle of proportion
- The principle of equivalence
- The relativity principle

In brief, they help us to accept the limits of medicine and the resources of a patient. The patient's perception of our efforts as a prolongation of dying, rather than an enhancement of living, justifies discontinuing life-prolonging techniques. Moreover, stopping a treatment is ethically not different from never starting it. The principle of relativity affirms that life is not an absolute good and that even death should be accepted as a "normal" event. Medicine should respect personal values and life-prolonging therapies should give way to other kinds of care.

A frequently raised ethical dilemma concerns euthanasia. Palliative care is a strong and modern answer to this problem: reducing physical and psychosocial suffering is surely a practicable alternative to euthanasia. Efforts then should be made to implement national palliative care programs, rather than requesting legalization of euthanasia.

FURTHER READING

1. Batel-Copel LM, Kornblith AB, Batel PC, Holland JC (1997) Do oncologists have an increasing interest in the Quality of life of their patients? A literature review of the last 15 years. *Eur J Cancer* 33:29–32.
2. WHO QOL Group (1993) Study protocol for the World Health Organization project to develop a quality of life assessment instrument. *Qual Life Res* 2:143–159.

3. Aaronson NK, Ahmedzai S, Bergman B, et al. (1993) The European Organization for the Research and Treatment of Cancer: A quality of life instrument for use in international clinical trials in oncology. *J Natl Cancer Inst* 85:365–376.

4. Cella DF, Tulsky DS, Gray G, et al. (1993) The Functional Assessment of Cancer Therapy (FACT) Scale: Development and validation of the general version. *J Clin Oncol* 11:570–579.

5. Schipper H, Clinch J, McMurray A, et al. (1984) Measuring the quality of life of cancer patients: The Functional Living-Index Cancer: development and validation. *J Clin Oncol* 2:472–483.

6. Padilla GV, Presant C, Grant MM, Metter G, Lipsett J, Heide F (1983) Quality of life index for patients with cancer. *Res Nurs Health* 3:117–126.

7. World Health Organization (1997) Annual Report 1996. WHO, Geneva.

8. World Health Organization (1990) Cancer Pain Relief and Palliative Care. Technical Report Series, No. 804, WHO, Geneva. p. 16.

9. Vainio A, Auvinen A (1996) Prevalence of symptoms among patients with advanced cancer: An international collaborative study. *J Pain Symp Manage* 12:3–10.

10. Waller A, Caroline NL (1996) *Handbook of Palliative Care in Cancer*. Butterworth-Heinemann, Boston.

ABCDE mnemonic, 329
Acetaminophen, 750
Acoustic Schwannomas, 613–614
Actinomycin D, chemotherapy, 284–285
Acute lymphoblastic leukemia, 654
Acute lymphocytic leukemia, 669–673
   allogeneic BMT/PBPC transplant, 296
   biology, 669–671
   clinical features, 671
   differential diagnosis, 671
   laboratory features, 671
   treatment, 671–672
Acute myeloid leukemia, 664–669
   allogeneic BMT/PBPC transplant, 295–296
   autologous BMT/PBPC transplant, 300–301
   classification, 664–666
   differential diagnosis, 666–667
   laboratory manifestations, 666
   pathophysiology, 664
   remission induction, 667
   signs and symptoms, 666
   treatment, 667–669
Acute promyelocytic leukemia, 668–669
Acyclovir, immunocompromised patients,
   734
Adeno-associated viruses, 117
Adenomas, colorectal cancer, 478
Adenoviruses, 117
Adjuvant therapies, 14, 752, 754
Adjuvant trials, endpoints, 317
Adrenal cancer, 370–373
Adrenal insufficiency, 738
Adult T-cell leukemia, viral infection, 663
Adult T-cell leukemia/lymphoma,
   smoldering/chronic, 652
Advanced disease trials, endpoints, 317
Agnogenic myeloid metaplasia, 684–685
AIDS related malignancies, 709–717
   Kaposi's sarcoma, 709–713
   lymphoma, 713–717
Alcohol consumption
   cancer risk, 144
   carcinogenesis and, 39
   esophageal carcinoma and, 426
Alkylating agents, chemotherapy, 280–282
Allele, mechanism of loss of function, 71–72
All-*trans*-retinoic acid, acute promyelocytic
   leukemia therapy, 668–669
α-tocopherol, β-carotene, trial, 167
Amino acids
   improving efficacy of feeding regiments,
      773
   metabolism, 761
      cytokine effects, 764
Amputation, rehabilitation, 787
Analgesics
   nonopioid, 750–751
   opioid, 751–753
Anaplastic large-cell lymphoma, 653
Anemia, use of transfusions, 741
Anesthesia, history, 236
Angiocentric lymphoma, 653
Angiography, pancreatic cancer, 464
Angioimmunoblastic lymphoma, 653
Animal models, genetic predisposition, 71
Animal studies, 2-year rodent bioassay, 24
Anorexia, 758, 760
Anthracyclines, chemotherapy, 286
Antibodies, 101–102
Anticonvulsants, 752
   symptomatic control of brain edema and
      increase intracranial pressure, 618
Antidepressants, 752
Antimetabolites, chemotherapy, 283–284
Antimicrotubule agents, chemotherapy,
   288–289
Antisense gene therapy, 124–125
Antiseptic techniques of Lister, 236–237
APC syndrome, colorectal cancer, 479
Apoptosis, 55–56
Ascites, malignant, 739–740
Aspirin, 750
   chemoprevention, 169–170
Astrocytomas, 610–611

Bacterial infections, following autologous
    bone marrow transplantation
    transplant, 303
Balkan nephropathy, 588
Barium enema, colorectal cancer, 484
Basal cell carcinomas, 325–326, 328
    surgery, 332–333
B cells, 101
Benzene, increased incidence of leukemias,
    663
β-carotene, chemoprevention, 174
Bethesda system, 519–520
Bioassay, 2-year rodent, 24
Biological carcinogens, 22
Biologic cancer therapy, 102, 105–125
    cellular therapy, 110–112
    cytokines, 105–108
    LAK cell therapy, 110–111
    monoclonal antibodies, 108–110
    TIL therapy, 111
    vaccines, 112–116
    see also Gene therapy
Biologic progression, 2
Biologic response modifiers, 290–291
Biopsy, 241–242
    laparoscopy and needle, liver cancer,
      412
    lymph node, esophageal carcinoma, 430
    open lung, 391
    soft tissue sarcomas, 624–625
    transthoracic needle, 390–391
Biostatistics, role in clinical trial, 307
Biotherapy, liver cancer, 419
Blackledge staging system, primary
    gastrointestinal lymphomas, 645
Bladder carcinoma, 581–588
    chemoprevention, 176
    chemotherapy, 587
    diagnosis, 583
    etiology, 581–582
    follow-up, 588
    metastatic, 587
    multimodality treatment, 585
    muscle-invasive, 586
    organ preservation, 587–588
    pathology, 582–583
    presentation and natural history, 582
    prevention, 588
    radiotherapy, 586
    screening, 582
    staging and prognosis, 583–585
    superficial, 585–586
    surgery, 586
Bleomycin, chemotherapy, 285

Body image, altered, 783
    dealing with, 788–789
Bone marrow, nonproliferating cells,
    reentering cell cycles, 4
Bone marrow transplantation, 293–304
    acute lymphocytic leukemia, 672–673
    acute myeloid leukemia, 668
    allogeneic, 293
      future, 304
      indications, 295–296
      phases, 297–299
    autologous, 294–295, 300–302
      future, 304
      phases, 302–303
    chronic myelogenous leukemia therapy, 676
    neuroblastoma, 695
    secondary malignancies, 300
    syngeneic, 293–294
Brachytherapy, 255–256
    brain tumors, 617
    clinical, 272–273
    intracavitary, cervical cancer, 528, 528–529
    prostate cancer, 569
Brain lymphoma, primary, 614
Brain metastasis, 615–616
Brainstem tumors, 613
Brain tumors, 607–618
    gliomas, 610–612
    imaging, 610
    metastases, 734–735
    neurotoxicity, 618
    pediatric, 703–705
    pediatric neurooncology, 612–616
    signs and symptoms, 608–609
    symptomatic control of edema and
      increased intracranial pressure,
      617–618
    therapy, 616–617
Breast cancer, 491–511
    adjuvant treatment by nodal status, 509
    autologous BMT/PBPC transplant, 301–302
    chemoprevention, 175–176
    diagnostic work-up, 501
    ductal and lobular carcinomas in situ,
      492–493
    epidemiology, 491–492
    geographical variation, 137–138
    hereditary, 495, 498
    invasive, 493–494
      surgical treatment, 502–504
    management of high-risk subjects, 498–500
    node-negative, risk categories, 508
    nonpalpable lesions, management, 501–502
    pathology, 492–495

prognostic factors, 495–497
risk
    after benign breast biopsy, 499
    hormonal contraceptive use, 145–147
screening, 150–151, 192–193, 500
systemic treatment, 504–511
    adjuvant prolonged chemotherapy, 506
    chemoendocrine therapies, 507
    high-dose chemotherapy, 507
    immunotherapy, 507–509
    metastatic disease treatment, 508–511
    ovarian ablation, 505–506
    perioperative and preoperative
        chemotherapy, 506
    tamoxifen, 506–507
variations in outcome of treatment, 153–154
Breast examination, clinical, 192–193
Breast lesions, nonpalpable, management,
    501–502
Bronchoscopy
    esophageal carcinoma, 430
    lung cancer, 390
Burkitt's lymphoma, 654

Cachexia, *see* Cancer cachexia
Calcium, chemoprevention, 169
Camptothecins, chemotherapy, 287
Cancer
    in ancient civilizations, 1–2
    cells, genetic changes, 63–64
    as cellular disease, 2–4
    definition, 45–46
    as multistage disease, 7–11
    as temporal disease, 4–6
Cancer cachexia, 757
    causes and consequences, 760–761
    clinical manifestations, 758–760
    cytokines as mediators, 762–764
    etiologies, 761
    glutamine, 762
Cancer predisposition genes
    carriers, demonstrating non-cancer-related
        phenotypic changes, 72, 74
    characteristics suggestive of presence, 74
    chemoprevention and, 88–89
    classes, 68–69
    early onset induced by, 74–75
    identification, 65, 68
    multiple primaries, 75
    regulating normal cell growth, cell survival,
        or genomic stability, 68–70
    techniques for identifying mutations,
        83–84
    variation in penetrance, 88–90

Cancer predisposition syndromes
    founder effects, 75
    management, 77–78
Cancer treatments, problem of undetected
        metastatic disease, 58
Carboplatin, 282
Carcinogen-DNA adducts, 27, 29–30
Carcinogenesis, 7, 19–43
    definition, 20
    electrophile theory, 20
    field, 165
    historical perspective, 19–20
    modifying factors, 38–39
    multistage, 33–38
        concept, 33–34
        human cancer, 37–38
        initiation, 35
        mouse skin model, 34–37
        progression, 37
        promotion, 35–36
    multistep, chemoprevention and,
        164–165
    stages, 7–11
Carcinogens
    biological, 22
    chemical. *See* Chemical carcinogens
    listing, 25
    major groups, 24
    mutations and, 29–30
    nongenotoxic, 20
    physical, 21–22
Care economic aspects, 223
Carotene and Retinol Efficacy Trial, 167
CA-125 tests, ovarian cancer, 544
Cells
    cycle, 2–3, 54–55
    fusion experiments, 50
    exponential and Gompertzian growth, 2–3
    growth, control, 48
    intrinsic radiation sensitivity, 265
    nonproliferating, 2, 4
    normal growth, regulation by predisposition
        genes, 68–70
    survival, regulation by predisposition genes,
        68–70
    terminally differentiated, 2
    transformed, properties, 46
Cellular disease, cancer as, 2–4
Cellular immunity, 100–101
Cellular therapy, biologic cancer therapy,
        110–112
Central nervous system. *See* Brain tumors
Central nervous system lymphoma,
        AIDS-related, 654, 716–717

Central nervous system metastases, testis
 cancer, 600–601
Cervical cancer, 515–534
 chemoprevention, 176–177
 diagnosis, 519–522
 epidemiology, 516–517
 etiology, 515–517
 geographical variation, 138–139
 multimodality treatment, 524–532
  invasive cervical cancer, 526–529
  microinvasive cervical cancer, 526
  preinvasive lesions, 524–526
  recurrent cervical cancer, 529–532
 preinvasive lesions, 519–521
 prevention, 534
 radical hysterectomy, complications,
  532–533
 radiotherapy, complications, 533–534
 rehabilitation, 532–534
 screening, 148–150, 191–192
  for neoplasias, 517–519
 signs and symptoms, 521
 spread patterns, 522
 staging, 522–524
Chemical carcinogenesis, inhibition, 40–43
Chemical carcinogens, 22–23
 direct, 26
 environmental factors, 20–21
 multistage carcinogenesis, 37–38
 DNA reactive intermediates, 28
 identification and classification, 23–25
 indirect, 26
 metabolic activation and, 26–28
Chemical modifiers, radiation sensitivity,
 271–272
Chemoendocrine therapies, breast cancer, 507
Chemoprevention, 40–42, 163–177
 agents, 167–173
  aspirin/NSAIDs, 169–170
  calcium, 169
  finasteride, 171
  lycopene, 171
  micronutrient supplements, 171–173
  retinoids, 167–168
  selenium, 170
  tamoxifen and raloxifene, 170–171
 biology, 164–165
 clinical trials, 173–177
  bladder cancer, 176
  breast cancer, 175–176
  cervical cancer, 176–177
  colorectal cancer, 174–175
  esophageal and stomach cancer, 176
  head and neck cancer, 173

  lung cancer, 174
  prostate cancer, 177
  skin cancer, 175
 definition, 163
 in individuals with abnormalities in cancer
  predisposition genes, 88–89
 multistep carcinogenesis and
  premalignancy, 164–165
 preinvasive lesions, cervical, 525
 trial designs, 165–167
Chemoradiation
 colorectal cancer, 486–487
 localized soft tissue sarcomas, preoperative,
  633
 locally advanced pancreatic cancer,
  471–472
 pancreatic cancer, 464–467
Chemotherapy
 acute lymphocytic leukemia, postremission,
  672
 acute myeloid leukemia
  postremission, 667
  relapsed patients, 667–668
 as adjuvant therapy, 14–15
 agents, 280–290
  alkylating agents and platinum
   coordination compounds, 280–282
  antimetabolites, 283–284
  antimicrotubule agents, 288–289
  antitumor antibiotics, 284–285
  hormonal agents, 289–290
  topoisomerase inhibitors and agents
   with pleiotropic mechanisms,
   286–287
 AIDS-related Kaposi's sarcoma, 713
 bladder carcinoma, 587
 brain tumors, 705
 breast cancer
  adjuvant prolonged, 506
  high-dose, 507
  perioperative and preoperative, 506
 cancer in the elderly, 726
 colorectal cancer, 487
 combined with radiation, 270–271
  esophageal carcinoma, 434
 drug resistance, 277
 enteritis, 766, 769–770
 esophageal carcinoma, 433–434
 Ewing's sarcoma, 701
 gastric cancer, 449
 gliomas, 612
 gynecologic cancer, 556
 head and neck cancer, 354–355
 hepatic tumors, 697

hyperuricemia and tumor lysis syndrome, 737
implications for rehabilitation, 781
infection risk, 732
intra-arterial, cervical cancer, 529
liver cancer, 419
localized soft tissue sarcomas
  postoperative, 631–632
  preoperative, 632–633
locally recurrent soft tissue sarcomas, 635
lung cancer, 399–401
metastatic soft tissue sarcoma, 636–637
neoadjuvant, cervical cancer, 529
neuroblastoma, 695
osteosarcoma, 703
ovarian cancer, 547
pancreatic and intestinal neuroendocrine tumors, 380
parathyroid cancer, 370
primary soft tissue sarcoma of retroperitoneum, 634
prostate cancer, 572–573
recurrent cervical cancer, 531
renal cell carcinomas, 580
rhabdomyosarcoma, 699
skin and melanoma cancer, 338–339
testis cancer, 601
vulvar cancer, 552
Wilms' tumor, 692
Chlorambucil, chronic lymphocytic leukemia therapy, 679
2-Chlorodeoxyadenosine, chronic lymphocytic leukemia therapy, 679
Choriocarcinoma, 554, 556
Chromosomal tumor translocations, associated with non-Hodgkin's lymphomas, 646
Chronic irritation, 22
Chronic lymphocytic leukemia, 651, 676–680
  biology, 676–677
  clinical features, 678
  differential diagnosis, 678–679
  laboratory features, 678
  treatment, 679–680
Chronic myelogenous leukemia, 673–676
  biology, 673–674
  clinical features, 674
  differential diagnosis, 675
  laboratory features, 674–675
  therapy, 675–676
Chronic myeloid leukemia, allogeneic BMT/PBPC transplant, 296
Chronic myeloproliferative diseases, 681, 683–685
Cisplatin, toxicity, 282

Classification, 215–217
Clinical phase, 6
Clinical trial, 307–323
  definition, 308
  endpoints, 317–318
  inclusion/exclusion of patients from analyses, 321–322
  intent to treat principle, 321–322
  meta-analyses, 322
  number of patients required, 319–320
  patient eligibility, 321
  patient selection, 315–316
  phase I, 309–310
  phase II, 310–313, 315
    feasibility trials, 313–314
  phase III, 315
  protocol, 308
  quality control, 322
  randomization and stratification, 316–317
  reporting results, 322–333
  statistical analyses, 320
  therapeutic approaches other than cytotoxic drugs, 314–315
  types, 308–315
Clonal nature of cancer, 46–47
Cocarcinogens, 20
Colony-stimulating factors, 108
Colorectal cancer, 477–489
  chemoprevention, 174–175
  chemotherapy, 487
  diagnosis, 483–485
  early detection, 480
  epidemiology, 477
  etiology, 478–480
  family history, 480
  follow up, local and distant recurrences, 487–489
  gastrointestinal obstruction, 799
  malignant ascites, 739–740
  pathology, 481
  preoperative evaluation, 484–485
  prevention, 480
  prognosis, 489
  progression, 481
  radiotherapy, 486–487
  rehabilitation, 489
  screening, 151–152, 193–195, 480
  signs and symptoms, 483
  staging, 481–483
  surgical oncology, 485–486
Colposcopy, 521
Communication
  disorder, rehabilitation, 785–786
  potential barriers, 224

Computed tomography
  esophageal carcinoma, 428
  liver cancer, 412
  pancreatic cancer, 457–458, 461–463
Conformal radiation therapy, 273
Constipation, management, 797
Contraceptives, hormonal, breast cancer risk,
  145–147
Control programs
  efficacy and staging, 222–223
  managing, staging role, 228–231
Conversion, 10
Corticosteroids, 752
Cost, screening tests, 190–191
Costimulatory molecules-B7, gene therapy,
  124
Cryoablation, prostate cancer, 571
Cyclin-dependent kinases, 54
Cytochrome P450 enzymes, metabolic
  activation of chemical carcinogens,
  26–27
Cytokines, 102–104
  biologic cancer therapy, 105–108
  cancer cachexia mediators, 762–764
  colony-stimulating factors, 108
  effects on glucose metabolism, 763
  fat metabolism effects, 764
  in gene therapy, 119–123
  inflammatory/T-cell reactive, 105–108
  protein/amino acid metabolism effects, 764
  use, 741–742
Cytoreductive surgery, 243–244
Cytosarcoma phylloides, 495
Cytosine arabinoside, chemotherapy, 284
Cytotoxic agents, breast cancer, 510–511
Cytotoxic T lymphocytes, 100–101

Daily living, rehabilitation, 787–788
Daunorubicin, chemotherapy, 286
Decision making, autonomous, staging role in
  promoting, 227–228
Deleted in Pancreatic Cancer tumor suppressor
  genes, 455–456
Delirium, management, 797–798
2-Deoxycoformycin, chronic lymphocytic
  leukemia therapy, 679
Depth-dose curves, 254–255
Diagnosis, 201–213
  bladder carcinoma, 583
  brain tumors, 704–705
  cancer in the elderly, 724–725
  colorectal cancer, 483–485
  differential
    acute lymphocytic leukemia, 671

  acute myeloid leukemia, 666–667
  chronic lymphocytic leukemia, 678–679
  chronic myelogenous leukemia, 675
  liver cancer, 412–413
endometrial cancer, 539
esophageal carcinoma, 427–430
Ewing's sarcoma, 700
gastric cancer, 445, 447
head and neck cancer, 343–345
hepatic tumors, 696
history taking, 201–202
Hodgkin's disease, 655–656
liver cancer, 410–412
lung cancer, 386–388
  evaluation techniques, 388–392
molecular markers, 210, 212
neuroblastoma, 693–694
osteosarcoma, 702
ovarian cancer, 544–545
pancreatic and intestinal neuroendocrine
  tumors, 378–379
pancreatic cancer, importance of
  pretreatment studies, 461–464
parathyroid cancer, 368
pathological analysis, 207–208, 210,
  212–213
pheochromocytoma, 374
physical examination, 202, 205–206
prostate cancer, 566–567
renal cell carcinomas, 577–578
rhabdomyosarcoma, 698
skin and melanoma cancer, 328–331
soft tissue sarcomas, 624–626
surgical oncology, 241–242
systemic metastases, 207, 211
testis cancer, 593–595
tumor localization, 206–207, 209–210
vulvar cancer, 549
Wilms' tumor, 690–691
Diagnostic imaging, 209–210
Dietary factors
  cancer risk, 143
  carcinogenesis and, 39
  colorectal cancer, 478
  pancreatic cancer, 454
Dietary intervention, 40
Differentiation, 53
Diffuse large B-cell lymphoma, 653
Digital rectal examination
  colorectal cancer, 484
  prostate cancer screening, 195–196
Disability
  assessment, 783
  definition, 779

rehabilitation, 785–787
DNA adducts, 27, 29–30
DNA repair, cancer risk and, 39
DNA testing
    limitation, 96
    risks associated with, 95–96
Docetaxel, 288–289
Doxorubicin, chemotherapy, 286
Drug activating genes, 59
Drugs
    delivery and dose intensity, 278–279
    discovery, 58
    resistance, 277
Ductal carcinoma in situ, 492–493
Duodenum, neuroendocrine tumors, 376–377
Dyspnea, management, 796

Economic aspects of cancer care, studies and
        staging, 223
Edema, brain, symptomatic control, 617–618
Education, patient, rehabilitation, 785
Elderly, cancer in, 723–729
    diagnosis, 724–725
    etiology and epidemiology, 724
    therapeutic decision making, 727
    treatment, 726–728
Electromagnetic spectrum, 252
Electrophile theory of chemical
        carcinogenesis, 20
Emergencies. *See* Oncological emergencies
Employment, returning to, rehabilitation, 788
Endocrine therapy
    hypercalcemia, 736
    metastatic prostate cancer, 571–572
    thrombosis and thrombophlebitis and, 736
Endocrine tumors, 359–380
    adrenal cancer, 370–373
    pancreatic and intestinal neuroendocrine
        tumors, 375–380
    parathyroid cancer, 368–370
    pheochromocytoma, 373–375
    thyroid cancer, 363–368
Endometrial cancer, 537–542
    diagnosis, 539
    epidemiology, 537–538
    etiology, 537–538
    incidence, 537
    pathology, 538–539
    postsurgical treatment, 541–542
    prognosis, 542
    screening, 538
    staging, 539–541
Endoscopic ultrasound, esophageal carcinoma,
        430

Enteral nutrition, 765–769
Enteritis, acute radiation and chemotherapy,
        766, 768–770
Environmental factors, 20–21
Ependymomas, 612–613, 705
Epidemiology, 131–155
    AIDS-associated lymphoma, 713–714
    AIDS-related Kaposi's sarcoma, 709
    brain tumors, 704
    breast cancer, 491–492
    cancer in the elderly, 724
    cervical cancer, 516–517
    colorectal cancer, 477
    deaths attributable to factors, 139
    endometrial cancer, 537–538
    esophageal carcinoma, 425–427
    Ewing's sarcoma, 699–700
    gastric cancer, 439–441
    geographic and temporal variation in risk,
        134–140
    gestational trophoblastic disease, 553
    global burden, 132–134
    head and neck cancer, 342
    hepatic tumors, 696
    history, 131–132
    Hodgkin's disease, 654–655
    leukemias, 662–663
    liver cancer, 407–408
    neuroblastoma, 693
    non-Hodgkin's lymphomas, 642–643
    osteosarcoma, 701–702
    ovarian cancer, 542–543
    pancreatic and intestinal neuroendocrine
        tumors, 375
    prevention, 141–143, 141–148
        alcohol consumption, 144
        diet, 143
        endogenous hormones, 145–148
        infective processes, 145
        occupational exposures, 145
        sunlight exposure, 144
    prostate cancer, 564
    rhabdomyosarcoma, 697
    screening, 148–153
        breast cancer, 150–151
        cervical cancer, 148–150
        colorectal cancer, 151–152
        for other forms of cancer, 152–153
    skin and melanoma cancer, 325–327
    staging, 223
    thyroid cancer, 363–364
    variations in outcome of cancer treatment,
        153–154
    vulvar cancer, 548

Epidemiology (*cont.*)
  Wilms' tumor, 689–690
Epigenetic processes, 71–72
Esophageal carcinoma, 425–437
  chemoprevention, 176
  chemotherapy, 433–434
  diagnosis and staging, 427–430
  epidemiology, 425–427
  geographical variation, 135
  multimodality therapy, 434–435
  palliation, advanced disease, 435
  postoperative follow-up, 436–437
  prevention, 437
  radiation, 433
  screening, 427
  surgery, 431–433
  survival by stage, 431
  treatment and prognosis, 431–435
Esophagectomy, 431–432
Essential thrombocythemia, 683–684
Etiology, 6–7
Ewing's sarcoma, 699–701
External-beam radiotherapy, 255
  cervical cancer, 527–528
  pancreatic cancer, 464–467
  prostate cancer, 569
  treatment planning, 256

FAB classification, myelodysplastic
    syndromes, 682
Familial adenomatous polyposis, colorectal
    cancer, 479
Familial cancer syndromes, with identified
    genetic mediators, 66–67
Familial medullary thyroid cancer, 360
Family history
  questionnaire, 76
  validation, 72
Fat, metabolism, cytokine effects, 764
Fecal occult blood testing, 193–194
  colorectal cancer, 480, 483
Fever, evaluation in neutropenic patient, 732
Fibroadenoma, 494
Fibroblasts, as gene therapy target cells, 118
Fibrocystic mastopathy, 494
Field cancerization, 42
FIGO staging
  cervical cancer, 523
  gestational trophoblastic disease, 555
  vulvar cancer, 549–550
Finasteride, chemoprevention, 171
Fludarabine, chronic lymphocytic leukemia
    therapy, 679
Fluoropyrimidines, chemotherapy, 283–284

Fluoroquinolones, prophylactic use, 734
5-Fluorouracil
  locally advanced pancreatic cancer,
    471–472
  pancreatic cancer, 464–467
Flutamide, chemotherapy, 289–290
Follicle center cell lymphoma, 652
Follicle center lymphoma, 651
Founder effects, 75
Fractionation, radiation oncology, 269–270

Gardner syndrome, colorectal cancer, 479
Gastric cancer, 439–452
  chemoprevention, 176
  chemotherapy, 449
  diagnosis and staging, 445, 447
  differences in Western and Asian
    populations, 447
  epidemiology and etiology, 439–441
  follow-up, 451
  geographical variation, 135
  hypothesis, 440–441
  immunochemosurgery, 450
  malignant ascites, 739–740
  natural history and spread, 442, 445–446
  palliative therapy, 450–451
  pathology, 442–444
  prevention, 451–452
  prognosis, 451
  radiation, 449
  signs and symptoms, 445
  staging, 442–445, 447–448
  surgery, 447–449
Gastrointestinal manifestations, multiple
    endocrine neoplasia type II, 363
Gastrointestinal obstruction, management,
    799–800
Gastrointestinal tumors, in the elderly, 728
Gemcitabine, 284
  pancreatic cancer, 473–474
Genes. *See* Cancer predisposition genes
Gene therapy, 58–61, 116–125
  antisense, 124–125
  costimulatory molecules-B7, 124
  cytokines, 119–123
  research, 246
  strategies, 61
  suicide, 124
  target cells, 118–119
  tumor suppressor genes, 123–124
Genetic abnormalities, multiple endocrine
    neoplasia type I, 359–360
Genetic changes
  cancer cells, 63–64

tumors, inherited in germline or acquired by somatic cells, 64
Genetic counseling
in high-risk clinic, 76–82
reasons dissuading individuals from obtaining, 82
Genetic predisposition, 63–97
animal models, 71
colorectal cancer, 478–479
future, 91–93
genetic counseling, 76–82
genetic testing, 82–86
identification of individuals at risk, 72–76
impact on management of sporadic cancer, 64–67
mechanism of loss of function of normal allele, 71–72
outcome, 89–91
tumor types, 70
Genetic tagging, 58
Genetic testing, 82–86
interpretation and presentation of test results, 86–87
interpretation of results, 85
potential benefits, 96–97
psychosocial consequences, 87–88
Genitourinary cancer, 575–603
kidney, 575–581
penis, 601–603
renal pelvis and ureter, 588–590
testis cancer, 592–601
urethral cancer, 590–592
urinary bladder, 581–588
see also Prostate cancer
Genomic instability, 53–54
Genomic stability, regulation by predisposition genes, 68–70
Geographical pathology, 135
Germ cell tumors, 614–615
nonseminomatous, 598–600
Germline, inherited genetic changes, 64
Gestational trophoblastic disease, 552–558
choriocarcinoma, 554, 556
classification, 553
complete mole, 553
EMA/CO protocol, 558
epidemiology and etiology, 553
high-risk protocol, 557
invasive mole, 554
partial mole, 553–554
placental site trophoblast tumor, 554
prognosis, 554, 556
staging, 554–555
treatment, 554–558

Glioblastoma multiforme, 611
Gliomas, 610–612
Glucocorticoids, symptomatic control of brain edema and increase intracranial pressure, 617–618
Glucose, metabolism, 761
cytokine effects, 763
Glucose-6-phosphate dehydrogenase gene, 46–47
Glutamine
cancer cachexia, 762
improving efficacy of feeding regiments, 773
Gompertzian curve, 15
Gompertzian growth, 2–3
tumor doubling, 5–6
Good medical practice, staging role in promoting, 227
Graft failure, autologous bone marrow transplantation transplant, 303
Graft-versus-host-disease, allogeneic bone marrow transplantation, 298–299
Granulocyte colony-stimulating factor, 108, 741–742
Granulocyte-macrophage colony-stimulating factor, 108, 741–742
in gene therapy, 122–123
Granulocytopenia, use of transfusions, 741
Growth, 8, 15
Growth curve of hypothetical cancer, 4–5
Growth factors, use, 741–742
Growth hormone, improving efficacy of feeding regiments, 772–773
Gynecologic cancer, 537–558
endometrial, 537–542
gestational trophoblastic disease, 552–558
ovarian cancer, 542–548
vulvar cancer, 548–552

Hairy cell leukemia, 651, 685–686
Halsted, William S., 237–238
Handicap, definition, 779–780
Head and neck cancer, 341–357
chemoprevention, 173
diagnosis, 343–345
etiology and epidemiology, 342
follow-up, 356–357
lymph node localization, 349–350
multimodality treatment, 350–356
chemotherapy, 354–355
organ preservation, 355
philosophy, 350–351
radiation, 353–354
retreatment, 355–356

Head and neck cancer (*cont.*)
  supportive treatment, 356
  surgery, 351–353
  natural history, 344–345
  pathology, 343–345
  prevention, 357
  screening, 343
  staging, 346–351
  symptoms by common sites of origin, 343
  tNM classification, 346–348
Health care reform, nutrition support and, 773
Hematopoietic growth factors, 741–742
  as biologic response modifiers, 291
Hematopoietic progenitor cells, 294
Heparin, use with hypercoagulability, 736
Hepatic metastases, surgical therapy, 487
Hepatic tumors
  diagnosis, 696
  epidemiology, 696
  genetics, 696
  pathology, 697
  pediatric, 695–697
  treatment, 697
Hereditary cancer syndromes, 203–204
Hereditary nonpolyposis colorectal cancer,
    479–480
High-risk clinic
  genetic counseling, 76–82
  multidisciplinary team, 76, 79
  triage, 76, 80
History taking, 201–202
Hodgkin's disease, 654–657
  autologous BMT/PBPC transplant, 301
  classification and diagnosis, 655–656
  epidemiology, etiology, and pathogenesis,
    654–655
  presentation, investigation, and staging,
    655–656
  treatment, 656–657
Homosexual men, AIDS related Kaposi's
    sarcoma, 711
Hormonal agents, chemotherapy, 289–290
Hormonal therapy, improving efficacy of
    feeding regiments, 772–773
Hormone replacement therapy, cancer risk,
    147–148
Hormones
  as carcinogens, 23
  endogenous, cancer risk, 145–148
Host factors, 279
Human Genome Project, 68
Human papilloma virus, cervical cancer risk,
    150
Humoral immunity, 101–102

Hydromorphone, 751
Hydroxyzine, 752, 754
Hypercalcemia, 736–737
Hypercoagulability, 735–736
Hyperfractionation, 269–270
Hyperparathyroidism, multiple endocrine
    neoplasia type I, 359–360
Hyperuricemia, 737–738
Hysterectomy, cervical cancer
  invasive, 526–527
  radical, complications, 532–533

Ibuprofen, 750
Imaging
  brain, 610
  liver cancer, 411–412
Immune adjuvants, 112–113
Immune system, 100–102
Immunochemosurgery, gastric cancer, 450
Immunogenicity, enhancing, 59
Immunoglobulin, high-dose intravenous,
    chronic lymphocytic leukemia therapy,
    679–680
Immunology. *See* Tumor immunology
Immunomodulators, 112–113
Immunotherapy
  breast cancer, 507–509
  renal cell carcinomas, 580
  skin and melanoma cancer, 338–339
Immunotoxins, 109
Impairments
  assessment, 783
  definition, 780
  rehabilitation, 785–787
Indirect carcinogens, oxidation, 27
Indolent lymphomas, 651–652
Infection
  cancer risk, 145
  as oncological emergency, 732–724
  surgery and, history, 236–237
Inflammatory bowel diseases, colorectal
    cancer, 478
Initiating event, irreversibility, 9
Initiation, 8
Insulin, improving efficacy of feeding
    regiments, 772
Intensity modulated radiation, 273
Interferon-α, 106
  AIDS-related Kaposi's sarcoma, 712
Iterferon-γ, 106
Interferons
  as biologic response modifiers, 290
  chronic myelogenous leukemia therapy,
    675–676

Interleukin-1, 107
Interleukin-2, 105–106
  biologic response modifiers, 291–292
  in gene therapy, 119–120
Interleukin-3, 108
Interleukin-4, 106
  in gene therapy, 120–121
Interleukin-6, 107
Interleukin-7, 107
  in gene therapy, 121–122
Interleukin-12, 107–108
  in gene therapy, 122
Interleukins, as biologic response modifiers,
    291–292
International Union against Cancer staging
    system, 396–397
Intestinal neuroendocrine tumors, 375–380
Intestinal T-cell lymphoma, 653
Intracranial pressure, symptomatic control,
    617–618
Intraductal papilloma, 494–495
Invasion, 11–12
Ionizing radiation, 253
Irinotecan, 287
Irritation, chronic, 22
Isolated limb perfusion, 335
Isotope therapy, 256
Ivor-Lewis esophagectomy, 431–432

Kaposi's sarcoma, AIDS related, 709–713
  chemotherapy, 713
  clinical manifestations, 711
  epidemiology, 709
  pathogenesis, 710
  pathology, 711
  prognosis, 712
  treatment, 712
Kidney. *See* Renal cell carcinomas
Kiel classification, comparison with REAL
    classification and working formulation
    non-Hodgkin's lymphomas, 647–649
Knowledge, disseminating, staging role,
    223–225

Laboratory examinations, 204, 207–208
Laparoscopy
  liver cancer, 412
  pancreatic cancer, 464
Leptomeningeal metastases, 616
Lesions, preinvasive, cervical cancer, 519–521
  multimodality treatment, 524–526
  staging, 522
Leukemias, 661–686
  acute lymphocytic, 669–673

acute myeloid, 664–669
chemical and drug exposure, 663–664
chronic lymphocytic, 676–680
chronic myelogenous, 673–676
chronic myeloproliferative diseases, 681,
    683–685
definition and categorization, 661–662
epidemiology, 662–663
genetic predisposition, 663
myelodysplastic syndromes, 680–682
radiation, increased incidence and, 663
viruses, 663
Life-prolonging treatments, ethical aspects,
    801
Lipids, metabolism, cancer patients, 762
Lister, Joseph, 236–237
Liver cancer, 407–423
  biotherapy, 419
  chemotherapy, 419
  clinical findings, 410–411
  comparison between small and large
      hepatocellular carcinoma, 419
  conversion of large into small hepatocellular
      carcinoma, 420
  diagnosis, 410–412
    differential, 412–413
  epidemiology and etiology, 407–408
  geographical variation, 135–136
  imaging, 411–412
  laboratory findings, 411
  laparoscopy and needle biopsy, 412
  pathology and molecular biology, 409–410
  postoperative complications, 416
  prevention, 422
  prognosis, 421–422
  radiotherapy, 418–419
  recurrence and metastases, 420–421
  regional cancer therapies, 418
  screening, 408–409
  staging, 413–414
  surgery, 415–417
  transcatheter arterial chemoembolization,
      417–418
  treatment, 414–419
  See also Hepatic tumors
Lobular carcinoma in situ, 492–493
Local anesthetics, 752
Loop electrosurgical excision procedure, 525
Loss of heterozygosity, 50
Lung cancer, 385–404
  bronchoscopy, 390
  chemoprevention, 174
  diagnosis, 386–388
    evaluation techniques, 388–392

Lung cancer (*cont.*)
  etiology, 386
  follow-up, for local, regional, or distant
      recurrence, 403–404
  geographical variation, 136
  management and survival, 397
  mediastinoscopy, 391
  natural history, 393–396
  non-small-cell, management, 397–400
    stage I, 397–398
    stage II, 398
    stage III, 399–400
  open lung biopsy, 391
  palliative therapy, 401–402
  pathologic cell type characteristics,
      388–389
  pathology, 393–396
  prevention, 404
  radiotherapy, 385
  rehabilitation, 402–403
  screening, 386–388
  search for extrathoracic metastases, 391
  sputum cytology, 388, 390
  staging, 392, 394–396
    prognosis and, 396–397
  superior vena caval syndrome, 738
  syndrome of inappropriate antidiuretic
      hormone secretion, 736
  in the elderly, 728
  thoracoscopy, 391
  transthoracic needle biopsy, 390–391
Lycopene, chemoprevention, 171
Lymph nodes
  axillary, breast cancer, 502, 504
  enlargement, non-Hodgkin's lymphomas,
      644
  localization, head and neck cancer, 349–350
  malignant pleural effusions, 739
  metastases, 12
  pathologic analysis, staging accuracy,
      246–247
  ureteral obstruction, 738
Lymphoblastic lymphomas, 654
Lymphocytes, as gene therapy target cells, 118
Lymphokine-activated killer cells, therapy,
      110–111
Lymphomas, 641–657
  aggressive, 652–654
  AIDS-related, 713–717
    clinical manifestations, 715
    epidemiology, 713–714
    pathogenesis, 714
    pathology, 715
    primary CNS, 716–717

  prognosis, 715–716
  treatment, 716
Hodgkin's disease, 654–657
indolent, 651–652
malignant, 495
non-Hodgkin's, 642–650
proposed clinical schema, 650
very aggressive, 654

MACOP-B regimen, AIDS-associated
    lymphoma, 716
Magnetic resonance imaging, liver cancer,
    412
Malignancy, clinical sequela, 16
Malignant effusions, 739–740
Malnutrition, 757
Mantle cell lymphoma, 652
Marginal zone lymphoma, 651
Mastectomy, prophylactic, 79, 499–500
MAXI model, 94–97
Maximum tolerated dose, 24
Mediastinal large B-cell lymphoma, 653
Mediastinoscopy, lung cancer, 391
Medical oncology, 275–291
  biologic response modifiers, 290–291
  drug delivery and dose intensity, 278–279
  drug resistance, 277
  most factors, 279
  multimodality therapy, 279–280
  tumor burden and tumor cell heterogeneity,
      276–277
Medullary thyroid carcinoma, multiple
    endocrine neoplasia type II, 362–363
Medulloblastomas, 613, 705
Melanoma cancer. *See* Skin and melanoma
    cancer
Meningiomas, 614
Meperidine, 752
Merkel cell tumors, 328, 337
Meta-analyses, clinical trial, 322
Metabolism
  intermediary, alterations, 761–762
  relationship with nutrition in cancer
      patients, 757–758
Metastasis, 11–15
  breast cancer, treatment, 508–511
  definition, 11
  development mechanisms, 14
  extrathoracic, search for, 391
  liver cancer, 420–421
  patterns of sites, 14
  stages, 13
Methadone, 752
Methotrexate, chemotherapy, 283

Micronutrients
  chemoprevention, 171–173
  in food, 40
Misoprostol, 751
Missense mutations, 85
Mitomycin C, chemotherapy, 285
Mitotic phase, 54
Model informed consent form, 94–97
Molecular basis, 45–61
  apoptosis, 55–56
  cell cycle, 54–55
  clinical applications, 56–58
  differentiation, 53
  field cancerization, 42
  gene therapy, 58–61
  genomic instability, 53–54
  oncogenes, 48–50
  prognosis, 57
  screening, 57
  treatment, 58
    tumor suppressor genes, 50–53
Molecular biology, liver cancer, 409–410
Molecular markers, 210, 212
Monitoring, follow-up, surgical oncology,
    244–245
Monoclonal antibodies
  biologic cancer therapy, 108–110
  biospecific, 109
  clinical results, 109–110
  conjugates, 109
  production, 108–109
Monooxygenases, metabolic activation of
    chemical carcinogens, 26–27
Morphine
  dyspnea management, 796
  gastrointestinal obstruction, 800
Mucosa-associated lymphoid tissue,
    lymphomas, 643
Multimodality therapy
  esophageal carcinoma, 434–435
  pancreatic cancer, potentially resectable
    disease, 464–471
Multiple endocrine neoplasia type I, 359–362
  familial medullary thyroid cancer, 360
  genetic abnormalities, 359–360
  hyperparathyroidism, 359–360
  pancreatic endocrine tumors, 376–377
  pancreatic islet cell tumors, 360–361
  pituitary tumors, 361–362
  screening, 359
Multiple endocrine neoplasia type II, 362–363
  gastrointestinal manifestations, 363
  gene defect, 362
  medullary thyroid carcinoma, 362–363

parathyroid disease, 363
pheochromocytoma, 363
Multiple myeloma, BMT/PBPC transplant
  allogeneic, 296
  autologous, 301
Mutagenicity, correlation with carcinogenicity,
    29–30
Mutations, accumulation and sporadic cancers,
    74
Mycosis fungoides, 652
Myelodysplastic syndromes, 680–682

Nasopharyngeal carcinoma, chemotherapy,
    354–355
Natural history, 2
  lung cancer, 393–396
  staging, 223
Natural killer cells, 101
Nausea
  chemotherapy and radiotherapy induced,
    740
  management, 798–799
Neck cancer. *See* Head and neck cancer
Necrolytic migratory erythema, 379
Neovascularization, 63
Nephrectomy, 579
Nephroblastoma, 689
Neuroblastoma, 692–695
  diagnosis, 693–694
  epidemiology, 693
  genetics, 693
  pathology, 694
  recurrent, 695
  staging, 694–695
  treatment, 695
Neurological paraneoplastic syndromes, 206
Neurooncology. *See* Pediatric neurooncology
Neurotoxicity, brain tumors, 618
NIH classification, malignant gestational
    trophoblastic disease, 555
Nitrosoureas, chemotherapy agent, 281
Non-Hodgkin's lymphomas, 642–650
  BMT/PBPC transplant
    allogeneic, 296
    autologous, 301
  classification and diagnosis, 646–649
  epidemiology, etiology, and pathogenesis,
    642–643
  presentation, investigation, and staging,
    643–645
  treatment, 650
Nonopioid analgesics, 750–751
Nonsteroidal anti-inflammatory agents,
    chemoprevention, 169–170

NSAIDS, 750–751
Nuclide imaging, liver cancer, 412
Nutrition, 757–773
    intermediary metabolism alterations,
        761–762
    relationship with metabolism in cancer
        patients, 757–758
    support of cancer patient, 764–773
        enteral nutrition, 765–769
        glutamine, 773
        health care reform, 773
        hormonal therapy, 772–773
        nutritional assessment, 765
        peripheral intravenous feedings, 766
        rationale, 764–765
        total parenteral nutrition, 766–770
        tumor growth and, 772
    see also Cancer cachexia
Nutritional epidemiology, 143

Occupational exposures, cancer risk, 145
Oncogenes, 30–32, 48–50
    functional classes, 49–50
    as intracellular messengers, 49
    prognosis, 57
    viral, 48
    suppressing expression, 59–60
Oncological emergencies, 731–742
    adrenal insufficiency, 738
    hypercalcemia, 736–737
    hypercoagulability, 735–736
    hyperuricemia and tumor lysis syndrome,
        737–738
    infection, 732–724
    malignant effusions, 739–740
    metastases to brain and spinal cord,
        734–735
    nausea and vomiting, 740
    superior vena caval syndrome,
        738–739
    syndrome of inappropriate antidiuretic
        hormone secretion, 736–737
    ureteral and urethral obstruction, 738
Open lung biopsy, lung cancer, 391
Opioid analgesics
    constipation, 797
    nausea and vomiting, 798
    pain management, 751–753
Organ preservation
    bladder carcinoma, 587–588
    head and neck cancer, 355
    penile cancer, 603
    renal cell carcinomas, 580–581
Osteosarcoma, 701–703

Outcomes
    defining based on treatment decisions, 247
    studies, types, 189
Ovarian ablation, 505–506
Ovarian cancer, 542–548
    autologous BMT/PBPC transplant, 302
    cell line, gene expression, 92–93
    epidemiology and etiology, 542–543
    gastrointestinal obstruction, 799
    malignant ascites, 739–740
    pathology, 543–544
    prognosis, 548
    screening and diagnosis, 544–545
    staging, 545–547
    treatment, 545, 547
Oxycodone, 751–752

Paclitaxel, chemotherapy, 288
Pain
    acute, 746
    assessment, 749–750
    barriers to relief, 747–748
    chronic, 746–747
    intensity, 749
    mechanisms, 746–7474
    as multidimensional phenomenon, 747
    problem of, 745–746
Pain management, 745–755
    adjuvant drugs, 752, 754
    gastrointestinal obstruction, 800
    inadequate, 747
    medications, patient noncompliance,
        747–748
    nonopioid analgesics, 750–751
    nonpharmacologic strategies, 754
    opioid analgesics, 751–753
    quality of life, 794–795
Palliative surgery, 244
Palliative therapy
    colorectal cancer, 487–488
    gastric cancer, 450–451
    lung cancer, 401–402
    pancreatic cancer, 462–463
    prostate cancer, 573
    quality of life, 793–795
    recurrent cervical cancer, 531–532
    see also Pain management
Pancreatic and intestinal neuroendocrine
        tumors, 375–380
Pancreatic cancer, 453–474
    etiologic factors, 453–455
    locally advanced disease, treatment,
        471–472
    management algorithm, 462–463

metastatic and recurrent, treatment, 473–474

molecular pathogenesis, 455–456

multimodality therapy, potentially resectable disease, 464–471

pancreaticoduodenectomy, 467–471

pretreatment diagnostic study importance, 461–464

signs and symptoms, 456

staging, 457–461

tumor progression patterns, 457

Pancreatic endocrine tumors, multiple endocrine neoplasia type I, 376–377

Pancreatic islet cell tumors, multiple endocrine neoplasia type I, 360–361

Pancreaticoduodenectomy, 467–471

specimen, pathology, 459–460

Papilledema, brain metastases, 734

Papilloma, intraductal, 494–495

Pap smear, 191–192, 517–519

Bethesda system, 519–520

Paraneoplastic syndromes, 202

neurological, 206

skin, 205

Parathyroid cancer, 368–370

Parathyroid disease, multiple endocrine neoplasia type II, 363

Parent carcinogen, 26

Pathology, 207–208, 210, 212–213

adrenal cancer, 370–371

gastric cancer, 442–444

head and neck cancer, 343–345

liver cancer, 409–410

lung cancer, 393–396

pancreatic and intestinal neuroendocrine tumors, 375–378

parathyroid cancer, 368, 370

pheochromocytoma, 373–374

skin and melanoma cancer, 328

thyroid cancer, 364–365

Patient education, rehabilitation, 785

Pediatric malignancies, 689–706

brain tumors, 703–705

Ewing's sarcoma, 699–701

hepatic tumors, 695–697

long-term follow-up, 706

neuroblastoma, 692–695

osteosarcoma, 701–703

rhabdomyosarcoma, 697–699

Wilms' tumor, 689–692

Pediatric neurooncology, 612–616

acoustic Schwannomas, 613–614

brain metastasis, 615–616

brainstem tumors, 613

ependymomas, 612–613

germ cell tumors, 614–615

leptomeningeal metastases, 616

medulloblastoma, 613

meningiomas, 614

metastatic spinal cord compression, 616

pituitary adenomas, 615

primary brain lymphoma, 614

primitive neuroectodermal tumors, 613

spinal cord tumors, 615

Pedigree

importance, 72–76

questionnaire, 76

significance, 79

Pelvic exenteration, cervical cancer, 530–531

Penetrance, variation in, 88–90

Penile cancer, 601–603

Percutaneous fine-needle biopsy, liver cancer, 412

Pericardial effusions, malignant, 739

Pericardiocentesis, 739

Peripheral blood progenitor stem cells, transplant, 294–295

allogeneic, 295–296

Peripheral intravenous feedings, 766

Peripheral T-cell lymphoma, 653

Pesticides, increased incidence of leukemias, 663

Phase 1 trials, 309–310

Phase II trials, 315

feasibility trials, 313–314

single-agent, 310–313

Phase III trials, 315

Pheochromocytoma, 373–375

malignant, 374–375

multiple endocrine neoplasia type II, 363

Physical carcinogens, 21–22

Physical examination, 202, 205–206

Physical function, rehabilitation, 786–787

Pituitary adenomas, 615

Pituitary tumors, multiple endocrine neoplasia type I, 361–362

Platinum coordination compounds, chemotherapy, 280–282

Pleural effusions, malignant, 739

Pneumonectomy, 399

Podopyllotoxins, chemotherapy, 287

PolarProbe, 149

Polycythemia vera, 683

Population screening, 57

Preclinical phase, 4–5

Premalignancy

chemoprevention and, 164–165

lung, chemoprevention, 174

Premalignancy (*cont.*)
oral, chemoprevention, 173
Preoperative considerations, 242–243
Preoperative lymph node biopsies, esophageal
carcinoma, 430
Preoperative preparation, pheochromocytoma,
374
Pretransplant phase
allogeneic, 297
autologous, 302–303
Prevention, 141–148
bladder carcinoma, 588
cervical cancer, 534
colorectal cancer, 480
endogenous hormones, 145–148
esophageal carcinoma, 437
gastric cancer, 451–452
head and neck cancer, 357
infective processes, 145
lung cancer, 404
occupational exposures, 145
prostate cancer, 564–565
skin and melanoma cancer, 339–340
surgical oncology and, 240
Primaries, multiple, 75
Primitive neuroectodermal tumors, 613
Progestational agents, chemotherapy, 290
Prognosis
acute lymphocytic leukemia, 673
acute myeloid leukemia, 668
AIDS-associated lymphoma, 715–716
AIDS-related Kaposi's sarcoma, 712
bladder carcinoma, 583–585
brain metastasis, 615–616
cancers in high-risk individuals, 89–91
endometrial cancer, 542
gastric cancer, 451
gliomas, 612
impact on rehabilitation, 780–781
liver cancer, 421–422
ovarian cancer, 548
prostate cancer, 567–568
renal cell carcinomas, 577–578
vulvar cancer, 552
Progression, 10–11, 217
Prolymphocytic leukemias, 652
Promotion, 8–10
Promyelocytic leukemia, 53
Propagation, 10
Prophylactic cranial irradiation, lung cancer,
401
Prostate cancer, 563–573
advanced disease, 571
chemoprevention, 177
diagnosis, 566–567
epidemiology and natural history, 564
etiology and prevention, 564–565
metastatic disease, 571–573
palliative treatment, 573
pathology, 565–566
screening, 152–153, 195–197, 566–567
staging and prognosis, 567–568
treatment, 568–571
Prostatectomy, 569
Prostate-specific antigen, 196–197
Prostrate cancer, geographical variation,
139–140
Proteins
metabolism, 761
cytokine effects, 764
oncogene-encoded, 48
Proto-oncogenes, 30, 48
Proximate carcinogen, 26
Psychological functioning, assessing, 783
Psychological support, rehabilitation, 788–789

Quality assurance, radiation oncology, 274
Quality control, clinical trial, 322
Quality management, staging and, 229–231
Quality of life, 791–801
definitions, 791–792
measuring, 792–793
palliative care, 793–795
symptom management, 795–796
constipation, 797
delirium, 797–798
dyspnea, 796
ethical aspects, 800–801
gastrointestinal obstruction, 799–800
nausea and vomiting, 798–799
terminal phase, 800

Radiobiology, normal tissue, 265, 267–268
Radiographic staging, pancreatic cancer,
458–459
Radiologic imaging, pancreatic and intestinal
neuroendocrine tumors, 379–380
Radiosensitizers, 271–272
cervical cancer, 529
Radiosurgery, brain tumors, 617
Radiotherapy, 251–274
advanced technologies and, 273
AIDS-associated lymphoma, 717
biology, 261–262
bladder carcinoma, 586
brain metastases, 734
brain tumors, 617, 705
cervical cancer, 527–529

complications, 533
clinical use, 268–273
   chemical modifiers of radiation
     sensitivity, 271–272
   clinical brachytherapy, 272–273
   combining with surgery, 270–271
   dose and fractionation principles,
     269–270
   indications, 268–269
   palliative role, 272
combined with chemotherapy, 270–271
   esophageal carcinoma, 434
colorectal cancer, 486–487
delivery, 255–256, 258, 260–261
dose
   distribution, 253–255
   measurement, 253
effects at cellular level, 262–263
effects at molecular level, 263–264
enteritis, 766, 768, 770
esophageal carcinoma, 433
external-beam. *See* External-beam
   radiotherapy
Ewing's sarcoma, 701
gastric cancer, 449
head and neck cancer, 353–354
implications for rehabilitation, 781
increased incidence of leukemia, 663
interaction with matter, 252–253
isodose distributions, 254–255
liver cancer, 418–419
localized soft tissue sarcomas, 629–631
locally recurrent soft tissue sarcomas, 635
lung cancer, 385
nature of, 252
neuroblastoma, 695
non-small-cell, lung cancer, 397–400
ovarian cancer, 547
parathyroid cancer, 370
primary soft tissue sarcoma of
   retroperitoneum, 634
quality assurance, 274
renal cell carcinomas, 579
rhabdomyosarcoma, 699
simulation, 258–261
skin and melanoma cancer, 336–338
testis cancer, 601
therapeutic, production, 253
tumor radiobiology, 263–266
volume treated, 257
vulvar cancer, 552
Wilms' tumor, 692
Rai strategy system, chronic lymphocytic
   leukemia, 677

Raloxifene, chemoprevention, 171
Randomization, clinical trial, 316–317
Range-of-motion, rehabilitation, 787
REAL classification, comparison with
   Kiel classification and working
   formulation non-Hodgkin's
   lymphomas, 647–649
Rectal cancer. *See* Colorectal cancer
Recurrence, liver cancer, 420–421
Regimen-related toxicities, allogeneic bone
   marrow transplantation, 297
Rehabilitation, 779–790
   assessment and goal-setting, 782–784
   cervical cancer, 532–534
   colorectal cancer, 489
   impact of disease site, stage, and prognosis,
     780–781
   implications of cancer treatment,
     781–782
   lung cancer, 402–403
   patient education, 785
   physical function, 785–787
   psychological support, 788–789
   return to work, 788
   self-care and activities of daily living,
     787–788
   skin and melanoma cancer, 339
   social and leisure, 789
Renal cell carcinomas, 575–581
   diagnosis, 577–578
   etiology, 576
   follow-up, 581
   multimodality treatment, 578–580
   pathology, 577
   philosophy of management, 578–579
   presentation, 576–577
   prognosis, 577–578
   screening, 576
Renal pelvis cancer, 588–590
Research, surgical oncology, 245–246
Resources, allocation and staging, 229
Resting energy expenditure, 761
Retinoblastoma, 51–52
Retinoids, chemoprevention, 167–168
   bladder cancer, 176
   breast cancer, 175–176
   head and neck cancer, 173
   lung cancer, 175
   skin cancer, 175
Retroperitoneum, primary soft tissue
   sarcomas, treatment, 634
Reverse transcriptase polymerase chain
   reaction, 246–247
Rhabdomyosarcoma, 697–699

Risk factors
  acute lymphocytic leukemia, 672
  acute myeloid leukemia, 667
  geographic and temporal variation, 134–140

Sarcoma, 495
Screening, 148–153, 181–197
  biases, 186–187
  biologic basis, 182–183
  bladder carcinoma, 582
  breast cancer, 150–151, 192–193, 500
  cervical cancer, 148–150, 191–192,
    517–519
  characteristics of test, 183–184
  colorectal cancer, 151–152, 193–195, 480
  cost and societal issues, 190–191
  efficacy, 188–190
  endometrial cancer, 538
  esophageal carcinoma, 427
  established tools, 185–186
  head and neck cancer, 343
  liver cancer, 408–409
  lung cancer, 386–388, 390
  models, 191–197
  multiple endocrine neoplasia type I, 359
  for other forms of cancer, 152–153
  ovarian cancer, 544–545
  principles, 182–191
  population, 57
  prostate cancer, 195–197, 566–567
  renal cell carcinomas, 576
  risks of, 188–190
  skin and melanoma cancer, 327–328
  surgical oncology and, 239–240
  test determinants, 183–186
  testis cancer, 593
Secondary malignancies, autologous bone
    marrow transplantation transplant, 303
Selenium, chemoprevention, 170
Self-care, rehabilitation, 787–788
Self-examination, 192
Seminoma, 595–598
Sepsis, 242–243
Sexuality, 783
  rehabilitation, 788
Sezary syndrome, 652
Sigmoidoscopy
  colorectal cancer, 484
  screening, 194–195
Signal transduction, oncogene-controlled, 49
Skin and melanoma cancer, 325–340
  chemoprevention, 175
  chemotherapy/immunotherapy, 338–339
  clinicopathologic types, 330–331

diagnosis, 328–331
epidemiology and etiology, 325–327
follow-up, 339
geographical variation, 136–137
incidence, 22
paraneoplastic syndromes, 205
prevention, 339–340
radiation oncology, 336–338
rehabilitation, 339
screening, 327–328
staging, 331–332
surgery, 332–336
Small lymphocytic lymphoma, 651
Smoking
  cancer risk, 141–143
  esophageal carcinoma and, 426
  pancreatic cancer and, 453–454
Social activities, rehabilitation, 789
Soft tissue sarcomas, 621–637
  anatomic distribution, 622
  biopsy, 624–625
  clinical presentation, 624
  diagnosis, 624–626
  etiology, 621–622
  histologic classification, 622–623
  histologic grading, 623–624
  localized, treatment, 627–633
    combined preoperative chemotherapy and
      radiotherapy, 633
    postoperative chemotherapy, 631–632
    preoperative chemotherapy, 632–633
    pre- or postoperative radiotherapy,
      629–631
    surgery, 628–629
  locally recurrent, treatment, 634–635
  metastatic, treatment, 635–637
  pathology, 622–624
  radiologic staging, 626
  retroperitoneum, treatment, 634
  staging, 626–627
  urethral obstruction, 738
Somatic cells, genetic changes acquired by, 64
Spinal cord compression, metastatic, 616, 735
Spinal cord tumors, 615
Splenectomy, septicemia risk, 733
Sporadic cancer
  accumulation of mutations, 74
  management, genetic predisposition and,
    64–67
Sputum cytology, screening for lung cancer,
    388, 390
Squamous cell carcinomas, 325, 327–330
  chemotherapy, 354
  surgery, 332–333

Stage, migration, 224–225
Staging, 14, 215–231
  adrenal cancer, 371
  bladder carcinoma, 583–585
  brain tumors, 705
  cervical cancer, 522–524
  classification, 215–217
  colorectal cancer, 481–483
  control program efficacy, 222–223
  definition, 215
  design of system, 218–219
  endometrial cancer, 539–541
  epidemiology, 223
  esophageal carcinoma, 427–430
  Ewing's sarcoma, 700
  gastric cancer, 442–445, 447–448
  gestational trophoblastic disease, 554–555
  graft-versus-host-disease, 299
  head and neck cancer, 346–351
  Hodgkin's disease, 655–656
  liver cancer, 413–414
  lung cancer, 392, 394–396
    prognosis and, 396–397
  natural history, 223
  neuroblastoma, 694–695
  non-Hodgkin's lymphomas, 644–645
  osteosarcoma, 703
  ovarian cancer, 545–547
  pancreatic cancer, 457–461
  problem of diversity, 215–216
  prostate cancer, 567–568
  quality management and, 229–231
  radiologic, soft tissue sarcomas, 626
  renal cell carcinomas, 577–578
  resource allocation and, 229
  rhabdomyosarcoma, 699
  role
    clinical practice, 226–228
    in disseminating knowledge, 223–225
    guiding treatment decisions, 226–227
    managing cancer control programs, 228–231
    promoting autonomous decision making, 227
    promoting good medical practice, 227
    research, 221–223
  skin and melanoma cancer, 331–332
  soft tissue sarcomas, 626–627
  strategic planning and, 228–229
  surgical oncology and, 242–243
  testis cancer, 595–597
  thyroid cancer, 366–367
  TNM system, 219–221
  treatment efficacy studies and, 221–222

  use, 216
  vulvar cancer, 549–551
  what is involved in, 226
  Wilms' tumor, 691–692
State, as a language, 223–224
Statistical analyses, clinical trial, 320
Stereotactic radiation therapy, 273
Stomach cancer. *See* Gastric cancer
Stratification, clinical trial, 316–317
Suicide gene therapy, 124
Sunlight, exposure and cancer risk, 144
Superior vena caval syndrome, 738–739
Supportive treatment, head and neck cancer, 356
Surgical oncology, 235–249
  adrenal cancer, 372
  bladder carcinoma, 586
  brain tumors, 617, 705
  cancer in the elderly, 726–728
  cancer prevention and screening, 239–240
  colorectal cancer, 485–486
  combined with radiation, 270–271
  diagnosis, 241–242
  esophageal carcinoma, 431–433
  follow-up monitoring, 244–245
  future, 248–249
  gastric cancer, 447–449
  head and neck cancer, 351–353
  hepatic tumors, 697
  history, 235–237
  implications for rehabilitation, 782
  interim analyses, 321
  invasive breast cancer, 502–504
  liver cancer, 415–417
  localized soft tissue sarcomas, 628–629
  locally recurrent soft tissue sarcomas, 635
  metastatic soft tissue sarcoma, 635–637
  milestones in evolution, 238–239
  neuroblastoma, 695
  non-small-cell, lung cancer, 397–401
  novel technologies, 246–248
  osteosarcoma, 703
  ovarian cancer, 545
  parathyroid cancer, 370
  preoperative considerations and staging, 242–243
  primary soft tissue sarcoma of retroperitoneum, 634
  prostate cancer, 569
  renal cell carcinomas, 579
  research, 245–246
  rhabdomyosarcoma, 699
  skin and melanoma cancer, 332–336
  spinal cord compression, 735

Surgical oncology (*cont.*)
  testis cancer, 595
  training and education, 237–238
  vulvar cancer, 551–552
  Wilms' tumor, 692
Surrogate endpoint biomarkers, 166
Swallowing disorders, rehabilitation, 786
Syndrome of inappropriate antidiuretic
      hormone secretion, 736–737
Syndromes, inherited, predisposing to cancer,
      51–53
Synthetic phase, 54
Systemic metastases, 207, 211

Tamoxifen
  breast cancer prevention, 500
  breast cancer treatment, 506–507
  chemoprevention, 170–171, 176
  chemotherapy, 289
Taxanes, chemotherapy, 288–289
T-cells, 100–101
Teletherapy. *See* External beam radiotherapy
Temporal disease, cancer as, 4–6
Terminal phase, quality of life, 800
Testis cancer, 592–601
  chemotherapy, 601
  CNS metastases, 600–601
  diagnosis, 593–595
  etiology, 592–593
  follow-up, 601
  geographical variation, 140
  multimodality treatment, 595
  nonseminomatous germ cell tumors,
      598–600
  radiotherapy, 601
  salvage therapy, 600
  screening, 593
  seminoma, 595–598
  staging, 595–597
  toxicity, 601
Therapy
  efficacy and staging, 221–222
  multimodality, 279–280
  staging role in guiding decisions, 226–227
  surgical oncology, 243–244
  variations in outcome, 153–154
  see also Biologic cancer therapy
Thoracoscopy, lung cancer, 391
Thrombocythemia, essential, 683–684
Thrombocytopenia, use of transfusions, 741
Thrombophlebitis, 735–736
Thyroid cancer, 363–368
  epidemiology, 363–364
  pathology, 364–365

  staging, 366–367
  thyroid nodule, 365–366
  treatment, 366–368
Thyroid nodule, 365–366
TNF-α, 106
  in gene therapy, 121
TNM classification, 219–221
  bladder carcinoma, 584
  clinical and pathologic classifications,
      221
  colorectal cancer, 482
  cutaneous T-cell lymphoma, 645
  elements, 219–220
  endometrial cancer, 540
  head and neck cancer, 346–348
  liver cancer, 413
  lung cancer, 394–396
  ovarian cancer, 546
  pancreatic cancer, 458
  penile cancer, 602
  prostate cancer, 568
  renal cell carcinomas, 578
  renal pelvis and ureter cancers, 589
  stomach cancer, 447–448
  testis tumors, 596–597
  urethral cancer, 591
Tobacco. *See* Smoking
Topoisomerase inhibitors, chemotherapy,
      286–287
Topotecan, 287
Total parenteral nutrition, 766–770
  complications, 771–772
  formulations, 771–772
  perioperative, 770–771
Transcatheter arterial chemoembolization,
      417–418
Transformed cells, properties, 46
Transfusions
  allogeneic bone marrow transplantation,
      298–299
  use, 741
Transplant phase
  allogeneic, 297–298
  autologous, 303
Transrectal ultrasound, 196–197
Transthoracic needle biopsy, lung cancer,
      390–391
Tumor antigen vaccines, 115–116
Tumor burden, 276
Tumor cells
  as gene therapy target cells, 119
  heterogeneity, 276–277
Tumor immunology, 99–125, *see also*
      Biologic cancer therapy

Tumor-inflating lymphocytes, therapy, 111–112
Tumor lysis syndrome, 737–738
Tumor markers, 204, 208
Tumor progression, 37
Tumor promoting agents, 20
Tumor promotion, targeting in chemoprevention, 42
Tumor radiobiology, 263–266
Tumors
    enhancing immunogenicity, 59
    genetic changes, inherited in germline or acquired by somatic cells, 64
    grading, 208, 210
    growth and nutrition, 772
    local extension of growth, 12–13
    localization, 206–207
    neovascularization, 63
    radiation therapy sites, 269
    sanctuaries, 278
    solid, autologous BMT/PBPC transplant, 302
    types, 70
    vectoring cytokines to, 59
Tumor suppressor genes, 31–33, 50–53
    gene therapy, 123–124
    inherited cancer syndromes, 51–53
    replacing defective, 60–61
    retinoblastoma, 51–52

UICC/AJCC staging system, soft tissue sarcomas, 627
UICC stage grouping, colorectal cancer, 482–483
Ultimate carcinogen, 26
Ultrasonography, liver cancer, 411
Ureteral obstruction, 738
Ureteral tumors, 588–590
Urethral cancer, 590–592
Urethral obstruction, 738
Urinary bladder. *See* Bladder cancer
Urinary tract, upper, cancer, 588–590
Uterine cervix, cancer. *See* Cervical cancer

Vaccines
    biologic cancer therapy, 112–116
    immune adjuvants and immunomodulators, 112–113
    tumor antigen, 115–116
    viral oncolysates, 114–115
    whole tumor cell, 113–114
Vancomycin, infection use, 733
Vinca alkaloids, chemotherapy, 288
Viral infection
    adult T-cell leukemia, 663
    cancer risk, 48, 145
    non-Hodgkin's lymphomas, 642
Viral oncolysates vaccines, 114–115
Viral vectors, 117
Vomiting
    chemotherapy and radiotherapy induced, 740
    management, 798–799
Vulvar cancer, 548–552
    diagnosis, 549
    epidemiology and etiology, 548
    pathology, 548–549
    prognosis, 552
    staging, 549–551
    treatment, 551–552

Waldenstrom's macroglobulinemia, 651
Weakness, 760
Weight loss, 758–759
WHO classification, ovarian cancer, 544
Whole tumor cell vaccines, 113–114
WHO prognostic index score, gestational trophoblastic disease, 556
Wilms' tumor, 689–692
    diagnosis, 690–691
    epidemiology, 689–690
    genetics, 690
    pathology, 691
    recurrent, 692
    staging, 691–692
    treatment, 692